Pathophysiology and Management of Thyroid

Pathophysiology and Management of Thyroid

Editor: Joaquin Noah

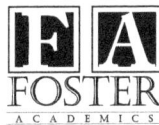

FOSTER
ACADEMICS

www.fosteracademics.com

www.fosteracademics.com

FA
FOSTER
ACADEMICS

Cataloging-in-Publication Data

Pathophysiology and management of thyroid / edited by Joaquin Noah.
    p. cm.
Includes bibliographical references and index.
ISBN 978-1-63242-651-2
    1. Thyroid gland--Pathophysiology. 2. Thyroid gland--Diseases. 3. Thyroid gland--Diseases--Prevention.
4. Thyroid gland--Diseases--Treatment. I. Noah, Joaquin.
RC655 .P38 2019
6164--dc23

Foster Academics,
118-35 Queens Blvd., Suite 400,
Forest Hills, NY 11375, USA

ISBN 978-1-63242-651-2 (Hardback)

Contents

Preface

The world is advancing at a fast pace like never before. Therefore, the need is to keep up with the latest developments. This book was an idea that came to fruition when the specialists in the area realized the need to coordinate together and document essential themes in the subject. That's when I was requested to be the editor. Editing this book has been an honour as it brings together diverse authors researching on different streams of the field. The book collates essential materials contributed by veterans in the area which can be utilized by students and researchers alike.

The medical condition which affects the functioning of the thyroid gland is known as thyroid disease. Its diagnosis is obtained through blood tests, radioiodine scanning, ultrasound and biopsy. The activity of the thyroid gland can be determined by the measurement of the levels of the thyroid hormones triiodothyronine, thyroxine and thyroid-stimulating hormone in blood. In case of diseases, anti-thyroid antibodies may be detected in blood such as anti-thyroid peroxidase antibodies, anti-thyroglobulin antibodies and TSH receptor antibodies. The detection of these can allow diagnosis of the specific condition. Radioactive iodine is used in thyroid scintigraphy to detect any irregularity in the size of the gland and determine its activity. Based on the condition diagnosed, the treatment may vary. While most conditions are treatable through the appropriate prescription of medications, surgery and radioiodine therapy may also be required. The thyroid gland may also be partly or completely removed to treat the condition. This book contains some path –breaking studies related to the functioning of the thyroid gland. It unravels the recent studies in the diagnosis, prevention and management of thyroid disease. For all readers who are interested in this domain, the case studies included in this book will serve as an excellent guide to develop a comprehensive understanding.

Each chapter is a sole-standing publication that reflects each author's interpretation. Thus, the book displays a multi-facetted picture of our current understanding of application, resources and aspects of the field. I would like to thank the contributors of this book and my family for their endless support.

Editor

Phylogenetic analysis of the human thyroglobulin regions

Abdelaziz Belkadi[1,2,3*], Caroline Jacques[1,2], Frédérique Savagner[1,2] and Yves Malthièry[1,2]

Abstract

Thyroglobulin is a large protein present in all vertebrates. It is synthesized in the thyrocytes and exported to lumen of the thyroid follicle, where its tyrosine residues are iodinated . The iodinated thyroglobulin is reintegrated into the cell and processed (cleaved to free its two extremities) for thyroid hormone synthesis. Thyroglobulin sequence analysis has identified four regions of the molecule: Tg1, Tg2, Tg3 and ChEL. Structural abnormalities and mutations result in different pathological consequences, depending on the thyroglobulin region affected. We carried out a bioinformatic analysis of thyroglobulin, determining the origin and the function of each region. Our results suggest that the Tg1 region acts as a binding protein on the apical membrane, the Tg2 region is involved in protein adhesion and the Tg3 region is involved in determining the three-dimensional structure of the protein. The ChEL domain is involved in thyroglobulin transport, dimerization and adhesion. The presence of repetitive domains in the Tg1, Tg2 and Tg3 regions suggests that these domains may have arisen through duplication.

Introduction

Thyroglobulin is the precursor of the thyroid hormones triiodothyronine (T3) and thyroxine (T4). In humans, thyroglobulin is synthesized by thyroid follicle cells, which are also known as thyrocytes [1]. Thyroglobulin molecules form dimers, which are exported to the lumen of the thyroid follicles [2]. There, the thyroglobulin is immobilized on the apical membrane. The thyroid hormones process starts by the iodination of tyrosine residues. Thyroperoxidaseis activated by H_2O_2, leading to the oxidation of iodide, followed by the iodination and conjugation of some of the tyrosine residues present in the thyroglobulin molecule. The iodinated and conjugated thyroglobulin is then returned to the cell via an endocytosis process that may involve histone H1 [3], megalin (gp330) [4] and/or the N-acetylglucosamine receptor [5]. Only a very small number of iodinated tyrosine residues are involved in thyroid hormone synthesis. T4 is formed by the conjugation of two residues of diiodotyrosine followed by cleavage. T3 is formed in a similar manner, but through the conjugation of diiodotyrosine with monoiodotyrosine [6,7]. T3 is the functional form; it is generated principally by T4 deiodinases in

the peripheral organs, with only 13% being formed in the thyroid gland [8]. Thyroid hormones reach their target organs via the bloodstream. Thyroglobulin has been reported to regulate some thyroid genes and the growth of epithelial cells [9,10]. It acts as both a hormone and an iodine reservoir [11].

In humans, mice and fish, thyroid hormone levels determine the basal rate of metabolism and overall energy expenditure [12-14]. In other species, such as Senegalese sole [15], amphibians [16], urochordatas [17], amphioxus [18] and lamprey [19], thyroid hormones play a critical role in the metamorphosis from larvae to juveniles. Thyroglobulin protein structure has been studied in detail [20-22]. This protein is present in all vertebrates and always has the same structure, consisting of four regions: the Tg1 (~ 10 repetitive domains), Tg2 (3 repetitive domains), Tg3 (5 repetitive domains) and ChEL regions (Figure 1-a and 1-b). The Tg1, Tg2 and Tg3 regions (moving along the molecule from its N-terminal end) consist of repetitive domains. All three regions are rich in cysteine residues, allowing them to form disulfide bonds [23]. The presence of these repetitive domains suggests their possible evolution through the duplication of source domains. The C-terminus of the molecule includes a 581-amino acid sequence displaying a high degree of similarity to the sequence of acetylcholinesterase (28% identity) [24,25]. One previous study identified the ChEL domain as the

* Correspondence: abdelaziz.belkadi@etud.univ-angers.fr
[1]INSERM U694, Institut Biologie Santé (IBS), rue des Capucins, F-49100 Angers, France
[2]University of Angers, rue de Rennes, F-49045 Angers, France
Full list of author information is available at the end of the article

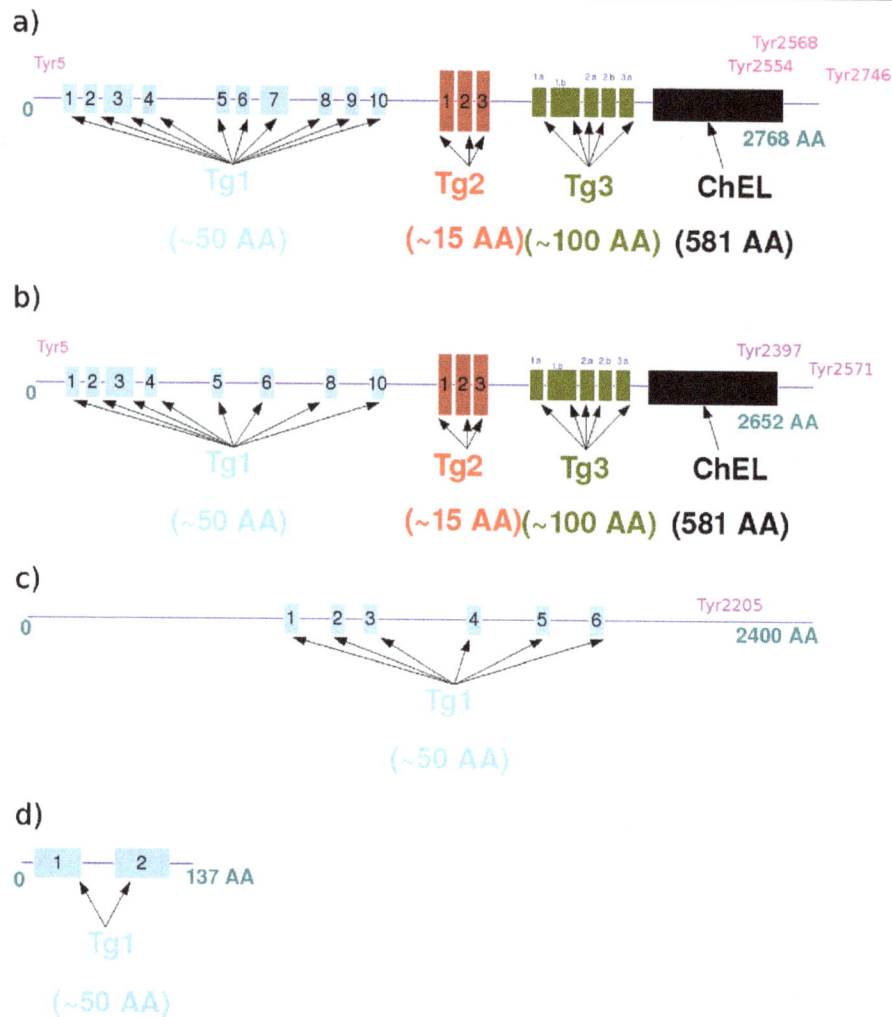

Figure 1 The structure of the thyroglobulin protein. a) Structure of the human thyroglobulin protein. **b)** Structure of the zebrafish thyroglobulin protein. **c)** Structure of the amphioxus thyroglobulin-like protein. **d)** Structure of the sea urchin thyroglobulin-like protein. Blue: Tg1 domains, red: Tg2 domains, green: Tg3 domains, black: the ChEL domain. Magenta: the location of the thyroid hormone synthesis sites on the proteins (tyrosine residues).

origininal source of thyroglobulin [26]. Thyroglobulin contains about 140 tyrosine residues, but only about 30 of these residues are iodinated and a very small number of these iodinated tyrosines undergo conjugation to form T3 and T4 [27]. Only four major thyroid hormone synthesis sites have been clearly identified in the human thyroglobulin molecule and these sites are located at either end of the protein: Tyr5, Tyr2554, Tyr2568 and Tyr2747 [21].

Thyroglobulin may thus be seen as a huge precursor of two very small products. Additional studies of its other, as yet unexplored functions in the cell may be useful. For example, this protein could potentially be involved in the trafficking of iodinefrom the thyrocyte to the follicle lumen and its storage. Many studies have made use of bioinformatics tools to analyze the evolution of proteins and genes, and such tools may be useful in this context [28,29].

We performed a phylogenetic analysis of the thyroglobulin molecule with the sequenced genomes of species corresponding to key steps in animal evolution. Our results provide clues to the evolution of thyroglobulin and potential functional roles for theTg1, Tg2, Tg3 and the ChEL regions.

Materials and methods

Sequence extraction

We extracted the available DNA and protein sequences for thyroglobulin (Tg) from the NCBI databank www.ncbi.nlm. nih.gov for four species: human [GenBank:CAA29104],rat [GenBank:AAF34909], mouse [GenBank:AAB53204], pig [GenBank:ACY66900]. We also extracted six predicted sequences: cattle [GenBank:NP_ 776308] horse [GenBank: XP 001916622] marmoset [GenBank:XP 002759270], panda [Gen-Bank:XP 002917659], zebrafish [GenBank:XP 694292] and zebra finch [GenBank:XP 002188056]. For other species, for which the amino-acid sequence of is unknown, such as opossum, and fugu, we used the human thyroglobulin genomic sequence in Blast searches of the UCSC website genome.ucsc.edu; We first translated the DNA sequence to obtain a putative amino-acid sequence. We then used Blast to check whether the predicted sequence was present in the database (chr3:411,623,333-412,004,486 and chrUn:270,007,531-270,025,053 for opossum and fugu, respectively). Homologous sequences from amphioxus [GenBank:XP 002607132] and sea urchin [Gen-Bank:XP 001202473] were also identified by BLAT analysis (chrUn:353,044,426-353,083,914 and Scaffold82420:233-1, 088 in the amphioxus and sea urchin genomes, respectively).

Sequence similarity

We searched for regions presenting sequence similarities to the constituent domains of thyroglobulin - Tg1 Tg2, Tg3 and ChEL - with the Blastall command ftp://ftp.ncbi.nlm. nih.gov/blast/db/, version 2.2.19. Pairs of sequences were compared on the basis of their global alignment with the Myers & Millers algorithm manpages.ubuntu.com/ manpages/karmic/man1. Results were generated in a separate text file containing alignment diagrams, scores, degrees of identity, similarity and gaps. We used ClustalX software ftp://ftpigbmc.u-strasbg.fr/pub/ClustalX/. for analysis of multiple alignments of three or more sequences. The results were output to a separate text file, but without information about score, because it was not possible to use more than two sequences for score calculation with Compositional Matrix Adjust.

Phylogeny

We used the neighbor-joining (NJ) method in PHYLIP [30] and mega 5 [31] for phylogenetic analysis. A range of analyses, from simple p distance to multiparameter models with gamma correction, were used. The significance of the phylogenetic tree was assessed by bootstrapping, with 10,000 iterations. The Jones-Taylor- Thornton (JTT) model of amino-acid sequence evolution, with gamma correction, was used for distance estimation [32]. In each case, the distance was validated with 10,000 bootstrap replications.

Results

The N-terminal Tg1 region

In humans, the first region of thyroglobulin consists of 10 Tg1 repeat domains, each containing 50 amino acids and displaying 14% identity. However, Molina, et al. identified an 11th domain located after the Tg2 region [33]. A comparison of this region in all the thyroglobulin protein sequences extracted (13 species) indicated that the fish thyroglobulins (zebrafish and fugu) lacked Tg1-7 and Tg1-9 (Additional file 1: Figure S1). We used mega 5 software to calculate the distance of the whole thyroglobulin protein sequences and of each of the component regions (Additional file 2: Tables S2, Additional file 3: Table S3, Additional file 4: Table S4 and Additional file 5:Table S5). We performed a phylogenetic analysis on the thyroglobulin Tg1 domains of four vertebrate species - (human (10 Tg1 domains), mouse (10 Tg1 domains), zebra finch (10 Tg1 domains) and zebrafish (8 Tg1 domains)) - six Tg1 domains from amphioxus (a cephalochordate) and two Tg1 domains from sea urchin (an echinoderm) (Figure 2). The sixth amphioxus Tg1 domain clusteredwith the second sea urchin domain in the phylogenetic tree. With a lower bootstrap percentage, we observed two big major branches of the phylogenetic tree, the first corresponding to the sea urchin and amphioxus Tg1 domains, which clustered with the thyroglobulin Tg1-8, Tg1-2, Tg1-1 and Tg1-10 domains, and the second corresponding to the Tg1-3, Tg1-4, Tg1-7, Tg1-5, Tg1-9 and Tg1-6 domains. For confirmation of these results, we performed a phylogenetic analysis on the thyroglobulin Tg1 domains of 13 vertebrate species (human (10 Tg1 domains), marmoset (10 Tg1 domains), pig (10 Tg1 domains), horse (10 Tg1 domains), dog (10 Tg1 domains), panda (10 Tg1 domains), rat (10 Tg1 domains), mouse (10 Tg1 domains), cow (10 Tg1 domains), opossum (10 Tg1 domains), zebra finch (10 Tg1 domains), zebrafish (8 Tg1 domains) and fugu (8 Tg1 domains)) together with six Tg1 domains from amphioxus and two from sea urchin. This new tree also had two major branches (Additional file 6: Figure S2). The fish Tg1-10 domains did not cluster with the other Tg1-10 domains in either of the trees. We also investigated the genome of the urochordate Ciona intestinalis. The protein with the largest number of Tg1 motifs was a predicted protein (rather than one for which the amino-acid sequence was actually known similar to entractin/nidogen (XP_ 002125504.1) and containing three Tg1 motifs. We generated two phylogenetic trees, one based on 13 vertebrate Tg1 regions (human, marmoset, pig, horse, dog, panda, rat, mouse, cow, opossum, zebra finch, zebrafish and fugu) (Figure 3) and the second based on 13 vertebrate thyroglobulin proteins (human, marmoset, pig, horse, dog, panda, rat, mouse, cow, opossum, zebra finch, zebrafish and fugu) together with the sequences of Thyroglobulin homologs from Ciona intestinalis, amphioxus and sea urchin (Figure 4).

We investigated the function of the Tg1 region of thyroglobulin, by investigating proteins containing domains similar to the Tg1 domain with cutoff e-value = 0.15 as recommended by the software. For the Tg1-1 domain, 107 proteins were selected (15 thyroglobulins, 15 nidogens, 18 testicans, 16 secreted proteins, acidic, cysteine-rich (SPARC) proteins, 13 invariant chains and 30 unnamed or hypothetical proteins). For the Tg1-2 domain, 49 proteins were

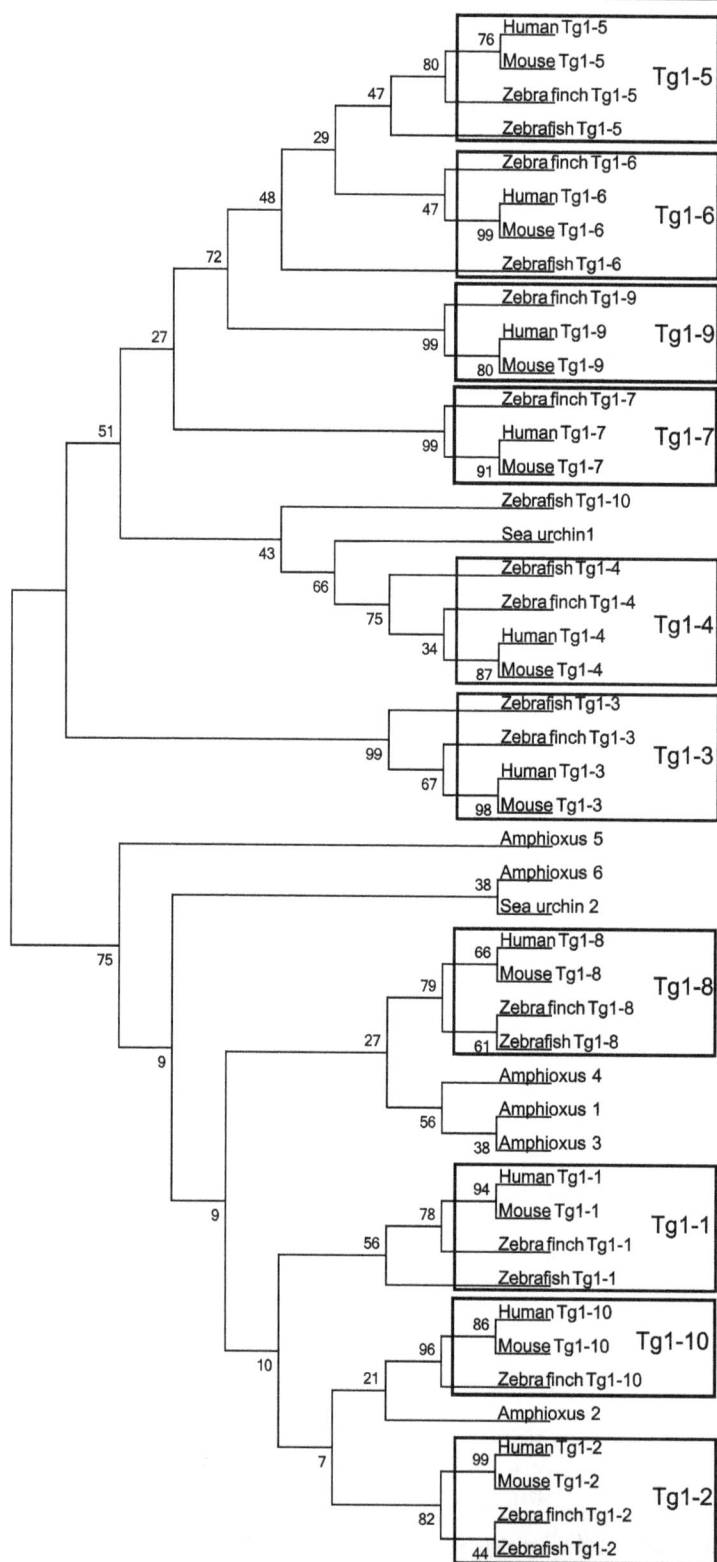

Figure 2 Phylogenetic analysis of thyroid hormone precursor Tg1 domains for six species. Phylogenetic analysis of thyroglobulin Tg1 domains from 4 species (human, mouse, zebra finch and zebrafish) and the amphioxus and sea urhin thyroglobulin-like Tg1 domains. Evolutionary history was inferred by the neighbor-joining method. The bootstrap consensus tree inferred from 1000 replicates is taken to represent the evolutionary history of the taxa analyzed. The numbers at nodes representing bootstrap support scores.

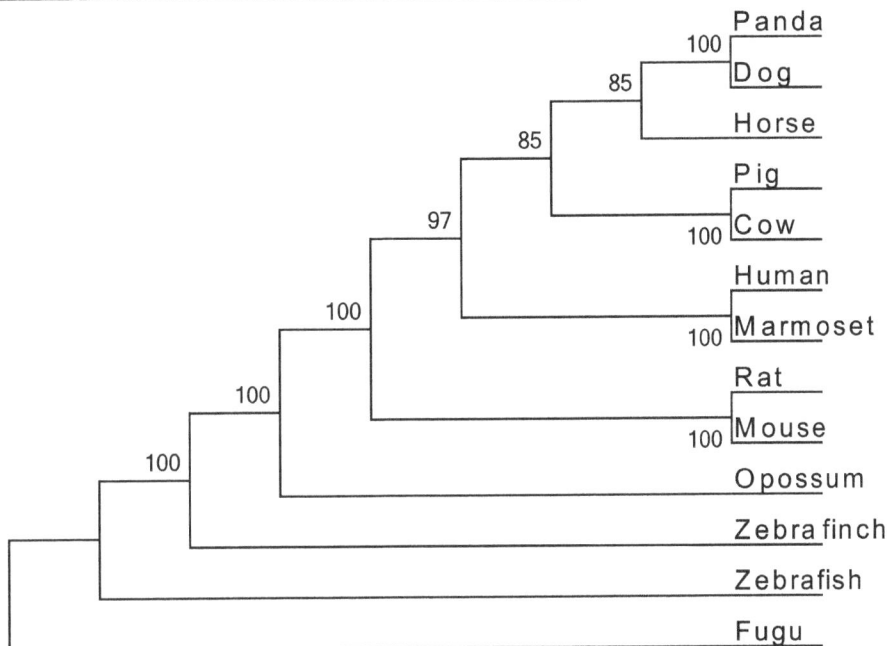

Figure 3 Phylogenetic analysis of thyroglobulin Tg1 regions from 13 species. Phylogenetic analysis of thyroglobulin Tg1 regions from 13 species (human, marmoset, rat, mouse, panda, dog, horse, pig, cow, opossum, zebra finch, zebrafish and fugu). Evolutionary history was inferred by the neighbor-joining method. The bootstrap consensus tree inferred from 1000 replicates is taken to represent the evolutionary history of the taxa analyzed. The numbers at nodes representing bootstrap support scores.

retained (15 thyroglobulins, 13 nidogens, 3 testicans, 2SPARC proteins, 3 invariant chains and 13 unnamed or hypothetical proteins). For the Tg1-3 domain, 16 proteins were found (thyroglobulins only). For the Tg1-4 domain, we retained 97 proteins (16 thyroglobulins, 13 nidogens, 10 testicans, 13 SPARC proteins, 4 invariant chains, 1 insulin-like growth factor binding protein (IGFBP) and 40 unnamed or hypothetical proteins). For the Tg1-5 domain, 103 proteins were retained (18 thyroglobulins, 6 nidogens, 11 testicans, 19 SPARC proteins, 3 invariant chains,2 IGFBPs and 44 unnamed or hypothetical proteins). For the Tg1-6 domains, 49 proteins were identified (17 thyroglobulins, 14 nidogens, 3 invariant chains and 15 unnamed or hypothetical proteins). For the Tg1-7 domain, 30 proteins were retained (10 thyroglobulins, 11 nidogens and 9 unnamed or hypothetical proteins). For the Tg1-8 domain, 105 proteins were retained (17 thyroglobulins, 13 nidogens, 9 testicans, 17 SPARC proteins, 5 invariant chains and 44 unnamed or hypothetical proteins). For the Tg1-9 domain, 11 proteins were found (thyroglobulins only). For the Tg1-10 domain, 100 proteins were retained (17 thyroglobulins, 13 nidogens, 7 testicans, 15 SPARC proteins, 3 invariant chains and 45 unnamed or hypothetical proteins). The number of thyroglobulin proteins displaying sequence similarity to the human Tg1 domains varied from 15 to 17, essentially due to the presence of incomplete thyroglobulin protein sequences in the databases we used, particularly for bears. The abovementioned proteinsdisplayed sequence

similarities to the Tg1 regions of proteins from five families [34]: testicans, SPARC-related modular calcium binding (SMOC) proteins, nidogens, IGFBPs and invariant chains. Testican proteins are involved in the regulation of cell attachment, cysteine protease and metalloprotease activities [35-38]. SMOC proteins are glycoproteins present principally at the basement membrane and involved in the regulation of calcium binding [39,40]. SMOC and testican proteins are present in metazoans. Proteins of the nidogen family are known to control the three-dimensional structure of the basal membrane [41]. Nidogen proteins arealso involved in cell attachment, neutrophil chemotaxis and nervous system development [42,43]. IGFBP belongs to a family of seven proteins with high affinity for IGF with different functions in several tissues [44]. Nidogen and IGFBP are present in both tunicates and craniates. The invariant chain is involved in MHC-II cell formation [45]. This protein, like the thyroglobulin protein, is present only in vertebrates.

The Tg2 region

The second region consists of three Tg2 repetitive domains of 15 amino acids each, presenting 24% identity. The phylogenetic analysis of this region was less robust than that of the Tg1 region, due to the small size of these domains. However, we identified 33 proteins displaying sequence similarity to the Tg2 region. Nine were thyroglobulins: Bos taurus, Mus musculus, Rattus norvegicus,

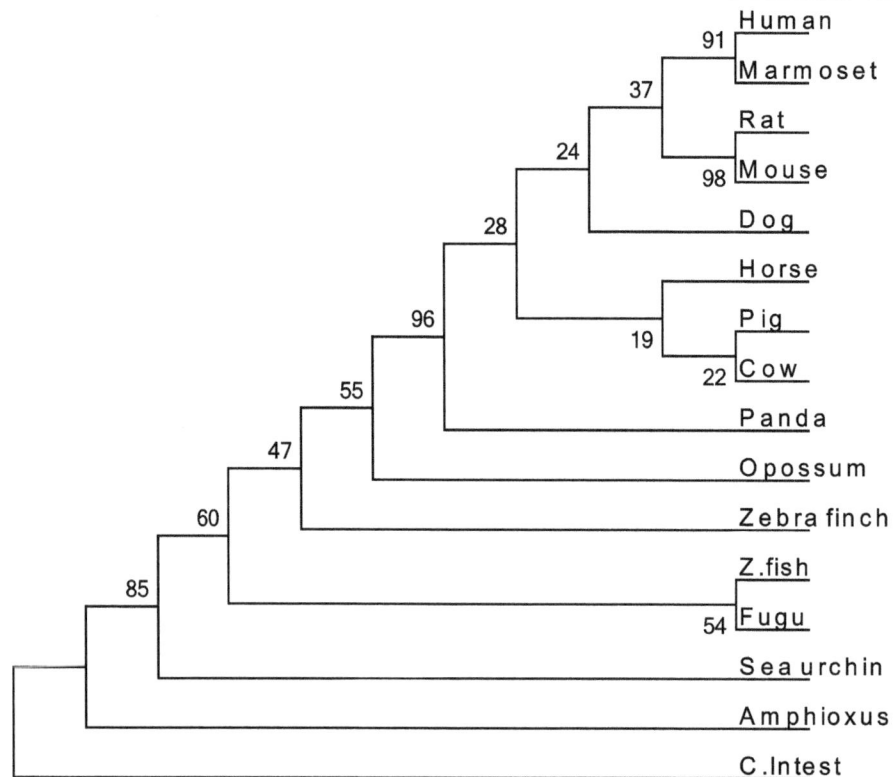

Figure 4 The phylogenetic analysis of thyroglobulins from 13 species. Phylogenetic analysis of thyroglobulins from 13 species (human, marmoset, rat, mouse, panda, dog, horse, pig, cow, opossum, zebra finch, zebrafish and fugu) and of thyroglobulin-like proteins from Ciona intestinalis, amphioxus and sea urchin. Evolutionary history was inferred by the neighbor-joining method. The bootstrap consensus tree inferred from 1000 replicates is taken to represent the evolutionary history of the taxa analyzed. The numbers at nodes representing bootstrap support scores.

Macaca mulatta, Canis lupus familiaris, Equus caballus, Sus scrofa, Taeniopygia guttata and Danio rerio. Eleven were signal peptide - CUB domain - EGF-like (SCUBE) proteins (SCUBE3: Canis familiaris, Mus musculus, Homo sapiens, Macaca mulatta, Sus scrofa and Danio rerio and/ or SCUBE1: Homo sapiens, Canis familiaris, Rattus norvegicus, Bos taurus and Danio rerio). The other 13 proteins were unnamed or hypothetical proteins. SCUBE proteins are known to involved in adhesion. Queries of the PFAM databas http://pfam.sanger.ac.uk identified a GCC2-GCC3 domain conserved in the Tg2 region of mouse and human thyroglobulins. The GCC2-GCC3 domain is also present in the human SVEP1 and mouse SCUB2 proteins.

The Tg3 region

In humans, the Tg3 region consists of five repetitive domains that can be classified into two subgroups: three domains in subgroup a (Tg3-a1: 111 AA, Tg3-a2: 98 AA, Tg3-a3: 58 AA) and two domains in subgroup b (Tg3-b1: 163 AA, Tg3-b2: 130 AA). TheseTg3 domains are 9% identical (Figure 5-a and 5-b). A search for proteins displaying sequence similarity to Tg3 domains identified only thyroglobulin proteins. Interestingly, the best conservation of

cysteine residues between domains was observed in humans, with perfect conservation (100%) for Tg3-a domains and very high levels of conservation (87%) for Tg3-b domains. Furthermore, the five amino acids perfectly conserved in all Tg3 domains were cysteine residues (Figure 5-c). Cysteine residues account for 6% of all the amino acids present in the human Tg3 region and these residues were remarkably conserved in the thyroglobulin Tg3 regions of all the species studied; 100% of the 34 cysteine residues were perfectly conserved between the Tg3 regions of 12 species (human, rat, panda, marmoset, mouse, horse, dog, cow, zebra finch, zebrafish and fugu). In the opossum, two of the 34 cysteine residues in the Tg3 region were displaced (Additional file 1: Figure S1).

Tg3 domains were found only in vertebrate thyroglobulins. We investigated the origin of the Tg3 region domains, by comparing the sequences of the zebrafish Tg3 domains with the amphioxus protein. We found a similar sequence in region 413–441 of the amphioxus protein. Phylogenetic analysis including this region with the human and zebrafish thyroglobulin Tg3 domains clustered the 413–441 region of the amphioxus protein with the Tg3-2b domain of the human and the zebrafish

a)

```
Tg3-a2   CLSRCVQEHSFCQLAEITESASLYFTCTLYP---EAQVCD------DIMESN------AQ   45
Tg3-a3   CLSECS-QHEACLITTLQTQPG-AVRCMFYA---DTQSCT------HSLQG--------Q   41
Tg3-a1   CLTDCT-EDEACSFFTVSTTEP-EISCDFYAWTSDNVACMTSDQKRDALGNSKATSFGSL  58
         **: *  :,. * :  :   .  * :*.  :   *    , : *
```

```
Tg3-a2   GCRLILP---QMPKALFRKKVI-LEDKVKNFYTRLPFQKLMGISIRNKVPMSEKSIS     98
Tg3-a3   NCRLLLR---EEATHIYRKP------------------------------------     58
Tg3-a1   RCQVKVRSHGQDSPAVYLKKGQGSTTTLQKRFEPTGFQNMLSG-LYNPIVFSAS---    111
         *.. .       ,     .. *
```

b)

```
Tg3-b1   CLLACDRDLCCDGF---VLTQVQGGAIICGLLSSPSVLLCNVKDWMDPSEAWANATCPGV   57
Tg3-b2   CERRCDADPCCTGFGFLNVSQLKGGEVTCLTLNSLGIQMCSE----ENGGAWR-------  49
         *   ** * ** **     ::*::** : *  *.* .: :*.    : , **
```

```
Tg3-b1   TYDQESHQVILRLGDQEFIKSLTPLEGTQDTFTNFQQVYLWKDSDMGSRPESMGCRKDTV  117
Tg3-b2   ---------ILDCGSPDIEVHTYPFG--------------WYQKPIAQNNAPSFCPLVVL   86
                  ** *, ::      *:             * :, :... , *    .:
```

```
Tg3-b1   PRPASPTEAGLTTELFSPVDLNQVIVNGNQSLSSQKHW--LFKHLFSA  163
Tg3-b2   P---SLTEK-VSLDSWQSLALSSVVVDPSIRHFDVAHVSTAATSNFSA  130
         *   * ** ::: : :,.: *.,*:*:. , * ,  ***
```

c)

```
Tg3-a2   CLSRCVQEHSFCQLA---EITESASLYFTCTLYP---EAQVCD--------DIMESN---  43
Tg3-a3   CLSECS-QHEACLIT---TLQTQPG-AVRCMFYA---DTQSCT--------HSLQG----  40
Tg3-a1   CLTDCT-EDEACSFF---TVSTTEP-EISCDFYAWTSDNVACMTSDQKR--DALGNSKAT  53
Tg3-b1   CLLACD-RDLCCDGF---VLTQVQGGAIICGLLS-SPSVLLCNVKDWMDPSEAWANATCP  55
Tg3-b2   CERRCD-ADPCCTGFGFLNVSQLKGGEVTCLTLN-SLGIQMCSEENGG-----------  46
         *   *  ,  *     :           , *          *
```

```
Tg3-a2   -----AQGCRLILP------------QMPKALFR---------------KKVI-LEDKV  69
Tg3-a3   ------QNCRLLLR------------EEATHIYR---------------KP--------  58
Tg3-a1   --SFGSLRCQVKVRSHG----------QDSPAVYL---------------KKGQGSTTTL  86
Tg3-b1   GVTYDQESHQVILRLGDQEFIKSLTPLEGTQDTFTNFQQVYLWKDSDMGSRPESMGCRKD  115
Tg3-b2   -------AWRILDCGSP----------DIEVHTYPFG---------WYQKPIAQNNAPS   79
                 ::                  :      :              :
```

```
Tg3-a2   KNFYTRLP-FQKLMGISIRNKVPMSEKSIS--------------------   98
Tg3-a3   --------------------------------------------------
Tg3-a1   QKRFEPTG-FQNMLSG-LYNPIVFSAS-----------------------  111
Tg3-b1   TVPRPASP-TEAGLTTELFSPVDLNQVIVNGNQSLSSQKHW--LFKHLFSA  163
Tg3-b2   FCPLVVLPSLTEKVSLDSWQSLALSSVVVDPSIRHFDVAHVSTAATSNFSA  130
```

Figure 5 Alignment of the Tg3 domains in human thyroglobulin. a) The alignment of Tg3-a domains in human thyroglobulin: 83% of the cysteine residues are conserved in Tg3-a1, Tg3-a2 and Tg3-a3; 100% of the cysteine residues are conserved between Tg3-a1 and Tg3-a2. 55% of the conserved amino acids in Tg3-a domains are cysteine residues. **b)** The alignment of Tg3-b domains in human thyroglobulin: 100% of the cysteine residues are conserved in Tg3-b1 and Tg3-b2; 23% of the conserved amino acids in Tg3-b domains are cysteine residues. **c)** The alignment of all Tg3 domains in human thyroglobulin: 44% of the cysteine residues are conserved in all Tg3 domains; 100% of the conserved amino acids in Tg3 domains are cysteine residues.

thyroglobulins, albeit witha low bootstrap percentage (data not shown).

The C-terminal ChEL domain

The ChEL domain of human thyroglobulin consists of 581 amino acids. This region displays a high level of similarity to acetylcholinesterase, hence its name. Acetylcholinesterase catalyzes the degradation of acetylcholine in the regulation of neurotransmission [46]. Blastall analyses of the ChEL domain identified 992 proteins displaying sequence similarity to this domain: 30 thyroglobulin proteins, 598 esterases (either carboxylesterases (n = 205) or cholinesterases (n = 150)) and 35 neuroligins. Cholinesterase-like regions have previously been identified in both enzymes and structural proteins [25]. When present in structural proteins, this region is thought to be related to cell movement, as a first sign of cell differentiation [47]. The function of the ChEL domain in thyroglobulin was recently linked to its transport throughout the endoplasmic reticulum [48]. Furthermore, ChEL-truncated thyroglobulin has been shown to be unable to form homodimers [49].

Thyroid hormone synthesis sites

We determined the number of thyroid hormone synthesis sites in the thyroglobulin proteins studied here. The human thyroglobulin protein contains four major thyroid hormone synthesis sites [21]; An alignment of thyroglobulin sequences showed that the zebra finch, zebrafish and fugu proteins contained only three of the human thyroid hormone synthesis sites (Additional file 1: Figure S1). The first site (Tyr5) is the main site of hormone synthesis (more than 50%) [50] and was found to be present in all the thyroglobulin proteins studied. In amphioxus, the tyrosine residue in this position was replaced by a phenylalanine residue. Sequence alignment data showed that only the third site was present in amphioxus and that the Ciona intestinalis protein contained no thyroid hormone synthesis sites.

Discussion

The Tg1 region of thyroglobulin may be involved in binding

In vertebrates, iodination of the tyrosine residues of thyroglobulin requires the protein to be present in the lumen of the thyroid follicle. The iodinated thyroglobulin is then returned to the cell via a process called pinocytosis, which involves histone H1 [3], megalin (gp330) [4] and/or the N-acetylglucosamine receptor [5]. Our study of the thyroglobulin Tg1 region showed this region to be structurally related to proteins with binding functions from five families. Novinec et al [34] also described another protein with sequence similarity to the Tg1 domain, trophinin. This membrane protein has been shown to mediate the adhesion of homophilic cells [51]. We think the Tg1 region

may mediate the binding of thyroglobulin to the thyrocyte apical membrane. The region of the H1 histone binding to thyroglobulin remains unidentified, whereas two regions of the N-acetylglucosamine receptor have been reported to bind thyroglobulin: RHL-1 subunit (N1-A500) [5] and (S789-M1,172) [52]. These receptors bind to the N-terminal end (Tg1 region) of the thyroglobulin protein. By contrast, megalin has been shown to interact with the carboxy-terminal domain of thyroglobulin, at R2,489-E2,503 [53], although the authors of this study were themselves critical of this work [54]. They reported that the region of interaction was poorly conserved between human and rat thyroglobulins and their finding that a rabbit antibody raised against R2,489-E2,503 reduced heparin-binding to rat Tg by only 70% led them to conclude that other heparin-binding sites must be involved in binding. These data, including the similarity of the Tg1 region to the extracellular matrix proteins nidogen and testican, provide support for our hypothesis that the Tg1 region is involved in the attachment and endocytosis of thyroglobulin.

Phylogeny of the Tg1 region

The function of thyroglobulin seems to depend strongly on the follicle structure of the thyroid. This follicular structure is observed only in vertebrates. Nonetheless, although it remains unclear whether a colloid is present in the endostyle of the invertebrates of the chordate group, such as cephalochordates and urochordates, the endostyle is widely considered to be homologous to the follicle of the vertebrate thyroid gland [55]. This is not consistent with the detection of a thyroglobulin protein in Eisenia fetida by Wilhelm [56]. In annelids, hormones are produced exclusively by the central nervous system. No sequence that could be unambiguously identified as corresponding to a thyroglobulin was found in the amphioxus genome [57], but a large protein (about 2,400 amino acids) with biochemical properties similar to those of thyroglobulin has been described in this organism [58]. Both T3 and T4 have also been described in this cephalochordate [59]. The 2,400-amino acid thyroglobulin-like protein of this species contains six domains displaying sequence similarity to the Tg1 region but not to the Tg2, Tg3 and ChEL domains (Figure 1-c).

Another smaller protein of about 137 amino acids that clusters with vertebrate thyroglobulin in phylogenetic analysis was identified in sea urchin (Figure 4). This protein contains two Tg1 domains but has no Tg2, Tg3 or ChEL domains (Figure 1-d). Phylogenetic analysis of a large number of sequences [60] classified the urochordates as more closely related to vertebrates than the cephalochordates (amphioxus) and echinoderms (sea urchin). On the basis of these data, we looked for a protein homologous to thyroglobulin in urochordates. Patricolo et al. demonstrated the presence of thyroid hormones and their involvement in metamorphosis in ascidian larvae from the Urochordata [17]. However, the genome of another urochordate, Ciona intestinalis, was found to contain no sequence homologous to thyroglobulin despite the presence of thyroid hormones. These data suggest that ascidians use other precursor proteins for iodotyrosine synthesis [61]. Together, these data suggest that the origins of the thyroglobulin protein lie in the Echinodermata.

We investigated the origin of the Tg1 region domains, by studying the phylogeny of the Tg1 domains in an analysis including the sea urchin protein (Echinodermata), the amphioxus protein (Cephalochordata), and the zebrafish (Teleostei), zebra finch (Aves) and human thyroglobulins. Our results suggest that the second Tg1 domain of the sea urchin protein is the ancestor of the sixth Tg1 domains of the amphioxus protein, while Tg1 domains 1, 2, 3, 4 and 5 of the amphioxus protein probably resulting from the duplication of domain 6. The phylogenetic analysis suggested that the Tg1-1, Tg1-2, Tg1-8 and Tg1-10 domains ofthyroglobulin were derived directly from the Tg1 domains of the amphioxus protein (Figure 2). The separation of thyroglobulin domains into two major branches may indicate two different origins of thyroglobulin Tg1 domains. The thyroglobulin Tg1 domains clustering with the amphioxus protein Tg1 domains are located at the end of the Tg1 region. We suggest that the thyroglobulin Tg1 domainsduplicated from the two ends to the center of the Tg1 region. The number of Tg1 domains presence increases with the number of evolutionary steps, suggesting that the evolution of thyroglobulin function may be dependent on number of Tg1 domains. However,the branching of the tree for Tg1 domains has only weak bootstrap support. (Figure 2 and Additional file 6: Figure S2), probably due to the length of time over which evolution has been occurring. Each Tg1 domain is free to evolve by itself, but the overall structure of the Tg1 region is conserved (Figure 3).

Involvement of the Tg2 region in cell adhesion

The presence of the Tg2 region in the SCUBE protein of many species suggests that these proteins may have a common function. SCUBE is a protein found in many embryonic tissues [62]. In zebrafish, mutations in the SCUBE2 gene are associated principally with developmental deficits [63]. A recent study showed that SCUBE1 was an adhesive molecule mediating platelet-matrix interaction and ristocetin-induced platelet agglutination [64]. On the basis of its secretory nature, SCUBE3 is thought to function locally or at distance, in a paracrine or endocrine fashion [65]. However, the exact functions of SCUBE3 remain elusive. On the basis of these and

published results, we suggest the Tg2 region isinvolved in thyroglobulin-mediated cell adhesion. The conservation of the GCC2-GCC3 domain in the Tg2 region highlights the structural conservation of this region. The function of the GCC2-GCC3 domain remains unknown, but this domain is present in the human SVEP1 protein. The functional annotation of this protein indicates a role in cell adhesion. This is potentially consistent with our hypothesis that the Tg2 region is involved in cell adhesion.

The Tg3 region may have a structural function

Cysteine is important for the correct three-dimensional structure of a protein, through its role in the formation of disulfide bonds. Misfolded proteins are recognized as abnormal and disposed of by a non lysosomal proteolytic pathway. Hishinuma et al [66] showed that replacement of the cysteine residues of (C1236R) (C1995S) thyroglobulin prevent the protein from forming the disulfide bonds required for thyroglobulin monomer production. As a result, intracellular transport is blocked and both these mutated thyroglobulins are retained in the endoplasmic reticulum. The high degree of cysteine residue conservation in Tg3 domains and in Tg3 regions from the 13 species used to generate the phyogenetic tree, from Actinopterygii to humans, highlights the importance of correct disulfide bond formation to the the tertiary structure of thyroglobulin. In a recent study, Targovenik et al [67] reviewed the cysteine mutations in thyroglobulin andshowed that more than half these mutations (55%) occurred in the Tg3 region. They also reported changes to the three-dimensional structure of thyroglobulin in the presence of cysteine mutations in the Tg3 region. The presence of Tg3 regions only in thyroglobulin proteins may be explained by a structural function, the disulfide bonds being essential to the three-dimensional structure of the molecule. The region of homology highlighted here between the zebrafish Tg3 region and the amphioxus protein suggests that this best conserved region between Tg3 domains may be the origin of these domains. There are two Tg3 subgroups, a and b. We therefore suggest that the original sequence duplicated twice initially, to generate the Tg3-a and Tg3-b domains. The Tg3-a domain duplicated three times, generating Tg3-a1, Tg3-a2 and Tg3-a3, and the Tg3-b domain duplicated twice, giving rise to Tg3-b1 and Tg3-b2.

The ChEL domain is involved in protein transport

The two studies mentioned above [48,49] demonstrated that a role for the ChEL domain in the dimerization and transport of thyroglobulin. Kim et al [68] indicated that mutations affecting the ChEL domain of mouse thyroglobulin resulted in the synthesis of a full-length thyroglobulin that folded abnormally, preventing its transport to the Golgi complex. However, the ChEL domain is present in structural proteins, as described by Krejci et al [25]. We demonstrated the similarity of this domain between thyroglobulin, esterase and neuroligin proteins, neuroligins being heterophilic cell adhesion proteins [69]. We suggest that the ChEL domain is involved in thyroglobulin transport (thyrocyte to apical membrane) and dimerization, with a possible additional function in cell adhesion. Phylogenetic studies of esterase domains from less evolved species have indicated that the thyroglobulin ChEL and esterase domains have a common ancestor [26]. Additional file 2: Tables S2, Additional file 3: Table S3, Additional file 4: Table S4 and Additional file 5:Table S5 show the pairwise distances between whole thyroglobulin protein sequences and each region of thyroglobulin. The ChEL domain is the region of thyroglobulin for which distances were lowest between different species. This suggests that the thyroglobulin ChEL domain may have been less subject to rearrangement during evolution than the other domains.

Existence of other thyroid hormone synthesis sites

We show here that not all the thyroid hormone synthesis sites characterized to date are systematically present in all species with a thyroglobulin protein. The lack of some thyroid hormone synthesis sites in some more highly evolved species (3 in zebra finch, zebrafish and fugu), the presence of only one site in the amphioxus protein and the total absence of thyroid hormone synthesis sites in the sea urchin protein may be explained by the relocation of these sites. Thyroid hormone synthesisrequires tyrosine residue iodination. The sea urchin protein has five tyrosine residues (positions 3, 24, 31, 34 and 102) and at least one of these residues is a thyroid hormone synthesis site. The lack of sites in amphioxus, zebrafinch, zebrafish and fugu may be explained by an absence of need for large thyroid hormone production or the use of other tyrosine residues as thyroid hormone synthesis sites.

We explored the function of thyroglobulin by phylogeny; we compared the thyroglobulin regions of echinoderms and vertebrate species. Our results suggest that the Tg1 region may have been the first to appear in the thyroglobulin protein. The Tg1 regionwas also subject to the largest number of rearrangements during evolution. The Tg2, Tg3 and ChEL regions are present only in the thyroglobulin of vertebrates, suggesting a link between these regions and an adaptive function of thyroglobulin. The thyroglobulin protein seems to result from the assembly of the four regions. We found no precursor of thyroid hormones with only two or three of these regions in databases. We therefore suggest that the Tg2, Tg3 and ChEL regions appeared in thyroglobulin at the same time. These data support the hypothesis of potential additional functions of thyroglobulin in the cell, as an iodine reservoir, in cell-cell adhesion and in binding. As each

thyroglobulin region may have a specific function in the protein, a mutation in one region may have consequences for the specific function of this region, resulting in a different pattern of phenotypic expression.

Note

A recent study raised the question of human DNA contamination in genomic databases [70], The first 5477 bp of chromosome 11 in zebrafish is 100% identical to human chromosome 4. We verified the zebrafish thyroglobulin located on chromosome 16 at position chr16:33,835,318-33,852,335, and the human thyroglobulin located on chromosome 8 at position chr8:133,909,894-134,147,141.

Additional files

Additional file 1: Figure S1. The phylogenetic analysis of Tg1 domains from the thyroglobulins of 13 species. The phylogenetic analysis of thyroglobulin Tg1 domains from 13 species (human, marmoset, rat, mouse, panda, dog, horse, pig, cow, opossum, zebra finch, zebrafish and fugu) and the Tg1 domains of thyroglobulin-like proteins from Ciona intestinalis, amphioxus and sea urchin. Evolutionary history was inferred by the neighbor-joining method. The bootstrap consensus tree inferred from 1000 replicates is taken to represent the evolutionary history of the taxa analyzed. The numbers at nodes representing bootstrap scores.

Additional file 2: Table S1. Estimation of evolutionary divergence between the thyroglobulin protein sequences of 13 species + the thryoglobulin-like sequences of Ciona intestinalis, amphioxus and sea urchin. The number of amino-acid substitutions per site between sequences is shown. Standard error estimates are shown above the diagonal and were obtained by a bootstrap procedure (10000 replicates). Analyses were conducted with the Jones-Taylor-Thornton matrix-based model. The rate variation between sites was modeled with a gamma distribution (shape parameter = 1).

Additional file 3: Table S2. Estimation of evolutionary divergence between the Tg1 region sequences of thyroglobulins from 13 species. The number of amino acid substitutions per site between sequences is shown. Standard error estimates are shown above the diagonal and were obtained by a bootstrap procedure (10000 replicates). Analyses were conducted with the Jones-Taylor-Thornton matrix-based model. The rate variation between sites was modeled with a gamma distribution (shape parameter = 1).

Additional file 4: Table S3. Estimation of evolutionary divergence between the Tg3 region sequences of thyroglobulins from 13 species. The number of amino acid substitutions per site between sequences is shown. Standard error estimates are shown above the diagonal and were obtained by a bootstrap procedure (10000 replicates). Analyses were conducted with the Jones-Taylor-Thornton matrix-based model. The rate variation between sites was modeled with a gamma distribution (shape parameter = 1).

Additional file 5: Table S4. Estimation of evolutionary divergence between the ChEL region sequences of thyroglobulins from 13 species. The number of amino acid substitutions per site between sequences is shown. Standard error estimates are shown above the diagonal and were obtained by a bootstrap procedure (10000 replicates). Analyses were conducted with the Jones-Taylor-Thornton matrix-based model. The rate variation between sites was modeled with a gamma distribution (shape parameter = 1).

Additional file 6: Figure S2. ClustalX sequence alignment for thyroglobulins from 13 species. The ClustalX sequence alignment of thyroglobulins from 13 species (human, marmoset, rat, mouse, panda, dog, horse, pig, cow, opossum, zebra finch, zebrafish and fugu) and the amphioxus and sea urchin thyroglobulin-like proteins. Red: the four humanthyroid hormone synthesis sites; in green, the 10 human Tg1 domains; in yellow, the human Tg2 region; in blue, the 5 human Tg3 domains.

Competing interests

The authors declare that they have no competing interests.

Authors' contributions

YM AB conceived the analysis. CJ FS contributed to discussion and edited the manuscript. AB analyzed data and wrote the manuscript. All authors read and approved the final manuscript.

Acknowledgements

This work was supported by the regional organization BioInformatique Ligérienne (BIL) directed by Rémi Houlgatte. We would like to thank Laurent Abel for his help. We would also like to thank La région Pays de Loire, the Institut National de Recherche Médical (INSERM) and the University of Angers.

Author details

[1]INSERM U694, Institut Biologie Santé (IBS), rue des Capucins, F-49100 Angers, France. [2]University of Angers, rue de Rennes, F-49045 Angers, France. [3]Laboratory of human genetics of infectious diseases. Necker Branch, INSERM, U980 Paris, France.

References

1. Kotlarz G, Wegrowski Y, Martiny L, Declerck P, Bellon G: **Enhanced expression of plasminogen activator inhibitor-1 by dedifferentiated thyrocytes**. *Biochem Biophys Res Commun* 2002, **295**:737–743.
2. Delom F, Mallet B, Carayon P, Lejeune P: **Role of extracellular molecular chaperones in the folding of oxidized proteins, Refolding of colloidal thyroglobulin by protein disulfide isomerase and immunoglobulin heavy chain-binding protein**. *J Biol Chem* 2001, **276**:21337–21342.
3. Brix K, Summa W, Lottspeich F, Herzog V: **Extracellularly occurring histone H1 mediates the binding of thyroglobulin to the cell surface of mouse macrophages**. *J Clin Invest* 1998, **102**:283–293.
4. Zheng G, Marino' M, Zhao J, McCluskey R: **Megalin (gp330): a putative endocytic receptor for thyroglobulin (Tg)**. *Endocrinology* 1998, **139**:1462–1465.
5. Montuori N, Pacifico F, Mellone S, Liguoro D, Jeso BD, Formisano S, Gentile F, Consiglio E: **The rat asialoglycoprotein receptor binds the amino-terminal domain of thyroglobulin**. *Biochem Biophys Res Commun* 2000, **268**:42–46.
6. Dunn J, Anderson P, Fox J, Fassler C, Dunn A, Hite L, Moore R: **The sites of thyroid hormone formation in rabbit thyroglobulin**. *J Biol Chem* 1987, **262**:16948–16952.
7. Dunn J, Dunn A: **The importance of thyroglobulin structure for thyroid hormone biosynthesis**. *Biochimie* 1998, **81**:505–509.
8. Schimmel M, Utiger R: **Thyroidal and peripheral production of thyroid hormones, Review of recent findings and their clinical implications**. *Ann Intern Med* 1977, **87**:760–768.
9. Suzuki K, Lavaroni S, Mori A, Ohta M, Saito J, Pietrarelli M, Singer D, Kimura S, Katoh R, Kawaoi A, Kohn L: **Autoregulation of thyroid-specific gene transcription by thyroglobulin**. *Proc. Natl. Acad. Sci. USA* 1998, **95**:8251–8256.
10. Hayashi M, Shimonaka M, Matsui K, Hayashi T, Ochiai D, Emoto N: **Proliferative effects of bovine and porcine thyroglobulins on thyroid epithelial cells**. *Endocr J* 2009, **56**:509–519.
11. Monaco F, Roche J, Carducci C, Carlini F, Cataudella S, Felli P, Andreoli M, Dominici R: **Effect of change of habitat (sea and fresh water) on in vivo thyroglobulin synthesis in Atlantic glassed eels (Anguilla anguilla L.)**. *C R Seances Soc Biol Fil.* 1981, **175**:452–456.
12. Kim B: **Thyroid hormone as a determinant of energy expenditure and the basal metabolic rate**. *Thyroid* 2008, **18**:141–144.
13. Flamant F, Baxter J, Forrest D, Refetoff S, Samuels H, Scanlan T, Vennström B, Samarut J: **International Union of Pharmacology, LIX. The Pharmacology and Classification of the Nuclear Receptor Superfamily: Thyroid Hormone Receptors**. *Pharmacol Rev* 2006, **58**:705–711.
14. Power D, Llewellyn L, Faustino M, Nowell M, Björnsson B, Einarsdottir I, Canario A, Sweeney G: **Thyroid hormones in growth and developement of fish**. *Comp Biochem Physiol C Toxicol Pharmacol.* 2001, **130**:447–459.
15. Manchado M, Infante C, Asensio E, Planas J, Canavate J: **Thyroid hormones down-regulate thyrotropin beta subunit and thyroglobulin during**

16. metamorphosis in the flatfish Senegalese sole (Solea senegalensis Kaup). *Gen Comp Endocrino.* 2008, **155**:447–455.
16. Tata J: **Amphibian metamorphosis as a model for the developmental actions of thyroid hormone**. *Mol Cell Endocrinol* 2005, **246**:10–20.
17. Patricolo E, Cammarata M, D'Agati P: **Presence of thyroid hormones in ascidian larvae and their involvement in metamorphosis**. *J Exp Zool* 2001, **290**:426–430.
18. Paris M, Laudet V: **The history of developmental stages: metamorphosis in chordates**. *Genesis* 2008, **46**:657–672.
19. Manzon R, Holmes J, Youson J: **Variable effects of goitrogens in inducing precocious metamorphosis in sea lampreys (Petromyzon marinus)**. *J Exp Zool* 2001, **289**:290–303.
20. Mercken L, Simons M, Swillens S, Massaer M, Vassart G: **Primary structure of bovine thyroglobulin deduced from the sequence of its 8,431-base complementary DNA**. *Nature* 1985, **316**:647–651.
21. Malthiéry Y, Lissitzky S: **Primary structure of human thyroglobulin deduced from the sequence of its 8448-base complementary DNA**. *Eur J Biochem* 1987, **165**:491–508.
22. de Graaf SV, Ris-Stalpers C, Pauws E, Mendive F, Targovnik H, Vijlder J: **Up to date with human thyroglobulin**. *Endocr J* 2001, **170**:307–321.
23. Veneziani B, Giallauria F, Gentile F: **The disulfide bond pattern between fragments obtained by the limited proteolysis of bovine thyroglobulin**. *Biochimie* 1999, **81**:517–525.
24. Schumacher M, Camp S, Maulet Y, Newton M, MacPhee-Quigley K, Taylor S, Friedmann T, Taylor P: **Primary structure of Tropedo californica acetylcholinesterase deduced form its cDNA sequence**. *Nature* 1986, **319**:407–409.
25. Krejci E, Duval N, Chatonnet A, Vincens P, Massoulié J: **Cholinesterase-like domains in enzymes and structural proteins: functional and evolutionary relationships and identification of a catalytically essential aspartic acid**. *Proc Natl Acad Sci USA* 1991, **88**:6647–6651.
26. Takagi Y, Omura Y, Go M: **Evolutionary origin of thyroglobulin by duplication of esterase gene**. *FEBS Lett* 1991, **282**:17–22.
27. Izumi M, Larsen P: **Metabolic clearance of endogenous and radioiodinated thyroglobulin in rats**. *Endocrinology* 1978, **103**:96–100.
28. Rigden D, Mosolov V, Galperin M: **Sequence conservation in the chagasin family suggests a common trend in cysteine proteinase binding by unrelated protein inhibitors**. *Protein Sci* 2002, **11**:1971–1977.
29. Saverwyns H, Visser A, Durme JV, Power D, Morgado I, Kennedy M, Knox D, Schymkowitz J, Rousseau F, Gevaert K, Vercruysse J, Claerebout E, Geldhof P: **Analysis of the transthyretin-like (TTL) gene family in Ostertagia ostertagi - Comparison with other strongylid nematodes and Caenorhabditis elegans**. *Int J Parasitol* 2008, **38**:1545–1556.
30. Felsenstein J: **PHYLIP - Phylogeny Inference Package (Version 3.2)**. *Cladistics.* 1989, **5**:164–166.
31. Tamura K, Peterson D, Peterson N, Stecher G, Nei M, Kumar S: **MEGA5: Molecular Evolutionary Genetics Analysis using Maximum Likelihood, Evolutionary Distance, and Maximum Parsimony Methods**. *Mol Biol and Evol* 2011, **28**:2731-2739.
32. Jones D, Taylor W, Thornton J: **A mutation data matrix for transmembrane proteins**. *FEBS Lett* 1994, **339**:269–275.
33. Molina F, Bouanani M, Pau B, Granier C: **Characterization of the type-1 repeat from thyroglobulin, a cysteine-rich module found in proteins from different families**. *Eur J Biochem* 1996, **240**:125–133.
34. Novinec M, Kordis D, Turk V, Lenarcic B: **Diversity and evolution of the thyroglobulin type-1 domain superfamily**. *Mol Biol Evol* 2006, **23**:744–755.
35. Marr H, Edgell C: **Testican-1 inhibits attachment of Neuro-2a cells**. *Matrix Biol* 2003, **22**:259–266.
36. Bocock J, Edgell C, Marr H, Erickson A: **Human proteoglycan testican-1 inhibits the lysosomal cysteine protease cathepsin L**. *Eur J Biochem* 2003, **270**:4008–4015.
37. Nakada M, Yamada A, Takino T, Miyamori H, Takahashi T, Yamashita J, Sato H: **Suppression of membrane-type 1 matrix metalloproteinase (MMP)-mediated MMP-2 activation and tumor invasion by testican 3 and its splicing variant gene product**. *N-Tes. Cancer Res.* 2001, **61**:8896–8902.
38. Nakada M, Miyamori H, Yamashita J, Sato H: **Testican 2 abrogates inhibition of membrane-type matrix metalloproteinases by other testican family proteins**. *Cancer Res* 2003, **63**:3364–3369.
39. Vannahme C, Smyth N, Miosge N, Gösling S, Frie C, Paulsson M, Maurer P, Hartmann U: **Characterization of SMOC-1, a novel modular calcium-**

binding protein in basement membranes. *J Biol Chem* 2002, 277:37977–37986.

40. Vannahme C, Gösling S, Paulsson M, Maurer P, Hartmann U: **Characterization of SMOC-2, a modular extracellular calcium-binding protein.** *Biochem J* 2002, 373:805–814.

41. Aumailley M, Battaglia C, Mayer U, Reinhardt D, Nischt R, Timpl R, Fox J: **Nidogen mediates the formation of ternary complexes of basement membrane components.** *Kidney Int* 1993, 43:7–12.

42. Chakravarti S, Tam M, Chung A: **The basement membrane glycoprotein entactin promotes cell attachment and binds calcium ions.** *J Biol Chem* 1990, 265:10597–10603.

43. Kim S, Wadsworth W: **Positioning of longitudinal nerves in C. elegans by nidogen.** *Science* 2000, 288:150–154.

44. Rajaram S, Baylink D, Mohan S: **Insulin-like growth factor-binding proteins in serum and other biological fluids: regulation and functions.** *Endocr Rev* 1997, 18:801–831.

45. Holst P, Sorensen M, Jensen CM, Orskov C, Thomsen A, Christensen J: **MHC class II-associated invariant chain linkage of antigen dramatically improves cell-mediated immunity induced by adenovirus vaccines.** *J Immunol* 2008, 180:3339–3346.

46. Tsim K, Leung K, Mok K, Chen V, Zhu K, Zhu J, Guo A, Bi C, Zheng K, Lau D, Xie H, Choi R: **Expression and Localization of PRiMA-linked globular form acetylcholinesterase in vertebrate neuromuscular junctions.** *J Mol Neurosci* 2009, 40:40–46.

47. Layer P, Kaulich S: **Cranial nerve growth in birds is preceded by cholinesterase expression during neural crest cell migration and the formation of an HNK-1 scaffold.** *Cell Tissue Res* 1991, 265:393–407.

48. Lee J, Jeso BD, Arvan P: **The cholinesterase-like domain of thyroglobulin functions as an intramolecular chaperone.** *J Clin Invest* 2008, 118:2950–2958.

49. Lee J, Wang X, Jeso BD, Arvan P: **The cholinesterase-like domain, essential in thyroglobulin trafficking for thyroid hormone synthesis, is required for protein dimerization.** *J Biol Chem* 2009, 284:12752–12761.

50. Palumbo G, Gentile F, Condorelli G, Salvatore G: **The earliest site of iodination in thyroglobulin is residue number 5.** *J Biol Chem* 1990, 265:8887–8892.

51. Fukuda M, Sugihara K, Nakayama J: **Trophinin: what embryo implantation teaches us about human cancer.** *Cancer Biol Ther* 2008, 7:1165–1170.

52. Mezghrani A, Mziaut H, Courageot J, Oughideni R, Bastiani P, Miquelis R: **Identification of the membrane receptor binding domain of thyroglobulin, Insights into quality control of thyroglobulin biosynthesis.** *J Biol Chem* 1997, 272:23340–23346.

53. Marino M, Friedlander J, McCluskey R, Andrews D: **Identification of a Heparin-binding Region of Rat Thyroglobulin Involved in Megalin Binding.** *J Biol Chem* 1999, 274:30377–30386.

54. Lisi S, Pinchera A, McCluskey R, Chiovato L, Marino M: **Binding of heparin to human thyroglobulin (Tg) involves multiple binding sites including a region corresponding to a binding site of rat Tg.** *Eur J Endocrinol* 2002, 146:591–602.

55. Ogasawara M, Lauro RD, Satoh N: **Ascidian homologs of mammalian thyroid peroxidase genes are expressed in the thyroid-equivalent region of the endostyle.** *J Exp Zool* 1999, 285:158–169.

56. Wilhelm M, Koza A, Engelmann P, Németh P, Csoknya M: **Evidence for the presence of thyroid stimulating hormone, thyroglobulin and their receptors in Eisenia fetida: a multilevel hormonal interface between the nervous system and the peripheral tissues.** *Cell Tissue Res* 2006, 324:535–546.

57. Paris M, Brunet F, Markov G, Schubert M, Laudet V: **The amphioxus genome enlightens the evolution of the thyroid hormone signaling pathway.** *Dev Genes Evol* 2008, 218:667–680.

58. Monaco F, Dominici R, Andreoli M, Pirro RD, Roche J: **Thyroid hormone formation in thyroglobulin synthetized in the amphioxus (Branchiostoma lanceolatum Pallas.** *Comp Biochem Physiol* 1980, 70:341–343.

59. Covelli I, Salvador G, Sena L, Roche J: **Sur la formation des hormones thyroïdiennes et de leurs précursseurs par Branchiostoma lanceolatum.** *C R Soc Biol Paris* 1960, 154:1165–1169.

60. Delsuc F, Brinkmann H, Chourrout D, Philippe H: **Tunicates and not cephalochordates are the closest living relatives of vertebrates.** *Nature* 2006, 439:965–968.

61. Campbell R, Satoh N, Degnan B: **Piecing together evolution of the vertebrate endocrine system.** *Trends Genet* 2004, 20:359–366.

62. Grimmond S, Larder R, Hateren NV, Siggers P, Hulsebos T, Arkell R, Greenfield A: **Cloning, mapping, and expression analysis of a gene encoding a novel mammalian EGF-related protein (SCUBE1).** *Genomics* 2000, 70:74–81.

63. Woods I, Talbot W: **The you gene encodes an EGF-CUB protein essential for Hedgehog signaling in zebrafish.** *PLoS Biol* 2005, 3:e66.

64. Tu C, Su Y, Huang Y, Tsai M, Li L, Chen Y, Cheng C, Dai D, Yang R: **Localization and characterization of a novel secreted protein SCUBE1 in human platelets.** *Cardiovasc Res* 2006, 71:486–495.

65. Wu B, Su Y, Tsai M, Wasserman S, Topper J, Yang R: **A novel secreted, cell-surface glycoprotein containing multiple epidermal growth factor-like repeats and one CUB domain is highly expressed in primary osteoblasts and bones.** *J Biol Chem* 2004, 279:37485–37490.

66. Hishinuma A, Takamatsu J, Ohyama Y, Yokozawa T, Kanno Y, Kuma K, Yoshida S, Matsuura N, Ieiri T: **Two novel cysteine substitutions (C1263R and C1995S) of thyroglobulin cause a defect in intracellular transport of thyroglobulin in patients with congenital goiter and the variant type of adenomatous goiter.** *J Clin Endocrinol Metab* 1999, 84:1438–1444.

67. Targovnik H, Esperante S, Rivolta C: **Genetics and phenomics of hypothyroidism and goiter due to thyroglobulin mutations.** *Mol Cell Endocrinol* 2009, 322:44–55.

68. Kim P, Hossain S, Park Y, Lee I, Yoo S, Arvan P: **A single amino acid change in the acetylcholinesterase-like domain of thyroglobulin causes congenital goiter with hypothyroidism in the cog/cog mouse: a model of human endoplasmic reticulum storage diseases.** *Proc Natl Acad Sci USA* 1998, 95:9909–9913.

69. Jaco AD, Dubi N, Comoletti D, Taylor P: **Folding anomalies of neuroligin3 caused by mutation in the α/β -hydrolase fold domain.** *Chem Biol Interact* 2010, 187:56–58.

70. Longo M, O'Neil M, O'Neill R: **Abundant Human DNA Contamination Identified in Non-Primate Genome Databases.** *PLoS One* 2011, 6:e16410.

2

Rare thyroid non-neoplastic diseases

Katarzyna Lacka* and Adam Maciejewski

Abstract

Rare diseases are usually defined as entities affecting less than 1 person per 2,000. About 7,000 different rare entities are distinguished and, among them, rare diseases of the thyroid gland. Although not frequent, they can be found in the everyday practice of endocrinologists and should be considered in differential diagnosis. Rare non-neoplastic thyroid diseases will be discussed. Congenital hypothyroidism's frequency is relatively high and its early treatment is of vital importance for neonatal psychomotor development; CH is caused primarily by thyroid dysgenesis (85%) or dyshormonogenesis (10-15%), although secondary defects - hypothalamic and pituitary - can also be found; up to 40% of cases diagnosed on neonatal screening are transient. Inherited abnormalities of thyroid hormone binding proteins (TBG, TBP and albumin) include alterations in their concentration or affinity for iodothyronines, this leads to laboratory test abnormalities, although usually with normal free hormones and clinical euthyroidism. Thyroid hormone resistance is most commonly found in *THRB* gene mutations and more rarely in *THRA* mutations; in some cases both genes are unchanged (non-TR RTH). Recently the term 'reduced sensitivity to thyroid hormones' was introduced, which encompass not only iodothyronine receptor defects but also their defective transmembrane transport or metabolism. Rare causes of hyperthyroidism are: activating mutations in *TSHR* or *GNAS* genes, pituitary adenomas, differentiated thyroid cancer or gestational trophoblastic disease; congenital hyperthyroidism cases are also seen, although less frequently than CH. Like other organs and tissues, the thyroid can be affected by different inflammatory and infectious processes, including tuberculosis and sarcoidosis. In most of the rare thyroid diseases genetic factors play a key role, many of them can be classified as monogenic disorders. Although there are still some limitations, progress has been made in our understanding of rare thyroid diseases etiopathogenesis, and, thanks to these studies, also in our understanding of how normal thyroid gland functions.

Keywords: Rare disease, Thyroid gland, Congenital hypothyroidism, Thyroxin binding globulin, Transthyretin, Thyroid hormone resistance, Dysgenesis, Dyshormonogenesis, Mutation

Introduction

Rare diseases are usually defined as entities affecting 5 or fewer per 10,000 (1 person per 2,000), although different thresholds can also be found, e.g. in Japan - fewer than 4 cases per 10,000 or in the United States - fewer than 200,000 patients affected across the country. Despite this rarity, the total number of a people with diagnosis of rare diseases is estimated at 350 million all over the world. Approximately 7,000 distinct rare entities are described, most of them genetically determined [1]. Another term - ultra-rare diseases - is usually referred to diseases that affect less than 1 person per 50,000 [2].

On the basis of prevalence, some thyroid gland diseases can also be classified as rare. They have genetic origin in most cases, often as a result of single gene mutations (monogenic disorders). Rare thyroid diseases should be considered in differential diagnosis of commonly seen thyroid entities, their right diagnosis may be often of vital importance. The aim of this review is therefore to briefly present the spectrum of rare thyroid diseases and underling etiopathogenesis. Rare thyroid diseases can be classified into two main categories: neoplastic and non-neoplastic disorders. Rare thyroid non-neoplastic entities will be discussed further in this paper.

Review

Congenital hypothyroidism

Congenital hypothyroidism (CH) can be classified as primary or secondary. The causes of primary CH are thyroid dysgenesis or dyshormonogenesis. Secondary CH may be: 1) hypothalamic (also called tertiary CH) – *TRH*

* Correspondence: kktlacka@gmail.com
Department of Endocrinology, Metabolism and Internal Medicine, University of Medical Sciences, Poznan, Poland

gene mutations; 2) pituitary – congenital hypopituitarism with multihormonal insufficiency (some known mutations of transcription factors' genes such as *Pit 1, Prop 1, LHX 3, LHX 4, HESX1*, but 80-90% of idiopathic origin) or isolated TSH deficiency (*TSHB* or *rTRH genes* mutations). Some cases of congenital thyroid hormones deficiency are transient (the percentage varies between studies, up to 40%) and euthyroidism is achieved within the first months or years of life (maternal antithyroid drug intake, maternal TSHR blocking antibodies, iodine deficiency or excess, some heterozygous mutations of DUOX2 and DUOXA2, congenital liver hemangioma) [3]. Lack of thyroid hormone action at birth may also result from peripheral causes (peripheral congenital hypothyroidism), which will be discussed in subsequent paragraphs.

The general prevalence of CH, regardless of its etiology, is 1:2,000 to 1:4,000 of neonates (primary CH - 1:4,000, secondary CH – 1:66,000) with a female-to-male ratio of 2:1. These values vary between different regions (1:800 in the Greek Cypriot population, 1:2,000 in China, 1:2,300 in the US and 1:10,000 in France) or ethnic groups (highest prevalence in Asians) [3-5]. In Poland it is estimated that CH affects about 1:4,500 of all screened neonates [6]. In iodine sufficient regions, the vast majority of CH cases are caused by thyroid dysgenesis (up to 85%) and dyshormonogenesis (10-15%), while secondary CH is responsible for only 0.0015% of all cases [7]. The genes involved in CH etiopathogenesis are presented in Figure 1.

Dysgenesis

The term thyroid dysgenesis includes the ectopic location of the gland (thyroid ectopy), absence (athyreosis) and underdevelopment of the thyroid tissue (hypoplasia). Unilateral thyroid agenesis (hemiagenesis) is also classified as thyroid dysgenesis, although usually with clinical euthyroidism [8]. Within the group of thyroid dysgenesis, ectopy is found most commonly, with lingual, supra- and infrahyoid localization of the gland most frequently seen. Cases of thyroid dysgenesis are usually sporadic, inherited genetic defects are only recognized in about 2% of all cases and result from transcription factor genes mutations (*PAX8, NKX2-1/TITF1, NXK2-5, FOXE1/TITF-2*) [9]. As these transcription factors are also involved in extrathyroid development, different organs' congenital anomalies may coexist (Table 1). The thyroid gland is the only organ affected by *TSHR gene* (14q31.1) mutations, which account for about 1% of all CH cases. As more than 60 different *TSHR* loss-of-function mutations have been found (Y444X described for the first time in the Polish population), a variable degree of TSH resistance and ongoing clinical presentation are observed (from euthyroid hyperthyrotropinemia to hypoplasia with severe hypothyroidism) [10,11]. TSH resistance is also observed in mutations of *GNAS gene* (20q13.32), encoding the alpha subunit of G protein, downstream of TSH receptor in the signaling pathway. As G protein is also responsible for signal transduction of other peptide

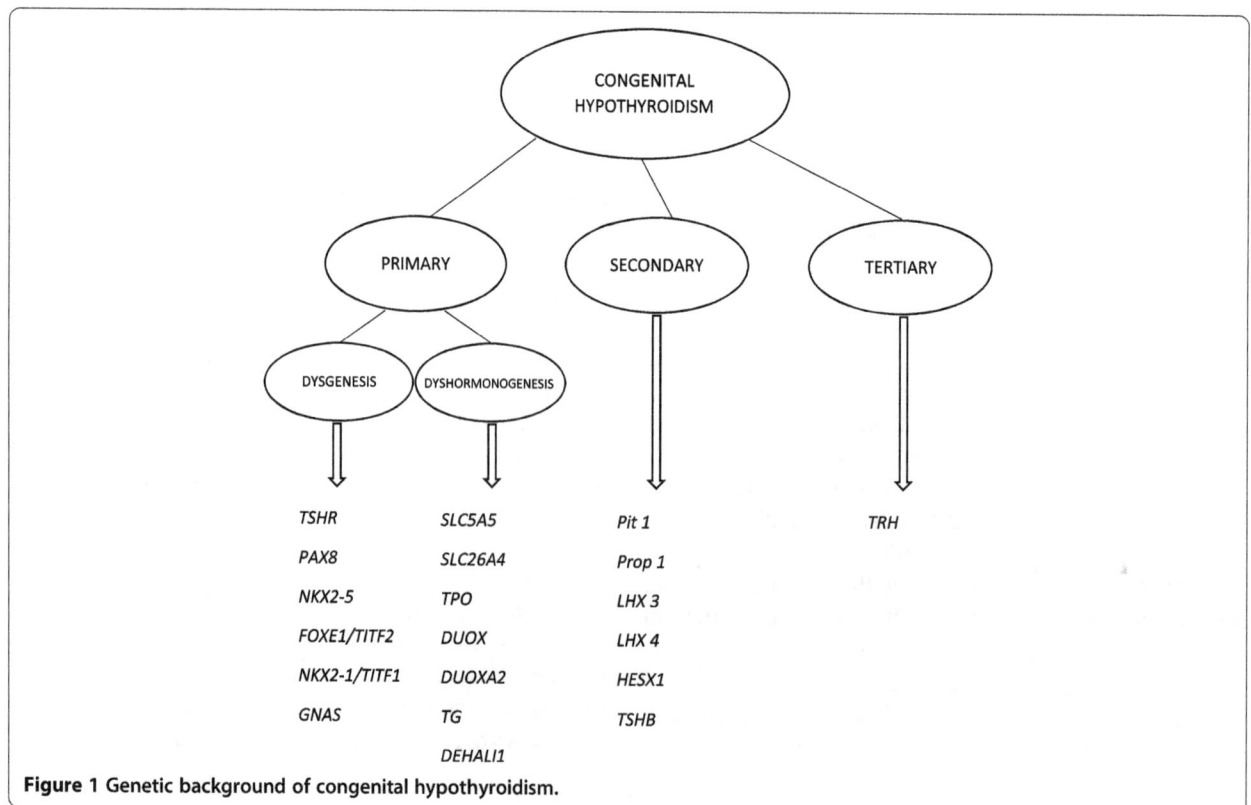

Figure 1 Genetic background of congenital hypothyroidism.

Table 1 Transcription factor genes responsible for thyroid dysgenesis

Gene	Locus	Type of inheritance	Expression	Clinical manifestation
PAX8	2q13	AD	Thyroid, kidney, CNS	Thyroid hypoplasia or athyreosis, agenesis/hemiagenesis of the kidneys
NKX2-5	5q35.1	AD	Thyroid, heart, pharynx	Thyroid ectopy, athyreosis, congenital cardiac malformations
FOXE1/TITF2	9q22.33	AR	Thyroid, pituitar, tongue, epiglottis, palate, pharynx, thymus and Rathke's pouch, choanae, hair follicles	Athyreosis, other forms of thyroid dysgenesis, cleft palate, cleft epiglottis, choanal atresia, spiky hair
NKX2-1/TITF1	14q13.3	AD	Thyroid, lung, trachea, CNS	Thyroid dysgenesis, dyshormonogenesis due to inhibited TG expression, choreoatetosis, hypotony, respiratory distress

hormones, in these cases resistance is multihormonal and the clinical picture is complex (pseudohypoparathyroidism type 1a) [12]. The role of environmental factors (e.g. intrauterine viral infections) in thyroid dysgenesis is also suggested [13].

Dyshormonogenesis

Another reason for primary CH – dyshormonogenesis – arises from defective thyroid hormone synthesis; all its stages may be affected (Figure 2). These monogenic defects are inherited predominantly with an autosomal recessive pattern. Clinically, in addition to the symptoms and signs of thyroid hormone deficiency (rarely euthyroidism), patients may present with goiter.

Mutations in the SLC5A5 gene (19p13.11) encoding sodium-iodide symporter (NIS) result in a defect in the active transport of iodide to thyrocytes. NIS glycoprotein is expressed not only in the thyroid follicular cells, but also in some non-thyroid tissues – salivary and lacrimal

glands, cancerous breast tissue, the breast during lactation, the intestines, stomach, testes and placenta. To data, at least 12 different loss-of-function mutations in the NIS gene have been described [14]. This relatively rare cause of dyshormonogenesis is characterized by an autosomal recessive pattern of inheritance. Diminished or completely inhibited iodine uptake by the thyroid is characteristic.

Pendrin, encoded by SLC26A4 gene (7q22.3), is an anion transporter expressed primarily in the thyroid (allows iodide efflux into the follicular lumen) but also in the inner ear, kidneys and lungs. Bi-allelic mutations of the SLC26A4 gene (about 470 mutations described to date) lead mainly to two different phenotypes: a) non-syndromic hearing loos with enlarged vestibular aqueduct (EVA) or b) Pendred syndrome (PDS) with congenital bilateral sensorineural hearing loss and thyroid defect (diffuse or multinodular goiter, thyroid hormone status is dependent on iodide intake, with dominance of

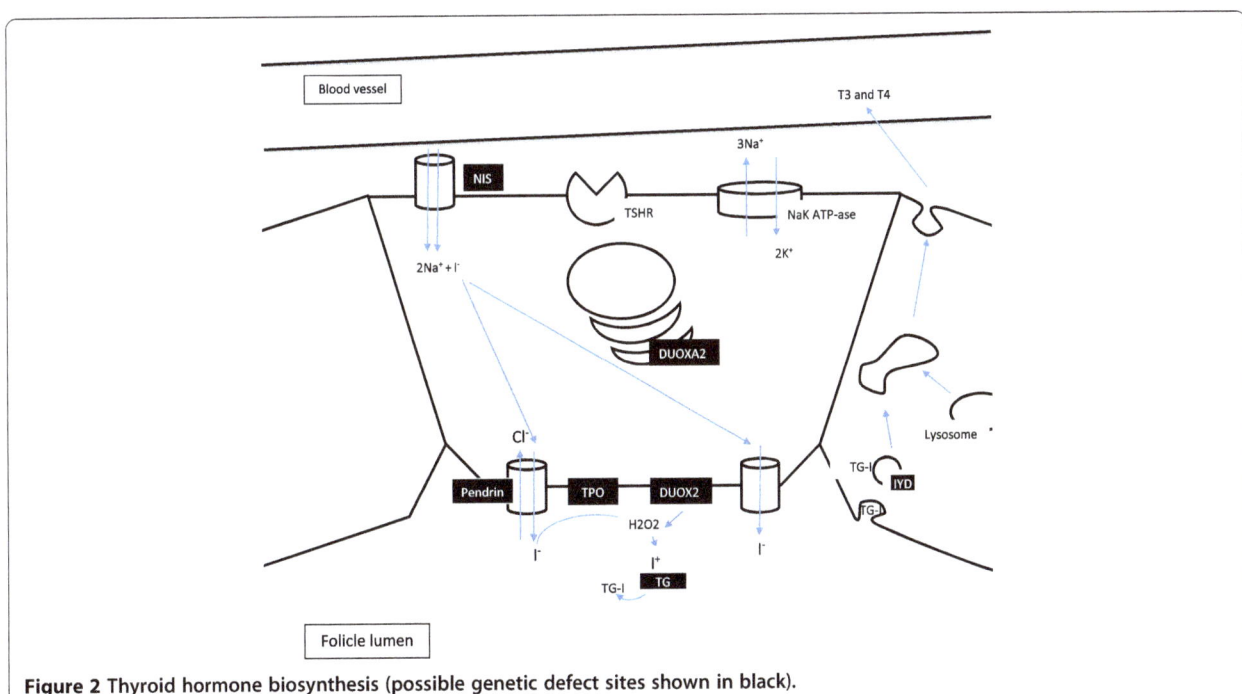

Figure 2 Thyroid hormone biosynthesis (possible genetic defect sites shown in black).

euthyroidism in iodide sufficient regions) [15-17]. PDS is a rare cause of CH (2-3%), goiter often occurs later, in childhood or early adolescence. Patients with PDS are at increased risk of thyroid cancer development (about 1%), most likely follicular carcinoma [18].

Thyroid peroxidase (TPO) catalyze iodide oxidation, tyrosyl residue iodination and their coupling to iodothyronines [19]. *TPO* (2p25.3) mutation is considered to be the most prevalent cause of dyshormonogenesis (24-46%), and is found in about 1:60,000 newborns, with about 90 different mutations already described [15,20]. The disease is generally inherited with an autosomal recessive manner, although monoallelic mutations may be a risk factor for transient hypothyroidism.

In the process of iodothyronine synthesis, H2O2 is required, which is produced by the dual oxidase enzyme (DUOX/ThOX). Two variants of DUOX can be distinguished, with type 2 being critical for thyroid hormone synthesis [21]. In the case of *DUOX2* (15q21.1), autosomal dominant mode of inheritance is observed, although homozygotes are usually affected more severely. Patients with mono-allelic mutations typically present with transient congenital hypothyroidism, but should be monitored in adulthood in situations characterized by an increased thyroid hormone requirement, such as pregnancy [22]. Defects in another thyroid protein - *DUOXA2* (15q21.1), which is indispensable for DUOX2 maturation and translocation, can also cause CH [23].

Thyroglobulin (TG) is essential in thyroid hormone synthesis as it provides tyrosyl residues and enable the storage of hormones and iodine. Since it was first described, more than 50 different mutations that lead to CH have been found [24]. *TG* (8q24.22) mutations are described as one of the most prevalent causes of dyshormonogenesis (1:67,000 to 1:100,000) [24,25]. A characteristically undetectable or very low TG level is observed in these patients, T4 concentration is found to be disproportionately lower than T3 (a result of increased type-2 iodothyronine deiodinase activity) [26].

Although the end products of hormonogenesis are T3 and T4, most iodine particles are embedded to mono- and diiodotyronines (MIT, DIT). Reuse of this iodine is possible due to MIT and DIT deiodination by an iodotyrosine deiodinase (IYD). Mutations in the *IYD* gene (6q25.1) may lead to goitrous hypothyroidism [27]. A characteristic feature is excessive urinary and blood MIT and DIT concentrations [28].

Inherited thyroid hormone binding protein abnormalities
TBG

Thyroxin binding globulin (TBG) is the main protein that binds T3 and T4 in the blood (70% and 70-80% respectively); other transporting particles (transthyretin and albumin) play a minor role. TBG is encoded by the *Serpina 7 gene* (Xq22.3) and expressed in the liver [29]. Three different congenital TBG abnormalities are distinguished according to its concentration: complete deficiency (TBG-CD), partial deficiency (TBG-PD) and excess (TBG-E). They are inherited in a X-linked recessive pattern (although a case of autosomal dominant inheritance of TBG-PD has been described) [30]. There are also some *TBG* polymorphic variants that do not alter the protein concentration.

TBG-CD is diagnosed when the protein level is undetectable by typically used assays (or is lower than 0.03% of the normal mean value), and can be found in hemizygous men and homozygous women. Heterozygous women usually have only a slightly diminished TBG concentration (carriers), although rarely, as a result of selective X chromosome inactivation, TBG-CD may develop [31]. Men with TBG-PD have a significantly decreased serum concentration of globulin, while women are found to have values that may even overlap the normal range. TBG deficiency is estimated to occur in 1:15,000 to 1:5,000 of all newborns in the Caucasian population (there is a higher frequency in the Japanese population), with TBG-CD in one-third of them [32]. At least 22 different TBG-CD and 8 TBG-PD mutations have been described (TBG-CD mutations shown on Figure 3) [33]. Laboratory tests in these generally euthyroid patients show normal TSH, fT3 and fT4 with a low T4, T3 and undetectable TBG level.

Excessive TBG concentration is typically observed in the course of elevated estrogen level (e.g. pregnancy). Congenital TBG-E occurs rarely, as a consequence of gene duplication or triplication (in 1:6,000 to 1:40,000 of all newborns) [34]. In such cases, the values measured are 2–3 times higher than normal in men and mildly elevated in heterozygous women [35].

TTR

About 20% of T4 and 10-20% of T3 is bound in serum by transthyretin (TTR)/thyroxine binding prealbumin (TBPA), a homotetrameric protein synthetized in the liver. Over 120 different disease-associated mutations have been found in *TTR gene* (18q12.1), with variable manifestation. Most commonly they lead to amyloid deposition in the cardiac tissue and/or peripheral nerves, without affecting the status of thyroid hormones [15,36]. There is also a group of mutations that lead to a considerably increased affinity for iodothyronines (predominantly T4) and may result in euthyroid dysprealbuminemic hyperthyroxinemia with an elevated serum total T4, rT3 and fT4 index (TSH, fT4, T3 and fT3 unaffected) [37]. Dysprealbuminemic hyperthyroxinemia is transmitted in an autosomal dominant manner and accounts for approximately 2% of all euthyroid hyperthyroxinemia cases [38]. Mutations associated with an increased concentration of

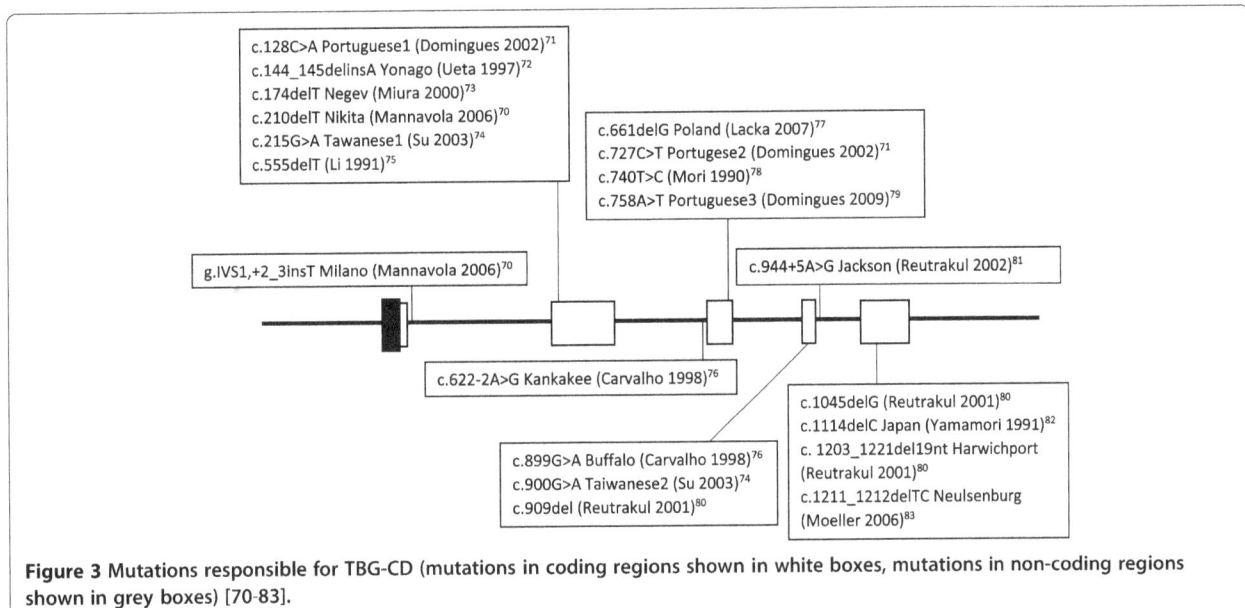

Figure 3 Mutations responsible for TBG-CD (mutations in coding regions shown in white boxes, mutations in non-coding regions shown in grey boxes) [70-83].

TTR do not cause euthyroid hyperthyroxinemia, as an observed augmentation in the protein level is not high enough (although in the course of some malignancies e.g. hepatocellular carcinoma, the TTR concentration may increase significantly and bring about the picture of euthyroid hyperthyroxinemia) [39]. Some of the *TTR* mutations lead to a decrease in protein blood concentration or a lesser affinity for iodothyronines, although without significant clinical or laboratory changes in thyroid hormones status.

Albumin

Familial dysalbuminemic hyperthyroxinemia (FDH) is another cause of inherited euthyroid hyperthyroxinemia. It results from *albumin gene* (4q13.3) mutations that lead to an increased affinity for fT4 and is inherited as an autosomal dominant disease. Although relatively rare, FDH is the most prevalent cause of inherited euthyroid hyperthyroxinemia in the Caucasian population (up to 12% of all cases, from 1:10,000 to 17:10,000) [40,41]. The following values are expected in laboratory tests: normal TSH (also after TRH stimulation) fT4, fT3, normal or slightly elevated T3, elevated T4, rT3 (in some cases) and an increased proportion of T4 bound to serum albumin (approximately four times higher than normally) [42]. The diagnostic problem may be falsely elevated fT4, as the laboratory techniques usually used are not accurate enough in that case, which may lead to unnecessary treatment [43]. In most cases, mutations at position 218 of the amino acid chain are present. However, another one was found in codon 66 (L66P) and leads to an increased affinity for fT3 and hypertriiodothyroninemia (FDH-T3) [44].

Thyroid hormone resistance (RTH)

Thyroid hormones act primarily via nuclear receptors (TR): 1) TRα1 encoded by *THRA* (17q21.1) and 2) TRβ1 or TRβ2 encoded by *THRB* (3p24.2) (different expression pattern of both subtypes). T3 forms a complex with TR, and subsequently binds to the promoter region of the target genes (thyroid hormone response elements), acting as a transcription factor.

Mutations in TR genes lead to thyroid hormone resistance (RTH), disorder transmitted in the majority of cases in an autosomal dominant manner. Although no precise data are available, the prevalence is estimated to be 1:40,000 newborns [45]. In approximately 85-90% of RTH cases, the disease is caused by *THRB* mutations that lead to a decreased affinity for T3 or impaired interactions with TRβ cofactors. In these cases, elevated fT4 (often also fT3 and rT3) associated with normal or elevated (non-suppressed) TSH level is observed [46]. As a consequence of the variable manifestations observed among patients, RTH was formerly classified into generalized, isolated peripheral and isolated pituitary resistance. Often some evidence of both hyper- and hypothyroidism can be found in one patient (goiter, sinus tachycardia etc. may be associated with learning disabilities and delayed growth or bone age). In rare cases of homozygous *THRB* mutations, more severe symptoms are observed with coexisting deaf-mutism and color blindness [47].

Mutations in *THRA* were also described, which lead to different symptoms and thyroid function test results than in *THRB* defects. The symptoms of thyroid hormone deficiency are restricted to those tissues in which TRα predominates (central nervous system, myocardium, striated muscles, the gastrointestinal tract, cartilages and bones) [48]. Laboratory tests show a decreased fT4, very low rT3 and elevated fT3.

In a group of RTH patients (up to 15%), neither *THRB* nor *THRA gene* mutations were found (non TR-RTH), although phenotypically they may be indistinguishable from those with TRβ alterations. This subtype is also inherited in an autosomal dominant manner and expected to result from some TRβ cofactors mutations or defects in receptor regulation, although undefined to date [49].

Recently, the term 'reduced sensitivity to thyroid hormones' (RSTH) was introduced, which encompasses RTH and decreased responsiveness to thyroid hormones caused by iodothyronine transmembrane transport defect (mutations of MCT8 gene - *SLC16A2* in Xq13.2) or T4 to T3 deiodination defect (mutations of *SBP2* gene - *SECISBP2* in 9q22.2) [50-52].

Rare causes of hyperthyroidism

Congenital hyperthyroidism, a generally rare disease (overt hyperthyroidism in 1:50,000 newborns), is most often transient and caused by the maternal thyroid stimulating antibodies in the course of Graves' disease, subsequently transferred to fetal circulation (hyperthyroidism in 0.6-1% of offspring born to GD mothers) [53]. However, in some neonates there are no thyroid antibodies in serum, the mother's disease is excluded and hyperthyroidism is persistent. This may suggest a condition called non-autoimmune hyperthyroidism (NAH). NAH develops as a result of gain-of-function germline mutation within the *TSH receptor gene (TSHR)*, leading to constitutive TSHR pathway activation. It can be divided into sporadic (SNAH) and familial (FNAH) with an autosomal dominant mode of inheritance [54,55]. To date, at least 21 different mutations of *TSHR* in FNAH and 12 in SNAH have been found. Similar mutations, but of a somatic type, can be found in toxic thyroid nodules [56]. Clinically, patients with NAH usually present with goiter and hyperthyroidism. Moreover, pharmacologic treatment may be ineffective (frequent relapses are observed) and total thyroidectomy or complete radioiodine ablation is usually necessary.

Hyperthyroidism is also observed in patients with McCune-Albright syndrome (MAS), as a result of the activating somatic mutation of the *GNAS gene*. As mentioned previously, GSα is a part of the TSHR signaling cascade and its constitutive activation is followed by a cAMP increase, which in turn results in thyrocyte hyperproliferation and iodothyronine excess. GSα is committed to extracellular signals transduction in different tissues as well. As *GNAS* mutations occur in MAS in the post-zygotic period and patients are mosaic, variable manifestations are observed. The classical triad of symptoms include bone fibrous dysplasia, café-au-lait spots and hyperfunctional endocrinopathies (most frequently peripheral precocious puberty, but also hyperthyroidism, hypercortisolism, hypophyseal hyperfunction and kidney phosphate wasting). MAS prevalence range from 1:100,000 to 1:1,000,000 [57], with functional or morphological changes in the thyroid in approximately 31% of cases [58].

Symptoms of hyperthyroidism may also be observed, albeit rarely, in the course of struma ovari (5-15% of cases), differentiated thyroid cancer (usually methastatic) and an gestational trophoblastic disease [59-61]. Furthermore, central (secondary) hyperthyroidism due to TSH secreting pituitary adenoma can be classified as a rare disease as it accounts for only about 1% of all pituitary adenomas (prevalence of 1:1,000,000) [62].

Rare thyroid inflammatory diseases

Thyroid gland tuberculosis is very rarely observed in the course of generalized disease (even in regions with a relatively high incidence of tuberculosis) and much less frequently as a change isolated or primarily localized in the thyroid. Analyses of surgically removed glands or fine needle aspiration biopsy (FNAB) materials showed a prevalence of 0.1-0.6% [63,64]. Thyroid tuberculosis may present as a single nodule, multinodular goiter or diffused swelling, it may be found as a cold abscess or rarely an acute abscess [65]. Some patients remain symptomless, while others develop dyspnea, dysphagia, hoarseness, pain or tenderness. Typically, the hormonal status of the thyroid gland is unaffected, although hyperthyroidism may occur in some cases, as a result of excessive release of thyroid hormones from damaged tissue. Hypothyroidism, which is extremely rarely observed, may be caused by extensive tissue destruction [66]. To establish the diagnosis, ultrasound-guided FNAB should be performed with Ziehl Neelsen staining, culture and cytological examination (caseating granulomas with epithelioid cells and Langhans giant cells).

Sarcoidosis - a noncaseating granulomatous disorder, may rarely affect the thyroid gland in the course of generalized disease. Usually, extrathyroidal manifestation of the disease precedes the diagnosis of thyroid involvement. Some rare cases of sarcoidosis limited to the thyroid gland can be also found in the literature [67]. In post-mortem studies of patients with previously found systemic sarcoidosis, the thyroid gland was affected in up to 4.5% [68]. Thyroid sarcoidosis usually presents as a progressive painless enlargement of the gland with unaffected hormonal status, although different manifestations are possible (hyperthyroidism, hypothyroidism, acute thyroiditis, multinodular goiter or solitary thyroid nodule, it may sometimes be painful). Cases of hyperthyroidism resistant to both pharmacological and radioiodine treatment were observed in the course of thyroid sarcoidosis, and in these cases surgical removal of the gland is required. Studies also suggest an increased prevalence of high antithyroid antibodies concentration and thyroid autoimmune diseases associated with sarcoidosis, regardless of thyroid gland involvement (an ATD frequency in patients with sarcoidosis 1.9-16,6%) [69].

Conclusions

Most of the rare thyroid diseases presented in this paper have a genetic origin, among them monogenic disorders can be found. Progress in our understanding of their etiology and pathogenesis has been observed in the past years, what also shed new light on how the normal thyroid gland functions and the role of different proteins in this process, although there are still some questions that need answers. Secondly, rare thyroid diseases may be a challenging problem for clinicians because of their rarity and variability in manifestations. They should be kept in mind as a differential diagnosis of other diseases more commonly seen in clinical practice. A correct and undelayed diagnosis is especially important in the case of congenital thyroid function disruptions, as untreated, they may lead to serious consequences.

Competing interests
The authors declare that they have no competing interests.

Authors' contribution
KL designed the study, wrote the manuscript and supervised preparation of the final version of the manuscript. AM was involved in literature review and drafting the manuscript. All authors read and approved the final manuscript.

References

1. Posada de la Paz M, Villaverde-Hueso A, Alonso V, János S, Zurriaga O, Pollán M, et al. Rare diseases epidemiology research. In: Posada de la Paz M, Groft SC, editors. Rare diseases epidemiology. London, New York: Springer Dordrecht Heidelberg; 2010. p. 17–40.
2. Hennekam RC. Care for patients with ultra-rare disorders. Eur J Med Genet. 2011;54(3):220–4.
3. Rastogi MV, LaFranchi SH. Congenital hypothyroidism. Orphanet J Rare Dis. 2010;5:17.
4. Harris KB. Pass KA Increase in congenital hypothyroidism in New York State and in the United States. Mol Genet Metab. 2007;91:268–77.
5. Zhan JY, Qin YF, Zhao ZY. Neonatal screening for congenital hypothyroidism and phenylketonuria in China. World J Pediatr. 2009;5(2):136–9.
6. Kumorowicz-Czoch M, Tylek-Lemanska D, Starzyk J. Thyroid dysfunctions in children detected in mass screening for congenital hypothyroidism. J Pediatr Endocrinol Metab. 2011;24(3–4):141–5.
7. Brown RS, Demmer LA. The etiology of thyroid dysgenesis-still an enigma after all these years. J Clin Endocrinol Metab. 2002;87(9):4069–71.
8. Ruchala M, Szczepanek E, Szaflarski W, et al. Increased risk of thyroid pathology in patients with thyroid hemiagenesis: results of a large cohort case–control study. Eur J Endocrinol. 2010;162(1):153–60.
9. Kırmızıbekmez H, Güven A, Yildiz M, Cebeci AN, Dursun F. Developmental defects of the thyroid gland: relationship with advanced maternal age. J Clin Res Pediatr Endocrinol. 2012;4(2):72–5.
10. Jeziorowska A, Pniewska-Siark B, Brzeziańska E, Pastuszak-Lewandoska D, Lewiński A. A novel mutation in the thyrotropin (thyroid-stimulating

hormone) receptor gene in a case of congenital hypothyroidism. Thyroid. 2006;16(12):1303–9.
11. Cassio A, Nicoletti A, Rizzello A, Zazzetta E, Bal M, Baldazzi L. Current loss-of-function mutations in the thyrotropin receptor gene: when to investigate, clinical effects, and treatment. J Clin Res Pediatr Endocrinol. 2013;5:29–39.
12. Persani L, Calebiro D, Cordella D, Weber G, Gelmini G, Libri D, et al. Genetics and phenomics of hypothyroidism due to TSH resistance. Mol Cell Endocrinol. 2010;322(1–2):72–82.
13. Miyai K, Inaoka K, Miyagi T. Further studies on episodic occurrence of congenital dysgenetic hypothyroidism in Osaka, Japan. Endocr J. 2005;52(5):599–603.
14. Spitzweg C, Morris JC. Genetics and phenomics of hypothyroidism and goiter due to NIS mutations. Mol Cell Endocrinol. 2010;322(1–2):56–63.
15. The Human Gene Mutation Database. Cardiff University. 2015. http://www.hgmd.cf.ac.uk/ac/index.php. Accessed 20 February 2015.
16. Maciaszczyk K, Lewiński A. Phenotypes of SLC26A4 gene mutations: Pendred syndrome and hypoacusis with enlarged vestibular aqueduct. Neuro Endocrinol Lett. 2008;29(1):29–36.
17. Kopp P. Mutations in the Pendred Syndrome (PDS/SLC26A) gene: an increasingly complex phenotypic spectrum from goiter to thyroid hypoplasia. J Clin Endocrinol Metab. 2014;99(1):67–9.
18. Nose V. Thyroid cancer of follicular cell origin in inherited tumor syndromes. Adv Anat Pathol. 2010;17:428–36.
19. Kimura S, Kotani T, McBride OW, Umeki K, Hirai K, Nakayama T, et al. Human thyroid peroxidase: complete cDNA and protein sequence, chromosome mapping, and identification of two alternately spliced mRNAs. Proc Natl Acad Sci USA. 1987;84:5555–9.
20. Avbelj M, Tahirovic H, Debeljak M, Kusekova M, Toromanovic A, Krzisnik C, et al. High prevalence of thyroid peroxidase gene mutations in patients with thyroid dyshormonogenesis. Eur J Endocrinol. 2007;156(5):511–9.
21. Moreno JC, Bikker H, Kempers MJ, van Trotsenburg AS, Baas F, de Vijlder JJ, et al. Inactivating mutations in the gene for thyroid oxidase 2 (THOX2) and congenital hypothyroidism. N Engl J Med. 2002;347(2):95–102.
22. Alexander EK, Marqusee E, Lawrence J, Jarolim P, Fischer GA, Larsen PR. Timing and magnitude of increases in levothyroxine requirements during pregnancy in women with hypothyroidism. N Engl J Med. 2004;351:241–9.
23. Grasberger H, Refetoff S. Identification of the maturation factor for dual oxidase. Evolution of an eukaryotic operon equivalent. J Biol Chem. 2006;281:18269–72.
24. Targovnik HM, Esperante SA, Rivolta CM. Genetics and phenomics of hypothyroidism and goiter due to thyroglobulin mutations. Mol Cell Endocrinol. 2010;322(1–2):44–55.
25. Hishinuma A, Fukata S, Nishiyama S, Nishi Y, Oh-Ishi M, Murata Y, et al. Haplotype analysis reveals founder effects of thyroglobulin gene mutations C1058R and C1977S in Japan. J Clin Endocrinol Metab. 2006;91:3100–4.
26. Kanou Y, Hishinuma A, Tsunekawa K, Seki K, Mizuno Y, Fujisawa H, et al. Thyroglobulin gene mutations producing defective intracellular transport of thyroglobulin are associated with increased thyroidal type 2 iodothyronine deiodinase activity. J Clin Endocrinol Metab. 2007;92:1451–7.
27. Moreno JC, Klootwijk W, van Toor H, Moreno JC, Klootwijk W, van Toor H, et al. Mutations in the iodotyrosine deiodinase gene and hypothyroidism. N Engl J Med. 2008;358:1811–8.
28. Afink G, Kulik W, Overmars H, de Randamie J, Veenboer T, van Cruchten A, et al. Molecular characterization of iodotyrosine dehalogenase deficiency in patients with hypothyroidism. J Clin Endocrinol Metab. 2008;93:4894–901.
29. Hayashi Y, Mori Y, Janssen OE, Sunthornthepvarakul T, Weiss RE, Takeda K, et al. Human thyroxine-binding globulin gene: complete sequence and transcriptional regulation. Mol Endocrinol. 1993;7:1049–60.
30. Kobayashi H, Sakurai A, Katai M, Hashizume K. Autosomally transmitted low concentration of thyroxine-binding globulin. Thyroid. 1999;9:159–63.
31. Okamoto H, Mori Y, Tani Y, Nakagomi Y, Sano T, Ohyama K, et al. Molecular analysis of females manifesting thyroxine-binding globulin (TBG) deficiency: selective X-chromosome inactivation responsible for the difference between phenotype and genotype in TBG-deficient females. J Clin Endocrinol Metab. 1996;81(6):2204–8.
32. Mandel S, Hanna C, Boston B, Sesser D, LaFranchi S. Thyroxine-binding globulin deficiency detected by newborn screening. J Pediatr. 1993;122:227–30.
33. Refetoff S. Abnormal thyroid hormone transport. In: Thyroid Disease Manager. South Dartmouth, Massachusetts: Endocrine Education; 2012.

http://www.thyroidmanager.org/chapter/abnormal-thyroid-hormone-transport/. Accesed 10.02.2015.

34. Griffiths KD, Virdi NK, Rayner PHW, Green A. Neonatal screening for congenital hypothyroidism by measurement of plasma thyroxine and thyroid stimulating hormone concentrations. Brit Med J. 1985;291:117–20.

35. Mori Y, Seino S, Takeda K, Flink IL, Murata Y, Bell GI, et al. A mutation causing reduced biological activity and stability of thyroxine-binding globulin probably as a result of abnormal glycosylation of the molecule. Mol Endocrinol. 1989;3:575–9.

36. Saraiva MJ. Transthyretin mutations in hyperthyroxinemia and amyloid diseases. Hum Mutat. 2001;17(6):493–503.

37. Moses AC, Lawlor J, Haddow J, Jackson IMD. Familial euthyroid hyperthyroxinemia resulting from increased thyroxine binding to thyroxine-binding prealbumin. N Engl J Med. 1982;306:966–9.

38. Scrimshaw BJ, Fellowes AP, Palmer BN, Croxson MS, Stockigt JR, George PM. A novel variant of transthyretin (prealbumin), Thr119 to Met, associated with increased thyroxine binding. Thyroid. 1992;2:21–6.

39. Alexopoulos A, Hutchinson W, Bari A, Keating JJ, Johnson PJ, Williams R. Hyperthyroxinaemia in hepatocellular carcinoma: relation to thyroid binding globulin in the clinical and preclinical stages of the disease. Br J Cancer. 1988;57:313–6.

40. Jensen IW, Faber J. Familial dysalbuminaemic hyperthyroxinemia: a review. J Royal Soc Med. 1988;81:34–7.

41. Arevalo G. Prevalence of familial dysalbuminemic hyperthyroxinemia in serum samples received for thyroid testing. Clin Chem. 1991;37:1430–1.

42. Mendel CM, Cavalieri RR. Thyroxine distribution and metabolism in familial dysalbuminemic hyperthyroxinemia. J Clin Endocrinol Metab. 1984;59(3):499–504.

43. Cartwright D, O'Shea P, Rajanayagam O, Agostini M, Barker P, Moran C, et al. Familial dysalbuminemic hyperthyroxinemia: a persistent diagnostic challenge. Clin Chem. 2009;55(5):1044–6.

44. Sunthornthepvarakul T, Likitmaskul S, Ngowngarmratana S, Angsusingha K, Sureerat K, Scherberg NH, et al. Familial dysalbuminemic hypertriiodothyroninemia: a new dominantly inherited albumin defect. J Clin Endocrinol Metab. 1998;83:1448–54.

45. Lafranchi SH, Snyder DB, Sesser DE, Skeels MR, Singh N, Brent GA, et al. Follow-up of newborns with elevated screening T4 concentrations. J Pediatr. 2003;143(3):296–301.

46. Refetoff S, Weiss RE, Usala SJ. The syndromes of resistance to thyroid hormone. Endocr Rev. 1993;14:348–99.

47. Ferrara AM, Onigata K, Ercan O, Woodhead H, Weiss RE, Refetoff S. Homozygous thyroid hormone receptor β-gene mutations in resistance to thyroid hormone: three new cases and review of the literature. J Clin Endocrinol Metab. 2012;97(4):1328–36.

48. Lazar MA. Thyroid hormone receptors: multiple forms, multiple possibilities. Endocr Rev. 1993;14:184–93.

49. Parikh S, Ando S, Schneider A, Skarulis MC, Sarlis NJ, Yen PM, et al. Resistance to thyroid hormone in a patient without thyroid hormone receptor mutations. Thyroid. 2002;12(1):81–6.

50. Friesema EC, Ganguly S, Abdalla A, Manning Fox JE, Halestrap AP, Visser TJ. Identification of monocarboxylate transporter 8 as a specific thyroid hormone transporter. J Biol Chem. 2003;278:40128–35.

51. Bianco AC, Salvatore D, Gereben B, Berry MJ, Larsen PR. Biochemistry, cellular and molecular biology and physiological roles of the iodothyronine selenodeiodinases. Endocr Rev. 2002;23:38–89.

52. Dumitrescu AM, Refetoff S. The syndromes of reduced sensitivity to thyroid hormone. Biochim Biophys Acta. 2013;1830(7):3987–4003.

53. Polak M, Legac I, Vuillard E, Guibourdenche J, Castanet M, Luton D. Congenital hyperthyroidism: the fetus as a patient. Horm Res. 2006;65(5):235–42.

54. Thomas JS, Leclere J, Hartemann P, Duheille J, Orgiazzi J, Petersen M, et al. Familial hyperthyroidism without evidence of autoimmunity. Acta Endocrinol (Copenh). 1982;100:512–8.

55. Kopp P, van Sande J, Parma J, Duprez L, Gerber H, Joss E, et al. Brief report: congenital hyperthyroidism caused by a mutation in the thyrotropin-receptor gene. New England Journal of Medicine. 1995;332:150–4.

56. Hébrant A, van Staveren WC, Maenhaut C, Dumont JE, Leclère J. Genetic hyperthyroidism: hyperthyroidism due to activating TSHR mutations. Eur J Endocrinol. 2011;164:1–9.

57. Dumitrescu CE, Collins MT. McCune-Albright syndrome. Orphanet J Rare Dis. 2008;19:3–12.

58. Tessaris D, Corrias A, Matarazzo P, De Sanctis L, Wasniewska M, Messina MF, et al. Thyroid abnormalities in children and adolescents with McCune-Albright syndrome. Horm Res Paediatr. 2012;78(3):151–7.

59. Dunzendorfer T. deLas Morenas A, Kalir T, Levin RM. Struma ovarii and hyperthyroidism. Thyroid. 1999;9(5):499–502.

60. Damle NA, Bal C, Kumar P, Soundararajan R, Subbarao K. Incidental detection of hyperfunctioning thyroid cancer metastases in patients presenting with thyrotoxicosis. Indian J Endocrinol Metab. 2012;16(4):631–6.

61. Narasimhan KL, Ghobrial MW, Ruby EB. Hyperthyroidism in the setting of gestational trophoblastic disease. Am J Med Sci. 2002;323(5):285–7.

62. Beck-Peccoz P, Persani L, Mannavola D, Campi I. Pituitary tumours: TSH-secreting adenomas. Best Pract Res Clin Endocrinol Metab. 2009;23(5):597–606.

63. Rankin FW, Graham AS. Tuberculosis of the thyroid gland. Annals of Surgery. 1932;96:625.

64. Das DK, Pant CS, Chachra KL, Gupta AK. Fine needle aspiration cytology diagnosis of tuberculous thyroiditis. A report of eight cases. Acta Cytol. 1992;36(4):517–22.

65. Majid U, Islam N. Thyroid tuberculosis: a case series and a review of the literature. J Thyroid Res. 2011;2011:359864.

66. Luiz HV, Pereira BD, Silva TN, Veloza A, Matos C, Manita I, et al. Thyroid tuberculosis with abnormal thyroid function–case report and review of the literature. Endocr Pract. 2013;19(2):e44–9.

67. Cabibi D, Di Vita G, La Spada E, Tripodo C, Patti R, Montalto G. Thyroid sarcoidosis as a unique localization. Thyroid. 2006;16(11):1175–7.

68. Manchanda A, Patel S, Jiang JJ, Babu AR. Thyroid: an unusual hideout for sarcoidosis. Endocr Pract. 2013;19(2):40–3.

69. Kmieć P, Lewandowska M, Dubaniewicz A, Mizan-Gross K, Antolak A, Wołyniak B, et al. Two cases of thyroid sarcoidosis presentation as painful, recurrent goiter in patients with Graves' disease. Arq Bras Endocrinol Metabol. 2012;56(3):209–14.

70. Mannavola D, Vannucchi G, Fugazzola L, Cirello V, Campi I, Radetti G, et al. TBG deficiency: description of two novel mutations associated with complete TBG deficiency and review of the literature. J Mol Med (Berl). 2006;84(10):864–71.

71. Domingues R, Bugalho MJ, Garrão A, Boavida JM, Sobrinho L. Two novel variants in the thyroxine-binding globulin (TBG) gene behind the diagnosis of TBG deficiency. Eur J Endocrinol. 2002;146(4):485–90.

72. Ueta Y, Mitani Y, Yoshida A, Taniguchi S, Mori A, Hattori K, et al. A novel mutation causing complete deficiency of thyroxine binding globulin. Clin Endocrinol (Oxf). 1997;47:1–5.

73. Miura Y, Hershkovitz E, Inagaki A, Parvari R, Oiso Y, Phillip M. A novel mutation causing complete thyroxine-binding-globulin deficiency (TBG-CD-Negev) among the Bedouins in southern Israel. J Clin Endocrinol Metab. 2000;85(10):3687–9.

74. Su CC, Wu YC, Chiu CY, Won JG, Jap TS. Two novel mutations in the gene encoding thyroxine-binding globulin (TBG) as a cause of complete TBG deficiency in Taiwan. Clin Endocrinol (Oxf). 2003;58(4):409–14.

75. Li P, Janssen OE, Takeda K, Bertenshaw RH, Refetoff S. Complete thyroxine-binding globulin (TBG) deficiency caused by a single nucleotide deletion in the TBG gene. Metabolism. 1991;40(11):1231–4.

76. Carvalho GA, Weiss RE, Refetoff S. Complete thyroxine-binding globulin (TBG) deficiency produced by a mutation in acceptor splice site causing frameshift and early termination of translation (TBG-Kankakee). J Clin Endocrinol Metab. 1998;83(10):3604–8.

77. Lacka K, Nizankowska T, Ogrodowicz A, Lacki JK. A novel mutation (del 1711 G) in the TBG gene as a cause of complete TBG deficiency. Thyroid. 2007;17(11):1143–6.

78. Mori Y, Takeda K, Charbonneau M, Refetoff S. Replacement of Leu227 by Pro in thyroxine-binding globulin (TBG) is associated with complete TBG deficiency in three of eight families with this inherited defect. J Clin Endocrinol Metab. 1990;70(3):804–9.

79. Domingues R, Font P, Sobrinho L, Bugalho MJ. A novel variant in Serpina7 gene in a family with thyroxine-binding globulin deficiency. Endocrine. 2009;36(1):83–6.

80. Reutrakul S, Janssen OE, Refetoff S. Three novel mutations causing complete T(4)-binding globulin deficiency. J Clin Endocrinol Metab. 2001;86(10):5039–44.

81. Reutrakul S, Dumitrescu A, Macchia PE, Moll Jr GW, Vierhapper H, Refetoff S. Complete thyroxine-binding globulin (TBG) deficiency in two families without mutations in coding or promoter regions of the TBG genes: in vitro demonstration of exon skipping. J Clin Endocrinol Metab. 2002;87(3):1045–51.

82. Yamamori I, Mori Y, Seo H, Hirooka Y, Imamura S, Miura Y, et al. Nucleotide deletion resulting in frameshift as a possible cause of complete thyroxine-binding globulin deficiency in six Japanese families. J Clin Endocrinol Metab. 1991;73(2):262–7.

83. Moeller LC, Fingerhut A, Lahner H, Grasberger H, Weimer B, Happ J, et al. C-terminal amino acid alteration rather than late termination causes complete deficiency of thyroxine-binding globulin CD-Neulsenburg. J Clin Endocrinol Metab. 2006;91(8):3215–8.

3

A solitary hyperfunctioning thyroid nodule harboring thyroid carcinoma

Sasan Mirfakhraee[1], Dana Mathews[2], Lan Peng[3], Stacey Woodruff[4] and Jeffrey M Zigman[1*]

Abstract

Hyperfunctioning nodules of the thyroid are thought to only rarely harbor thyroid cancer, and thus are infrequently biopsied. Here, we present the case of a patient with a hyperfunctioning thyroid nodule harboring thyroid carcinoma and, using MEDLINE literature searches, set out to determine the prevalence of and characteristics of malignant "hot" nodules as a group. Historical, biochemical and radiologic characteristics of the case subjects and their nodules were compared to those in cases of benign hyperfunctioning nodules. A literature review of surgical patients with solitary hyperfunctioning thyroid nodules managed by thyroid resection revealed an estimated 3.1% prevalence of malignancy. A separate literature search uncovered 76 cases of reported malignant hot thyroid nodules, besides the present case. Of these, 78% were female and mean age at time of diagnosis was 47 years. Mean nodule size was 4.13 ± 1.68 cm. Laboratory assessment revealed T_3 elevation in 76.5%, T_4 elevation in 51.9%, and subclinical hyperthyroidism in 13% of patients. Histological diagnosis was papillary thyroid carcinoma (PTC) in 57.1%, follicular thyroid carcinoma (FTC) in 36.4%, and Hurthle cell carcinoma in 7.8% of patients. Thus, hot thyroid nodules harbor a low but non-trivial rate of malignancy. Compared to individuals with benign hyperfunctioning thyroid nodules, those with malignant hyperfunctioning nodules are younger and more predominantly female. Also, FTC and Hurthle cell carcinoma are found more frequently in hot nodules than in general. We were unable to find any specific characteristics that could be used to distinguish between malignant and benign hot nodules.

Keywords: Hot nodule, Thyroid cancer, Malignancy

Introduction

Thyroid nodules are frequently-encountered entities in clinical practice, occurring with a prevalence of 4% by palpation [1], 33% to 68% by ultrasound examination [2,3], and 50% on autopsy series [4]. While approximately 95% of thyroid nodules are benign, certain historical, laboratory, and sonographic features raise the suspicion for malignancy [5]. As the initial step for evaluation of a thyroid nodule is measurement of serum thyroid stimulating hormone (TSH) [6,7], it is not uncommon for patients with a solitary thyroid nodule to be diagnosed with hyperthyroidism. In this setting, the thyroid nodule may represent a solitary hyperfunctioning thyroid nodule in an otherwise normal thyroid gland or it may represent a hyperfunctioning or nonfunctioning nodule occurring within a toxic multinodular goiter, within a Graves' disease or destructive thyroiditis milieu, or in an individual with a less common cause of thyrotoxicosis [8]. Thyroid scintigraphy employs radioiodine (^{123}I, ^{131}I) or technetium-99m-(^{99m}Tc) pertechnetate in order to differentiate these diagnostic possibilities. The distinction is important, because hyperfunctioning nodules – also referred to as "autonomous," "autonomously-functioning," or "hot" nodules – are thought to only rarely harbor malignancy, such that fine needle aspiration (FNA) is not traditionally indicated in this circumstance [6]. Per the 2009 revised American Thyroid Association Management Guidelines for Patients with Thyroid Nodules and Differentiated Thyroid Cancer, "Since hyperfunctioning nodules rarely harbor malignancy, if one is

* Correspondence: jeffrey.zigman@utsouthwestern.edu
[1]Department of Internal Medicine, Division of Endocrinology and Metabolism, The University of Texas Southwestern Medical Center, Dallas, Texas 75390, USA
Full list of author information is available at the end of the article

found that corresponds to the nodule in question, no cytologic evaluation is necessary" [6].

Here, we present the case of a woman with subclinical hyperthyroidism due to a hyperfunctioning thyroid nodule who was diagnosed with minimally-invasive follicular carcinoma after surgical resection. We also include our findings from a formal literature review on this topic, in which the historical, laboratory, and radiological features of similarly-documented cases were scrutinized to determine if there are features that differentiate hyperfunctioning thyroid carcinomas from solitary toxic adenomas. The results of a separate literature review aimed at estimating the prevalence of thyroid cancer within hot thyroid nodules are also presented. Our goal is to call attention to the fact that hyperfunctioning thyroid carcinomas are well-described in the literature (and also likely underreported), challenging the commonly-held notion that the hot thyroid nodule is very unlikely to be cancerous.

Materials and methods

A MEDLINE literature search of English-language studies published between 1950 and January 2012 with the terms, "thyroid cancer, hyperthyroidism, surgery," "thyroid cancer, hyperfunctioning nodule, surgery," and "thyroid cancer, hot nodule, surgery," was performed to determine the reported prevalence of thyroid carcinoma in patients undergoing resection of solitary hyperfunctioning thyroid nodules. Another literature search, using the terms, "hyperfunctioning thyroid carcinoma," "toxic adenoma, thyroid carcinoma," and "hot nodule, thyroid carcinoma" was performed using MEDLINE and by reviewing the citations of relevant articles in order to collect data on reported cases of patients with a solitary thyroid nodule found to harbor thyroid carcinoma. Case series were included provided that at least some demographic and clinical details of individual subjects were described. A third MEDLINE literature search, using the terms "hot nodule," "hyperfunctioning thyroid nodule," and "autonomous thyroid nodules," was performed to establish the demographic characteristics and nodule sizes of subjects with solitary hyperfunctioning thyroid nodules. In this third group, the available studies analyzed the group of hyperfunctioning nodules en masse and did not make a distinction between hyperfunctioning nodules that were benign and those that may have been malignant. Therefore, while the aggregate data from these studies most likely involved predominantly benign cases, a small number of malignant cases also may have been included. For this reason, we will subsequently refer to this group as "predominantly-benign" hyperfunctioning (or hot) nodules.

Weighted averages of data were calculated by assigning a "weight" to each study (based on the number of subjects in the study divided by the total number of

subjects for all studies), multiplying each weight by the subject mean in the corresponding study, and then taking the sum of these products.

Results

Patient case

A 29-year-old teacher was referred to her local endocrinologist to evaluate a palpable left thyroid nodule. While she did not report thyrotoxic symptoms at that time, she was found to have a suppressed TSH. Thyroid scintigraphy revealed a hyperfunctioning left-sided thyroid nodule, and ultrasonography revealed it to be 2.4 cm in greatest dimension, isoechoic, and in the left lower lobe. A follow-up ultrasound one year later revealed an essentially unchanged nodule measuring 2.5 cm.

The patient presented to our institution the next year, at which time she endorsed tremors, anxiety, insomnia, and oligomenorrhea. She denied local compressive symptoms, history of radiation exposure, or family history of thyroid malignancy. Her only medication was a daily multivitamin. Her weight was 106 kg with a height of 1.7 m, blood pressure of 117/73 mmHg, and heart rate of 79 beats per minute. A 1.5 cm, firm, slightly tender nodule was palpated in the left lower lobe of the thyroid; it moved with swallowing. There was no evidence of cervical lymphadenopathy or thyroid bruit. The patient had a slight, fine tremor of the hands with normal biceps deep-tendon reflexes bilaterally.

Thyroid function tests revealed a suppressed TSH (0.005 mcIU/mL, normal 0.4 - 4.5 mcIU/mL) but normal free T4 (1.1 ng/dL, normal 0.9 - 1.8 ng/dL) and free T3 (3.5 pg/mL, normal 2.3 - 4.2 pg/mL). Thyroid peroxidase antibody testing was negative (0.4 IU/mL, normal < 9 IU/mL), as were thyroglobulin antibody (< 20 IU/mL) and thyroid stimulating immunoglobulin (< 1.0) testing. Thyroid ultrasound revealed a 2.6 × 2.7 × 2.6 cm predominantly solid, isoechoic left lower lobe nodule with internal hypervascularity within a slightly enlarged but otherwise normal-appearing thyroid gland (Figure 1A and B). ^{123}I thyroid scintigraphy revealed a left lower lobe hyperfunctioning nodule with 24-hour uptake of 27% (Figure 1C).

After discussing with the patient the benefits and risks of radioiodine ablation versus surgical resection (left hemithyroidectomy), she elected for the latter, citing the reduced risk of permanent hypothyroidism as her main deciding factor. Histologic evaluation of the surgical specimen revealed a solitary, circumscribed, and well-encapsulated tumor measuring 2.5 × 2.5 × 2.2 cm without lymphovascular invasion or extra-thyroidal extension (Figure 1D). A focus was identified where the tumor penetrated and budded through the well-defined fibrous capsule, giving the diagnosis of minimally-invasive follicular thyroid carcinoma (Figure 1E) in the setting of background lymphocytic thyroiditis. Given the pathologic

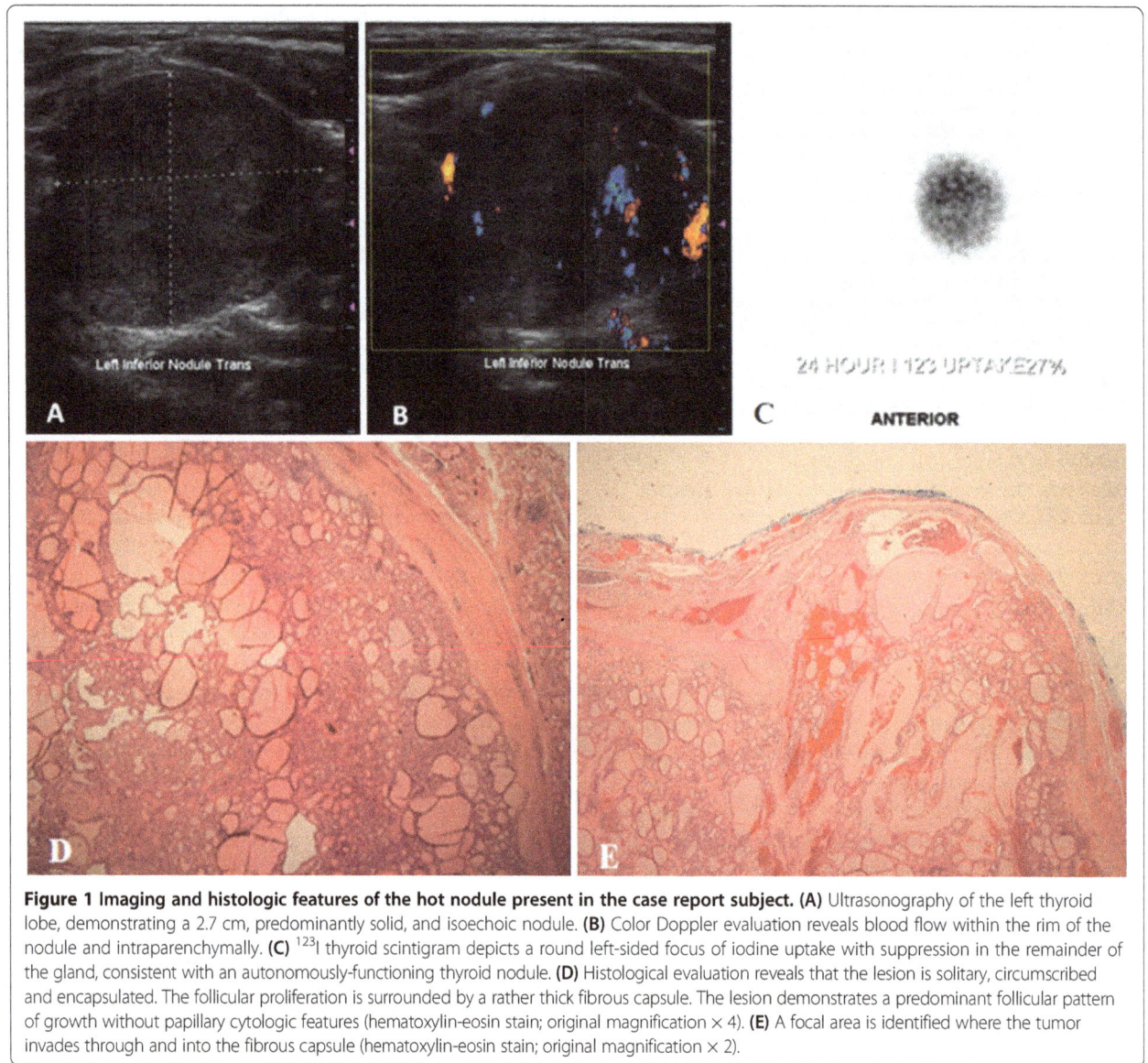

Figure 1 Imaging and histologic features of the hot nodule present in the case report subject. (A) Ultrasonography of the left thyroid lobe, demonstrating a 2.7 cm, predominantly solid, and isoechoic nodule. **(B)** Color Doppler evaluation reveals blood flow within the rim of the nodule and intraparenchymally. **(C)** [123]I thyroid scintigram depicts a round left-sided focus of iodine uptake with suppression in the remainder of the gland, consistent with an autonomously-functioning thyroid nodule. **(D)** Histological evaluation reveals that the lesion is solitary, circumscribed and encapsulated. The follicular proliferation is surrounded by a rather thick fibrous capsule. The lesion demonstrates a predominant follicular pattern of growth without papillary cytologic features (hematoxylin-eosin stain; original magnification × 4). **(E)** A focal area is identified where the tumor invades through and into the fibrous capsule (hematoxylin-eosin stain; original magnification × 2).

diagnosis, lobectomy was felt to be sufficient, and neither completion thyroidectomy nor radioactive iodine ablation was pursued in this patient. Molecular testing was performed on the surgical specimen for BRAF and KRAS mutations, both of which were negative. At her 6-month follow up appointment, the patient was symptomatically and biochemically euthyroid on low-dose levothyroxine replacement and showed no evidence of cancer recurrence.

Estimated prevalence of malignancy within hot thyroid nodules

In order to place the current case report in context, we have attempted to establish the prevalence of malignancy within hot thyroid nodules. This involved a literature search for surgical case series of solitary hyperfunctioning nodules managed by thyroid resection. A total of

14 relevant case series were uncovered. The earliest we found was from 1967 and included 79 hot nodules that underwent surgical resection; none of those cases were found to harbor thyroid carcinoma. Among the 14 case series, carcinoma rates of intranodular carcinoma ranging from 0 – 12.5% were noted, with a weighted total of 3.1% (Table 1). Of note, some of those case series also included cases in which thyroid carcinoma occurred outside of the hot nodule; however for the purposes of our review, such extranodular cases were not included in our estimated prevalence determination.

Search for distinctive features of malignant hot thyroid nodules

We next sought to establish historical and/or clinical features that may help to differentiate malignant,

Table 1 Intranodular thyroid carcinoma prevalence in patients undergoing resection of solitary, hyperfunctioning thyroid nodules

Author	Cases of hyperfunctioning nodule (n)	Cases of thyroid carcinoma within the hyperfunctioning nodule (n)	Thyroid carcinoma prevalence (%)
Giles [9]	176	4	2.3
Cakir [10]	63	4	6.3
Cappelli [11]	207	3	1.4
Foppiani [12]	16	2	12.5
Sahin [13]	77	2	2.6
Gabriele [14]	120	2	1.7
Harach [15]	73	6	8.2
Vaiana [16]	153	3	2
Zanella [17]	41	3	7.3
Terzioglu [18]	25	2	8
Pacini [19]	40	1	2.5
Smith [20]	30	2	6.7
Hamburger [21]	24	1	4.2
Horst [22]	79	0	0
Total	1124	35	3.1

Only cases of intra-nodular malignancy are included. Studies are arranged in order of ascending date of publication.

n = number of case.

hyperfunctioning thyroid nodules from benign, toxic adenomas, especially since hyperfunctioning thyroid carcinoma is generally an ex post facto diagnosis. Using the search criteria listed in the Methods Section, we discovered 76 cases (in addition to the current case) of malignant hot thyroid nodules, in which autonomy was highly suggested by both biochemical parameters of hyperthyroidism and scintigraphic evidence of increased radioiodine or labeled technetium uptake. All possibly-relevant features of the 77 cases were extracted and are displayed in Table 2, and a further analysis of these features appears in Table 3. An additional 27 cases with scintigraphic evidence suggestive of nodular autonomy but with normal thyroid function tests, absent thyroid function testing, or uninterpretable laboratory results (e.g., patients already on levothyroxine therapy at time of laboratory collection) were also found in the literature search (Table 4); these cases were excluded from subsequent analyses since autonomy seemed less certain.

Demographic characteristics

We compared age at diagnosis and female: male ratio of individuals with malignant, hyperfunctioning thyroid nodules to those with benign, toxic adenomas. Data on the latter group was compiled from a separate literature search which identified several surgical case series of

predominantly-benign hot nodules, as described in the Methods section (Table 5). Subjects with malignant hot nodules were younger at the time of diagnosis than those listed in multiple case series of predominantly-benign hot nodules [47.0 vs. 57.6 years, respectively (Tables 3 and 5)]. Additionally, a greater percentage of subjects with malignant hot nodule were female as compared to those with predominantly-benign hot nodules [3.53:1 vs. 1.65:1 female to male ratio, respectively (Tables 3 and 5)].

Size

The sizes of the malignant hot nodules (Table 2) and predominantly-benign hot thyroid nodules are compared in Figure 2A. Of note, the clinical use of ultrasonography began in the late 1960s, so that the sizes listed in the early case reports of malignant hot nodule were estimated by palpation. We include tumors that were noted to encompass the entirety of the hot nodule as well as microcarcinomas embedded within a larger hot nodule. The actual size of the tumor within the thyroid nodule determined by pathological review was occasionally provided in the literature and is listed in Tables 2 and 4. The mean nodule size among the subjects with thyroid carcinoma was 4.13 ± 1.68 cm, which closely approximates the mean size of the predominantly-benign hyperfunctioning nodules.

Biochemical profile

The majority of subjects with a malignant hot nodule demonstrated elevation of triiodothyronine (76.5%), whereas closer to half of the subjects had elevation of thyroxine (51.9%) (Table 3). Note that these percentages represent the number of subjects with an elevated thyroid hormone level (total and/or free value, depending on the particular study) divided by the total number of subjects with a hyperfunctioning thyroid nodule. Far fewer subjects had subclinical hyperthyroidism (13%) (Table 3). In comparison, with the exception of 3 studies, similar data on the biochemical profiles of subjects with benign, toxic adenoma in the collected case series were only sparsely included. In a study of 35 subjects with toxic adenoma, Hamburger found 16 with elevations in both T_3 and T_4 levels, 16 with elevations of only T_3, 3 with isolated T_4 excess, and 7 with subclinical hyperthyroidism [77]. In a study of 63 patients with solitary toxic adenoma, Langer found that mean free T_3 level was significantly higher (8.8 ± 3.5 pg/mL, normal range $4 - 6.8$ pg/mL) than mean free T_4 level (16.9 ± 6.6 pg/mL, normal range $7 - 17.5$ pg/mL) [78]. Blum evaluated 35 patients with solitary autonomous thyroid nodule and found that 65% had elevated T_3 levels, 54 % had elevated T_4 levels, and 31% were biochemically euthyroid [72]. Thus, hypersecretion of T_3 appears to be a common factor among both benign and malignant hyperfunctioning

Table 2 Reported cases of biochemically-hyperthyroid patients with a reported hyperfunctioning nodule discovered to harbor thyroid carcinoma on pathological review

#	Age	Sex	Tumor growth (cm)	High risk history[a]	Suspicious U/S[b]	Nodule size[c] (cm)	Tumor size[d] (cm)	TFTs[e]	Toxic sx?	Compression sx?	Scan type	FNA	Surgical path	Reference (1st author)
1	29	F		-	IV	2.7	2.5	SHT	+	-	^{123}I		FTC	Current case
2	43	F		-	-	6.5	5	fT$_3$,fT$_4$	+	-	Tc		Hurthle	Karanchi [23]
3	13	F		-	IV	3.5	5	TT$_3$	-	-	^{123}I		Hurthle	Yalla [24]
4	63	M		-	-	4		fT$_4$	-	+	^{123}I	Suspicion of FVPTC	FVPTC	Bommireddipalli [25]
5	68	F		-	HE	5.3		fT$_3$	+	+	Tc,^{123}I		FTC	Giovanella [26]
6	11	F		-	-	3.5		TT$_3$	-	-	^{123}I	Nonspecific	PTC	Tfayli [27]
7	47	F		-	-	2.6	3	TT$_3$,fT$_4$	-	-	^{131}I	PTC	FVPTC	Azevedo [28]
8	36	M	1.4→1.8 in 11mo	-	HE,IV	1.8	1.5	SHT	+	-	^{131}I	PTC	PTC	Uludag [29]
9	62	F		-	-		2	fT$_3$,fT$_4$	+	-	Tc	PTC	PTC	Nishida [30]
10	32	M		-	-	4.3		fT$_3$,fT$_4$	+	-	Tc	Benign	FVPTC	Kim [31]
11	64	F		-	-	6		TT$_3$	-	-	^{131}I		FTC	Niepomniszcze [32]
12	57	F		-	-	6		High[f]	+	-	Tc	Nondiagnostic	FTC	Bitterman [33]
13	59	F		-	-	5		High	+	-	Tc		FTC	Bitterman [33]
14	59	F		-	HE,PD,Cal	1.5	1.5	fT$_3$,fT$_4$	+	+	Tc,^{123}I	PTC	PTC	Majima [34]
15	NA	F		-	-	5	5	fT$_3$,fT$_4$	+	+	Tc		PTC	Gozu [35]
16	67	F		-	-	2.5	3	fT$_4$	+	-	Tc	Benign	Hurthle	Wong [36]
17	39	F	Subjective ↑	-	-	2		NI→SHT	-	-→+	^{123}I		PTC	Yaturu [37]
18	36	M	2x size in 5yrs	-	-	2.8	2.3	SHT	-	+		Follicular neoplasm	FVPTC	Logani [38]
19	11	F		-	-		4	TT$_3$,fT$_4$	+	-	Tc,^{131}I		PTC	Mircescu [39]
20	49	F			-	4	3.5	fT$_4$	+	-	^{123}I		FTC	Camacho [40]
21	47	M				3.5	3.5	fT$_3$	+	-	^{123}I	Suspicious	PTC	Bourasseau [41]
22	36	M				2.5	2.5	SHT	-	-	^{123}I	Nondiagnostic	FTC	Bourasseau [41]
23	56	M				5.5	5.5	fT$_4$	+	-	^{123}I		FTC	Bourasseau [41]
24	39	F				1	1	fT$_3$,fT$_4$	+	-	^{123}I	Suspicious	PTC	Bourasseau [41]
25	33	F				3	3	SHT	-	-	^{123}I	Nondiagnostic	PTC	Bourasseau [41]
26	42	F	4.5→7.4 (no interval given)	-	-	7.4		SHT	-	-	^{123}I	Benign	Hurthle	Russo [42]
27	17	F		-	HE	2.1	2.1	TT$_3$	-	-	Tc,^{123}I		PTC	Cirillo [43]
28	60	F			-	5	6	TT$_3$	+	-	^{131}I		Insular	Russo [44]
29	16	F		-	-	2		TT$_4$	+	-	^{123}I	Colloid	Hurthle	Siddiqui [45]

Table 2 Reported cases of biochemically-hyperthyroid patients with a reported hyperfunctioning nodule discovered to harbor thyroid carcinoma on pathological review (*Continued*)

No.	Age	Sex	Growth	Size	Duration	Nodule	Thyroid function			Isotope	Cytology	Pathology	Reference
30	64	F		4			High			123I		FTC	Mizukami [46]
31	25	F		4.2		-	TT_3,TT_4	+	+	131I		PTC/FTC	De Rosa [47]
32	72	M		2.8			TT_3,TT_4	+		Tc		PTC	Ikekubo [48]
33	52	M		5			TT_3			Tc		PTC	Ikekubo [48]
34	55	F		1.6			SHT			Tc		PTC	Ikekubo [48]
35	67	F		3	2.5	-	TT_3,fT_4	+	-	123I	Malignant node	PTC	Sandler [49]
36	11	F		3.5		-	TT_3	+	-	123I		FTC	Nagai [50]
37	45	F		3.5	3	-	High	+	-	123I		FVPTC	Nagai [50]
38	70	F		4	4	-	fT4	-	-	131I	PTC	PTC	Fukata [51]
39	27	F		3		-	TT_4	+	-	131I		PTC	Sobel [52]
40	14	M		4			TT_3	+	-	131I		PTC	Sobel [52]
41	32	F		2.5		-	TT_4	+	-	131I		FVPTC	Sobel [52]
42	29	F			1	-	TT_4	+	-	131I		PTC	Hoving [53]
43	44	F		2.5	0.3	irregular	TT_4	+	-	131I		PTC	Khan [54]
44	15	F		2.5	2.5		TT_3	+		123I		PTC	Hopwood [55]
45	6	F	↑ over 8mo	5-6x nl			High	+	-	131I		PTC/FTC	Sussman [56]
46	42	F	4→6 in 4 yrs	6	6		High		-	131I		FTC	Dische [57]
47	71	F					fT_3,fT_4			131I		FTC	Als [58]
48	62	M		8			fT_3			131I		FTC	Als [58]
49	62	F		7			fT_3			131I		FTC	Als [58]
50	71	F		4			fT_3,fT_4			131I		FTC	Als [58]
51	69	F		6			fT_3			131I		FTC	Als [58]
52	79	F					fT_3,fT_4			131I		FTC	Als [58]
53	65	M		6.5			fT_3			131I		FTC	Als [58]
54	56	M					fT_3			131I		FVPTC	Als [58]
55	75	M		5.5			fT_3			131I		FTC	Als [58]
56	77	F		4			fT_3			131I		PTC	Als [58]
57	71	F		6			fT_3			131I		FVC	Als [58]
58	63	M		6			fT_3,fT_4			131I		FVPTC	Als [58]
59	74	F		7			fT_3,fT_4			131I		FTC	Als [58]
60	68	M		6		HE	SHT	-		Tc	Follicular neoplasm	FTC	Foppiani [12]

Table 2 Reported cases of biochemically-hyperthyroid patients with a reported hyperfunctioning nodule discovered to harbor thyroid carcinoma on pathological review (Continued)

Case	Age	Sex	High-risk hx	HE	Nodule size	Tumor size	TFTs	SHT	Tc	Initial path	Final dx	Reference
61	38	F				2.7	SHT			Hyperplastic goiter	FTC	Foppiani [12]
62	35	F		-	>1cm		High	+	^{131}I	PTC	PTC	Sahin [13]
63	65	F		-	>1cm		High	+	^{131}I	PTC	PTC	Sahin [13]
64	19	F				5	TT_4, TT_3				PTC	Lin [59]
65	38	F		-		0.3	TT_3	+	^{131}I	no malignancy	PTC	Taneri [60]
66	44	F		Cal		1	TT_3	+	^{131}I	no malignancy	PTC	Taneri [60]
67	56	F		-		0.8	High		^{131}I		FTC	Gabriele [14]
68	21	F		IV		1.6	High		^{131}I		FTC	Gabriele [14]
69	57	F		-		0.7	High				PTC	Vaiana [16]
70	58	F		-		3	High				PTC	Vaiana [16]
71	51	F		-		0.6	High				PTC	Vaiana [16]
72	17	F		-		1	High	+			PTC	Pacini [19]
73	65	F	Subjective ↑			5	High	+			FTC	Terzioglu [18]
74	42	F					High	+			PTC	Terzioglu [18]
75	35	F		-		2.2	High				PTC	Zanella [17]
76	70	F		-		4.1	High				PTC	Zanella [17]
77	35	M		-		5.4	High				Hurthle	Zanella [17]

Abbreviations: + = yes; - = no; Cal = microcalcifications; FNA = fine needle aspiration; FTC = follicular thyroid carcinoma; HE = hypoechoic; FVPTC = follicular variant of papillary thyroid carcinoma; ^{123}I = Iodine-123; ^{131}I = Iodine-131; IV = internal vascularity; NA = not available; nl = normal; PD = poorly demarcated; PTC = papillary thyroid carcinoma; sx = symptoms; SHT = subclinical hyperthyroidism; fT_3 = free triiodothyronine; LT_4 = levothyroxine; T_4 = total thyroxine; T_3 = total triiodothyronine; fT_4 = free thyroxine; ^{99m}Tc = technetium-99m-pertechnetate; TFTs = thyroid function testing; U/S = ultrasound; XRT = external beam radiotherapy; as per Cooper et al. [6].

[a] High-risk history: ionizing radiation exposure as child/adolescent, prior personal history of thyroid cancer, and family history of thyroid cancer in one or more 1st-degree relatives; as per Cooper et al. [6].

[b] Suspicious ultrasound: hypoechoic, microcalcifications, increased nodular vascularity, poorly demarcated; as per Cooper et al. [6].

[c] Nodule size: The largest diameter of the thyroid nodule measured by ultrasonography, or if ultrasound not available, then by palpation.

[d] Tumor size: The largest diameter of the thyroid nodule measured grossly after surgical resection.

[e] TFTs: Indicates which thyroid hormone values (total T3, total T4, free T3, and/or free T4) were elevated at time of presentation, as opposed to SHT or euthyroidism. Of note, for many of these cases, no mention of one or more of these four standard thyroid hormone values was included.

[f] High: Indicates that the patient was biochemically hyperthyroid, though specific thyroid hormone levels were not given.

Table 3 Demographic and clinical characteristics of the reported cases of hyperthyroid patients with hyperfunctioning thyroid carcinoma from the literature and the current case (n = 77)

Characteristic	
Age	
Mean—yr	47.0 ± 19.8*
Distribution – no. (%)	
< 15 yr	6 (7.9%)
15-30 yr	10 (13.2%)
31-45 yr	20 (26.3%)
46-60 yr	15 (19.7%)
> 60 yr	25 (32.9%)
Sex – no. (%)	
Female	60 (77.9%)
Male	17 (22.1%)
High risk features	
Historical – no. (%)	0 (0%)
Ultrasonographical – no. (%)	11 (36.7%)
Thyroid nodule size (via ultrasound or palpation) (cm)	4.13 ± 1.68
Thyroid carcinoma size on pathological review	
Mean (cm)	2.48 ± 1.70
No. (%) with size < 1cm	8 (20.5%)
Biochemical hyperthyroidism	
T_3 elevated – no. (%)	39 (76.5%)
T_4 elevated – no. (%)	27 (51.9%)
Subclinical hyperthyroidism – no. (%)	10 (13.0%)
Thyrotoxic symptoms – no. (%)	37 (78.7%)
Compression symptoms – no. (%)	5 (14.7%)
Thyroid scintigraphy	
Technetium-99m-pertechnetate – no. (%)	16 (24.2%)
Iodine-123 or −131 – no. (%)	53 (80.3%)
Fine-needle aspiration	
Benign – no. (%)	7 (30.4%)
Malignant (or suspicious findings) – no. (%)	10 (43.5%)
Follicular neoplasm – no. (%)	2 (8.7%)
Nondiagnostic sample – no. (%)	4 (17.4%)
FNA accordant with final pathological diagnosis – no. (%)	12 (60%)
FNA not accordant with final pathological diagnosis – no. (%)	9 (39.1%)
Type of thyroid carcinoma on surgical pathological review	
Follicular thyroid carcinoma	28 (36.4%)
Papillary thyroid carcinoma	44 (57.1%)
Follicular variant of papillary thyroid carcinoma	8 (18.2%)
Hurthle cell carcinoma	6 (7.8%)
Insular cell carcinoma	1 (1.3%)

* Mean ± standard deviation.
no. = Number of subjects with this characteristic, % = percentage of subjects with this characteristic.

thyroid nodules. Of interest, a greater prevalence of frank biochemical hyperthyroidism can be seen in patients with malignant hyperfunctioning thyroid nodules who have larger nodules (Figure 2B).

Historical and sonographic features

We next turned our attention to high-risk historical features and suspicious sonographic features to determine if these were present in cases of malignant hot nodule (Table 3). These features are described in Cooper et al. [6] and are listed in the Tables 2 and 3 legend. None of the 77 subjects with malignant hot nodules was noted to have high-risk historical features. Eleven subjects (36.7%) had suspicious features on ultrasonography, which is likely an underestimate, as some of the more newly-recognized high-risk sonographic features (e.g., taller than wide on transverse view) were not utilized in the earlier published reports. It was difficult to assess cases for nodule growth as a risk factor for malignancy, since the vast majority of the subjects were referred to surgery for immediate resection. However in seven cases, nodules were noted to grow over time. While an increase in nodule size is an indication for biopsy, the specificity of this finding for malignancy is limited, as 9-89% of benign nodules have been shown to grow over time depending on which definition for significant growth is used [21,73,77,79].

Histologic subtype

The majority of malignant hot nodules were proven to be PTC (57.1%), and of these, 18.2% were the follicular variant of PTC (FVPTC). Follicular thyroid carcinoma (as seen in our patient) comprised 36.4% of cases, while Hurthle cell carcinoma was found in 7.8% of samples. By comparison, in the U.S. National Cancer Data Base (1985–1995), which includes histologic information on all thyroid nodules as a group, the prevalence of PTC was approximately 85%, FTC was 10%, and Hurthle cell carcinoma was nearly 3% [80]. Thus, there does seem to be a higher prevalence of both FTC and Hurthle cell carcinoma in the hyperfunctioning thyroid carcinoma cases.

Of note, within the 77 identified cases of malignant hot nodule, only 23 subjects received FNA of their thyroid nodule prior to resection. FNA enabled a preoperative diagnosis of thyroid carcinoma in 43.5% of cases. However, 30.4% of subjects undergoing FNA were erroneously characterized as having benign lesions, and 17.4% of samples were nondiagnostic. Of the subjects with false negative biopsies, surgical pathology eventually revealed PTC in 3 cases (one of these was FVPTC), FTC in 1 case, and Hurthle cell carcinoma in 3 cases. Tumor size was given in only 3 instances of false negative biopsies. Two of these were of subcentimetric PTC,

Table 4 Additional cases with scintigraphic evidence suggestive of an autonomous thyroid nodule without documented hyperthyroidism (or already on levothyroxine replacement therapy) discovered to harbor thyroid carcinoma on pathologic review

#	Age	Sex	Tumor growth (cm)	High risk history[a]	Suspicious U/S[b]	Nodule size[c] (cm)	Tumor size[d] (cm)	TFTs[e]	Toxic sx?	Compression sx?	Scan type	FNA	Surgical path	Reference (1st author)
1	51	F	2.7→5.3 in 2yrs	-	-	5.3	5	on LT$_4$	-	+	Tc,131I	Follicular neoplasm	Poor diff cancer	Low [61]
2	44	F		-		3.5	3.7	nl	-	-→+	Tc	Benign	FTC	Schneider [62]
3	47	M				1.4	1	nl	-		123I		PTC	Bourasseau [41]
4	34	F				1	1	nl	-		123I	"Cancer"	PTC	Bourasseau [41]
5	37	F				1.5	1.5	nl	-		123I	Nondiagnostic	FTC	Bourasseau [41]
6	39	M				3		nl			123I		FVPTC	Mizukami [46]
7	69	F		Prior PTC		4	3.3	on LT$_4$	+	-	131I		Hurthle	Caplan [63]
8	39	M			HE,PD,Cal		1.5	nl	-	-	123I		PTC	Michigishi [64]
9	65	F				4.3		nl			Tc		PTC	Ikekubo [48]
10	37	F				2.5		nl			Tc		PTC	Ikekubo [48]
11	39	F				3.5		nl			Tc		PTC	Ikekubo [48]
12	38	F				4.5		nl			Tc		PTC	Ikekubo [48]
13	35	F		-		1	0.4	nl	-	-	123I		PTC	Rubenfeld [65]
14	51	M		XRT		"large"		on LT$_4$			123I		FTC	Nagai [50]
15	19	F	4x2→4x3 in 1 yr	-		4	4	nl	-	-	131I		PTC/FTC	Abdel-Razzak [66]
16	15	F		-				nl	-	-	Tc		PTC	Scott [67]
17	27	F			-	4	2.3	nl	+	-	131I		PTC	Fujimoto [68]
18	21	F				3	1	NA	+	+	131I		PTC	Becker [69]
19	23	F				1.5	1	NA	-	-	131I		PTC	Becker [69]
20	28	M				4.5	0.5	NA	+	-	131I		PTC	Molnar [70]
21	54	M				8.5		NA			131I		FTC	Als [58]
22	62	F						NA			131I		PTC	Als [58]
23	61	M						NA			131I		FTC	Als [58]
24	50	M				10		NA			131I		FTC	Als [58]
25	65	F				5		NA			131I		FTC	Als [58]
26	55	F				5.5		NA			131I		FTC	Als [58]

Table 4 Additional cases with scintigraphic evidence suggestive of an autonomous thyroid nodule without documented hyperthyroidism (or already on levothyroxine replacement therapy) discovered to harbor thyroid carcinoma on pathologic review (*Continued*)

27	66	F	-	Cal	+	-	nl		Tc,^{131}I	Colloid goiter	PTC	Bitterman [33]
77	35	M	-	5.4	0.5	High^f	High^f				Hurthle	Zanella [17]

Abbreviations: + = yes; - = no; Cal = microcalcifications; FNA = fine needle aspiration; FTC = follicular thyroid carcinoma; FVPTC = follicular variant of papillary thyroid carcinoma; HE = hypoechoic; ^{123}I = Iodine-123; ^{131}I = Iodine-131; IV = internal vascularity; LT$_4$ = levothyroxine; NA = not available; nl = normal; PD = poorly demarcated; PTC = papillary thyroid carcinoma; sx = symptoms; SHT = subclinical hyperthyroidism; fT$_3$ = free triiodothyronine; fT$_4$ = free thyroxine; TT$_3$ = total triiodothyronine; TT$_4$ = total thyroxine; ^{99m}Tc = technetium-99m-pertechnetate; TFTs = thyroid function testing; U/S = ultrasound; XRT = external beam radiotherapy.

^{a} High-risk history: ionizing radiation exposure as child/adolescent, prior personal history of thyroid cancer, and family history of thyroid cancer in one or more 1st-degree relatives; as per Cooper et al. [6].

^{b} Suspicious ultrasound: hypoechoic, microcalcifications, increased nodular vascularity, poorly demarcated, or if ultrasound not available, then by palpation.

^{c} Nodule size: The largest diameter of the thyroid nodule measured by ultrasonography, or if ultrasound not available, then by palpation.

^{d} Tumor size: The largest diameter of the thyroid nodule measured grossly after surgical resection.

^{e} TFTs: Indicates which thyroid hormone values (total T3, total T4, free T3, and/or free T4) were elevated at time of presentation, as opposed to SHT or euthyroidism. Of note, for many of these cases, no mention of one or more of these four standard thyroid hormone values was included.

^{f} High: Indicates that the patient was biochemically hyperthyroid, though specific thyroid hormone levels were not given.

Table 5 Demographic characteristics of patients with solitary hyperfunctioning thyroid nodules

Author	Mean age (years)	Female: male (n)
Bransom [71]	49.7±13.4	33:35
Blum [72]	50.9±17.5	31:4
Burch [73]	45.8±16.8	42:13
Cappelli [11]	61.8	445:381
Giles [9]	48.5±11.4	147:29
Hamburger [21]	60±15	19:5
Iwata [74]	48.8±15.4	44:0
Landgarten [75]	49.3	106:11
Linos [76]	40	53:9
Sahin [13]	58.3±13.7	50:27
Smith [20]	34.8	24:6
Vaiana [16]	61.8	340:290
Weighted average	**57.6**	**1.65:1**

and it is presumed that small size was likely a chief factor leading to misdiagnosis. However, the other was a 3 cm nodule comprised wholly of Hurthle cell carcinoma.

Discussion

To our knowledge, the current data set is the largest and most detailed to date of patients with malignant hot thyroid nodule. In that regard, this study complements the informative and excellent 2012 review by Pazaitou-Panayiotou and colleagues examining the association of thyroid carcinoma with a broader spectrum of hyperthyroid states, including Graves' disease and toxic multinodular goiter in addition to hyperfunctioning thyroid nodule [81]. Of note, although it was not the focus of the Pazaitou-Panayiotou et al. review to perform a detailed analysis of the historical and clinical features of malignant hot nodule cases, as we did here, Pazaitou-Panayiotou and colleagues did include an evaluation of thyroid carcinoma prevalence. The reported percentages of thyroid carcinoma in their collected case series of patients with hot nodules, which overlapped but did not mirror exactly those case series evaluated here and which also included some cases of thyroid carcinoma occurring in extranodular thyroid tissue, ranged between 2.5 – 12.0%. This corresponds to a weighted average of 6.9% and thus is similar to the 3.1% prevalence estimated here. In its discussion of thyroid carcinoma in patients with hyperfunctioning nodules, the Pazaitou-Panayiotou et al. review also included several other important commentaries. For instance, they draw attention to two studies suggestive of a higher prevalence of thyroid carcinoma in hot nodules occurring in children [82,83], though the latter study included children from an iodine-deficient region. In addition, they discuss several

reports in which activating mutations of the TSH receptor gene were identified within malignant hot nodules [81].

There are several noteworthy discussion points and implications to the findings presented here. The first relates to the prevalence of malignancy within solitary hot nodules. As mentioned, in the available surgical case series that addressed this topic, a varied prevalence was noted, ranging from 0 – 12.5%, with a weighted average of 3.1%. Only a minority of the patients who underwent surgery in those series did so because of concerning findings from FNA, and as such, we do not believe that the data set is biased towards cases in which a postoperative diagnosis of malignancy was expected. We realize that this collection of case series includes only a small fraction of the total number of solitary hot nodules that have occurred, and also that the vast majority of malignant hot nodules likely have gone unreported. Furthermore, it is likely that malignancy goes undiagnosed in many cases of hot nodules treated with radioiodine, especially those harboring microcarcinomas. Despite these limitations, we do believe there are sufficient numbers of cases included among the collected 14 surgical case series of subjects to cite the 3.1% figure as being a fair and representative estimate of malignancy prevalence amongst solitary hyperfunctioning nodules. While this 3.1% prevalence figure is low – and in fact is lower than the estimated 5 - 15% prevalence of malignancy among all thyroid nodules [6] – it is not trivial. Thus, the possibility of malignancy within a hot nodule must not be overlooked by a managing clinician, particularly if management other than surgical resection is chosen.

Another important discussion point regards the limitations resulting from the retrospective nature of this analysis, including incomplete data and differing methodology used in many of the collected case reports and case series of malignant hot nodule. While some of the primary sources were meticulous in their case descriptions, others included less-thorough descriptions. For example, tumor size was frequently not reported, and thus it was unclear if a PTC tumor was simply an incidental microcarcinoma embedded within a larger hot nodule or a large, follicular variant of PTC comprising the entirety of the nodule. While we have included some cases in which the malignancy was a microcarcinoma and thus of uncertain clinical significance [84], these cases are clearly in the minority (only 8 of the 77 reported tumors were less than one centimeter in size). Other factors affecting the data set are the evolution of technology and our understanding of risk factors for thyroid carcinoma. For instance, thyroid ultrasound began clinical use in the late 1960s, and prior to this, nodule size was estimated by palpation. Earlier reports would not have commented on some of the suspicious

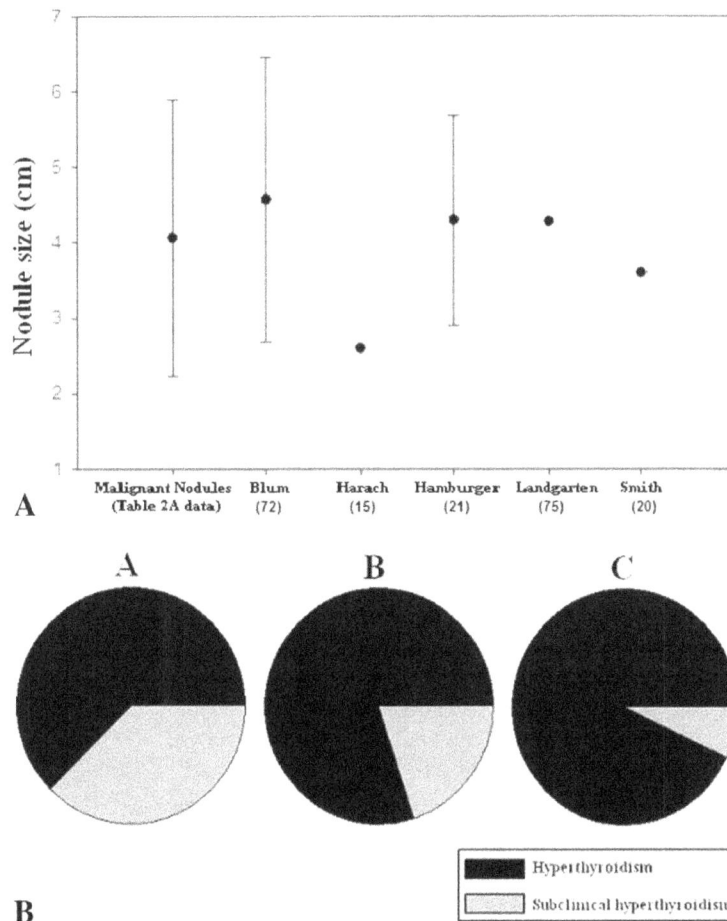

Figure 2 Size and biochemical assessment of hyperfunctioning thyroid nodules. (**A**) The mean greatest dimension of the malignant hot thyroid nodules from our case series is compared with that from five published surgical cases series of solitary, hyperfunctioning thyroid nodules. (**B**) The proportion of subjects with scintigraphically-determined hyperfunctioning thyroid carcinoma (Tables 2) who have frank biochemical hyperthyroidism vs. subclinical hyperthyroidism, based on varying nodule size. Subjects are characterized as having nodules < 2.5 cm (**A**), 2.5 – 4.5 cm (**B**), and > 4.5 cm (**C**) in diameter.

sonographic features recognized today. Additionally, the radioimmunoassays used to measure TSH have undergone many generations of refinement over the past several decades, and thus the presence and degree of hyperthyroidism may have been underestimated in earlier studies.

Also worth discussing are the differential prevalences of thyroid carcinoma histologic subtype found in hot nodules as compared to nodules as a group. As mentioned, there was a much higher prevalence of both FTC and Hurthle cell carcinoma in hot nodules (36.4% and 7.8%, respectively) as compared to in all nodules (10% and nearly 3%, respectively). Additionally, a substantial percentage of the PTC cases found in hot nodules were the follicular variant. This may have bearing on the current algorithm for evaluation of patients with thyroid nodules as recommended in the 2009 thyroid nodule and thyroid carcinoma management guidelines [6]. In

particular, for those nodules found by biopsy to have follicular neoplasm by histology, the guidelines recommend consideration be made for performing an ^{123}I thyroid scan, if not already done, especially if the serum TSH is in the low-normal range; if the nodule is found to be hyperfunctioning, it can then be followed [6]. However, the high prevalence of both FTC and FVPTC reported for malignant hot nodules suggests that a biopsy diagnosis of follicular neoplasm within a hot nodule may not be as reassuring as previously thought. Also of interest, in a 2009 study, Sundaraiya and colleagues reported a case of metastatic FTC occurring in the setting of thyrotoxicosis, in which high-grade extrathyroidal uptake of technetium-99m-pertechnetate was observed; in a literature search, they found 74 other cases of thyrotoxicosis resulting from well-differentiated thyroid cancer metastatic lesions, most of which demonstrated histologic evidence of FTC [85].

As a final point of discussion, since none of the historical, biochemical or radiologic characteristics that were assessed seems to predict malignancy in the collected cases of hot nodules, one might ask if there is any utility in biopsying hot nodules. Such would be a shift from the current thyroid nodule management guidelines which views an increased nodular radiotracer uptake pattern as a reassuring characteristic from a cancer perspective [6]. Given the estimated 3.1% prevalence of malignancy within hot nodules, and also taking into account the difficulty in predicting whether a particular hot nodule is malignant, we recommend that hot nodules that are not treated surgically (as is an option to manage the hyperthyroidism) be considered for biopsy if high-risk historical and/or suspicious sonographic features are present or if these nodules grow over time, just as is currently recommended for nodules that are not hyperfunctioning [6]. This should also include previously hyperfunctioning nodules treated with radioiodine, although the known occurrence of dystrophic calcification and cystic degeneration as sequelae of radioiodine ablation should be taken into account when assessing their sonographic features [86]. Future prospective studies could help determine if biopsying at the time of diagnosis all hot nodules with suspicious sonographic characteristics and/or associated high-risk historical features versus biopsying hot nodules only if the initial sonographic characteristics worsen over time would result in better outcomes.

Competing interests
The authors declare that they have no competing interests.

Authors' contributions
SM performed the literature review and drafted the manuscript. DM provided the radiology images and participated in drafting/revising the manuscript. LP provided the pathology images and participated in drafting/revising the manuscript. SW helped to provide the surgery perspective and edited the manuscript. JZ assisted with the literature review and drafting of the manuscript. All authors read and approved the final manuscript.

Acknowledgements
The authors would like to acknowledge Jeffrey R. Garber, M.D. for helpful discussions. We also acknowledge the support of the Diana and Richard C. Strauss Professorship in Biomedical Research and the Mr. and Mrs. Bruce G. Brookshire Professorship in Medicine at UTSW Medical Center.

Author details
[1]Department of Internal Medicine, Division of Endocrinology and Metabolism, The University of Texas Southwestern Medical Center, Dallas, Texas 75390, USA. [2]Department of Radiology, Neurology and Neurotherapeutics, The University of Texas Southwestern Medical Center, Dallas, TX 75390, USA. [3]Department of Pathology, The University of Texas Southwestern Medical Center, Dallas, TX, USA75390. [4]Department of Surgery, The University of Texas Southwestern Medical Center, Dallas, TX 75390, USA.

References
1. Vander JB, Gaston EA, Dawber TR: The significance of nontoxic thyroid nodules. Final report of a 15-year study of the incidence of thyroid malignancy. Ann Intern Med 1968, 69:537–540.
2. Reiners C, Wegscheider K, Schicha H, Theissen P, Vaupel R, Wrbitzky R, Schumm-Draeger PM: Prevalence of thyroid disorders in the working population of Germany: ultrasonography screening in 96,278 unselected employees. Thyroid 2004, 14:926–932.
3. Guth S, Theune U, Aberle J, Galach A, Bamberger CM: Very high prevalence of thyroid nodules detected by high frequency (13 MHz) ultrasound examination. Eur J Clin Invest 2009, 39:699–706.
4. Mortensen JD, Woolner LB, Bennett WA: Gross and microscopic findings in clinically normal thyroid glands. J Clin Endocrinol Metab 1955, 15:1270–1280.
5. Hegedus L: Clinical practice. The thyroid nodule. N Engl J Med 2004, 351:1764–1771.
6. Cooper DS, Doherty GM, Haugen BR, Kloos RT, Lee SL, Mandel SJ, Mazzaferri EL, McIver B, Pacini F, Schlumberger M, et al: Revised American Thyroid Association management guidelines for patients with thyroid nodules and differentiated thyroid cancer. Thyroid 2009, 19:1167–1214.
7. Garber JR: Thyroid nodules 2006: managing what has been known for over 50 years. Hormones (Athens) 2006, 5:179–186.
8. Bahn RS, Burch HB, Cooper DS, Garber JR, Greenlee MC, Klein I, Laurberg P, McDougall IR, Montori VM, Rivkees SA, et al: Hyperthyroidism and other causes of thyrotoxicosis: management guidelines of the American Thyroid Association and American Association of Clinical Endocrinologists. Endocr Pract 2011, 17:456–520.
9. Senyurek Giles Y, Tunca F, Boztepe H, Kapran Y, Terzioglu T, Tezelman S: The risk factors for malignancy in surgically treated patients for Graves' disease, toxic multinodular goiter, and toxic adenoma. Surgery 2008, 144:1028–1036. discussion 1036–1027.
10. Cakir M, Arici C, Alakus H, Altunbas H, Balci MK, Karayalcin U: Incidental thyroid carcinoma in thyrotoxic patients treated by surgery. Horm Res 2007, 67:96–99.
11. Cappelli C, Braga M, De Martino E, Castellano M, Gandossi E, Agosti B, Cumetti D, Pirola I, Mattanza C, Cherubini L, Rosei EA: Outcome of patients surgically treated for various forms of hyperthyroidism with differentiated thyroid cancer: experience at an endocrine center in Italy. Surg Today 2006, 36:125–130.
12. Foppiani L, Del Monte P, Marugo A, Arlandini A, Sartini G, Marugo M, Bernasconi D: Heterogeneous malignancy in toxic thyroid nodules. J Endocrinol Invest 2005, 28:294–295.
13. Sahin M, Guvener ND, Ozer F, Sengul A, Ertugrul D, Tutuncu NB: Thyroid cancer in hyperthyroidism: incidence rates and value of ultrasound-guided fine-needle aspiration biopsy in this patient group. J Endocrinol Invest 2005, 28:815–818.
14. Gabriele R, Letizia C, Borghese M, De Toma G, Celi M, Izzo L, Cavallaro A: Thyroid cancer in patients with hyperthyroidism. Horm Res 2003, 60:79–83.
15. Harach HR, Sanchez SS, Williams ED: Pathology of the autonomously functioning (hot) thyroid nodule. Ann Diagn Pathol 2002, 6:10–19.
16. Vaiana R, Cappelli C, Perini P, Pinelli D, Camoni G, Farfaglia R, Balzano R, Braga M: Hyperthyroidism and concurrent thyroid cancer. Tumori 1999, 85:247–252.
17. Zanella E, Rulli F, Muzi M, Sianesi M, Danese D, Sciacchitano S, Pontecorvi A: Prevalence of thyroid cancer in hyperthyroid patients treated by surgery. World J Surg 1998, 22:473–477. discussion 477–478.
18. Terzioglu T, Tezelman S, Onaran Y, Tanakol R: Concurrent Hyperthyroidism and Thyroid-Carcinoma. Brit J Surg 1993, 80:1301–1302.
19. Pacini F, Elisei R, Di Coscio GC, Anelli S, Macchia E, Concetti R, Miccoli P, Arganini M, Pinchera A: Thyroid carcinoma in thyrotoxic patients treated by surgery. J Endocrinol Invest 1988, 11:107–112.
20. Smith M, McHenry C, Jarosz H, Lawrence AM, Paloyan E: Carcinoma of the thyroid in patients with autonomous nodules. Am Surg 1988, 54:448–449.
21. Hamburger JI: Solitary autonomously functioning thyroid lesions. Diagnosis, clinical features and pathogenetic considerations. Am J Med 1975, 58:740–748.
22. Horst W, Rosler H, Schneider C, Labhart A: 306 cases of toxic adenoma: clinical aspects, findings in radioiodine diagnostics, radiochromatography and histology; results of 131-I and surgical treatment. J Nucl Med 1967, 8:515–528.
23. Karanchi H, Hamilton DJ, Robbins RJ: Hurthle cell carcinoma of the thyroid presenting as thyrotoxicosis. Endocr Pract 2012, 18:e5–9.
24. Yalla NM, Reynolds LR: Hurthle cell thyroid carcinoma presenting as a "hot" nodule. Endocr Pract 2011, 17:e68–72.

25. Bommireddipalli S, Goel S, Gadiraju R, Paniz-MondolFi A, DePuey EG: Follicular variant of papillary thyroid carcinoma presenting as a toxic nodule by I-123 scintigraphy. *Clin Nucl Med* 2010, 35:770–775.

26. Giovanella L, Fasolini F, Suriano S, Mazzucchelli L: Hyperfunctioning solid/trabecular follicular carcinoma of the thyroid gland. *J Oncol* 2010, 2010.

27. Tfayli HM, Teot LA, Indyk JA, Witchel SF: Papillary thyroid carcinoma in an autonomous hyperfunctioning thyroid nodule: case report and review of the literature. *Thyroid* 2010, 20:1029–1032.

28. Azevedo MF, Casulari LA: Hyperfunctioning thyroid cancer: a five-year follow-up. *Arq Bras Endocrinol Metabol* 2010, 54:78–80.

29. Uludag M, Yetkin G, Citgez B, Isgor A, Basak T: Autonomously functioning thyroid nodule treated with radioactive iodine and later diagnosed as papillary thyroid cancer. *Hormones (Athens)* 2008, 7:175–179.

30. Nishida AT, Hirano S, Asato R, Tanaka S, Kitani Y, Honda N, Fujiki N, Miyata K, Fukushima H, Ito J: Multifocal hyperfunctioning thyroid carcinoma without metastases. *Auris Nasus Larynx* 2008, 35:432–436.

31. Kim TS, Asato R, Akamizu T, Harada D, Nakashima Y, Higashi T, Yamamoto N, Tamura Y, Tamaki H, Hirano S, et al: A rare case of hyperfunctioning papillary carcinoma of the thyroid gland. *Acta Otolaryngol Suppl* 2007, 127:55–57.

32. Niepomniszcze H, Suarez H, Pitoia F, Pignatta A, Danilowicz K, Manavela M, Elsner B, Bruno OD: Follicular carcinoma presenting as autonomous functioning thyroid nodule and containing an activating mutation of the TSH receptor (T620I) and a mutation of the Ki-RAS (G12C) genes. *Thyroid* 2006, 16:497–503.

33. Bitterman A, Uri O, Levanon A, Baron E, Lefel O, Cohen O: Thyroid carcinoma presenting as a hot nodule. *Otolaryngol Head Neck Surg* 2006, 134:888–889.

34. Majima T, Doi K, Komatsu Y, Itoh H, Fukao A, Shigemoto M, Takagi C, Corners J, Mizuta N, Kato R, Nakao K: Papillary thyroid carcinoma without metastases manifesting as an autonomously functioning thyroid nodule. *Endocr J* 2005, 52:309–316.

35. Gozu H, Avsar M, Bircan R, Sahin S, Ahiskanali R, Gulluoglu B, Deyneli O, Ones Y, Narin Y, Akalin S, Cirakoglu B: Does a Leu 512 Arg thyrotropin receptor mutation cause an autonomously functioning papillary carcinoma? *Thyroid* 2004, 14:975–980.

36. Wong CP, AuYong TK, Tong CM: Thyrotoxicosis: a rare presenting symptom of Hurthle cell carcinoma of the thyroid. *Clin Nucl Med* 2003, 28:803–806.

37. Yaturu S, Fowler MR: Differentiated thyroid carcinoma with functional autonomy. *Endocr Pract* 2002, 8:36–39.

38. Logani S, Osei SY, LiVolsi VA, Baloch ZW: Fine-needle aspiration of follicular variant of papillary carcinoma in a hyperfunctioning thyroid nodule. *Diagn Cytopathol* 2001, 25:80–81.

39. Mircescu H, Parma J, Huot C, Deal C, Oligny LL, Vassart G, Van Vliet G: Hyperfunctioning malignant thyroid nodule in an 11-year-old girl: pathologic and molecular studies. *J Pediatr* 2000, 137:585–587.

40. Camacho P, Gordon D, Chiefari E, Yong S, DeJong S, Pitale S, Russo D, Filetti S: A Phe 486 thyrotropin receptor mutation in an autonomously functioning follicular carcinoma that was causing hyperthyroidism. *Thyroid* 2000, 10:1009–1012.

41. Bourasseau I, Savagner F, Rodien P, Duquenne M, Reynier P, Guyetant S, Bigorgne JC, Malthiery Y, Rohmer V: No evidence of thyrotropin receptor and G(s alpha) gene mutation in high iodine uptake thyroid carcinoma. *Thyroid* 2000, 10:761–765.

42. Russo D, Wong MG, Costante G, Chiefari E, Treseler PA, Arturi F, Filetti S, Clark OH: A Val 677 activating mutation of the thyrotropin receptor in a Hurthle cell thyroid carcinoma associated with thyrotoxicosis. *Thyroid* 1999, 9:13–17.

43. Cirillo RL Jr, Pozderac RV, Caniano DA, Falko JM: Metastatic pure papillary thyroid carcinoma presenting as a toxic hot nodule. *Clin Nucl Med* 1998, 23:345–349.

44. Russo D, Tumino S, Arturi F, Vigneri P, Grasso G, Pontecorvi A, Filetti S, Belfiore A: Detection of an activating mutation of the thyrotropin receptor in a case of an autonomously hyperfunctioning thyroid insular carcinoma. *J Clin Endocrinol Metab* 1997, 82:735–738.

45. Siddiqui AR, Karanauskas S: Hurthle cell carcinoma in an autonomous thyroid nodule in an adolescent. *Pediatr Radiol* 1995, 25:568–569.

46. Mizukami Y, Michigishi T, Nonomura A, Yokoyama K, Noguchi M, Hashimoto T, Nakamura S, Ishizaki T: Autonomously functioning (hot) nodule of the thyroid gland. A clinical and histopathologic study of 17 cases. *Am J Clin Pathol* 1994, 101:29–35.

47. De Rosa G, Testa A, Maurizi M, Satta MA, Aimoni C, Artuso A, Silvestri E, Rufini V, Troncone L: Thyroid carcinoma mimicking a toxic adenoma. *Eur J Nucl Med* 1990, 17:179–184.

48. Ikekubo K, Hino M, Ito H, Otani M, Yamaguchi H, Saiki Y, Ui K, Habuchi Y, Ishihara T, Mori T: Thyroid carcinoma in solitary hot thyroid lesions on Tc-99m sodium pertechnetate scans. *Ann Nucl Med* 1989, 3:31–36.

49. Sandler MP, Fellmeth B, Salhany KE, Patton JA: Thyroid carcinoma masquerading as a solitary benign hyperfunctioning nodule. *Clin Nucl Med* 1988, 13:410–415.

50. Nagai GR, Pitts WC, Basso L, Cisco JA, McDougall IR: Scintigraphic hot nodules and thyroid carcinoma. *Clin Nucl Med* 1987, 12:123–127.

51. Fukata S, Tamai H, Matsubayashi S, Nagai K, Hirota Y, Matsuzuka F, Katayama S, Kuma K, Nagataki S: Thyroid carcinoma and hot nodule. *Eur J Nucl Med* 1987, 13:313–314.

52. Sobel RJ, Liel Y, Goldstein J: Papillary carcinoma and the solitary autonomously functioning nodule of the thyroid. *Isr J Med Sci* 1985, 21:878–882.

53. Hoving J, Piers DA, Vermey A, Oosterhuis JW: Carcinoma in hyperfunctioning thyroid nodule in recurrent hyperthyroidism. *Eur J Nucl Med* 1981, 6:131–132.

54. Khan O, Ell PJ, Maclennan KA, Kurtz A, Williams ES: Thyroid carcinoma in an autonomously hyperfunctioning thyroid nodule. *Postgrad Med J* 1981, 57:172–175.

55. Hopwood NJ, Carroll RG, Kenny FM, Foley TP Jr: Functioning thyroid masses in childhood and adolescence. Clinical, surgical, and pathologic correlations. *J Pediatr* 1976, 89:710–718.

56. Sussman L, Librik L, Clayton GW: Hyperthyroidism attributable to a hyperfunctioning thyroid carcinoma. *J Pediatr* 1968, 72:208–213.

57. Dische S: The radioisotope scan applied to the detection of carcinoma in thyroid swellings. *Cancer* 1964, 17:473–479.

58. Als C, Gedeon P, Rosler H, Minder C, Netzer P, Laissue JA: Survival analysis of 19 patients with toxic thyroid carcinoma. *J Clin Endocrinol Metab* 2002, 87:4122–4127.

59. Lin JD, Huang MJ, Chao TC, Weng HF, Hsueh C: Prevalence of thyroid cancer in 1894 patients with surgically treated thyroid nodules. *Cancer J* 1997, 10:217–221.

60. Taneri F, Kurukahvecioglu O, Ege B, Yilmaz U, Tekin EH, Cifter C, Onuk E: Clinical presentation and treatment of hyperthyroidism associated with thyroid cancer. *Endocr Regul* 2005, 39:91–96.

61. Low SC, Sinha AK, Sundram FX: Detection of thyroid malignancy in a hot nodule by fluorine-18-fluorodeoxyglucose positron emission tomography. *Singapore Med J* 2005, 46:304–307.

62. Schneider PW, Meier DA, Balon H: A clear cell variant of follicular carcinoma presenting as an autonomously functioning thyroid nodule. *Thyroid* 2000, 10:269–273.

63. Caplan RH, Abellera RM, Kisken WA: Hurthle cell neoplasms of the thyroid gland: reassessment of functional capacity. *Thyroid* 1994, 4:243–248.

64. Michigishi T, Mizukami Y, Shuke N, Satake R, Noguchi M, Aburano T, Tonami N, Hisada K: An autonomously functioning thyroid carcinoma associated with euthyroid Graves' disease. *J Nucl Med* 1992, 33:2024–2026.

65. Rubenfeld S, Wheeler TM: Thyroid cancer presenting as a hot thyroid nodule: report of a case and review of the literature. *Thyroidology* 1988:63–68.

66. Abdel-Razzak M, Christie JH: Thyroid carcinoma in an autonomously functioning nodule. *J Nucl Med* 1979, 20:1001–1002.

67. Scott MD, Crawford JD: Solitary thyroid nodules in childhood: is the incidence of thyroid carcinoma declining? *Pediatrics* 1976, 58:521–525.

68. Fujimoto Y, Oka A, Nagataki S: Occurrence of papillary carcinoma in hyperfunctioning thyroid nodule. Report of a case. *Endocrinol Jpn* 1972, 19:371–374.

69. Becker FO, Economou PG, Schwartz TB: The occurrence of carcinoma in "hot" thyroid nodules. Report of two cases. *Ann Intern Med* 1963, 58:877–882.

70. Molnar GD, Childs DS Jr, Woolner LB: Histologic evidence of malignancy in a thyroid gland bearing a hot nodule. *J Clin Endocrinol Metab* 1958, 18:1132–1134.

71. Bransom CJ, Talbot CH, Henry L, Elemenoglou J: Solitary toxic adenoma of the thyroid gland. *Br J Surg* 1979, 66:592–595.

72. Blum M, Shenkman L, Hollander CS: **The autonomous nodule of the thyroid: correlation of patient age, nodule size and functional status.** *Am J Med Sci* 1975, **269:**43–50.

73. Burch HB, Shakir F, Fitzsimmons TR, Jaques DP, Shriver CD: **Diagnosis and management of the autonomously functioning thyroid nodule: the Walter Reed Army Medical Center experience, 1975–1996.** *Thyroid* 1998, **8:**871–880.

74. Iwata M, Kasagi K, Hatabu H, Misaki T, Iida Y, Fujita T, Konishi J: **Causes of appearance of scintigraphic hot areas on thyroid scintigraphy analyzed with clinical features and comparative ultrasonographic findings.** *Ann Nucl Med* 2002, **16:**279–287.

75. Landgarten S, Spencer RP: **A study of the natural history of "hot" thyroid nodules.** *Yale J Biol Med* 1973, **46:**259–263.

76. Linos DA, Karakitsos D, Papademetriou J: **Should the primary treatment of hyperthyroidism be surgical?** *Eur J Surg* 1997, **163:**651–657.

77. Hamburger JI: **Evolution of toxicity in solitary nontoxic autonomously functioning thyroid nodules.** *J Clin Endocrinol Metab* 1980, **50:**1089–1093.

78. Langer M, Madeddu G, Costanza C: **Free thyroxine (FT4) and free triiodothyronine (FT3) in autonomous thyroid nodules.** *Clin Endocrinol (Oxf)* 1979, **11:**461–464.

79. Alexander EK, Hurwitz S, Heering JP, Benson CB, Frates MC, Doubilet PM, Cibas ES, Larsen PR, Marqusee E: **Natural history of benign solid and cystic thyroid nodules.** *Ann Intern Med* 2003, **138:**315–318.

80. Hundahl SA, Fleming ID, Fremgen AM, Menck HR: **A National Cancer Data Base report on 53,856 cases of thyroid carcinoma treated in the U.S., 1985–1995 [see commetns].** *Cancer* 1998, **83:**2638–2648.

81. Pazaitou-Panayiotou K, Michalakis K, Paschke R: **Thyroid cancer in patients with hyperthyroidism.** *Horm Metab Res* 2012, **44:**255–262.

82. Croom RD 3rd, Thomas CG Jr, Reddick RL, Tawil MT: **Autonomously functioning thyroid nodules in childhood and adolescence.** *Surgery* 1987, **102:**1101–1108.

83. Niedziela M, Breborowicz D, Trejster E, Korman E: **Hot nodules in children and adolescents in western Poland from 1996 to 2000: clinical analysis of 31 patients.** *J Pediatr Endocrinol Metab* 2002, **15:**823–830.

84. Pacini F: **Thyroid microcarcinoma.** *Best Pract Res Clin Endocrinol Metab* 2012, **26:**421–429.

85. Sundaraiya S, Dizdarevic S, Miles K, Quin J, Williams A, Wheatley T, Zammitt C: **Unusual initial manifestation of metastatic follicular carcinoma of the thyroid with thyrotoxicosis diagnosed by technetium Tc 99m pertechnetate scan: case report and review of literature.** *Endocr Pract* 2009, **15:**458–462.

86. Kim JH, Park JH, Kim SY, Bae HY: **Symptomatic calcification of a thyroid lobe and surrounding tissue after radioactive iodine treatment to ablate the lobe.** *Thyroid* 2011, **21:**203–205.

4

Negative correlation between bone mineral density and TSH receptor antibodies in long-term euthyroid postmenopausal women with treated Graves' disease

Monica A Ercolano[1*], Monica L Drnovsek[1], Maria C Silva Croome[1], Monica Moos[1], Ana M Fuentes[1], Fanny Viale[1], Ulla Feldt-Rasmussen[2] and Alicia T Gauna[1]

Abstract

Background: Thyrotoxicosis is a cause of secondary osteoporosis. High concentrations of triiodotironine (T3) in Graves' disease stimulate bone turnover, but it is unclear if euthyroidism will always normalize bone metabolism. Thyrotropin (TSH) is known to affect directly the bone metabolism through the TSH receptor and TSH receptor antibodies (TRAb) may have an important role in bone turn-over.
The aim of our study was to determine, in pre and postmenopausal euthyroidism patients with previous overt hyperthyroidism due to Graves' disease the bone mineral density (BMD) as well as factors that could affect BMD in each group, including TRAb.

Methods: Cross-sectional, non-interventional study. Fifty-seven patients with previous hyperthyroidism due to Graves' disease (premenopausal: 30, postmenopausal: 27) that remained euthyroid for at least 6 months prior to study were included and compared with fifty- two matched respective controls. Thyrotoxine (T4), TSH, TRAb and BMD were measured.

Results: Only euthyroid postmenopausal patients with a history of hyperthyroidism due to Graves' disease showed lower whole body BMD than matched controls. The BMD expressed as Z-score was less in whole body and lumbar spine in postmenopausal in relation to premenopausal women with previous overt hyperthyroidism due to Graves' disease.
In the postmenopausal patients, the Z-score of lumbar spine BMD correlated negatively with TRAb ($r = -0,53$, $p < 0.008$), positively with the time of evolution of the disease ($r = +0.42$, $p < 0.032$) and positively with the time of euthyroidism ($r = + 0.50$, $p < 0.008$), but neither with serum T4 nor TSH. In a multiple regression analysis TRAb was the only significant independent variable in relation to lumbar spine BMD ($F = 3. 90$, $p < 0.01$).

Conclusions: In euthyroid women with a history of Graves' hyperthyroidism, BMD was only affected in the postmenopausal group. The negative correlation of Z-score of lumbar spine BMD with TRAb suggests that this antibody may affect the bone metabolism.

Introduction

Thyroid hormones exert their effect on osteoblasts via nuclear receptors stimulating osteoclastic bone resorption [1-3]. Hyperthyroidism is thus one of the major causes of secondary osteoporosis.

Reduction in bone mineral density (BMD) following hyperthyroidism in female subjects has been described in many reports [4-10]. A bone histomorphometric study in patients with hyperthyroidism has shown that the increase in osteoclastic resorption was more prominent in cortical than in cancellous bone [9,11] and that normalization of thyroid function was associated with an increase in lumbar spine BMD, which was preceded by a significant attenuation of bone turnover [12]. However, discrepancy exists in the results of studies to determine whether antithyroid treatment can completely normalize bone metabolism [13,14]. In those studies, the time of follow up varied considerably, the populations were heterogeneous with reference to etiology of hyper-

* Correspondence: aoyacobi@intramed.net
[1]Endocrinology Division, Hospital Ramos Mejía, Buenos Aires, Argentina
Full list of author information is available at the end of the article

thyroidism, osteoporosis risk factors and menopausal status.

Furthermore, it has recently been demonstrated that TSH affects bone metabolism through the TSH receptor found on osteoblast and osteoclast precursors in mice [15]. On the other hand, both higher serum TSH receptor antibodies (TRAb) and thyroid stimulating antibodies had a significant correlation with a reduction in BMD at the distal radius in male patients with untreated Graves'disease. In addition, higher TSAb significantly correlated with higher urinary N-terminal telopeptide of type I collagen [16].

Previous studies have suggested that the past history of Graves' disease itself, and not the current state of thyroid function, was responsible for bone loss in women receiving long-term levothyroxine therapy [17]. These results suggested some deleterious effects of TRAb and TSAb on bone metabolism, probably via TSH receptors on osteoblasts or osteoclasts.

The aim of our study was to determine BMD in pre and postmenopausal euthyroid female patients with previous overt hyperthyroidism due to Graves' disease as well as the factors that could affect BMD in each group, including TRAb.

Materials and methods
Subjects
One hundred and twenty-two patients with personal history of Graves' disease and euthyroidism attended consecutively in our endocrine Division between 2006 and 2008 were evaluated. Fifty seven patients who fulfilled the inclusion criteria were consecutively enrolled in this study after informed consent. The study was carried out in compliance with the Helsinki Declaration. Sixty five patients were excluded by previous bone fracture (n = 3); non-thyroidal illness (n = 16); intake of drugs that could influence bone metabolism (n = 18); incomplete follow up (n = 21); early menopause (n = 1) and refused to participate (n = 6).

Inclusion criteria were: personal history of Graves' disease and persistent euthyroidism for at least 6 months before entering the study. Exclusion criteria were: personal history of fracture prior to the beginning to the disease, non-thyroidal illness (liver disease, renal dysfunction, malignancy, diabetes mellitus, hyperparathyroidism, hypercortisolism, or hypogonadism) or intake of drugs (active vitamin D3, bisphosphonates, calcitonin, testosterones, steroids, diuretics, heparin, or anticonvulsants) that could influence bone metabolism and early menopause. All subjects underwent plain x-ray (antero-posterior and lateral views) of the lumbar spine, and those found to have scoliosis, compression fractures, or ectopic calcifications that could interfere with the bone mineral results were also excluded.

The diagnosis of Graves' disease had been established by the presence of symptoms and signs of hyperthyroidism, diffuse goitre, ophthalmopathy and/or positive TRAb, high serum concentrations of thyroxine (T4) and triiodothyronine (T3) and suppressed TSH. Ultimate treatment was achieved with antithyroid drugs in five patients and radioiodine in fifty-two patients. All patients had at least two T4 and TSH values within the normal range for at least 6 months prior to this study.

The patients were divided into two groups according to their menopausal status at the moment of the study (Premenopausal n = 30 and Postmenopausal n = 27) and were compared with 52 euthyroid controls mathed according to age, gender, and anthropometrical status (Premenopausal controls n = 36 and Postmenopausal controls n = 16). Menopause was defined as one year of amenorrhea and high levels of FSH.

All subjects completed a questionnaire administered by the physician or nurse and underwent laboratory blood tests. The questionnaire determined risk factors of osteoporosis, calcium intake and score of activity (0 = immobile, 1 = normal daily activity, 2 = programmed physical activity 2 times per week, 3 = programmed physical activity 3 times per week and 4 = programmed physical activity > three times per week.

Total time of hyperthyroidism was calculated as the sum of all the periods in which the patient had high levels of thyroid hormones and suppressed TSH (including relapses). Time of euthyroidism was considered since the moment the patient permanently normalized T4 and TSH levels postreatment until inclusion in the study. The total time of evolution of the disease includes the sum of both periods: hyperthyroidism and euthyroidism.

Biochemical measurements
Blood samples were drawn after an overnight fast in all the patients and matched controls of this study. The thyroid function variables: T4 and TSH were measured using commercially available kits (Solid phase competitive chemiluminescent enzyme inmumoasay-Immulite 2000, interassay coefficient of variation (CV): 10% and 5% respectively). TRAb was measured by radioreceptor assay [18] using a commercial kit (Radioreceptor assay; this method is based on the ability of TRAb to inhibit the binding of 125 I b-TSH to detergent-solubilized TSH-receptors from porcine thyroids cells. Results are expressed as the percentage of inhibition of 125I b-TSH binding, interassay CV: 10%). Control values were (mean +/– SD) 2.4+/–6.1% and results higher than 14.6% were considered positive [18-20]. Briefly, total calcium, phosphorus and creatinine were measured in serum using standard laboratory methods. Serum intact parathyroid hormone was measured by an Immulite 1000 with intra- and interassay CVs of 5.5% and 7.9%, respectively. Serum

total 25-hydroxyvitamin D (25OHD) was measured by a DiaSorin RIA with inter- and intra-assay CVs 12,8% and 8,4%, respectively.

BMD measurements

BMD measurements were performed at the Lumbar spine (L2-L4), hip and whole body by dual energy X-ray absorptiometry (DPX-L; Lunar, Madison, WI). Values of BMD were expressed as the mean in g/cm2 and Z-scores on the basis of normal reference values of an age and gender-matched group provided by the DXA system manufacturer. The same operator measured all the subjects. The phantom precision expressed as the CV (%) was 0.82.

Statistical analysis

Results are expressed as percentage, mean ± SD when data passed a normality test of Kolmogorov-Smirnov or median and range when they did not. Differences between groups were analyzed using the Student T-test (when the distribution was normal) or Mann–Whitney's U test for assessment of non-parametric median values. Correlation coefficients and multiple regression analyses were calculated. A p-value <0.05 was considered statistically significant. Statistical analysis was performed with the GraphPad Instat software program and SPSS 17.0. Advanced Calculus. Statistical Software. SPSS Inc, Chicago. 2008.

A post hoc study was applied in order to evaluate the power calculation with a 0.5 difference between the Z- score medians.

Results

The euthyroid patients with a history of hyperthyroidism due to Graves' disease did not differ in relation to their respective controls in demographic and anthropometric characteristics, osteoporosis risk factors nor in biochemical data (Table 1). The euthyroid patients with a history of hyperthyroidism due to Graves' disease evaluated in premenopause presented BMD similar to their respective controls in all the regions studied and postmenopausal women only presented a lower whole body BMD than controls (Table 1). Furthermore, both whole body and lumbar spine BMD Z-scores were significantly lower in postmenopausal compared to premenopausal women (Figure 1).

In order to investigate which variable could account for the smaller BMD expressed as Z-score in posmenopausal patients in relation to the premenopausal ones, both groups with previous hyperthyroidism due to Graves' disease were compared. No significant differences were found in osteoporosis risk factors nor in biochemical data of mineral metabolism. Calcium intake was higher in the postmenopausal than in the

premenopausal group (p < 0.003). The posmenopausal euthyroid Graves' disease patients presented the beginning of their disease at an older age, had a longer time of evolution of the disease, a longer time of euthyroidism and a higher percentage of patients with L-T4 treatment than the premenopausal group. No differences were found in the levels of T4, TSH, TRAb or the percentage of patients with persistently positive TRAb at the time of the study (Table 2). In the premenopausal group, no correlation was found between the Z-score of L2-L4 with time of evolution of the disease, time of euthyroidism, nor with TRAb at the moment of study. However, in the posmenopausal group, the Z-score of lumbar spine correlated negatively with TRAb (r = –0,53, p <0.008) and positively with time of evolution of the disease (r = +0.42, p < 0.032) and with time of euthyroidism (r = 0.50, p < 0.008) (Figures 2 and 3). On the other hand, TRAb correlated negatively with the time of evolution of the disease (r = –0.45, p <0.02) (Figure 4). There was no correlation between BMD and T4 or TSH (r = +0.14 and –0.19 respectively, p:.ns). In the multiple regression analysis using the Z-Score of BMD in L2-L4 as the dependent variable and TRAb, T4, TSH and time of evolution of the disease as independent variables, the TRAb was the only significant variable in relation to L2L4 BMD, accounting for 45.2% of the variation in L2L4 BMD (F = 3,90, p <0.01).

Discussion

Hyperthyroidism has been shown to accelerate bone turnover [11] and shorten the normal bone remodelling cycle [21]. Thus, active thyrotoxicosis resulted in a 12–15% reduction of BMD, predominantly in cortical bone [22]. Several small studies have been devised to assess the change in bone mass after treatment of hyperthyroidism. Although all of these studies have demonstrated improvement in bone density after restoration of the euthyroid state, the amount of improvement and the time frame evaluated varied considerably, the populations studied on the different surveys were heterogeneous with reference to etiology of hyperthyroidism, osteoporosis risk factors and menopausal status [23-27]. The long-term effects of treated thyrotoxicosis remain uncertain, but most studies suggest a persistent two to three-fold increased relative risk for hip fracture, mainly in postmenopausal women [28-32].

In the present study only women with previous Graves' disease hyperthyroidism were investigated, and they were analyzed in two groups according to the menopausal status at the time of evaluation. It was demonstrated that the population of premenopausal patients with a previous history of hyperthyroidism due to Graves' disease and long time of euthyroidism, showed no differences in BMD in relation to their matched controls; while postmenopausal patients at the time of

Table 1 Data of pre and post-menopausal patients with history of hyperthyroidism by Graves' disease

	GD-Pre-MP (n = 30)	C-Pre-MP (n = 36)	p	GD-Pos-MP (n = 27)	C-Pos-MP (n = 16)	p
Age (years)	38,8 ± 9,7	36,3 ± 10,6	ns	56,6 ± 5,5	54,8 ± 7,4	ns
Age of menarche (years)	12,7 ± 1,1	12,6 + 1,2	ns	12,9 + 0,6	12,8 + 0,9	ns
Age of menopausal (years)	-	-	ns	47,6 ± 4,6	47,5 ± 4,7	ns
BMI	25,2 ± 3,8	23,2 ± 4,2	ns	26,1 ± 4,5	28,6 ± 4,7	ns
Maternal hip fracture (%)	0	0	ns	0	0	ns
Fracture (%)	0	0	ns	1 (4)	0	ns
Tobacco (%)	3 (10)	4 (11)	ns	2 (7,4)	4 (25)	ns
Alcohol (%)	0	0	ns	0	0	ns
Physical activity	1,3 ± 0,6	1,1 ± 0,5	ns	1,3 + 0,7	1,2 ± 0,5	ns
Calcium intake (gr/day)	240 (23–1113)	416 (117–1277)	ns	795 (194–1562)	280 (51–886)	<0.003
Serum calcium (mg/dL)	9.4 ± 0.5	9.4 ± 0.4	ns	9.4 ± 0.4	9.4 ± 0.4	ns
Serum phosphorous (mg/dL)	3.4 ± 0.6	3.7 ± 0.6	ns	4.0 ± 0.5	4.0 ± 0.5	ns
Serum creatinine (mg/dL)	0.7 ± 0.1	0.8 ± 0.1	ns	0.7 + 0.1	0.8 + 0.1	ns
PTH (ug/mL)	59.8 ± 30.7	45.9 ± 15.8	ns	48.3 ± 17.9	62.8 ± 24.2	ns
25OHD (ng/mL)	26,7 ± 11,5	50,3 ± 20,5	ns	29,7 ± 17,2	37,1 ± 12,4	ns
BMD L2-L4 (gr/cm²)	1,19 ± 0,15	1,17 ± 0,12	ns	1,001 ± 0,17	1,06 ± 0,13	ns
BMD L2-L4 (z-score)	0,11 ± 1,19	0,04 ± −1,0	ns	−0,43 ± 1,17	−0,51 ± 0,83	ns
BMD FN (gr/cm²)	0,96 ± 0,10	0,95 ± 0,12	ns	0,852 ± 0,14	0,84 ± 0,13	ns
BMD FN (z-score)	0,11 ± 0,8	0,00 ± 0,89	ns	−0,04 ± 0,87	−0,53 ± 0,81	ns
BMD W-B (gr/cm²)	1,13 ± 0,08	1,15 ± 0,06	ns	0,99 ± 0,14	1,12 ± 0,10	<0,003
BMD W-B (z-score)	0,24 ± 0,91	0,61 ± 0,74	ns	−0,79 + 1,03	0,40 ± 0,90	<0,0007

Data are presented as means ± SD, median or percentages. The power calculation with a 0.5 difference between the Z- score medians for Lumbar spine (L2-L4), femoral neck (FN) and whole body (W-B) were between 0.32 and 0.58. GD-Pre-MP Premenopausal Graves Disease, GD-Post-MP Postmenopausal Graves Disease, C-Pre-MP Premenopausal controls, C-Pos-MP Post-menopausal controls.

evaluation presented a lower whole body BMD in relation to their matched controls. Whole body BMD represents predominantly cortical bone, and it is known that thyroid hormone excess causes mainly cortical bone loss [22]. This was in keeping with results obtained in hyperthyroid patients of non-autoimmune origin such as multinodular goitre [33]. Since only three patients were

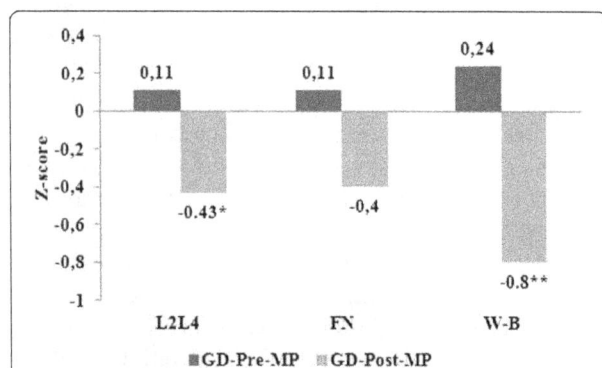

Figure 1 Bone mineral density expressed as Z-score in W-B, FN and L2-L4 in premenopausal (n = 30) vs postmenopausal patients (n = 27) with a history of hyperthyroidism due to Graves' disease. *: p < 0,005, **: p < 0,0002. W-B: whole body; FN: femoral neck; L2-L4: lumbar spine; Pre-MP: premenopausal; Post-MP: postmenopausal.

excluded for prior fractures, it is improvable that exclusion of patients with more severe bone disease may have resulted in a bias of this study.

When comparing the euthyroid postmenopausal to euthyroid premenopausal Graves' disease patients, not only did they have a lower whole body BMD Z-score but also a lower lumbar spine BMD Z-score.. The BMD difference between pre- and postmenopausal patients at the time of evaluation with a previous history of hyperthyroidism due to Graves' disease is remarkable. This difference cannot be due to posmenopausal status per se, since it was avoided using Z score (on the basis of normal reference values of an age- and gender-matched group provided by the DXA system manufacturer), or to the duration of hyperthyroidism which was similar in both groups, or to the time of euthyroidism which was even longer in the posmenopausal group. T4, TSH and TRAb values were similar at the time of evaluation in both groups. Despite the fact that the inclusion criteria of persistent euthyroidism for 6 months or more before entering the study may have introduced a bias due to the short time interval for re-establishing normal BMD-levels, medium time of persistent euthyroidism was 70.6 and 146.8 months for pre and posmenopausal respectively.

Negative correlation between bone mineral density and TSH receptor antibodies in long-term euthyroid...

41

Table 2 Graves' disease characteristics in euthyroid premenopausal vs postmenopausal patients

	G-Pre-MP (n = 30)	G-Pos-MP (n = 27)	p
Age of beginning of the disease (years)	30.0 ± 7.7	40.9 ± 11.0	0,0007
Time of hyperthyroidism (months)	38,5 ± 44,9	53,7 ± 88,0	ns
Time of euthyroidism (months)	70,6 ± 68,2	146,8 ± 126,9	0,007
Time of evolution of disease (months)	98,8 ± 80,5	198,9 ± 130,0	0,002
Euthyroid patients with T4 (%)	60	93	0,003
T4 (ug/dL)	9,2 ± 2,2	9,8 ± 1,8	ns
TSH (uUI/mL)	1,4 ± 1,4	1,6 ± 1.3	ns
TRAb (%)	22,4 ± 19,0	21,5 ± 21,7	ns
PositiveTRAb patients (%)	45	34	ns

Data are presented as means ± SD, median or percentages. *GD-Pre-MP* Premenopausal Graves Disease, *GD-Post-MP* Postmenopausal Graves Disease.

The main difference between these groups was the ten-year later onset of hyperthyroidism in the postmenopausal group compared to the premenopausal group at the moment of the evaluation, the former starting during their perimenopause. This would reaffirm that the beginning of hyperthyroidism during this period of great vulnerability of bone mass [34] has a more deleterious effect on bone or does not allow a complete recovery of BMD.

This study shows that postmenopausal patients at the time of evaluation with a previous history of perimenopausal hyperthyroidism due Graves' disease, despite a long time of euthyroidism, had a lower bone mass than matched controls. In contrast, those patients studied in premenopause with a previous history of hyperthyroidism due Graves' disease did not show any difference from matched controls.

In the correlation analyses, only the postmenopausal population showed an inverse correlation between L2-L4 Z-score and the level of TRAb as well as a positive correlation with the time of evolution of the disease and time of euthyroidism. On the other hand, as expected, TRAb and time of evolution of the disease showed a negative correlation. So with longer time of evolution of

the disease, lower TRAb levels and better BMD were seen. TRAb was the only significant variable in relation to lumbar spine BMD in the multiple regression analysis. This result suggested a deleterious effect of TRAb on bone metabolism. To our knowledge, only a few studies conducted to date have suggested an effect of TRAb on BMD in patients with Graves' disease [16,35]. To our knowledge, no similar analyses were performed in women with a history of toxic multinodular goitre, i.e. subjects negative for TRAb.

A recent study on TSH receptor in null mice found evidence for direct effects of TSH on osteoblastic bone formation and osteoclastic bone resorption, mediated by the receptor on osteoblast and osteoclast precursors. These animals were found to be osteoporotic despite thyroid extract replacement therapy, linking directly the bone phenotype to the lack of action of TSH on bone [15]. Consequently, the authors suggested that the skeletal loss occurring in hyperthyroidism was due to the low TSH rather than thyroid hormone excess. In this way, the receptor antibodies could play a direct role on BMD by a similar mechanism to TSH, but the present results seem to be opposite to those reported about effect of TSH on bone turnover. This difference could be

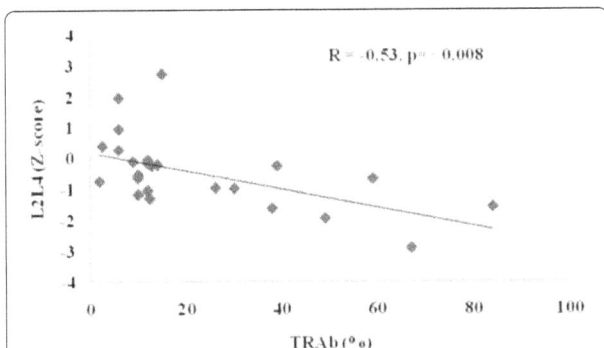

Figure 2 Negative correlation between bone mineral density Z-score of L2-L4 and TRAb in postmenopausal patients with Graves' disease (n = 27). (R = −0, 3, p < 0,008).

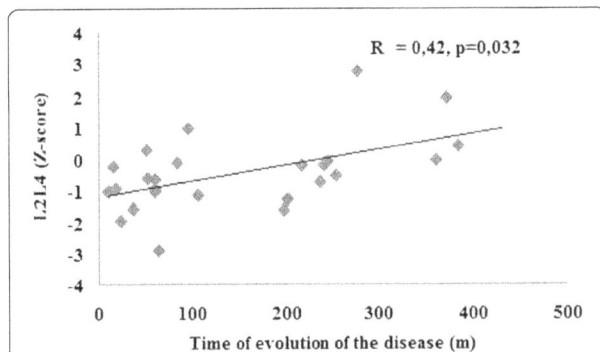

Figure 3 Positive correlation between L2-L4- Z score and time of evolution of the disease (months) in postmenopausal patients with Graves' disease (n = 27). (R = 0, 42, p < 0,032).

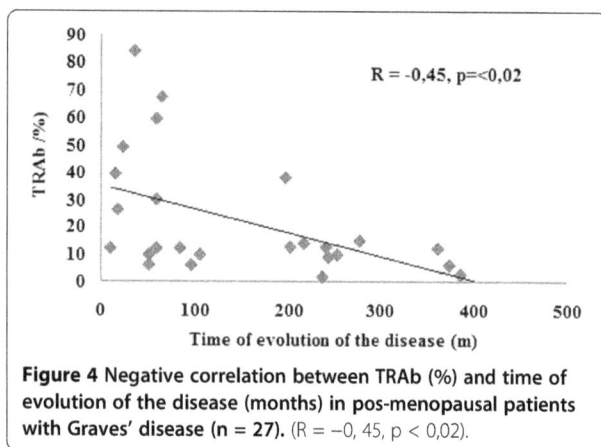

Figure 4 Negative correlation between TRAb (%) and time of evolution of the disease (months) in pos-menopausal patients with Graves' disease (n = 27). (R = −0, 45, p < 0,02).

explained by different sites of action for TSH and antibodies on the TSH receptor [36]; switches in the pool of antibodies with predominance of blocking antibodies that would not allow TSH action, which cannot be discriminated with the TRAb assay performed in this study [37] or regulation of the TSH receptor by stimulating TSH autoantibodies [38]. In relation to TRAb on DMO, the study by Majima et al. [16] is in line with our results. They found that both higher serum TSH receptor antibodies (TRAb) and thyroid stimulating antibodies (TSAb) had a significant correlation with a reduction in BMD at the distal radius in male patients with untreated Graves' disease. In addition, higher TSAb significantly correlated with higher urinary N-terminal telopeptide of type I collagen. On the other hand, Belsing et al. [39] showed that the best predictors for BMD were a negative association with free T4 and a positive one with TRAb. However, they included only premenopausal women and the follow-up was shorter than in this study.

More recently, Morimura et al. [40] showed that TSH positively regulated intracellular T3 production by controlling type 2 iodothyronine deiodinase in human osteoblasts. It is, therefore, tempting to hypothesize that TSH receptor antibodies might overproduce intracellular T3 to decrease bone mass by accelerating bone turnover.

Previous studies have suggested that the past history of Graves' disease itself, not the current state of thyroid function, is responsible for bone loss in women receiving long-term levothyroxine therapy [17] indicating some autoimmune effects of TRAb on bone metabolism. It is known that normalization of the autoimmune abnormality comes much later than euthyroidism and the disappearance of TRAb in serum came gradually over a considerable period of time [41]. A decreased fracture risk in patients with hyperthyroidism treated with surgery and an increased fracture risk in patients treated with radioiodine [31,42] could also support this hypothesis of TRAb being involved in bone metabolism, considering that surgical treatment of Graves' disease was associated with less pronounced or shorter elevation of TRAb, whereas radioiodine treatment was associated with a higher elevation [41].

It is not clear why the estrogen status influences thyroid hormones and TSH effects on bone mass. Both T3 and estradiol are essential for normal bone turnover in vivo, as demonstrated by the skeletal phenotypes of aromatase-deficient mice, human aromatase deficiency and postmenopausal women [43]. One recent study showed that acute TSH administration in postmenopausal women resulted in an increase of serum N-terminal propeptide of type-I procollagen, an index of osteoblastic activity, associated with an increase of serum RANKL. Lack of this response in premenopausal women suggested an influence of estrogen status on bone reactivity to TSH [44].

In our cross-sectional study, postmenopausal patients with history of Graves' disease hyperthyroidism, with normal TSH and T4 and longstanding euthyroidism, TRAb exhibited a significant negative correlation with the Z-score of lumbar spine, suggesting that TRAb might affect bone metabolism in these patients.

The present study has several limitations, such as the small number of patients, the lack of BMD at the distal radius measurement and the fact that there were no data about bone status prior to the beginning of the disease, but patients with other causes of BMD loss were excluded. The radioreceptor assay used to assess TRAb concentrations in this study, based on inhibition of binding of ^{125}I, could reflect stimulating as well as blocking activities. Assays that detect cAMP production could be useful to discriminate the antibodies activity [45,46].

The strengths include that it is the first study in Graves' disease patients with longstanding euthyroidism, which has analyzed homogeneous subpopulations in menopausal status and osteoporosis risk factors. These results show, in relation to respective matched controls, a normal BMD in premenopausal patients with previous hyperthyroidism, but a diminished BMD in postmenopausal patients with a previous history of perimenopausal hyperthyroidism due to Graves' disease, despite a long time of euthyroidism. They also show, in the last group of patients, an association between TRAb and BMD regardless of hyperthyroidism. We consider that these results suggest that the past history of Graves' disease itself, and not the current state of thyroid function, could be responsible for bone loss in postmenopausal women.

This study does not show a direct causal relationship nor does it elucidate the mechanisms by which serum TRAb could affect bone measurements. Further studies will be needed to understand the differential actions of thyroid hormones, TSH and TRAb on osteoblasts and osteoclasts and their relationship with estrogens.

Competing interests
The authors declare that they have no competing interests.

Authors' contributions
MAE, MLD, MCSC and ATG contributed to conception and design, acquisition of data, analysis and interpretation of data; has been involved in drafting the manuscript and revising it critically for important intellectual content; and has given final approval of the version to be published. AMF MM and FV contributed to acquisition of data, analysis and interpretation of data; has been involved in drafting the manuscript and revising it critically for important intellectual content; and has given final approval of the version to be published. UF-R has contributed analysis and interpretation of data; has been involved in drafting the manuscript and revising it critically for important intellectual content; and has given final approval of the version to be published. All authors read and approved the final manuscript.

Acknowledgments
We thank J. Laguna, our Densitometry Technique.

Author details
[1]Endocrinology Division, Hospital Ramos Mejía, Buenos Aires, Argentina. [2]Department of Medical Endocrinology, Rigshospitalet, Copenhagen University, Copenhagen, Denmark.

References
1. Rizzoli R, Poser J, Bürgi U: Nuclear thyroid hormone receptors in cultured bone cells. *Metabolism* 1986, 35:71–74.
2. Coindre JM, David JP, Rivie'Re L, Goussot JF, Roger P, De Mascarel A, Meunier PJ: Bone loss in hyperthyroidism with hormone replacement. *Arch Intern Med* 1986, 146:48–53.
3. Britto JM, Fenton AJ, Holloway WR, Nicolson GC: Osteoblasts mediate thyroid hormone stimulation of osteoclastic bone resorption. *Endocrinology* 1994, 134:169–176.
4. Campos-Pastor MM, Munoz-Torres M, Escobar-Jimenez F, Ruiz De Almodovar M, Jodar Gimeno E: Bone mass in females with different thyroid disorders: influence of menopausal status. *Bone Miner* 1993, 21:1–82.
5. Diamond T, Vine J, Smart R, Butler P: Thyrotoxic bone disease in women: a potentially reversible disorder. *Ann Intern Med* 1994, 120:8–11.
6. Gomez Acotto C, Schott AM, Hans D, Niepomniszcze H, Mautalen CA, Meunier PJ: Hyperthyroidism influences ultrasound bone measurement on the Os calcis. *Osteoporos Int* 1998, 8:455–459.
7. Olkawa M, Kushida K, Takahashi M, Ohishi T, Hoshino H, Suzuki M, Ogihara H, Ishigaki J, Inoue T: Bone turnover and cortical bone mineral density in the distal radius in patients with hyperthyroidism being treated with antithyroid drugs for various periods of time. *Clin Endocrinol (Oxf)* 1999, 50:171–176.
8. Mora S, Pitukcheewanont P, Kaufman FR, Nelson JC, Gilsanz V: Biochemical markers of bone turnover and the volume and the density of bone in children at different stages of sexual development. *J Bone Miner Res* 1999, 14:1664–1671.
9. Ben-Shlomo A, Hagag P, Evans S, Weiss M: Early postmenopausal bone loss in hyperthyroidism. *Maturitas* 2001, 39:19–27.
10. Karga H, Papapetrou PD, Korakovouni A, Papandroulaki F, Polymeris A, Pampouras G: Bone mineral density in hyperthyroidism. *Clin Endocrinol (Oxf)* 2004, 1:466–472.
11. Mosekilde L, Eriksen EF, Charles P: Effects of thyroid hormones on bone and mineral metabolism. *Endocrinol Metab Clin North Am* 1990, 19:35–63.
12. Jódar E, Muñoz-Torres M, Escobar-Jiménez F, Quesada M, Luna JD, Olea N: Antiresorptive therapy in hyperthyroid patients: longitudinal changes in bone and mineral metabolism. *J Clin Endocrinol Metab* 1997, 82:1989–1994.
13. Langdahl BL, Loft AGR, Eriksen EF, Mosekilde L, Charles P: Bone mass, bone turnover, body composition, and calcium homeostasis in former hyperthyroid patients treated by combined medical therapy. *Thyroid* 1996, 6:161–168.
14. Mudde AH, Houben AJ, Nieuwenhuijzen Kruseman AC: Bone metabolism during anti-thyroid drug treatment of endogenous subclinical hyperthyroidism. *Clin Endocrinol (Oxf)* 1994, 41:421–424.
15. Abe E, Marians RC, Yu W, Wu XB, Ando T, Li Y, Iqbal J, Eldeiry L, Rajendren G, Blair HC, Davies TF, Zaidi M: TSH is a negative regulator of skeletal remodeling. *Cell* 2003, 115:151–162.
16. Majima T, Komatsu Y, Doi K, Takagi C, Shigemoto M, Fukao A, Morimoto T, Corners J, Nakao K: Negative correlation between bone mineral density and TSH receptor antibodies in male patients with untreated Graves' disease. *Osteoporos Int* 2006, 7:1103–1110.
17. Greenspan SL, Greenspan FS, Resnick NM, Block JE, Friedlander AL, Genant HK: Skeletal integrity in premenopausal and postmenopausal women receiving longterm L-thyroxine therapy. *Am J Med* 1991, 91:5–14.
18. Rees Smith B, McLachlan SM, Furmaniak J: Autoantibodies to the thyrotropin receptor. *Endocr Rev* 1988, 9(1):106–121.
19. Takasu N, Oshiro C, Akamine H, Komiya I, Nagata A, Sato Y, Yoshimura H, Ito K: Thyroid-stimulating antibody and TSH-binding inhibitor immunoglobulin in 277 Graves' patients and in 686 normal subjects. *J Endocrinol Invest* 1997, 20(8):452–461.
20. Gauna AT, Guillén CE, Sartorio GC, Soto RJ: Graves' disease: evolution and prognosis after eight months of treatment with methimazole. *Medicina (B Aires)* 1992, 52(3):207–212.
21. Eriksen EF: Normal and pathological remodeling of human trabecular bone: three dimensional reconstruction of the remodeling sequence in normals and in metabolic bone disease. *Endocr Rev* 1986, 7:379–408.
22. Ross DS: Hyperthyroidism, thyroid hormone therapy, and bone. *Thyroid* 1994, 4:319–326.
23. Udayakumar N, Chandrasekaran M, Rasheed MH, Suresh RV, Sivaprakash S: Evaluation of bone mineral density in thyrotoxicosis. *Singapore Med J* 2006, 47(11):947–950.
24. Nagasaka S, Sugimoto H, Nakamura T, Kusaka I, Fujisawa G, Sakuma N, Tsuboi Y, Fukuda S, Honda K, Okada K, Ishikawa S, Saito T: Antithyroid therapy improves bony manifestations and bone metabolic markers in patients with Graves' thyrotoxicosis. *Clin Endocrinol (Oxf)* 1997, 47(2):215–221.
25. Grant DJ, McMurdo ME, Mole PA, Paterson CR: Is previous hyperthyroidism still a risk factor for osteoporosis in post-menopausal women? *Clin Endocrinol (Oxf)* 1995, 43(3):339–345.
26. Krølner B, Jørgensen JV, Nielsen SP: Spinal bone mineral content in myxoedema and thyrotoxicosis. effects of thyroid hormone(s) and antithyroid treatment. *Clin Endocrinol (Oxf)* 1983, 18(5):439–446.
27. Rosen CJ, Adler RA: Longitudinal changes in lumbar bone density among thyrotoxic patients after attainment of euthyroidism. *J Clin Endocrinol Metab* 1992, 75(6):1531–1534.
28. Cummings SR, Nevitt MC, Browner WS, Stone K, Fox KM, Ensrud KE, Cauley J, Black D, Vogt TM: Risk factors for hip fracture in white women. study of osteoporotic fractures research group. *N Engl J Med* 1995, 23(12):767–773.
29. Wejda B, Hintze G, Katschinski B, Olbricht T, Benker G: Hip fractures and the thyroid: a case–control study. *J Intern Med* 1995, 237(3):241–247.
30. Vestergaard P, Rejnmark L, Weeke J, Mosekilde L: Fracture risk in patients treated for hyperthyroidism. *Thyroid* 2000, 10(4):341–348.
31. Vestergaard P, Mosekilde L: Fractures in patients with hyperthyroidism and hypothyroidism: a nationwide follow-up study in 16,249 patients. *Thyroid* 2002, 12(5):411–419.
32. Solomon BL, Wartofsky L, Burman KD: Prevalence of fractures in postmenopausal women with thyroid disease. *Thyroid* 1993, 3(1):17–23.
33. Faber J, Jensen IW, Petersen L, Nygaard B, Hegedüs L, Siersbaek-Nielsen K: Normalization of serum thyrotrophin by means of radioiodine treatment in subclinical hyperthyroidism: effect on bone loss in postmenopausal women. *Clin Endocrinol (Oxf)* 1998, 48(3):285–290.
34. Finkelstein JS, Brockwell SE, Mehta V, Greendale GA, Sowers MR, Ettinger B, Lo JC, Johnston JM, Cauley JA, Danielson ME, Neer RM: Bone mineral density changes during the menopause transition in a multiethnic cohort of women. *J Clin Endocrinol Metab* 2008, 93(3):861–868.
35. Kumeda Y, Inaba M, Tahara H, Kurioka Y, Ishikawa T, Morii H, Nishizawa Y: Persistent increase in bone turnover in Graves' patients with subclinical hyperthyroidism. *J Clin Endocrinol Metab* 2000, 85(11):4157–4161.
36. Mizutori Y, Chen CR, Latrofa F, McLachlan SM, Rapoport B: Evidence that shed thyrotropin receptor A subunits drive affinity maturation of autoantibodies causing Graves' disease. *J Clin Endocrinol Metab* 2009, 94(3):927–935.
37. Weetman AP, McGregor AM: Autoimmune thyroid disease: further developments in our understanding. *Endocr Rev* 1994, 15:788–830.
38. Ando T, Latif R, Davies TF: Concentration-dependent regulation of thyrotropin receptor function by thyroid-stimulating antibody. *J Clin Inv* 2004, 113(11):189–195.
39. Belsing TZ, Tofteng C, Langdahl BL, Charles P, Feldt-Rasmussen U: Can bone loss be reversed by antithyroid drug therapy in premenopausal women with Graves' disease? *Nutr Metab (Lond)* 2010, 1(7):72–81.

40. Morimura T, Tsunekawa K, Kasahara T, Seki K, Ogiwara T, Mori M, Murakami M: **Expression of type 2 iodothyronine deiodinase in human osteoblast is stimulated by thyrotropin.** *Endocrinology* 2005, **146**(4):2077–2084.

41. Torring O, Tallstedt L, Wallin G, Lundell G, Ljunggren JG, Taube A, Saaf M, Hamberger B: **Graves' hyperthyroidism: treatment with antithyroid drugs, surgery, or radioiodine–a prospective, randomized study. thyroid study group.** *J Clin Endocrinol Metab* 1996, **81**:2986–2993.

42. Laurberg P, Wallin G, Tallstedt L, Abraham-Nordling M, Lundell G, Tørring O: **TSH-receptor autoimmunity in Grave' disease after therapy with antithyroid drugs, surgery, or radioiodine: a 5-year prospective randomized study.** *Eur J Endocrinol* 2008, **158**(1):69–75.

43. Duncan Bassett JH, Williams GR: **The molecular actions of thyroid hormone in bone.** *TRENDS Endocrinol Metab* 2003, **14**(8):356–364.

44. Martini G, Gennari L, De Paola V, Pilli T, Salvadori S, Merlotti D, Valleggi F, Stella C, Franci B, Nuti AA, Pacini F: **The effects of recombinant TSH on bone turnover markers and serum osteoprotegerin and RANKL levels.** *Thyroid* 2008, **18**(4):455–460.

45. Takasu N, Matsushita M: **Changes of TSH-stimulation blocking antibody (TSBAb) and thyroid stimulating antibody (TSAb) over 10 years in 34 TSBAb-positive patients with hypothyroidism and in 98 TSAb-positive Graves' patients with hyperthyroidism: reevaluation of TSBAb and TSAb in TSH-receptor-antibody (TRAb)-positive patients.** *J Thyroid Res* 2012, **2012**:1–11.

46. Barbesino G, Tomer Y: **Clinical review: clinical utility of TSH receptor antibodies.** *J Clin Endocrinol Metab* 2013, **98**(6):2247–2255.

5

The use of semi-quantitative ultrasound elastosonography in combination with conventional ultrasonography and contrast-enhanced ultrasonography in the assessment of malignancy risk of thyroid nodules with indeterminate cytology

Massimo Giusti[1,4]*, Claudia Campomenosi[1], Stefano Gay[1], Barbara Massa[2], Enzo Silvestri[3], Eleonora Monti[1] and Giovanni Turtulici[3]

Abstract

Background: The pre-surgical selection of thyroid nodules with indeterminate cytology (Thy 3 according to British Thyroid Association) after fine-needle aspiration biopsy (FNAB) is currently required in order to reduce unnecessary total thyroidectomy. The objective of our study was to use a surgical series of Thy 3 nodules to evaluate the predictive role of ultrasound elastosonography (USE) and contrast-enhanced ultrasonography (CEUS) in pre-surgical diagnoses of malignancy.

Subjects and methods: We enrolled 63 patients with Thy 3 nodules in which cytological–histological correlation was available. The ELX 2/1 strain index was obtained by means of semi-quantitative USE, which was performed before surgery in addition to conventional ultrasonography (US) and contrast-enhanced US (CEUS) on the Thy 3 nodules. The ELX 2/1 strain index, a five-item US score and both peak (P) index and time to peak (TTP) index from CEUS were correlated with the histological results. After surgical diagnosis, the data were analysed by using a receiver-operating characteristic (ROC) curve.

Results: Histology was benign in 50 and malignant in 13 Thy 3 nodules. No difference in maximal diameter was noted between benign (22.8 ± 1.6 mm) and malignant (18.9 ± 2.9 mm) nodules. Significant correlations were found between histology and cumulative US findings ($p=0.005$), ELX 2/1 index ($p=0.002$), P index ($p=0.01$) and TTP index ($p=0.02$). On analysing data from US, USE and CEUS, significant ROC areas under the curve were observed ($p<0.0001$). A cut-off value was set for US (>2), ELX 2/1 (>0.95), P index (<0.99) and TTP index (>0.98) scores. The diagnostic power of the cumulative pre-surgical analysis of Thy 3 nodules with US, USE and CEUS, considering the experimental cut-off points obtained from the ROC curves was: sensitivity 64%, specificity 92%, PPV 75% and accuracy 84%.

(Continued on next page)

* Correspondence: magius@unige.it
[1]Endocrine Unit, IRCCS Azienda Ospedaliera Universitaria San Martino – IST Istituto Nazionale per la Ricerca sul Cancro, Genoa, Italy
[4]UO Clinica Endocrinologica, Viale Benedetto XV, 6, I-16100 Genoa, Italy
Full list of author information is available at the end of the article

(Continued from previous page)

Conclusion: The ELX 2/1 index in conjunction with the US score can be useful in orienting surgical strategies in Thy 3 nodules. The information added by CEUS is less sensitive than that provided by US and USE. The use of a cut-off based on histology can reduce thyroidectomy. Observation should be the first choice when not all instrumental results are suspect.

Keywords: Thyroid nodules, Indeterminate cytology, Ultrasosonography, Ultrasound elastosonography, Strain index, Contrast-enhanced ultrasonography, Cytological–histological correlation, ROC analysis

Introduction

The prevalence of diagnoses of thyroid nodules often varies according to the method of examination used [1-3]. The current thyroid nodule and thyroid cancer epidemic can be explained by the worldwide diffusion of ultrasonography (US) equipment [4,5]. When a nodule is found, the most important clinical problem is to exclude malignancy, which accounts for approximately 5%-15% of all thyroid nodules [6-8]. A combination of clinical factors (age, sex, exposure to radiation, familial traits) and US features determines whether or not the clinician should proceed with further tests or observation. The accuracy of US in predicting thyroid cancer has recently been reviewed by Brito et al. [9]. Only two US findings – spongiform and cystic thyroid nodule features – seem to provide sufficient probability to help rule out cancer and to suggest observation at first, while all other US findings, when assessed individually, might not be able to rule in or rule out malignancy, owing to their modest likelihood ratio [9]. Therefore, in order to distinguish malignant from benign thyroid nodules, cytological investigation by means of fine-needle aspiration biopsy (FNAB) must be performed under US guidance in nodules larger than 10 mm or with suspicious US findings [10-13]. Thyroid cytology is usually reported both descriptively and as suggested categories with different risks of malignancy. Both the Bethesda system and the British Thyroid Association (BTA) category (Thy 1 – Thy 5) are used. The ultimate aim of FNAB is to reassure the patient and to avoid surgery if not otherwise indicated [13]. FNAB yields useful cytological results in about 80% of cases, but has several weaknesses, including false negative (about 1-2%), non-diagnostic (3-16%) and indeterminate (follicular lesions; 6-20%) results [13-16]. The low risk of underestimating a thyroid cancer supports the recommendation for repeat thyroid nodule evaluation 2–4 years after initial benign (Thy 2) FNAB [16], while the very high probability (77-100%) [17-21] of cancer in nodules "suspicious for malignancy" (Thy 4) obliges surgery, as in the case of findings that are "diagnostic of malignancy" (Thy 5). Core-needle biopsy seems more useful than FNAB repetition in reducing non-diagnostic (Thy 1) cytology [22], but its utility in cases of indeterminate cytology after FNAB is still debated [22,23]. As indeterminate

lesions (Thy 3) are associated with an approximately 25% risk of malignancy [12,17,19,24-27], histological examination is still required by the current guidelines of thyroid societies. Rago et al. [27] recently reported an overall good prognosis in Thy 3 lesions with malignant histology, which suggests the possibility that more exhaustive pre-surgical evaluation might reduce unnecessary (about 70% of cases) surgery. In this context, the role of US in distinguishing malignant from benign Thy 3 nodules is still uncertain, though in the large series of Thy 3 nodules examined in Rago's study, blurred nodule margins and spots of microcalcification were significantly associated with malignancy.

The introduction of novel diagnostic tools may provide a more reliable approach to assessing the risk of malignancy in Thy 3 nodules. Recently, the determination of somatic mutation in FNAB specimens from Thy 3 nodules has been proposed [17,28,29], and may also help in deciding the extent of surgery [30]. However, the role of molecular screening could be overestimated, as this technique increases FNAB sensitivity from 67% to only 75% in indeterminate lesions [31]. On the other hand, a search for several gene expressions conducted in 326 nodules with indeterminate cytology has demonstrated the substantial impact of this approach on clinical care recommendations, though site-to-site variation exists [32] and this evaluation is not yet universally available.

US elastography (USE) and contrast-enhanced US (CEUS) are another two innovative techniques under evaluation for the detection of malignancy in thyroid nodules, but they still need validation. USE has been likened to "electronic palpation" and provides reproducible stiffness measurements even in otherwise non-palpable thyroid lesions [33]. At present, heterogeneity among different USE technologies (difference in compression source, modality of processing, stiffness expression), equipment and applications explains why USE is not yet part of routine nodule management [19,33]. USE should primary be implemented in the pre-surgical differential diagnosis between benign and malignant nodules; however, its accuracy is debated and surgery has not always been taken as the reference in evaluating USE data [17-21,25]. In addition, a certain risk of false negative results has been reported, especially in cases of follicular [34,35] or medullary thyroid cancer [36]. CEUS is a dynamic evaluation which enables thyroid nodules to be characterized by studying vascular enhancement patterns, which it does better than conventional US. Some authors have reported that the absence of ring enhancement and the presence of heterogeneous enhancement [37-39] or a shorter time to peak of the perfusion curve [40] could characterize malignant nodules. However, these data are still controversial [19,41].

The pre-surgical diagnostic role of USE [17-19,21,25,42,43] and CEUS [19,37] in nodules with indeterminate cytology has been considered uncertain because of the low number of these nodules in the series analyzed. Two recently published studies have focused on USE in indeterminate nodules. In 169 patients in whom histology was available after qualitative USE, Rago et al. [27] reported that high elasticity is closely associated with benign histology, with a negative predictive value of 97%. In addition, in a series of 270 nodules with atypia of indeterminate significance evaluated by means of semi-quantitative USE, Cakir et al. [44] reported a higher median strain index in the malignant group than in the benign group. To our knowledge, no data are available in the literature on large series of Thy 3 nodules evaluated by CEUS in order to judge the pre-surgical role of this technique.

The aim of the present study was to retrospectively evaluate the pre-surgical role of both USE and CEUS together with US findings in our series of patients with indeterminate cytology and known histology. The construction of a validate cut-off for numerical indices could be used to avoid surgical procedures in Thy 3 patients in whom all tests (US, USE, CEUS) yield "benign" results. The cost and time consumption of these techniques could be lower than those of unnecessary thyroid surgery.

Materials and methods
Patients
This prospective study enrolled 78 consecutive patients (60 female, 18 male; age: 20–82 yrs; mean ± SD: 55.4 ± 14.7 yrs) with thyroid nodules observed at the out-patient Thyroid Cancer Unit. On FNAB, performed as previously reported [19], all patients had an indeterminate thyroid lesion (Thy 3) according to the 2009 BTA classification. These patients were considered candidates for surgery in accordance with the cytological result. In 47% of these patients, the Thy 3 nodule was found in a multinodular goitre, while 53% had a uninodular goiter. In 8 patients, laboratory data were compatible with Hashimoto's thyroiditis, while one patient had a single Thy 3 nodule in a diffuse toxic goiter. Levothyroxine was being taken by 20% of patients, either for hypothyroidism (n=3) or as a TSH-reducing therapy (n=13). Three patients were on methimazole therapy for pre-toxic goiter. All patients underwent laboratory evaluations. TSH and free-T4 (f-T4)

were measured by means of ultra-sensitive chemiluminescence immunoassay (Roche Diagnostics, Mannheim, Germany). Normal ranges are: 0.3-4.2 mIU/l for TSH and 12.0-22.0 pmol/l for f-T4. Thyroperoxidase antibodies (TPOAb) were evaluated by means of the Dia Sorin assay (Saluggia, Italy); concentrations <100 mIU/l were regarded as negative. Serum calcitonin (CT) was assayed by chemiluminescence immunoassay (Dia Sorin); in our laboratory, the upper limit of the normal CT range is 10 ng/l. All patients were invited to undergo further sonographic evaluation. All patients gave their informed consent to participate in the study. The collection of patient's data and subsequent analysis was performed in compliance with the Helsinki declaration and was approved by University of Genoa Ethical Committee.

Thyroid US, USE and CEUS
All patients were examined in the supine position with the neck extended. Scans of both thyroid lobes and isthmus were obtained in both transverse and longitudinal planes. The Thy 3 nodules were examined by means of conventional high-resolution US with a colour-Doppler module (MyLab40, Esaote Biomedica, Genoa) equipped with a 7.5 MHz linear probe. In 23 subjects, a further FNAB was performed with the aid of this equipment. As previously reported [19] and in accordance with US guidelines [45], the following parameters were investigated: echogenicity vs. non-nodular tissue, presence or absence of halo sign, presence or absence of microcalcifications, and flow pattern of the nodule. All USE examinations were performed by the same operator (GT) by means of a MyLab 70 XvG US scanner (Esaote Biomedica) equipped with an LA-522 linear probe working in the range of 7–12 MHz and software for the quantification of the USE features of the tissue. Static and moving images were recorded, as already reported by Lyshchik et al. [34], at least 3 times in order to obtain mean values. The elasticity score (ELX 2/1) index was calculated at the same depth as the ratio between the elasticity feature of the selected region-of-interest (ROI) located on US-normal thyroid tissue and the ROI of the nodule under investigation. As previously reported [19], we considered the ELX 2/1 index directly reported on the screen of the equipment, as this is a less operator-dependent variable than the elasticity colour-scale extrapolated from breast tissue to the thyroid gland by some authors [18,25,35,46]. CEUS images were acquired by the MyLab 70 US scanner, as previously reported [19], by using a non-destructive US mode after bolus injection of SonoVue (4.8 ml; Bracco, Milan). CEUS video-clips were digitally recorded and analysed by means of Q-Contrast software V.4.0. (Bracco). Time-intensity curves within selected ROI and colour maps were acquired. Nodule and healthy thyroid tissue values of peak

contrast enhancement (Peak) and time to peak (TTP) were calculated. Peak and TTP are reported as indexes (Peak index, TTP index) derived from the ratio between the values from the ROI of the nodule and the ROI of normal thyroid tissue [19].

Statistical analysis

Non-parametric tests were used to compare averages; the correlation coefficient r was calculated by means of Spearman correlation (Sr) (GraphPad 6.0 Software, San Diego, CA, USA). Data are reported as mean ± standard error of mean (SEM) if not otherwise reported. Significance was set at $p \leq 0.05$. A US score (from 0 to 5) was arbitrarily calculated for the nodule under evaluation, with one point being assigned for the presence of each of the following radiological findings: solid, hypo-echoic, microcalcification, internal vascularisation, and irregular shape [19]. All cytological and histology diagnoses were made by a pathologist (BM) with 10 years' experience in the pathologic analysis of thyroid cancer. After surgery, Thy 3 lesions were classified as malignant or benign. The diagnostic value of the ELX 2/1 index from USE or the P index and TTP index from CEUS in distinguishing between benign and malignant nodules was analysed by means of the receiver-operating characteristic (ROC) curve and calculated area under the curve. After using this curve to establish a cut-off point, we established sensitivity and specificity values and likelihood ratios. The cumulative results from US, USE and CEUS were evaluated for sensitivity, specificity, positive predictive value and accuracy. Thy 3 nodules that fitted all experimental cut-off points obtained from ROC curves were considered true positive if they proved malignant and false

positive if they proved benign on histological examination. In addition Thy 3 nodules that did not fit all experimental cut-off points obtained from ROC curves were considered true negative if they proved benign and false negative if they proved malignant on histology.

Results

At the time of FNAB evaluations, all patients had normal f-T4 (15.1 ± 0.3 pmol/l) and TSH (2.0 ± 0.2 mIU/l) levels. CT was in the normal range in all but two patients; in these two patients, CT levels above the upper limit of the normal range (20 ng/l and 27 ng/l) were recorded. Surgery was performed in 63 of the 78 patients (81%). Surgery was not performed in 19% of Thy 3 nodules for the following reasons: down-grading of BTA classification from Thy 3 to Thy 2 (benign lesion) after the second FNAB (n=6), patient lost (n=4), patient request for further follow-up (n=2), patient refusal (n=2) and severe comorbidity (n=1). After surgery, a benign histological diagnosis of the cytological Thy 3 nodule was found in 50 cases (25 hyperplastic nodules; 18 follicular adenomas; 6 Hürthle cell adenomas; 1 intra-thyroid parathyroid adenoma). In 9 of these 50 cases (18%) an extra-nodular focal lymphocytic thyroiditis pattern was found, and in 6 (12%) a micro-papillary carcinoma of the isthmus (n=1) or in the contralateral lobe (n=5) was incidentally found. In one patient, C-cell hyperplasia was described. A final diagnosis of malignancy in the cytological Thy 3 nodules was reported in 13 cases (21%) (5 papillary thyroid carcinomas; 5 follicular variants of papillary thyroid carcinomas; 2 follicular carcinomas; 1 medullary thyroid carcinoma). Table 1 reports the clinical details of patients with thyroid

Table 1 Clinical and instrumental data on Thy 3 nodules with proven malignancy on histology

#	Age (yrs)	Sex	Nodule size (mm)	US (score)	USE (ELX 2/1)	CEUS P index	TTP index	Histology (°)	Tumour stage (*)
1	23	m	25	3	1.10	0.75	0.90	FTC	1
2	34	m	9	3	1.90	0.86	1.10	MTC	1
3	36	f	20	3	1.53	0.69	1.07	FvPTC	1
4	40	f	15	1	1.50	1.00	1.00	FTC	1
5	45	f	30	4	3.00	0.69	1.25	FvPTC	3
6	45	f	44	4	ne	0.82	1.62	FvPTC	3
7	46	f	7	4	1.00	0.60	0.63	PTC	1
8	46	f	9	3	1.30	0.95	1.20	FvPTC	1
9	50	m	13	3	1.80	0.33	1.00	PTC	3
10	54	m	20	3	1.70	0.90	2.40	PTC	1
11	66	m	23	5	1.50	0.80	1.01	PTC	1
12	71	f	7	3	1.90	0.77	1.00	PTC	1
13	74	f	22	3	2.00	0.90	1.00	PTC	1

(°) FTC = follicular thyroid carcinoma; MTC = medullary thyroid carcinoma; FvPTC = follicular variant of papillary thyroid carcinoma; PTC = papillary thyroid carcinoma.
(*) Tumour stage on diagnosis according to AJCC/UICC 2010 Seventh Edition criteria.
ne = not evaluable owing to coarse calcification (case #6).

malignancy. No difference in maximal diameter was noted between Thy 3 nodules with benign (22.8 ± 1.6 mm) or malignant (18.9 ± 2.9 mm) histology.

A significant correlation was seen between cumulative US findings and histology (n=63, Sr 0.35; p=0.005). A ROC curve was obtained (Figure 1) with an area under the curve (AUC) of 0.97 ± 0.01 (p<0.0001). By establishing a cut-off level that classified Thy 3 nodules with a US score greater than 2 as malignant, we were able to achieve a sensitivity of 79.0% and a specificity of 100%, with a 5.0 likelihood ratio.

USE was available in 61 Thy 3 nodules before surgery. In the remaining 2 cases, the ELX 2/1 index was unobtainable owing to coarse calcification of a 44 mm malignant nodule and the loss of data in a 23 mm benign nodule. A significant correlation was seen between the ELX 2/1 index and histology (Sr 0.39; p=0.002). A ROC curve was obtained (Figure 2) with an AUC of 0.95 ± 0.02 (p<0.0001). By establishing a cut-off level that classified Thy 3 nodules with an ELX 2/1 index greater than 0.95 as malignant, we were able to achieve a sensitivity of 83.6% and a specificity of 80.3%, with a 4.2 likelihood ratio. No significant correlation was found between the ELX 2/1 index and nodule (maximal) size or cumulative US findings (score).

CEUS was performed on 53 Thy 3 nodules; no side effects were recorded during or immediately after injection of the contrast agent. CEUS could not be performed in 10 Thy 3 nodules owing to refusal of intravenous injection of the contrast agent (n=5), technical impossibility of recording adequate video-clips (n=3) and loss of data (n=2). All these Thy 3 nodules (size-range: 14–30 mm)

had benign histology. A significant inverse correlation was observed between histology and P index (Sr –0.37; p=0.01) while a significant positive correlation was found between histology and TTP index (Sr 0.32; p=0.02). ROC curves were obtained for the P index and TTP index, with an AUC of 0.83 ± 0.04 (p<0.0001) and 0.86 ± 0.04 (p<0.0001), respectively (Figure 3). By establishing a cut-off level that classified Thy 3 nodules with a P index lower than 0.99 as malignant, we were able to achieve a sensitivity of 37.7% and a specificity of 75.5%, with a 1.5 likelihood ratio. By establishing a cut-off level that classified Thy 3 nodules with a TTP index greater than 0.98 as malignant, we were able to achieve a sensitivity of 56.6% and a specificity of 75.5%, with a 2.3 likelihood ratio. A significant inverse correlation was found between P index and US findings (score) (Sr –0.44; p=0.001). The peak index was not related to nodule size, while the TTP index was not related to either US findings (score) or nodule size.

A cohort of 51 Thy 3 cases underwent US-guided FNAB, USE and CEUS before surgery. In 9 out of 12 (75%) histologically malignant Thy 3 nodules, all indictors were positive for malignancy, while they were all positive in 5 out of 39 (13%) histologically benign Thy 3 nodules. The diagnostic power of the cumulative pre-surgical analysis of Thy 3 nodules by means of US, USE and CEUS, considering the experimental cut-off points obtained from ROC curves was: sensitivity 64%, specificity 92%, PPV 75%, and accuracy 84%.

Discussion

The number of thyroid cancer diagnoses is currently increasing. This is probably the result of a reservoir

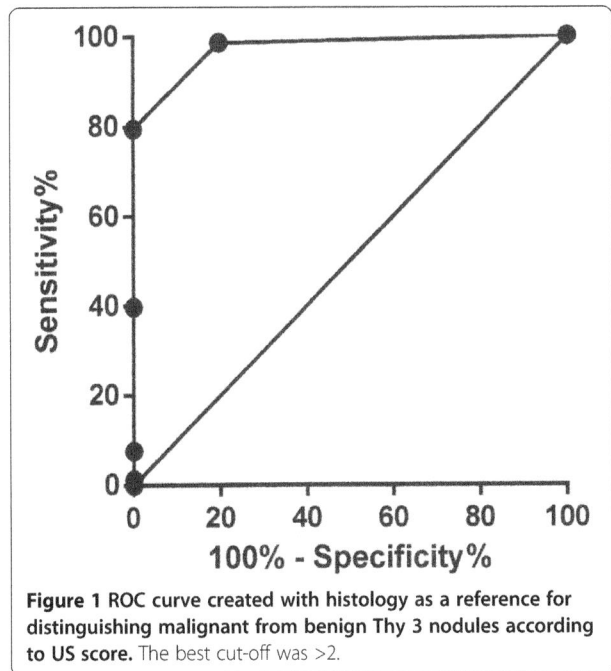

Figure 1 ROC curve created with histology as a reference for distinguishing malignant from benign Thy 3 nodules according to US score. The best cut-off was >2.

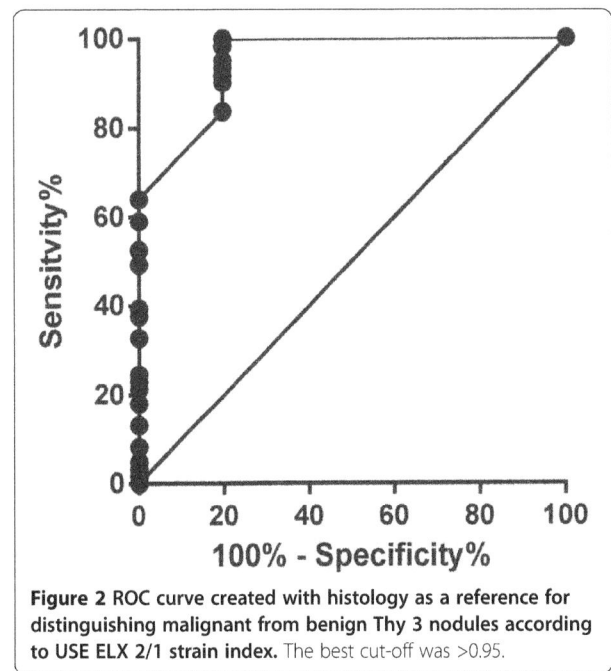

Figure 2 ROC curve created with histology as a reference for distinguishing malignant from benign Thy 3 nodules according to USE ELX 2/1 strain index. The best cut-off was >0.95.

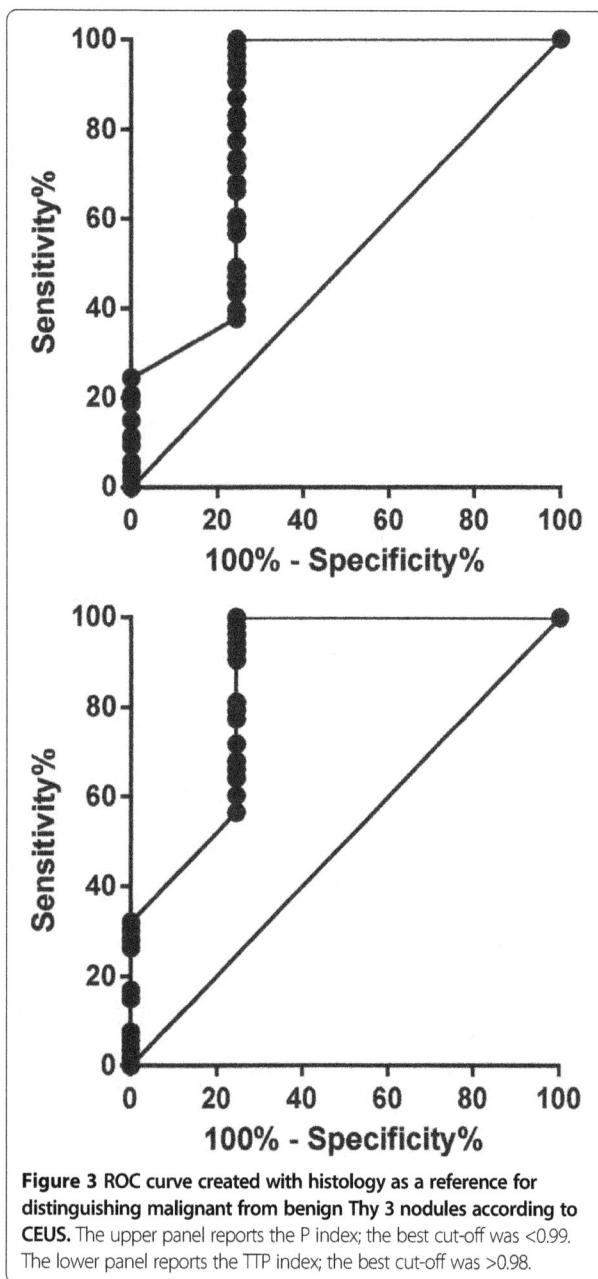

Figure 3 ROC curve created with histology as a reference for distinguishing malignant from benign Thy 3 nodules according to CEUS. The upper panel reports the P index; the best cut-off was <0.99. The lower panel reports the TTP index; the best cut-off was >0.98.

of asymptomatic (subclinical) malignant nodular thyroid disease which is disclosed in parallel with the "epidemic" of thyroid nodules due to the increase in instrumental, mainly US, diagnostics. Current clinical efforts should be aimed at defining the nature (malignant or benign) of a given nodule and identifying the relatively rare malignant nodules, in order to reduce unnecessary invasive surgical procedures.

US, which is the most sensitive means of evaluating thyroid morphology, can evaluate the size and characteristics of non-palpable nodules, reveal lymph-node metastases and guide FNAB. It is well known that no single US pattern can be used alone as a definite criterion of malignancy [45],

and individual US features are not now considered accurate predictors of thyroid cancer [9].

The present study demonstrates that, in Thy 3 nodules, nodule size is not a useful means of distinguishing malignant from benign nodules, as already reported by several other authors [12,27,47]. In a previous study involving five US parameters (hypoechogenic, solid, intra-nodular vascularization, microcalcifications, and irregular margins), we found that the diagnostic power of color-Doppler US was high; indeed, 100% of nodules in which four or five these parameters were positive proved to be malignant [19]. Similarly, on using the so-called "thyroid imaging reporting and data system", Horvath et al. [48] found malignancy in 80% of nodules classified as probably malignant on US. A limitation of these studies, however, was the 5-14% of false negative results in nodules with a low number of suspicious US features [19,48]. In a very large series of Thy 3 nodules, Rago et al. [27] recently reported a significant association of three suspicious US features (blurred margins, spot microcalcifications and hypoechogeneicity) with malignancy. Moreover, in the present study, a significant correlation was found between cumulative US findings and histology, and the ROC curve analysis indicated that the presence of more than two suspicious US findings in Thy 3 nodules reached a sensitivity of 82% and a specificity of 100%, with a 5.0 likelihood ratio. In a series of 40 Thy 3 nodules with US available for review, Matthey-Gie et al. [49] reported that high nodule vascularity associated with ill-defined borders was a suspicious US finding linked to malignancy. In a series of 78 indeterminate lesions, Batawil and Alkordy [50] found that solid structure and irregular border were the most suspicious findings. Yoo et al. [26] examined a selected series of 249 nodules which met the criteria of atypia or follicular lesion of indeterminate significance and in which core-biopsy or surgery were used as references; they observed that taller-than-wide shape and marked hypoechogenicity were highly suspicious US findings. In 61 follicular neoplasms and 99 Hürthle cell neoplasms, Tutuncu et al. [51] did not report the role of cumulative US findings; however, they indicated that hypoechogenicity and microcalcification had the highest odds ratios. In sum, in Thy 3 nodules, US is helpful to the initial decision-making process, but combination with other evaluations is needed.

More recently, USE machines able to measure tissue hardness qualitatively (colour score), semi- quantitatively (strain ratio), or quantitatively (elasticity index, shear-wave velocity) have been introduced into the clinical setting in order to overcome the limitations of FNAB and US in thyroid nodules [33]. The efficacy of USE in distinguishing benign from malignant thyroid nodules varies widely among studies [17-20,25,34,35,46,47,52]). In a 2013 meta-analysis by Razavi et al. [53], in which 24 studies comprising 3531 nodules were evaluated and the results were compared with those yielded by US, USE was reported to be more sensitive (colour score 82%; strain ratio 89%) and specific (colour score and strain ratio 82%) than each individual US feature. However, in a previous study in which we evaluated a subset of 27 Thy 3 nodules with cytological-histological correlation by means of semi-quantitative USE, we were unable to distinguish these nodules from cytological benign (Thy 2) or malignant (Thy 5) nodules on the basis of the ELX 2/1 strain index [19]. The only reported finding was an increasing trend in low-range ELX 2/1 strain index values from Thy 2 to Thy 5 nodules [19]. In the present study, which involved a higher number of Thy 3 nodules, the ELX 2/1 strain index showed a significant correlation with histology, and the established cut-off level, which classified Thy 3 nodules with an ELX 2/1 index greater than 0.95 as malignant, showed better sensitivity of 83.6% and specificity of 80.3%, with a 4.2 likelihood ratio. In the study by Rago et al. [27], qualitative USE was performed in 169 Thy 3 nodules in which cytological-histological correlation was available, and low stiffness was found in nodules with benign diagnoses, the negative predictive value of 97% increasing the predictivity of US features. In several other studies on the pre-surgical utility of USE in thyroid nodules, the number of indeterminate lesions was limited, ranging from 9 to 58 [17,21,43,47,53], and separate data analysis was either not done [17] or, when done, was poorly understandable [21] or revealed low sensitivity (78%) and specificity (44%) [47]. Similarly, a very low specificity (6%) was observed in a study by Lippolis et al. [46], which evaluated 103 nodules with indeterminate cytology. On the other hand, in 270 nodules cytologically classified as atypia of undetermined significance by means of qualitative and semi-quantitative USE, Cakir et al. [44] reported favourable conclusions, suggesting the use of this technique in the pre-surgical evaluation of indeterminate nodules. The best strain index value in distinguishing between cytologically benign and cytologically malignant nodules reaches a sensitivity of 99% and a specificity of 96%.

Overall, the diagnostic utility of USE in Thy 3 nodules remains under evaluation. However, qualitative and semi-quantitative methods and definite cut-off values obtained in large numbers of subjects have yielded promising results (present study, [27,44]), thus supporting a less aggressive strategy, especially when no suspicious features are noted on US.

The latest technique involving US for the study of thyroid vascularization uses a microbubble contrast agent. It is well known that the thyroid gland has an abundant microvasculature, and that the parenchyma of normal thyroid shows rapid and uniform enhancement after intravenous injection of contrast agents. By contrast, the vascular structure of nodules differs from the normal pattern, and hence enhancement differs from that of the normal parenchyma. Argalia et al. [54] have shown that CEUS time-intensity curves can provide an indirect description of intra-nodular vascularization, which seems to be anarchic in malignant nodules. Literature data on the utility of CEUS in distinguishing malignant from benign nodules are controversial. Zhang et al. [37] reported that heterogeneous enhancement rendered a thyroid nodule suspicious for malignancy, while Friedrich-Rust et al. [41] reported that the time-intensity CEUS curve did not prove useful in distinguishing between benign and malignant nodules. Moreover, in our previous report [19], the P index and TTP index were found to be unrelated to cytological and histological results. More recently, two studies involving Chinese patients examined the role of CEUS in distinguishing between malignant and benign thyroid nodules. In 175 nodules, without histological reference in all cases, Deng J et al. [39] reported a CEUS sensitivity of 82% and a specificity of 85%. Their study was based on the impression that hypo-enhancement could be regarded as an indicator of malignancy. Ma et al. [38] studied the preoperative diagnostic role of CEUS combined with US in 172 nodules, all surgically removed. Both US and CEUS areas under the ROC curves were significant, but the best sensitivity (89%) and specificity (94%) was reached by considering five positive features (ring enhancement, homogeneity of enhancement, arrival time of the nodule at CEUS, microcalcifications, and halo sign on US) on combining US and CEUS.

To our knowledge, no studies on CEUS have focused on the subpopulation of indeterminate nodules. In our previous study on CEUS in thyroid nodules, CEUS was available in 17 indeterminate nodules with cytological-histological correlation [19]. Regarding the indicators P index and TTP index, no differences were noted among the nodules scored according to the Thy classification [19]. The present study provided more interesting data. Significant correlations were noted between histology and both P index (negative) and TTP index (positive). The areas under the ROC curves for the P index and TTP index were significant at an established cut-off level that classified Thy 3 nodules as malignant when the P index was lower than 0.99 (sensitivity 37.7%; specificity 75.5%) and the TTP index was greater than 0.98 (sensitivity 56.6%; specificity 75.5%). Our experience of Thy 3 nodules seems to indicate a greater diagnostic role of semi-quantitative USE than of CEUS. In the study by Deng et al. [39], however, quantitative USE and CEUS displayed the same value in distinguishing between benign and malignant nodules.

The simultaneous evaluation of different indicators from US, USE and CEUS and the use of validated cut-off levels for interpreting data – without or with low subjectivity – is crucial in clinical decision-making when cytological results are indeterminate and lobectomy or thyroidectomy is indicated by the guidelines. In the 51 cases that were fully evaluable, our study indicates that the diagnostic power of the cumulative pre-surgical analysis of Thy 3 nodules by means of US, USE and CEUS does not increase sensitivity (64%) but improves specificity (92%); moreover, it showed interesting levels of PPV (75%) and accuracy (84%). While false negative (25%) and false positive (13%) results are limitations, these preliminary data on the combination of US, USE and CEUS with FNAB seem to provide promising indications that unnecessary lobectomy/thyroidectomy can be reduced. To our knowledge there are no studies on Thy 3 nodules in which results obtained from conventional US, USE and CEUS have been simultaneously scored in order to make a clinical decision. In our opinion, US-guided FNAB remains the gold standard in solid nodules. However, when an indeterminate response emerges from cytology, surgery may be postponed if no suspicious findings are observed (in our hands: US score ≤ 2, ELX 2/1 <0.95, P index >0.99 and TTP index <0.98).

There are some limitations to this study. First, the number of fully evaluable Thy 3 nodules was small. As the thyroid tissue adjacent to the Thy 3 nodule may not be normal, both USE and CEUS may sometimes be impracticable. Moreover, injection of the contrast agent before CEUS is sometimes refused by the patient. Second, we did not divide FNAB results into Thy 3 atypia and Thy 3 follicular neoplasm, as suggested by the BTA in 2014 [27,43]. Larger numbers of Thy 3 nodules could necessary in order to compare USE and CEUS data in these two Thy 3 subpopulations. Third, genetic markers were not considered in the present study; however, BRAF, the most frequent mutation in thyroid cancer, seems to be less important in follicular neoplasms [31]. Fourth, this was a single-centre study. However, pooling data from different centres for qualitative and semi-quantitative USE remains impracticable, since different devices may yield various types of strain indices, such as maximum ratio or simple ratio. While we used an average ELX 2/1 index from at least 3 measures, it is unclear whether the average index is truly representative of nodular stiffness. Among our Thy 3 lesions, medullary carcinomas and follicular carcinomas were rare (25% of Thy 3 nodules with histological malignancy). According to some authors [34-36,39], however, false negative results from these tumours should be taken into consideration when USE and CEUS data are evaluated.

In conclusion, in cytologically Thy 3 nodules, conventional US must be associated, when feasible, to the combined application of USE and CEUS. The use of a cut-off based on histology can reduce the surgical approach. Observation should be the first choice when not all instrumental results are suspect.

Competing interests
The authors declare that they have no competing interests.

Authors' contributions
MG and GT designed the initial study and prepared the final version of the paper. ST and EM provided patients data and analysis. BM carried out the cytological and histological examinations. CC. GT and ES carried out radiological examinations. All authors had read and approval the final manuscript.

Author details
[1]Endocrine Unit, IRCCS Azienda Ospedaliera Universitaria San Martino – IST Istituto Nazionale per la Ricerca sul Cancro, Genoa, Italy. [2]Cytopathology and Pathology Unit, IRCCS Azienda Ospedaliera Universitaria San Martino – IST Istituto Nazionale per la Ricerca sul Cancro, Genoa, Italy. [3]Radiology Unit, Ospedale Evangelico, Genoa, Italy. [4]UO Clinica Endocrinologica, Viale Benedetto XV, 6, I-16100 Genoa, Italy.

References
1. Mortensen JD, Woolner LB, Bennett WA: Cross and microscopic findings in clinically normal thyroid gland. *J Clin Endocrinol Metab* 1955, **15**:1270–1280.
2. Vander JB, Gaston EA, Dawber TR: The significance of nontoxic thyroid nodules. Final report of a 15-year study of the incidence of thyroid malignancy. *Ann Intern Med* 1968, **69**:537–540.
3. Guth S, Theune U, Aberle J, Galach A, Bamberger CM: Very high prevalence of thyroid nodules detected by high frequency (13 MHz) ultrasound examination. *Eur J Clin Invest* 2009, **39**:699–706.
4. Udelsman R, Zhang Y: The epidemic of thyroid cancer in the United States: the role of endocrinologists and ultrasounds. *Thyroid* 2014, **24**:472–479.
5. Van der Bruel A, Francart J, Dubois C, Adam A, Vlayen J, De Schutter H, Stordeur S, Decallonne B: Regional variation in thyroid cancer incidence in Belgium is associated with variation in thyroid imaging and thyroid disease management. *J Clin Endocrinol Metab* 2013, **98**:4063–4071.
6. Hegedus L: Clinical practice. The thyroid nodule. *N Engl J Med* 2004, **351**:1764–1771.
7. Jin J, McHenry CR: Thyroid incidentaloma. *Best Pract Res Clin Endocrinol Metab* 2012, **26**:83–96.
8. Frates MC, Benson CB, Doubilet PM, Kunreuther E, Contreras M, Cibas ES, Orcutt J, Moore FR Jr, Larsen PR, Marqusee E, Alexander EK: Prevalence and distribution of carcinoma in patients with solitary and multiple thyroid nodules on sonography. *J Clin Endocrinol Metab* 2006, **91**:3411–3417.
9. Brito JP, Gionfriddo MR, Al Nofal A, Boehmer KR, Leppin AL, Reading C, Callstrom M, Elraiyah TA, Prokop LJ, Stan MN, Murad MH, Morris JC, Montori VM: The accuracy of thyroid nodule ultrasound to predict thyroid cancer: systemic review and meta-analysis. *J Clin Endocrinol Metab* 2014, **99**:1253–1263.
10. Lee TI, Yang HJ, Lin SY, Lee MT, Lin HD, Braverman LE, Tang KT: The accuracy of fine-needle aspiration biopsy and frozen section in patients with thyroid cancer. *Thyroid* 2002, **19**:619–626.
11. Nam-Goong IS, Kim HY, Gong G, Lee HK, Hong SJ, Kim WB, Shong YK: Ultrasonography-guided fine-needle aspiration of thyroid incidentaloma: correlation with pathological findings. *Clin Endocrinol (Oxf)* 2004, **60**:21–28.
12. Sidoti M, Marino G, Resmini E, Augeri C, Cappi C, Cavallero D, Lagasio C, Ceppa P, Minuto F, Giusti M: The rational use of fine-needle aspiration biopsy (FNAB) in diagnosing thyroid nodules. *Minerva Endocrinol* 2006, **31**:159–172.
13. Castro MR, Gharib H: Thyroid fine-needle aspiration biopsy: progress, practice, and pitfalls. *Endocr Pract* 2003, **9**:128–136.
14. Gharib H, Papini E: Thyroid nodules: clinical importance, assessment, and treatment. *Endocrinol Metab Clin North Am* 2007, **36**:707–735.
15. Cibas ES, Ali SZ, NCI Thyroid FNA State of the Science Conference: The Bethesda system for reporting thyroid cytopathology. *Am J Clin Pathol* 2009, **132**:658–655.
16. Nou E, Kwong N, Alexander LK, Cibas ES, Marqusee E, Alexander EK: Determination of optimal time interval for repeat evaluation following a benign thyroid nodule aspiration. *J Clin Endocrinol Metab* 2014, **99**:510–516.
17. Nacamulli D, Nico L, Barollo S, Zambonin L, Pennelli G, Girelli ME, Casal Ide E, Pelizzo MR, Vianello F, Negro I, Watutantrige-Fernando S, Mantero F, Rugge M, Mian C: Comparison of the diagnostic accuracy of combined elastosonography

and BRAF analysis *vs* cytology and ultrasonography for thyroid nodule suspected of malignancy. *Clin Endocrinol (Oxf)* 2012, **77**:608–614.

18. Trimboli P, Guglielmi R, Monti S, Misischi I, Graziano F, Nasrollah N, Amendola S, Morgante SN, Deiana MG, Valabrega S, Toscano V, Papini E: **Ultrasound sensitivity for thyroid malignancy is increased by real-time elastosonography: a prospective multicenter study.** *J Clin Endocrinol Metab* 2012, **97**:4524–4530.

19. Giusti M, Orlandi D, Melle G, Massa B, Silvestri E, Minuto F, Turtulici G: **Is there a real diagnostic impact of elastosonography and contrast-enhanced ultrasonography in the management of thyroid nodules?** *J Zhejiang Univ Sci B* 2013, **14**:195–206.

20. Magri F, Chytiris S, Capelli V, Gaiti M, Zerbini F, Carrara R, Malovini A, Rotondi M, Bellazzi R, Chiovato L: **Comparison of elastographic strain index and thyroid fine–needle aspiration cytology in 631 thyroid nodules.** *J Clin Endocrinol Metab* 2013, **98**:4790–4797.

21. Guazzaroni M, Spinelli A, Coco I, Del Giudice C, Girardi V, Simonetti G: **Value of strain-ratio on thyroid real-time sonoelastography.** *Radiol Med* 2014, **119**:149–155.

22. Na DG, Kim JH, Sung JY, Beak JH, Jung KC, Lee H, Yoo H: **Core-needle biopsy is more useful than repeat fine-needle aspiration in thyroid nodules read as nondiagnostic or atypia of undetermined significance by Bethesda system for reporting thyroid cytopathology.** *Thyroid* 2012, **22**:468–475.

23. Hakala T, Kholova I, Sand J, Saaristo R, Kellokumpu-Lehtinen P: **A core needle biopsy provides more malignancy-specific results than fine-needle aspiration biopsy in thyroid nodules suspicious for malignancy.** *J Clin Pathol* 2013, **66**:1046–1050.

24. Mihai R, Parker AJ, Roskell D, Sadler GP: **One in four patients with follicular thyroid cytology (THY 3) has a thyroid carcinoma.** *Thyroid* 2009, **19**:33–37.

25. Rago T, Scutari M, Santini F, Loiacono V, Piaggi P, Di Coscio G, Basolo F, Berti P, Pinchera A, Vitti P: **Real-time elastosonography: useful tool for refining the presurgical diagnosis in thyroid nodules with indeterminate or nondiagnostic cytology.** *J Clin Endocrinol Metab* 2010, **95**:5274–5280.

26. Yoo WS, Choi HS, Cho SW, Moon JH, Kim KW, Park HJ, Park SY, Choi SI, Choi SH, Lim S, Yi KH, Park Do J, Jang HC, Park YJ: **The role of ultrasound findings in the management of thyroid nodules with atypia or follicular lesions of undetermined significance.** *Clin Endocrinol (Oxf)* 2014, **80**:735–742.

27. Rago T, Scutari M, Latrofa F, Loiacono V, Piaggi P, Marchetti I, Romani R, Basolo F, Miccoli P, Tonacchera M, Vitti P: **The large majority of 1520 patients with indeterminate thyroid nodules at cytology have a favorable outcome and a clinical risk score has a high negative predictive value for a more cumbersome cancer disease.** *J Clin Endocrinol Metab* 2014, **99**:3700–3007.

28. Nikiforov YE, Steward DL, Robinson-Smith TM, Haugen BR, Klopper JP, Zhu Z, Fagin JA, Falciglia M, Weber K, Nikiforova MN: **Molecular testing for mutations in improving the fine-needle aspiration diagnosis of thyroid nodules.** *J Clin Endorinol Metab* 2009, **94**:2092–2098.

29. Ferraz C, Eszlinger M, Paschke R: **Current state and future perspective of molecular diagnosis of fine-needle aspiration biopsy of thyroid nodules.** *J Clin Endocrinol Metab* 2011, **96**:2016–2026.

30. Gomberawalla A, Elaraj DM: **How to use molecular testing to guide surgery: a surgeon's perspective.** *Curr Opin Oncol* 2014, **26**:14–21.

31. Eszlinger M, Krogdahl A, Munz S, Rehfeld C, Precht Jensen EM, Ferraz C, Bosenberg E, Drieschner N, Scholz M, Hegedus L, Paschke R: **Impact of molecular screening for point mutations and rearrangements in routine air-dried fine-needle aspiration samples of thyroid nodules.** *Thyroid* 2014, **24**:305–313.

32. Alexander EK, Schorr M, Klopper J, Kim C, Sipos J, Nabhan F, Parker C, Steward DL, Mandel SJ, Haugen BR: **Multicenter clinical experience with the Afirma gene expression classifier.** *J Clin Endocrinol Metab* 2014, **99**:119–125.

33. Andrioli M, Persani L: **Elastographic techniques of thyroid gland: current status.** *Endocrine* 2014, **46**:455–461.

34. Lyshchik A, Higashi T, Asato R, Tanaka S, Ito J, Mai JJ, Pellot-Barakat C, Insana MF, Brill AB, Saga T, Hiraoka M, Togashi K: **Thyroid gland tumor diagnosis at US elastography.** *Radiology* 2005, **237**:202–2011.

35. Vorlander C, Wolff J, Saalabian S, Lienenluke RH, Wahl RA: **Real-time ultrasound elastography – a non invasive diagnostic procedure for evaluating dominant thyroid nodules.** *Langenbecks Arch Surg* 2010, **395**:865–871.

36. Andrioli M, Trimboli P, Amendola S, Valabrega S, Fukunari N, Mirella M, Persani L: **Elastographic presentation of medullary thyroid carcinoma.** *Endocrine* 2013, **45**:153–155.

37. Zhang B, Jiang YX, Liu JB, Yang M, Dai Q, Zhu QL, Gao P: **Utility of contrast-enhanced ultrasound for evaluation of thyroid nodules.** *Thyroid* 2010, **20**:51–57.

38. Ma JJ, Ding H, Xu BH, Xu C, Song LJ, Huang BJ, Wang WP: **Diagnostic performances of various gray-scale, color Doppler, and contrast-enhanced ultrasonography findings in predicting malignant thyroid nodules.** *Thyroid* 2014, **24**:355–363.

39. Deng J, Zhou P, Tian SM, Zhang L, Li JI, Qian Y: **Comparison of diagnostic efficacy of contrast-enhanced ultrasound, acoustic radiation force impulse imaging, and their combined use in differentiating focal solid thyroid nodules.** *PLoS One* 2014, **9**:e90674.

40. Spiezia S, Farina R, Cerbone G, Assanti AP, Iovino V, Siciliani M, Lombardi G, Colao A: **Analysis of color Doppler signal intensity variation after levovist injection: a new approach to the diagnosis of thyroid nodules.** *J Ultrasound Med* 2001, **20**:223–231.

41. Friedrich-Rust M, Sperber A, Holzer K, Diener J, Grunwald F, Badenhoop K, Weber S, Kriener S, Herrmann E, Bechstein WO, Zeuzem S, Bojunga J: **Real-time elastography and contrast-enhanced ultrasound for the assessment of thyroid nodules.** *Exp Clin Endocrinol Diabetes* 2010, **118**:602–609.

42. Ragazzoni F, Deandrea M, Mormile A, Ramunni MJ, Garino F, Magliona G, Motta M, Torchio B, Garberoglio R, Limone P: **High diagnostic accuracy and interobserver reliability of real-time elastography in the evaluation of thyroid nodules.** *Ultrasound Med Biol* 2012, **38**:1154–1162.

43. Mehrotra P, McQueen A, Kolla S, Johnson SJ, Richardson DL: **Does elastography reduce the need for thyroid FNAs?** *Clin Endocrinol (Oxf)* 2013, **78**:942–949.

44. Cakir B, Ersoy R, Cuhaci FN, Aydin C, Polat B, Kilic M, Yazgan A: **Elastosonographic strain index in thyroid nodules with atypia of undetermined significance.** *J Endocrinol Invest* 2014, **37**:127–133.

45. Moon WJ, Baek JH, Jung SL, Kim DW, Kim EK, Kim JY, Kwak JY, Lee JH, Lee JH, Lee YH, Na DG, Park JS, Korean Society of Thyroid Radiology (KSThR); Korean Society of Radiology, Park SW: **Ultrasonography and the ultrasound-based management of thyroid nodules: consensus statement and recommendations.** *Korean J Radiol* 2011, **12**:1–14.

46. Lippolis PV, Tognini S, Materazzi G, Polini A, Mancini R, Ambrosini CE, Dardano A, Basolo F, Seccia M, Miccoli P, Monzani F: **Is elastography actually useful in the presurgical selection of thyroid nodules with indeterminate cytology?** *J Clin Endocrinol Metab* 2011, **96**:E1826–E1830.

47. Unluturk U, Erdogan MF, Demir O, Gullu S, Baskal N: **Ultrasound elastography is not superior to grayscale ultrasound in predicting malignancy in thyroid nodules.** *Thyroid* 2012, **22**:1031–1038.

48. Horvath E, Majlis S, Rossi R, Franco C, Niedmann JP, Castro A, Dominguez M: **An ultrasonogram reporting system for thyroid nodules stratifying cancer risk for clinical management.** *J Clin Endocrinol Metab* 2009, **94**:1748–1751.

49. Matthey-Gie ML, Walsh SM, O'Neill AC, Lowery A, Evoy D, Gibbson D, Prichard RS, Skehan S, McDermott EW: **Ultrasound predictors of malignancy in indeterminate thyroid nodules.** *Ir J Med Sci*, in press

50. Batawil N, Alkordy T: **Ultrasonographic features associated with malignancy in cytologically indeterminate thyroid nodules.** *Eur J Surg Oncol* 2014, **40**:182–186.

51. Tutuncu Y, Berker D, Isik S, Akbaba G, Ozuguz U, Kucukler FK, Gocmen E, Yalcin Y, Aydin Y, Guler S: **The frequency of malignancy and the relationship between malignancy and ultrasonographic features of thyroid nodules with indeterminate cytology.** *Endocrine* 2014, **45**:37–45.

52. Rivo-Vazquez A, Rodriguez-Lorenzo A, Rivo-Vazquez JE, Paramo-Fernandez C, Garcia-Lorenzo F, Pardellas-Rivera H, Casal-Nunez JE, Gil-Gil P: **The use of ultrasound elastography in the assessment of malignancy risk in thyroid nodules and multinodular goitres.** *Clin Endocrinol (Oxf)* 2013, **79**:887–891.

53. Razavi SA, Hadduck TA, Sadigh G, Dwamena BA: **Comparative effectiveness of elastographic and B-mode ultrasound criteria for diagnostic discrimination of thyroid nodules: a meta-analysis.** *AJR Am J Roentgenol* 2013, **200**:1317–1326.

54. Argalia G, De Bernardis S, Mariani D, Abbattista T, Taccaliti A, Ricciardelli L, Faragona S, Gusella PM, Giuseppetti GM: **Ultrasonographic contrast agent: evaluation of time-intensity curves in the characterisation of solitary thyroid nodules.** *Radiol Med* 2002, **103**:407–413.

High level of oxidized nucleosides in thyroid mitochondrial DNA; damaging effects of Fenton reaction substrates

Małgorzata Karbownik-Lewińska[1,3*], Jan Stępniak[1] and Andrzej Lewiński[2,3]

Abstract

Background: The mitochondrial DNA (mtDNA) lies in close proximity to the free radical-producing electron transport chain, thus, it is highly prone to oxidative damage. Oxyphilic type of follicular thyroid carcinoma consists of cells filled – almost exclusively – with aberrant mitochondria. In turn, bivalent iron (Fe^{2+}) and hydrogen peroxide (H_2O_2) are indispensable for thyroid hormone synthesis, therefore being available in physiological conditions presumably at high concentrations. They participate in Fenton reaction ($Fe^{2+}+H_2O_2 \rightarrow Fe^{3+}+{}^{\bullet}OH + OH^-$), resulting in the formation of the most harmful free radical – hydroxyl radical (${}^{\bullet}OH$). The same substrates may be used to experimentally induce oxidative damage to macromolecules. The aim of the study was to evaluate the background level of oxidative damage to mtDNA and the damaging effects of Fenton reaction substrates.

Methods: Thyroid mtDNA was incubated in the presence of either H_2O_2 [100, 10, 1.0, 0.5, 0.1, 0.001, 0.00001 mM] or $FeSO_4$ (Fe^{2+}) [300, 150, 30, 15, 3.0, 1.5 μM], or in the presence of those two factors used together, namely, in the presence of Fe^{2+} [30 μM] plus H_2O_2 [100, 10, 1.0, 0.5, 0.1, 0.001, 0.00001 mM], or in the presence of H_2O_2 [0.5 mM] plus Fe^{2+} [300, 150, 30, 15, 3.0, 1.5 μM]. 8-oxo-7,8-dihydro-2'-deoxyguanosine (8-oxodG) concentration, as the index of DNA damage, was measured by HPLC.

Results: Both Fenton reaction substrates, used separately, increased 8-oxodG level for the highest H_2O_2 concentration of 100 mM and in Fe^{2+} concentration-dependent manner [300, 150, and 30 μM].
When Fe^{2+} and H_2O_2 were applied together, Fe^{2+} enhanced H_2O_2 damaging effect to a higher degree than did H_2O_2 on Fe^{2+} effect.

Conclusions: The level of oxidized nucleosides in thyroid mtDNA is relatively high, when compared to nuclear DNA. Both substrates of Fenton reaction, i.e. ferrous ion and hydrogen peroxide, increase oxidative damage to mtDNA, with stronger damaging effect exerted by iron. High level of oxidative damage to mtDNA suggests its possible contribution to malignant transformation of thyroid oncocytic cells, which are known to be especially abundant in mitochondria, the latter characterized by molecular and enzymatic abnormalities.

Keywords: Mitochondrial DNA, Thyroid, Ferrous ion, Hydrogen peroxide, Oxidative damage

* Correspondence: MKarbownik@hotmail.com
[1]Department of Oncological Endocrinology, Medical University of Łódź, 7/9 Żeligowski St, 90-752, Łódź, Poland
[3]Polish Mother's Memorial Hospital - Research Institute, 281/289, Rzgowska St, 93-338, Łódź, Poland
Full list of author information is available at the end of the article

Background

Reactive oxygen species (ROS) are generated in animal cells as natural by-products of oxygen metabolism. They participate in numerous important life processes, like cell signaling or host defense against pathogens [1,2]. On the other hand, due to highly reactive nature, ROS are potentially very toxic and they can damage macromolecules, such as DNA, proteins and lipids. Normally, the cell is able to maintain an adequate balance between the formation and removal of ROS. However, when the levels of ROS increase, this balance may be disturbed, leading to oxidative stress, a condition involved in the pathogenesis of many diseases [1,3-5].

The most basic reaction of oxidative stress is Fenton reaction:

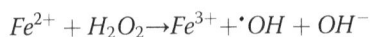

$$Fe^{2+} + H_2O_2 \rightarrow Fe^{3+} + {}^{\bullet}OH + OH^-$$

Hydroxyl radical ($^{\bullet}OH$) – being the most harmful free radical – is produced during the above reaction. Both substrates of Fenton reaction are normally present in thyroid cells and possess important physiological roles.

H_2O_2 is an indispensable factor in the process of thyroid hormone synthesis, acting as an electron acceptor at each step of this process, namely, at iodide oxidation, next, at its organification, as well as at iodotyrosine coupling reactions [6]. H_2O_2 is synthesized in the thyroid gland by certain enzymes of a dual oxidase/NADPH oxidase family (NOX/DUOX), with the most convincing experimental evidence found for DUOX2, acting mainly at the apical membrane or extracelluary – in the colloid [7] and for NOX4, acting intracellulary [8]. H_2O_2 availability is the rate-limiting step in thyroid hormone biosynthesis, although H_2O_2 is produced in large excess compared to the amount of iodide incorporated into proteins. This may be due to relatively high Michaelis-Menten constant of thyroperoxidase (TPO) for H_2O_2, which means that relatively high concentrations of H_2O_2, as a substrate, are required to properly activate the enzyme [9,10]. It should be stressed that the stimulated thyroid cell generates as much H_2O_2 as an activated leukocyte [11]. Large quantities and membrane permeable nature of H_2O_2 can lead to its diffusion from the luminal side of the apical membrane back to the cell, potentially creating conditions for a huge oxidative stress.

Iron is an essential element for normal metabolic processes, being a cofactor for many biological reactions. On the other hand, free ionic iron, as a potent generator of ROS, can enhance oxidative stress. In the thyroid gland, iron is bound to TPO and it is required for its biological activity. Activated TPO (hemoprotein) constitutes only approximately 2% of total TPO; it is located in the apical membrane and it exposes its heme-linked catalytic site facing the thyroid follicular lumen [12,13]. This kind of iron compartmentalization constitutes, in a certain sense, defense mechanisms against oxidative damage in the thyroid, caused by heme iron.

Bivalent iron (ferrous ion; Fe^{2+}) and/or H_2O_2 which – when used together – initiate Fenton reaction, are frequently used to experimentally induce oxidative damage to macromolecules [6,14-22]. Thus, the present study is the next approach to evaluate oxidative damage to macromolecules caused by Fenton reaction substrates but the first one, in which thyroid mtDNA has been used.

Mitochondria remain the main source of ROS, even in thyroid tissue. Furthermore, they are the only cellular organelles in cells that contain their own DNA. This mitochondrial DNA (mtDNA) lies in close proximity to the free radical-producing electron transport chain and it is not protected by histones and polyamines, thus it is highly prone to oxidative damage. Additionally, lack of buffering structures, such as introns, also renders mtDNA more prone to mutations [23]. Consistently, it has been reported that mtDNA is characterized by a higher level of oxidative DNA damage than nuclear DNA [24]. In human mtDNA, over 150 pathogenic mutations have been identified; there is evidence that these mutations lead to a wide variety of degenerative diseases, preferentially in tissues with high energy demands, such as the central nervous system, heart, skeletal muscles and endocrine system [25]. Accumulation of somatic mutations in mtDNA causes deficiencies in oxidative phosphorylation and the electron transport chain, which, in turn, cause both further increased production of ROS and their leakage into the cytoplasm.

The aim of the study was to evaluate the background level of oxidative damage to thyroid mtDNA and the damaging effects of Fenton reaction substrates. Since 8-oxo-7,8-dihydro-2'-deoxyguanosine (8-oxodG) is a major product of oxidatively damaged DNA, this oxidized nucleoside has been used to evaluate oxidative damage to mtDNA. It should be stressed that the level of 8-oxodG, resulting from oxidative mtDNA damage, has never been examined in the thyroid gland under any conditions.

Methods
Ethical approval
The procedures, used in the study, were approved by the Ethics Committee of the Medical University of Lodz, Poland.

Chemicals
Ferrous sulfate ($FeSO_4$), hydrogen peroxide (H_2O_2), alkaline phosphatase and nuclease P_1 were purchased from Sigma (St. Louis, MO). MilliQ-purified H_2O was used for preparing all solutions. All the used chemicals were of analytical grade and came from commercial sources.

Animals

Porcine thyroids were collected from sixty three (63) animals at a slaughter-house, frozen on solid CO_2, and stored at $-80°C$ until assay. Three independent experiments were performed. Therefore, three tissue pools were prepared, with twenty one (21) thyroid glands used for each experiment.

Mitochondrial DNA isolation

Mitochondrial DNA was isolated using an alkaline lysis method [26]. Thyroid tissue was homogenized in chilled homogenization buffer (0.25 M sucrose, 10 mM EDTA, 30 mM Tris–HCl, pH 7.5) and centrifuged at $1000 \times g$ for 3 min at $4°C$ in order to pellet the nuclei and cellular debris. The supernatant was centrifuged again at $12,000 \times g$ for 10 min at $4°C$, to obtain pellet of mitochondria. This pellet was resuspended in 10 mM Tris-EDTA buffer (containing 0.15 M NaCl and 10 mM EDTA, pH 8.0) and then two volumes of freshly prepared 0.18 M NaOH, containing 1% SDS, were added. After 5 min incubation on ice, solution of ice-cold potassium acetate (3 M potassium and 5 M acetate) was added. After another 5 min incubation on ice, mixture was centrifuged at $12,000 \times g$ for 5 min at $4°C$. The obtained supernatant was mixed with an equal volume of phenol/chloroform/isoamyl-alcohol (25:24:1) mixture. After centrifugation at $12,000 \times g$ for 5 min at room temperature, mtDNA was precipitated by the addition of five volumes of ethanol ($-20°C$).

Mitochondrial DNA incubation

Mitochondrial DNA was incubated in 10 mM potassium phosphate buffer (pH 7.4) at a final volume of 0.5 ml in the presence of either H_2O_2 [100, 10, 1.0, 0.5, 0.1, 0.001, 0.00001 or 0.0 mM] or $FeSO_4$ [300, 150, 30, 15, 3.0, 1.5, or 0.0 μM] or in the presence of those two agents used together, namely $FeSO_4$ [30 μM] + H_2O_2 [100, 10, 1.0, 0.5, 0.1, 0.001, 0.00001 or 0.0 mM] or H_2O_2 [0.5 mM] + $FeSO_4$ [300, 150, 30, 15, 3.0, 1.5, or 0.0 μM]. The reaction was carried out at $37°C$ for 1 hr in a water bath. Three independent experiments were performed, and in each experiment mtDNA was isolated from twenty one (21) different thyroid glands.

Evaluation of the 8-oxo-7,8-dihydro-2'deoxyguanosine/2'-deoxyguanosine (8-oxodG/dG) ratio

After incubation, 50 μl of sodium acetate (3 M, pH 5.0) and two volumes of ethanol (20°C) were added to each sample to terminate the reaction. DNA was precipitated by centrifugation ($13,000 \times g$, 5 min); DNA was washed once with 70% ethanol. Thereafter, the DNA sample was dried and dissolved in 20 mM sodium acetate (pH 5.0); the samples were denatured by heating at 95°C for 10 min and, then, cooled on ice for 5 min. The DNA

samples were digested to nucleotides by incubation with 8 units of nuclease P_1 at 37°C for 30 min. Next, pH was adjusted by adding 20 μl of 1 M Tris–HCl and the samples were treated with 4 units of alkaline phosphatase at 37°C for 1 hr. The resulting deoxynucleoside mixture was filtered through a Millipore filter (0.22 mm) and analyzed by HPLC with electrochemical (EC) detection. The HPLC system consisted of a Smartline Pump 1000, Smartline Autosampler 3800, 250 mm × 4 mm Eurosphere-100 C18 column and electrochemical detector EC3000 with measurement cell model Sputnik. An eluent (10% aqueous methanol containing 12.5 mM citric acid, 25 mM sodium acetate, 30 mM sodium hydroxide and 10 mM acetic acid) was used at a flow rate of 1 ml/min. The quantities of 8-oxo-7,8-dihydro-2'-deoxyguanosine (8-oxodG) and of 2'-deoxyguanosine (dG) were measured using two oxidative potentials (600 mV, 900 mV, respectively). The results are expressed as the ratio of 8-oxodG to dG $\times 10^5$.

Statistical analyses

Results represent means ± SE. Data were statistically analyzed, using a one-way analysis at variance (ANOVA), followed by the Student-Neuman-Keuls' test. The level of $p < 0.05$ was accepted as statistically significant.

Results

The incubation of mtDNA in the presence of either H_2O_2 (Figure 1) or ferrous ions (Figure 2) increased the level of oxidative damage, namely the level of 8-oxodG increased significantly when H_2O_2 was used in the highest concentration of 100 mM (Figure 1), and Fe^{2+} increased 8-oxodG level in concentration-dependent manner (for concentrations of 300, 150, 30 μM) (Figure 2).

When Fe^{2+} [30 μM] was used together with different concentrations of H_2O_2, 8-oxodG level in mtDNA increased significantly in H_2O_2 concentration-dependent manner (Figure 3). When comparing Figures 1 and 3, the damaging effect of both substrates used together has been much more stronger comparing to damaging effect of H_2O_2 alone. First, the range of H_2O_2 concentrations [100 mM, 10 mM and 1 mM], which have increased 8-oxodG level, is wider in the presence of Fe^{2+}. Second, 8-oxodG level is approximately 4 × higher in the presence of H_2O_2 [100 mM] plus Fe^{2+} when compared to the effect of H_2O_2 [100 mM] alone. This suggests that the addition of Fe^{2+} strongly enhanced the effect of H_2O_2.

In turn, when H_2O_2 [0.5 mM] was used together with different concentrations of Fe^{2+}, 8-oxodG level in mtDNA increased significantly in Fe^{2+} concentration-dependent manner (Figure 4). These effect was observed for exactly the same concentrations [300, 150 and 30 μM], as when ferrous ion was used separately (compare with Figure 2). However, 8-oxodG level was above

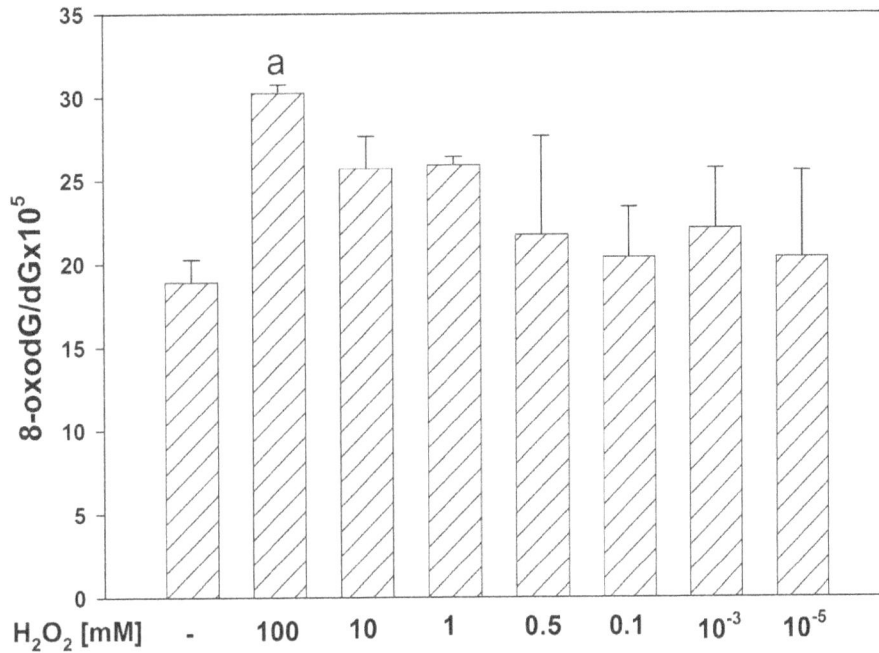

Figure 1 Oxidative damage to mitochondrial DNA in porcine thyroid. mtDNA was incubated in the presence of H_2O_2 alone [100, 10, 1.0, 0.5, 0.1, 0.001, 0.00001 mM]. Data are expressed as the ratio 8-oxodG/dGx10^5. Data are from three independent experiments. Values are expressed as mean ± SE (error bars). [a]p = 0.05 vs. control (in the absence of H_2O_2).

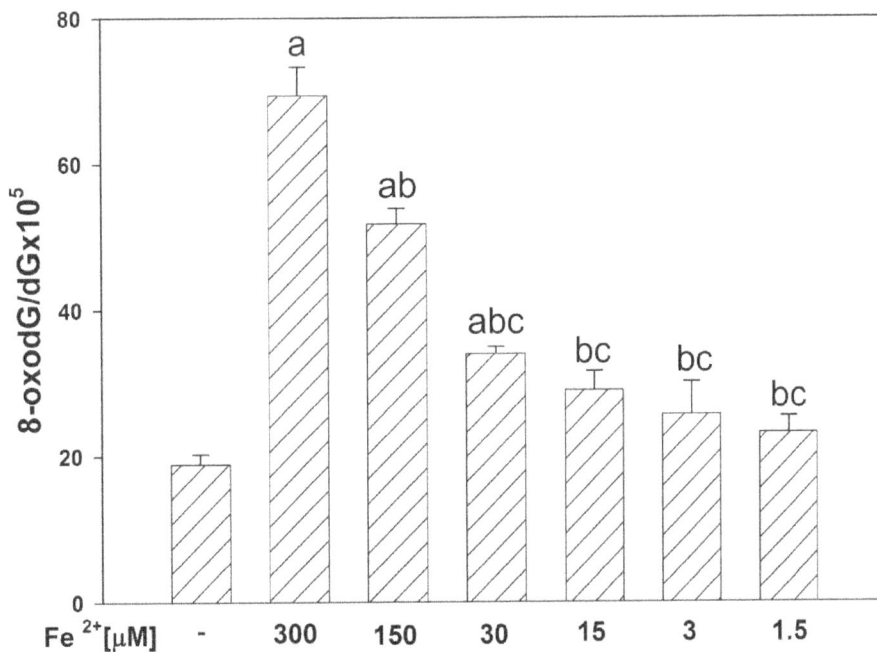

Figure 2 Oxidative damage to mitochondrial DNA in porcine thyroid. mtDNA was incubated in the presence of $FeSO_4$ (Fe^{2+}) alone [300, 150, 30, 15, 3.0, 1.5 µM]. Data are expressed as the ratio 8-oxodG/dGx10^5. Data are from three independent experiments. Values are expressed as mean ± SE (error bars). [a]p = 0.05 vs. control (in the absence of Fe^{2+}), [b]p = 0.05 vs. 300 µM, [c]p = 0.05 vs. 150 µM.

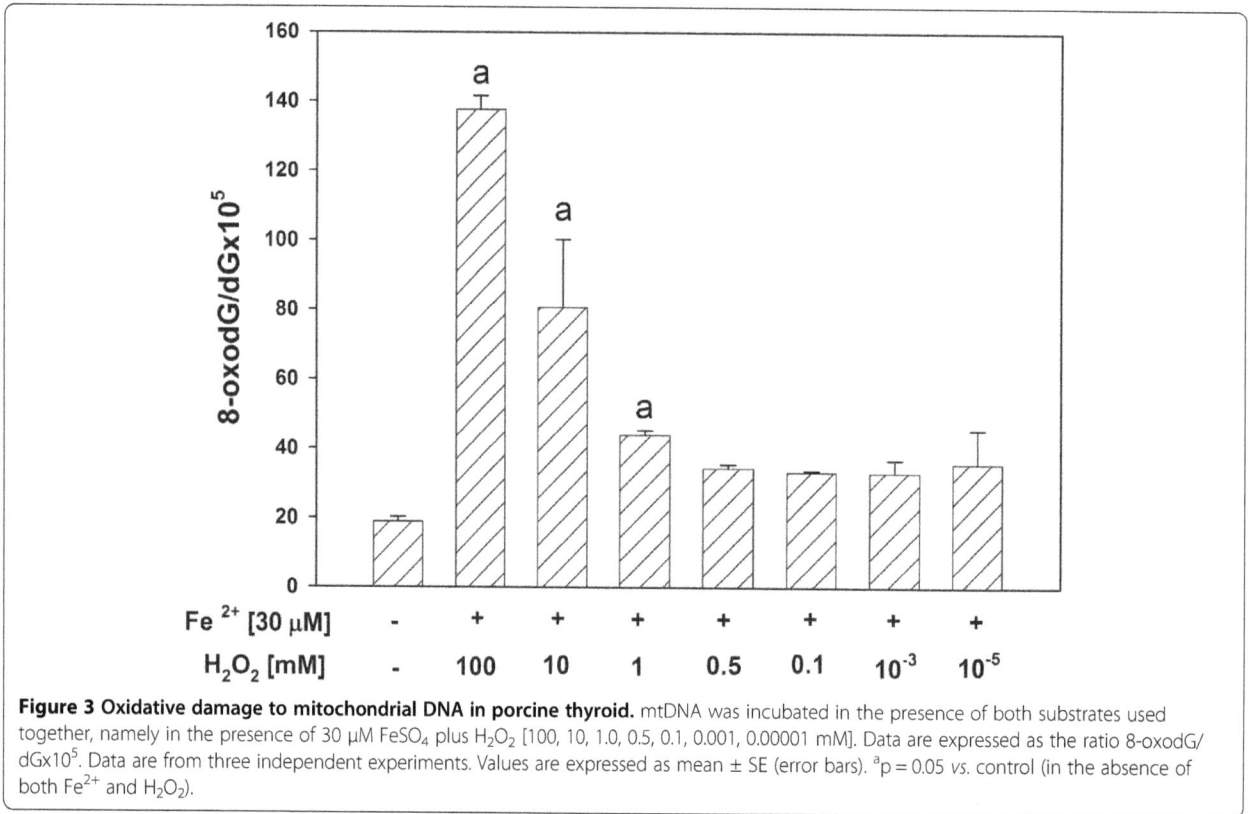

Figure 3 Oxidative damage to mitochondrial DNA in porcine thyroid. mtDNA was incubated in the presence of both substrates used together, namely in the presence of 30 μM FeSO$_4$ plus H$_2$O$_2$ [100, 10, 1.0, 0.5, 0.1, 0.001, 0.00001 mM]. Data are expressed as the ratio 8-oxodG/dGx10^5. Data are from three independent experiments. Values are expressed as mean ± SE (error bars). [a]p = 0.05 vs. control (in the absence of both Fe^{2+} and H$_2$O$_2$).

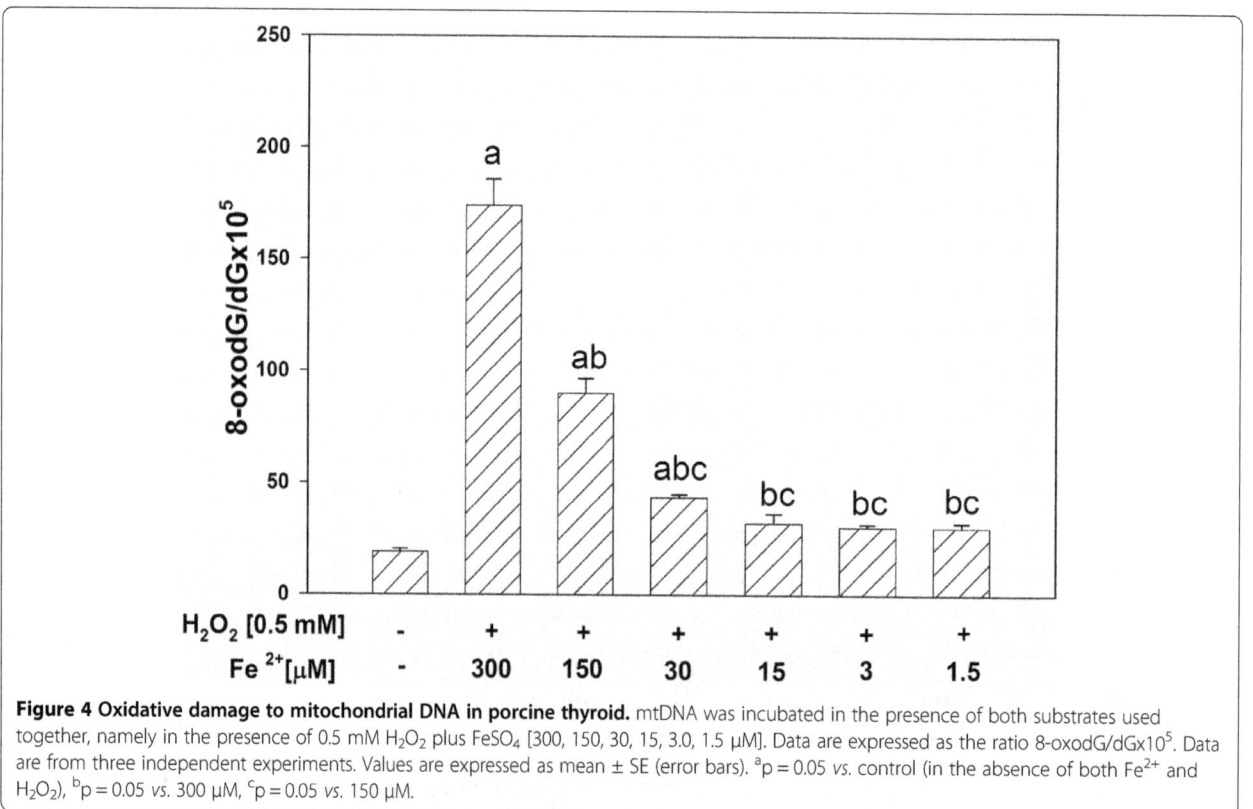

Figure 4 Oxidative damage to mitochondrial DNA in porcine thyroid. mtDNA was incubated in the presence of both substrates used together, namely in the presence of 0.5 mM H$_2$O$_2$ plus FeSO$_4$ [300, 150, 30, 15, 3.0, 1.5 μM]. Data are expressed as the ratio 8-oxodG/dGx10^5. Data are from three independent experiments. Values are expressed as mean ± SE (error bars). [a]p = 0.05 vs. control (in the absence of both Fe^{2+} and H$_2$O$_2$), [b]p = 0.05 vs. 300 μM, [c]p = 0.05 vs. 150 μM.

2 × higher in the presence of Fe^{2+} [300 μM] plus H_2O_2 [0.5 mM] (Figure 4) than in the presence of Fe^{2+} [300 μM] alone (Figure 2). The difference between damaging effects of $Fe^{2+} + H_2O_2$ and Fe^{2+} alone is not so obvious for two other lower Fe^{2+} concentrations, namely for 150 μM and 30 μM. The results suggest that the addition of H_2O_2 enhanced the effect of Fe^{2+}.

It should be stressed that Fe^{2+} intensified the damaging effect of H_2O_2 stronger than H_2O_2 intensified the damaging effect of Fe^{2+}.

Discussion

In mitochondrial and nuclear DNA, 8-oxodG is the most abundant oxidatively damaged product following the exposure to free radicals, and – therefore – it is widely used as a biomarker of oxidative stress and carcinogenesis. According to our knowledge, this study is the first one, in which the level of oxidized nucleosides in mtDNA in the thyroid gland has been measured. The fact that the attempt to measure oxidative damage to mtDNA in the thyroid has not been undertaken before may be due to technical difficulties occurring during mtDNA isolation from the thyroid. In the process of mtDNA isolation significant amount of the mtDNA is lost, especially at the step of isolation of the whole mitochondria; therefore, much more tissue is required and the procedure is more time-consuming, comparing to nuclear DNA isolation.

When designing this study, we expected that physiological damage to mtDNA would be much higher than that one to nuclear DNA. Expectedly, the background oxidative damage to mtDNA in the present study (8-oxodG/dG×10^5 = from 15.96 to 21.32) was approximately ten (10) times higher than to nuclear DNA, the latter being observed in our earlier study (8-oxodG/dG×10^5 = from 2.24 to 2.80) [27]. These results are in agreement with data already presented in numerous published studies concerning other tissues. Values for the ratio of mitochondrial to nuclear levels of 8-oxodG range from 2 (in human fibroblasts) [28] to 16 (in rat liver) [24]. That significantly higher background oxidative damage in mtDNA appears to represent evidence for more extensive oxidation of mtDNA comparing to nuclear DNA under physiological conditions. Main reasons for higher sensitivity to oxidative stress of mtDNA, comparing to nuclear DNA, comprise mentioned above such characteristics as proximity of mtDNA to the mitochondrial electron transport chain, being a site of superoxide anion ($O_2^{-\bullet}$) and H_2O_2 generation, as well as the lack of protective histones. It should be also stressed that mtDNA does not possess introns, therefore, the whole mtDNA – when exposed to free radicals – can be damaged.

It should be mentioned that in the last years certain doubts arose concerning the reliability of the measurement of mtDNA oxidation. The question to what extent mitochondrial 8-oxodG levels, measured in experimental conditions, correspond to those typical for physiological conditions (in the living organism) has not been yet adequately answered. Some authors argue, that additional oxidative damage might be induced during the procedure of mitochondria isolation. According to this hypothesis, during the process of mitochondria isolation, organelles may continue to generate oxygen radicals which can contribute to increase *ex vivo* oxidation. Moreover, mitochondria contain large quantities of heme protein with redox-active iron atom, which also may cause extensive oxidation during the isolation [29]. However, it should be underlined that the above hypothesis has not been univocally proved. In turn, even if any additional oxidation occurs during mitochondria isolation or, later on, before 8-oxodG measurement, it is still unknown to what extent such an oxidation contributes to the final result. High ratio of mitochondrial/nuclear 8-oxodG, mentioned above and described for different tissues [29], as well as the value of that ratio equal to 10, as observed by us in the thyroid in the present study, support the statement that oxidative damage to mtDNA is much stronger than that directed against nuclear DNA.

Another aspect which should be discussed in the present study is the sensitivity of thyroid mtDNA to Fenton reaction substrates. In our present study, addition of a single Fenton reaction substrate was sufficient to increase 8-oxodG level in mtDNA. The damaging effects of Fenton reaction substrates, when used separately, suggest that exogenous ferrous ion and exogenous H_2O_2 reacted with the other substrate present already (physiologically) in mtDNA. Thus, the exposure to only one of these factors can cause oxidative damage to mtDNA. When both Fenton reaction substrates were applied together, elevations in 8-oxodG levels were, expectedly, higher than those when they were used separately. It should be stressed that ferrous ion revealed stronger damaging effect than H_2O_2, both when the substrates were used separately or were applied together. The results on oxidative mtDNA damage suggest that in the thyroid gland iron is a more potent prooxidative factor, when compared to H_2O_2. These results are in agreement with our observation for nuclear DNA and also for membrane lipids in our previous study [27]. In turn, as regards the response of nuclear DNA [27] and mtDNA (the present study) to Fenton reaction substrates, mtDNA seems to be less vulnerable. Such results have been expected, as macromolecules with physiologically high oxidative damage are usually less sensitive to additional oxidative abuse. However, the differences in the oxidative response of mtDNA and nuclear DNA are not obvious enough to draw final conclusions as to which of these two kinds of DNA is more sensitive to Fenton reaction substrates.

What is a clinical significance of the present findings is not clear enough. Our results show that excessive amounts of Fe^{2+} or H_2O_2 contribute to the increased oxidative damage to mtDNA which, in turn, can lead to mutations, impairment of electron transport chain and loss of mitochondrial functions. Decline of the mitochondria respiratory functions is generally accepted as an important contributor to aging and wide range of degenerative diseases. Dysfunction of mitochondria are also suggested to be a predominant feature in oncocytic tumor transformation. Oncocytic neoplasms are the tumours composed of cells filled – almost exclusively – with mitochondria characterized by molecular and enzymatic abnormalities. They mainly occur in endocrine and exocrine tissues but also have been observed in other organs [23,30]. In the thyroid gland, oncocytic cells (also known as Hürtle cells or oxyphilic cells) are frequently observed in benign and malignant tumors, as well as in chronic inflammatory conditions or in hyperplastic lesions. Hürtle cells are characterized by blocked apoptosis, probably as a consequence of mitochondrial abnormalities. The main reason responsible for oncocytic transformation can be compensatory mechanism, in which the activation of mitochondrial biogenesis pathways constitutes the response to metabolic stress, caused by loss of mitochondrial function. This leads to increase of mitochondrial mass and further intensifies oxidative stress.

Oxidative stress is hypothesized to play a crucial role in thyroid cancer, especially in papillary thyroid carcinoma, initiation [31]. However, the present results allow to propose that oxidative processes substantially contribute to formation of tumors, with oxyphilic type of follicular thyroid carcinoma being of special significance. The frequency of this type of cancer is much lower than one should expect, taking into account huge oxidative damage to mtDNA under normal conditions. It is assumed that – due to enormous oxidative stress in mitochondria – defense mechanisms are perfectly developed in these organelles under physiological conditions, preventing serious consequences, such as cancer. However, with additional insult, the protective mechanisms may be disrupted and the formation of ROS may be even higher, leading to the initiation of thyroid cancer, composed of cells rich in abnormal mitochondria. Further studies are required to confirm such a hypothesis.

Conclusions

The level of oxidized nucleosides in thyroid mtDNA is relatively high, when compared to nuclear DNA. Both substrates of Fenton reaction, i.e. ferrous ion and hydrogen peroxide, increase oxidative damage to mtDNA,

with stronger damaging effect exerted by iron. High level of oxidative damage to mtDNA suggests its possible contribution to malignant transformation of thyroid oncocytic cells, which are known to be especially abundant in mitochondria, the latter characterized by molecular and enzymatic abnormalities.

Competing interests
Authors declare that they have no competing interests.

Authors' contributions
MK-L designed the study, supervised its conducting and prepared the final version of the manuscript. JS carried out the experiments, performed the statistical evaluation and prepared the draft of the manuscript. AL revised the final version of the manuscript. All authors read and approved the final manuscript.

Acknowledgement
The research was supported by the statutory funds No. 503/1-107-03/503-01 from the Medical University of Łódź.

Author details
[1]Department of Oncological Endocrinology, Medical University of Łódź, 7/9 Żeligowski St, 90-752, Łódź, Poland. [2]Department of Endocrinology and Metabolic Diseases, Medical University of Łódź, 281/289 Rzgowska St, 93-338, Łódź, Poland. [3]Polish Mother's Memorial Hospital - Research Institute, 281/289, Rzgowska St, 93-338, Łódź, Poland.

References
1. Halliwell B: Free radicals and antioxidants: updating a personal view. *Nutr Rev* 2012, **70:**257–265.
2. Ray PD, Huang BW, Tsuji Y: Reactive oxygen species (ROS) homeostasis and redox regulation in cellular signaling. *Cell Signal* 2012, **24:**981–990.
3. Lau AT, Wang Y, Chiu JF: Reactive oxygen species: current knowledge and applications in cancer research and therapeutic. *J Cell Biochem* 2008, **104:**657–667.
4. Valko M, Leibfritz D, Moncol J, Cronin MT, Mazur M, Telser J: Free radicals and antioxidants in normal physiological functions and human disease. *Int J Biochem Cell Biol* 2007, **39:**44–84.
5. Ziech D, Franco R, Pappa A, Panayiotidis MI: Reactive oxygen species (ROS)-induced genetic and epigenetic alterations in human carcinogenesis. *Mutat Res* 2011, **711:**167–173.
6. Karbownik M, Lewiński A: Melatonin reduces Fenton reaction-induced lipid peroxidation in porcine thyroid tissue. *J Cell Biochem* 2003, **90:**806–811.
7. Dupuy C, Ohayon R, Valent A, Noel-Hudson MS, Deme D, Virion A: Purification of a novel flavoprotein involved in the thyroid NADPH oxidase: cloning of the porcine and human cDNAs. *J Biol Chem* 1999, **274:**37265–37269.
8. Weyemi U, Caillou B, Talbot M, Ameziane-El-Hassani R, Lacroix L, Lagent-Chevallier O, Al Ghuzlan A, Roos D, Bidart JM, Virion A, Schlumberger M, Dupuy C: Intracellular expression of reactive oxygen species-generating NADPH oxidase NOX4 in normal and cancer thyroid tissues. *Endocr Relat Cancer* 2010, **17:**27–37.
9. Corvilain B, Laurent E, Lecomte M, Van Sande J, Dumont JE: Role of the cyclic adenosine 3,5-monophosphate and the phosphatidylinositol-Ca2+ cascades in mediating the effects of thyrotropin and iodide on hormone synthesis and secretion in human thyroid slices. *J Clin Endocrinol Metab* 1994, **79:**152–159.
10. Rousset B, Poncet C, Dumont JE, Mornex R: Intracellular and extracellular sites of iodination in dispersed hog thyroid cells. *Biochem J* 1980, **192:**801–812.
11. Song Y, Driessens N, Costa M, De Deken X, Detours V, Corvilain B, Maenhaut C, Miot F, Van Sande J, Many MC, Dumont JE: Roles of hydrogen peroxide in thyroid physiology and disease. *J Clin Endocrinol Metab* 2007, **92:**3764–3773.

12. Ruf J, Carayon P: Structural and functional aspects of thyroid peroxidase. *Arch Biochem Biophys* 2006, **445**:269–277.
13. Fayadat L, Niccoli-Sire P, Lanet J, Franc JL: Human thyroperoxidase is largely retained and rapidly degraded in the endoplasmic reticulum. Its N-glycans are required for folding and intracellular trafficking. *Endocrinology* 1998, **139**:4277–4285.
14. Cabrera J, Burkhardt S, Tan DX, Manchester LC, Karbownik M, Reiter RJ: Autoxidation and toxicant-induced oxidation of lipid and DNA in monkey liver: reduction of molecular damage by melatonin. *Pharmacol Toxicol* 2001, **89**:225–230.
15. Gitto E, Tan DX, Reiter RJ, Karbownik M, Manchester LC, Cuzzocrea S, Fulia F, Barberi I: Individual and synergistic antioxidative actions of melatonin: studies with vitamin E, vitamin C, glutathione and desferrioxamine (desferoxamine) in rat liver homogenates. *J Pharm Pharmacol* 2001, **53**:1393–1401.
16. Karbownik M, Reiter RJ, Garcia JJ, Tan D: Melatonin reduces phenylhydrazine-induced oxidative damage to cellular membranes: evidence for the involvement of iron. *Int J Biochem Cell Biol* 2000, **32**:1045–1054.
17. Karbownik M, Gitto E, Lewiński A, Reiter RJ: Relative efficacies of indole antioxidants in reducing autoxidation and iron-induced lipid peroxidation in hamster testes. *J Cell Biochem* 2001, **81**:693–699.
18. Karbownik M, Lewiński A, Reiter RJ: Anticarcinogenic actions of melatonin which involve antioxidative processes: comparison with other antioxidants. *Int J Biochem Cell Biol* 2001, **33**:735–753.
19. Karbownik-Lewińska M, Stępniak J, Krawczyk J, Zasada K, Szosland J, Gesing A, Lewiński A: External hydrogen peroxide is not indispensable for experimental induction of lipid peroxidation via Fenton reaction in porcine ovary homogenates. *Neuro Endocrinol Lett* 2010, **31**:343–347.
20. Mehta R, Dedina L, O'Brien PJ: Rescuing hepatocytes from iron-catalyzed oxidative stress using vitamins B1 and B6. *Toxicol In Vitro* 2011, **25**:1114–1122.
21. Natoli M, Felsani A, Ferruzza S, Sambuy Y, Canali R, Scarino ML: Mechanisms of defence from Fe(II) toxicity in human intestinal Caco-2 cells. *Toxicol In Vitro* 2009, **23**:1510–1515.
22. Qi W, Reiter RJ, Tan DX, Garcia JJ, Manchester LC, Karbownik M, Calvo JR: Chromium(III)-induced 8-hydroxydeoxyguanosine in DNA and its reduction by antioxidants: comparative effects of melatonin, ascorbate, and vitamin E. *Environ Health Perspect* 2000, **108**:399–402.
23. Gasparre G, Romeo G, Rugolo M, Porcelli AM: Learning from oncocytic tumors: Why choose inefficient mitochondria? *Biochim Biophys Acta* 2011, **1807**:633–642.
24. Richter C, Park JW, Ames BN: Normal oxidative damage to mitochondrial and nuclear DNA is extensive. *Proc Natl Acad Sci USA* 1988, **85**:6465–6467.
25. Wallace DC: Mitochondrial DNA mutations in disease and aging. *Environ Mol Mutagen* 2010, **51**:440–450.
26. Tamura K, Aotsuka T: Rapid isolation method of animal mitochondrial DNA by the alkaline lysis procedure. *Biochem Genet* 1988, **26**:815–819.
27. Stępniak J, Lewiński A, Karbownik-Lewińska M: Membrane lipids and nuclear DNA are differently susceptive to Fenton reaction substrates in porcine thyroid. *Toxicol In Vitro* 2013, **27**:71–78.
28. Yakes FM, Van Houten B: Mitochondrial DNA damage is more extensive and persists longer than nuclear DNA damage in human cells following oxidative stress. *Proc Natl Acad Sci USA* 1997, **94**:514–519.
29. Beckman KB, Ames BN: Endogenous oxidative damage of mtDNA. *Mutat Res* 1999, **424**:51–58.
30. Máximo V, Lima J, Prazeres H, Soares P, Sobrinho-Simões M: The biology and the genetics of Hurthle cell tumors of the thyroid. *Endocr Relat Cancer* 2012, **19**:R131–R147.
31. Detours V, Delys L, Libert F, Weiss Solís D, Bogdanova T, Dumont JE, Franc B, Thomas G, Maenhaut C: Genome-wide gene expression profiling suggests distinct radiation susceptibilities in sporadic and post-Chernobyl papillary thyroid cancers. *Br J Cancer* 2007, **97**:818–825.

7

Iodine intake as a risk factor for thyroid cancer: a comprehensive review of animal and human studies

Michael B. Zimmermann[1][*] and Valeria Galetti[2]

Abstract

Thyroid cancer (TC) is the most common endocrine malignancy and in most countries, incidence rates are increasing. Although differences in population iodine intake are a determinant of benign thyroid disorders, the role of iodine intake in TC remains uncertain. We review the evidence linking iodine intake and TC from animal studies, ecological studies of iodine intake and differentiated and undifferentiated TC, iodine intake and mortality from TC and occult TC at autopsy, as well as the case–control and cohort studies of TC and intake of seafood and milk products. We perform a new meta-analysis of pooled measures of effect from case–control studies of total iodine intake and TC. Finally, we examine the post-Chernobyl studies linking iodine status and risk of TC after radiation exposure. The available evidence suggests iodine deficiency is a risk factor for TC, particularly for follicular TC and possibly, for anaplastic TC. This conclusion is based on: a) consistent data showing an increase in TC (mainly follicular) in iodine deficient animals; b) a plausible mechanism (chronic TSH stimulation induced by iodine deficiency); c) consistent data from before and after studies of iodine prophylaxis showing a decrease in follicular TC and anaplastic TC; d) the indirect association between changes in iodine intake and TC mortality in the decade from 2000 to 2010; e) the autopsy studies of occult TC showing higher microcarcinoma rates with lower iodine intakes; and f) the case control studies suggesting lower risk of TC with higher total iodine intakes.

Keywords: Iodine deficiency, Iodine excess, Iodine status, Iodized salt, Iodine supplement, Urinary iodine, Goiter, Nodule, Thyroid cancer

Introduction

Thyroid cancer (TC) is the most common endocrine malignancy and in most countries, incidence rates have been steadily increasing over the past few decades, particularly in women. In 2012, the age standardized (world population) incidence rate was 6.1/100,000 women and 1.9/100,000 men [1]. Comparing populations around the world, there is a greater than ten-fold difference in incidence; high incidence areas (incidence rates greater than 10/100,000 women) are Japan and the Pacific Islands, Italy and several countries in the Americas. Incidence rates in developed countries are more than twofold higher than in developing countries (in women, 11.1/

100,000 versus 4.7/100,000) [1]. If recent trends continue, thyroid cancer will be the fourth most common cancer in the U.S. by 2030 [2]. Papillary thyroid cancer (PTC) is by far the most prevalent subtype, in most countries accounting for greater than 80 % of thyroid cancer, but anaplastic thyroid cancer (ATC), because of its poor prognosis, accounts for a large portion of the mortality. Increased screening and diagnostic testing is likely the major, but may not be the only, contributor to the rising incidence of thyroid cancer [3–7]. Suspected risk factors include radiation exposure during childhood (whether from nuclear accidents, natural radiation or medical imaging) [8–10], obesity and the metabolic syndrome [11, 12], environmental pollutants [13, 14], a family history of thyroid cancer or thyroid disorders [15], and possibly, iodine intake.

It is clear that variations in population iodine intake are a primary determinant of benign thyroid disorders,

* Correspondence: michael.zimmermann@hest.ethz.ch
[1]Laboratory of Human Nutrition, Department of Health Sciences and Technology, ETH Zürich, Schmelzbergstrasse 7, LFV D21, CH-8092 Zürich, Switzerland
Full list of author information is available at the end of the article

such as goiter, nodules, and hyper- and hypothyroidism [16]. In contrast, the role of iodine intake in thyroid cancer remains uncertain, despite decades of study and debate. At the 1927 International Conference on Goiter, the eminent pathologist Carl Wegelin argued that thyroid cancer was more common in areas of endemic goiter, with frequency at autopsy varying from 1.04 per cent in central Switzerland, an endemic goiter region, to 0.09 per cent in Berlin, a non-endemic region [17]. He predicted a drop in incidence of thyroid cancer as endemic goiter disappeared due to iodized salt, with a lag time of 30 to 40 years. Iodized salt was introduced into a handful of countries in the 1920s and then increasingly since the 1960s; in 2015, around 100 countries have national iodized salt programs [18]. Although there has been a decrease in the prevalence of ATC in many of these countries, at the same time the incidence of PTC has increased, particularly since the 1980s, as discussed below. Because of this temporal pattern, several authors have suggested increasing iodine intakes are contributing to the increase in PTC, while others disagree.

The prevalence of goiter and thyroid nodules is higher in iodine deficient populations [19] and goiter and nodularity, in many cases, precede the development of thyroid cancer [20]. In animal studies, chronic thyroid-stimulating hormone (TSH) stimulation produces thyroid tumors, and because an increase in TSH is an adaptation to iodine deficiency, one might expect this could be the mechanism for an increased incidence of thyroid cancer in iodine deficient populations [21]. However, mean TSH may be actually lower in mildly iodine deficient populations than in populations with higher iodine intakes [16], and the highest incidence rates for thyroid cancer are in Japan, where iodine intake is high [22]. On the other hand, mortality from thyroid cancer tends to be higher in regions of endemic goiter because of more frequent advanced tumor stages at diagnosis and an increased ratio of more aggressive subtypes. Clearly, the links between iodine intake and thyroid cancer are complex, and are discussed in detail in this review.

Recommended daily iodine intakes from WHO/UNICEF/ICCIDD are 90 µg for infants and young children (0–59 months), 120 µg for children 6–12 years, 150 µg for adolescents and adults, and 250 µg for pregnant and lactating women [23]. To assess iodine intakes and status of populations, WHO recommend the use of spot urine collections to measure the urinary iodine concentration (UIC), expressed as the median in µg/L. National UIC surveys are often done in school-aged children because they are easy to reach through school-based surveys and their iodine status can be used as a proxy for the non-pregnant adult population [23]. The median UIC is an excellent biomarker of recent exposure to iodine in populations, because it reflects intake from all dietary sources [24]. The

median UIC criteria for iodine nutrition are shown in Table 1 [23]. These WHO criteria are used throughout this review to describe iodine nutrition in populations as deficient, sufficient or excessive.

Review
Animal studies
Thyroid cancer in animals fed iodine deficient or iodine excessive diets
In female rats, provision of iodine deficient diets for 6 to 20 months increases serum TSH and causes thyroid tumors in 54–100 % of animals, mainly follicular adenomas and follicular carcinomas [25–28]. Similar effects were observed in hamsters [29], where the malignancies reported were both follicular and papillary carcinomas. Correa and Welsh [30] fed rats ($n = 30$) for 9 months a diet containing excess iodine ($\approx$120 mg of iodine per day) or a control diet. There was a 40 % increase in thyroid weight, and histologic changes included enlarged follicles with increased colloid lined by flattened epithelia, but no thyroid tumors were found.

Thyroid cancer in animals fed iodine deficient or iodine excessive diets and exposed to carcinogens
Thyroid tumor-promoting effects of iodine deficiency and excess have also been investigated in two-stage models in rats given carcinogens, such as N-bis(2-hydroxypropyl)-nitrosamine (DHPN) or N-nitrosomethylurea (NMU), and provided iodine deficient or excessive diets [31–33]. In iodine deficient rats, administration of NMU induces thyroid cancer after a shorter latency period and at higher incidence and multiplicity when compared to rats only iodine deficient or to rats that received NMU but were iodine sufficient [31, 32]. Kanno et al. [33] examined the potential thyroid tumor-promoting effects of iodine deficiency and excess for 26 weeks in a 2-stage model in rats given DHPN or saline. In saline-treated rats, iodine deficiency or excess alone was not carcinogenic,

Table 1 Epidemiological criteria for assessment of iodine nutrition in populations based on median urinary iodine concentration [23, 24].

Median urinary iodine concentration (UIC)	Iodine intake	Iodine nutrition
<20 µg/L	Insufficient	Severe iodine deficiency
20–49 µg/L	Insufficient	Moderate iodine deficiency
50–99 µg/L	Insufficient	Mild iodine deficiency
100–299 µg/L	Adequate or more-than-adequate	Sufficient
≥300 µg/L	Excessive	Risk of adverse health consequences (iodine-induced hyperthyroidism, autoimmune thyroid disease)

but in DHPN-treated rats, both iodine deficiency and excess increased thyroid follicular tumors, with iodine deficiency having a markedly stronger effect (Fig. 1a). In a similar 2-stage study that exposed rats to N-nitrosobis(2-hydroxypropyl)amine (BHP) and an excessive iodine diet [34], the incidence of thyroid cancer was 29 % in those fed the excessive iodine diet versus 33 % in those fed the iodine sufficient diet. To study the effects of iodine deficiency early in life on subsequent susceptibility to thyroid carcinogens, an iodine-free diet was fed to lactating rats and their weaned offspring until postnatal week 7, and then the offspring were exposed to DHPN [35], but this did not significantly increase thyroid tumors.

Boltze et al. [36] fed rats over a period of 110 weeks high (≈10 times normal), normal, and low (≈0.1 times normal) daily iodine intake and subjected them to single external radiation of 4 gray (Gy) or sham radiation. This study differed from the animal studies described above in that the induced iodine deficiency and excess were less severe and the experiments were done in younger rats. Iodine deficiency induced a doubling of serum TSH, while iodine excess had no effect on TSH. Alone, both iodine deficiency and excess increased the thyrocyte proliferation rate and induced thyroid adenomas, but induced no thyroid carcinomas. Combined with radiation, both iodine deficiency and iodine excess induced thyroid carcinomas (PTC and follicular thyroid cancer, FTC) in 50–80 % of animals, while iodine sufficient animals did not develop thyroid carcinomas (Fig. 1b). These data suggest both long-term iodine deficiency and excess are insufficient to stimulate thyroid carcinogenesis, but both promote thyroid carcinogenesis induced by radiation.

Conclusions

Overall, these animal studies suggest that iodine deficiency acts primarily as a promoter rather than as an initiator of thyroid carcinogenesis, or as a weak complete carcinogen. Iodine excess appears not to be an initiator, but may be a weak promoter. The relevance of the thyroid tumors produced in these animal experiments to human lesions is uncertain: most of the studies induced profound iodine deficiency and excess more severe than found in human diets, and, in general, the follicular tumors show a pattern of morphology and behavior different from human thyroid cancers.

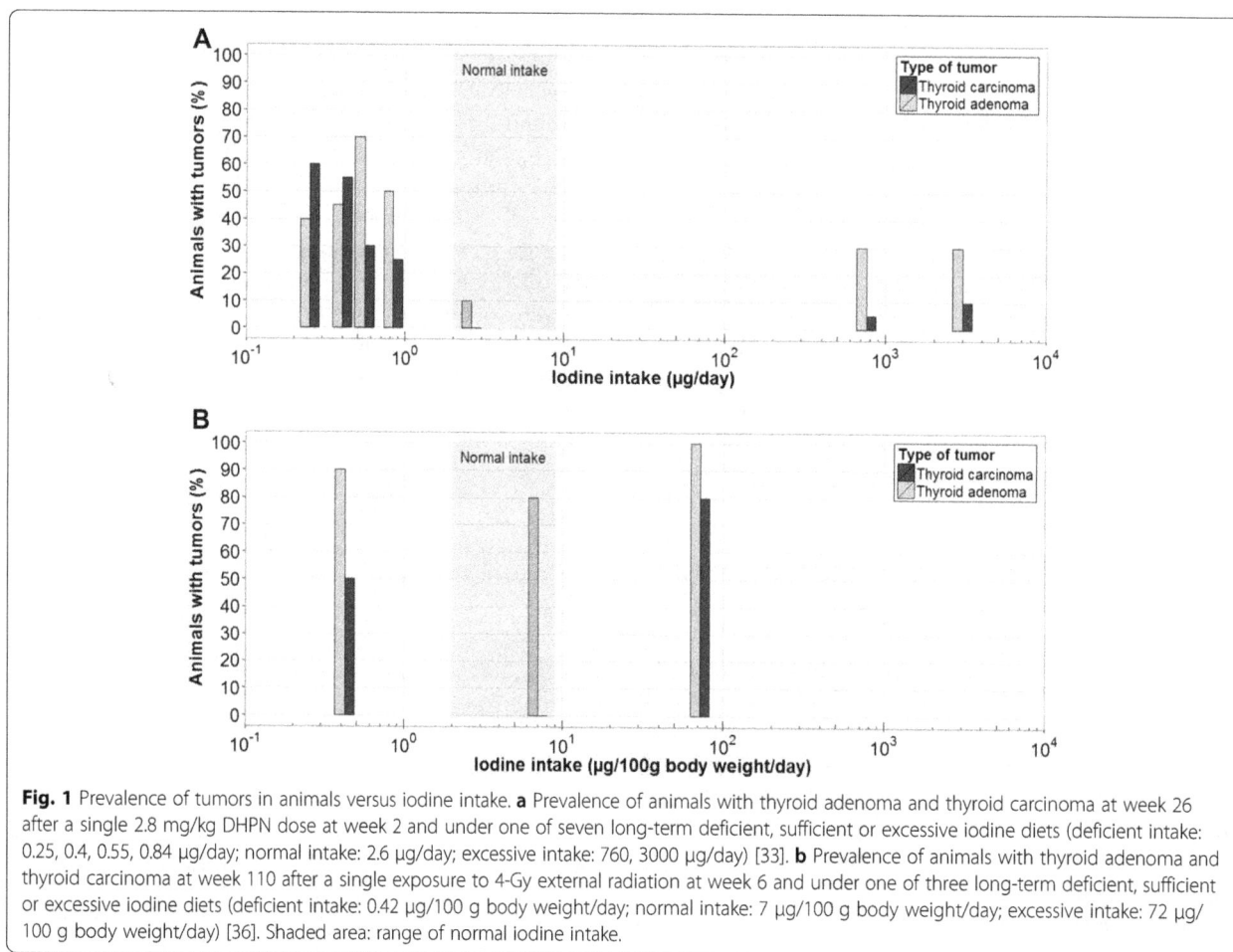

Fig. 1 Prevalence of tumors in animals versus iodine intake. a Prevalence of animals with thyroid adenoma and thyroid carcinoma at week 26 after a single 2.8 mg/kg DHPN dose at week 2 and under one of seven long-term deficient, sufficient or excessive iodine diets (deficient intake: 0.25, 0.4, 0.55, 0.84 µg/day; normal intake: 2.6 µg/day; excessive intake: 760, 3000 µg/day) [33]. b Prevalence of animals with thyroid adenoma and thyroid carcinoma at week 110 after a single exposure to 4-Gy external radiation at week 6 and under one of three long-term deficient, sufficient or excessive iodine diets (deficient intake: 0.42 µg/100 g body weight/day; normal intake: 7 µg/100 g body weight/day; excessive intake: 72 µg/ 100 g body weight/day) [36]. Shaded area: range of normal iodine intake.

Proposed mechanisms linking iodine intake and thyroid cancer

Chronic TSH stimulation in iodine deficiency

Thyroid follicular cells proliferate only slowly under normal conditions, but in iodine deficient animals, serum TSH increases and the proliferation rate of thyroid cells increases by 5 to 30-fold [36], leading to marked thyroid hyperplasia and hypertrophy. Rapidly proliferating thyrocytes are likely more vulnerable to mutagens such as radiation, chemical carcinogens and oxidative stress, and may accumulate a higher number of genetic alterations. Thyroid hyperplasia induced by iodine deficiency results in chromosomal changes in the rat thyroid, with an increased number of aneuploid cells [37]. Several authors have suggested that thyroid tumors caused by iodine deficiency are due to chronic TSH overstimulation, possibly working together with epidermal growth factor and insulin-like growth factor I [38–41]. Consistent with this hypothesis, rat studies have shown that chronic TSH stimulation induced by goitrogen-containing diets or partial thyroidectomy result in a transition from thyroid follicular adenomas to follicular carcinomas [42–44]. This hypothesis is also consistent with the findings of increased FTC and ATC in populations with severe endemic goiter, because serum TSH is increased in moderate-to-severe iodine deficiency in an effort to maintain euthyroidism [16].

Excess iodide, by inhibiting thyroid hormone production (the Wolff-Chaikoff effect), can transiently increase TSH. However, in animal studies, chronic iodine excess does not increase serum TSH [36], and, in cell studies, moderate doses of iodide inhibit thyroid cell proliferation [45]. Most humans escape from the Wolff-Chaikoff effect as intrathyroidal iodide suppresses further iodide uptake via Na/I symporter inhibition [46]. Thus, the mechanism by which iodine excess promotes thyroid tumorigenesis is uncertain. Some population studies have reported slightly higher mean serum TSH in populations with sufficient or excess iodine intakes, compared to mildly deficient populations, but this is likely due to increased toxic adenomas in mild iodine deficiency [16].

Iodine, oxidative damage and apoptosis

Other mechanisms besides chronic TSH stimulation may contribute to thyroid tumorigenesis during iodine deficiency. Iodine deficiency increases H_2O_2-mediated, reactive oxygen species (ROS) generation, which can damage DNA and result in mutations [47]. Activity of antioxidant enzyme systems, including superoxide dismutase-3, are increased in iodine deficient rat thyroids, and this is accompanied by an increase of uracil and oxidized purine or pyrimidine adducts in thyroid DNA [48]. In immortalized thyroid cell cultures (TAD-2) and primary cultures of human thyroid cells, excess molecular iodide, generated by oxidation of iodine by endogenous peroxidases, induces apoptosis through a mechanism involving generation of free radicals [49]. Providing additional iodide to human thyroid cell lines reduces generation of H_2O_2 [50]. Exposure to iodine can also cause apoptosis in human thyroid cells and thyroid carcinoma cell lines through generation of iodolactones (iodinated derivatives of fatty acids) [51, 52].

Iodine intake and the BRAF mutation in PTC

Molecular alterations identified in PTC result in the activation of proteins along the mitogen-activated protein kinase (MAPK) pathway and include point mutations of the BRAF and RAS genes and BRAF and RET rearrangements [53]. BRAF mutations or rearrangements are found in 29–83 % of PTC, but are rare in FTC [54]. Several cross-sectional studies have looked at the effects of varying iodine status on the prevalence of the BRAF mutation in PTC. A study in southern Italy compared the percentage of PTC containing the BRAF mutation in two regions, one iodine sufficient and one iodine deficient; the individual iodine status of the cases was not defined [55]. The prevalence of BRAF positive PTCs was 107 out of 270 (39.6 %) in the iodine sufficient area and 18 out of 53 (33.9 %) in the iodine deficient area (N.S.). In China the prevalence of the BRAF mutation in PTC was significantly higher (69.2 %) in cases from a region with excessive iodine intake due to iodine rich drinking water (median UIC in the population was >900 μg/L) compared to 53.3 % in PTC cases from regions with mildly deficient to sufficient iodine intakes from iodized salt (median UICs of 82–198 μg/L) [56]. The overall incidence of PTC in the different regions was not reported. In contrast, in thyroid cells expressing activated BRAF, excess iodine may exert protective effects, attenuating acute BRAF oncogene-mediated microRNA deregulation [57].

Iodine intake and RAS mutations in thyroid cancer

Mutations in the RAS genes are present in 40–53 % of FTC and 6–51 % of ATC, but are rare in PTC [54]. A cross-sectional study compared the frequency of RAS oncogene mutations in thyroid tumors (25 adenomas, 16 FTC, and 22 PTC) from cases in an iodine sufficient area in Canada to cases in a mildly iodine deficient region in Hungary [58]. The RAS oncogene mutation rate was significantly higher in adenomas (85 versus 17 %) and FTC (50 versus 10 %), from the iodine deficient area than the iodine sufficient area, with no RAS mutations detected in PTC.

Iodine and RET rearrangements in thyroid cancer

RET rearrangements are reported in 13–43 % of PTC, but are rare in ATC and have not been reported in FTC [54]. Fiore et al. [59] reported that excess iodine may play a protective role during RET/PTC3 oncogene activation in thyroid cells. They treated *RET/PTC3*-activated rat thyroid cells with 10^{-3} M sodium iodide, and found a reduction in cell proliferation and attenuation of the loss of Nis and Tshr genes and protein expression induced by *RET/PTC3* oncogene induction. When the human PTC cell line W3 and the FTC cell line FTC133 were incubated with excess iodine, progressively increasing iodine exposure first promoted (10^{-3} M iodine) and then inhibited (10^{-2} and 10^{-1} M iodine) growth and migration of thyroid cancer cells [60]. However, it should be remembered that the physiological concentration of iodine in the human thyroid is in the range of 10^{-5} to 10^{-6} M. Thus, thyrocyte exposure to iodine in these cell studies was several orders of magnitude above that encountered under physiological conditions resulting from varying dietary iodine intakes.

Iodine intake and thyroid cancer: ecological studies
Sources of potential bias
Many ecological studies have examined the relationship between iodine intake and thyroid cancer incidence and mortality. The results of these studies should be interpreted with caution, because of multiple sources of potential bias [21]. It is difficult to compare thyroid cancer incidence across cancer registries because data collection methods are usually not standardized. The rate of thyroid microcarcinomas depends largely on the frequency and intensity of histological investigation of surgical and autopsy specimens; the higher the number of sections investigated per case, the more microcarcinomas can be found [61]. There is considerable observer variation in histological typing of thyroid cancer subtypes, particularly for FTC and mixed PTC-FTC, and this limits comparisons from different studies [62]. Comparing thyroid cancer rates across different time periods is biased by differences in histological classification, due to changes in 1974 and 1988 in the WHO classification system for thyroid cancer [63]; in 1988, WHO specified that all FTC presenting a papillary component should be considered PTC, and this likely contributed to the increase in the ratio of PTC:FTC in many countries after the classification change [64].

Because of its relatively low incidence, comparing rates of thyroid cancer between populations requires long periods of observation and this increases the likelihood of confounding from other risk factors that may have changed over the same time period. Also, there is likely to be a latency period after exposure of susceptible individuals to iodine excess or deficiency and subsequent changes in the thyroid cancer incidence. The length of this latency period is not known, with experts suggesting it could be 15 to 40 years [17, 65, 66]. There is also a long latency period in the elimination of goiter in endemic populations: for example, in central Switzerland, after three

decades of salt iodization, the prevalence of goiter was <5 % in schoolchildren but was still 75 % in 50–60 year-olds [67]. An abrupt increase or decrease in population iodine intake might be expected to produce a period effect if all age groups were similarly affected, or a cohort effect if the effect were limited to a vulnerable age, such as childhood. Whether these effects confound longitudinal studies is uncertain.

It is particularly difficult to reliably compare thyroid cancer rates in populations with and without endemic goiter as a proxy for varying iodine intake. Ascertainment bias is high in these studies due to differences in the work-up of goiter and nodules, the frequency of surgical operations, and the indication for operation and preoperative diagnostic methods. The ratio of surgically removed goiters to non-operated goiters tends to be higher in non-endemic areas, because willingness of patients and physicians to perform operations is usually lower in endemic goiter areas. Also, because presence of a thyroid nodule has a higher likelihood of malignancy in iodine sufficient areas free of endemic goiter, there may be differences in diagnostic work-up [21].

Finally, in many countries, the introduction of iodized salt and an increase in iodine intake has coincided with the more widespread use of improved thyroid diagnostic tools (e.g., ultrasound, fine-needle biopsy and thyroid scintigraphy) and corresponding increases in incidence of PTC, often clinically silent. In France, an increase in the use of thyroid ultrasound in patients referred for evaluation of a thyroid disorder (from 3 to 85 %) and of cytology (from 4.5 to 23%) was associated with an increase in PTC incidence [68]. This introduces strong ascertainment bias in longitudinal or before and after studies favoring a higher incidence of PTC in more recent surveys. Thus, evidence from older longitudinal studies done before this increase in diagnostic intensity may be more valid than newer studies.

Iodine intake and differentiated thyroid cancer
Differentiated thyroid cancer, comprising PTC, FTC and, rarely, Hürthle cell thyroid cancer, makes up about 95 % of all thyroid cancers. The following section discusses the possible links between changes in iodine intake and changes in rates of differentiated thyroid cancer in selected countries. In this section, Fig. 2a-c that plot country data on median UIC as a proxy for iodine intake versus incidence of thyroid cancer use comparable data from the Cancer Incidence in Five Continents (CI5) up to 2007 [69].

The U.S.
Based on the national UIC data from successive National Health and Nutrition Examination Surveys (NHANES I-III), the U.S. population had excessive iodine intake in

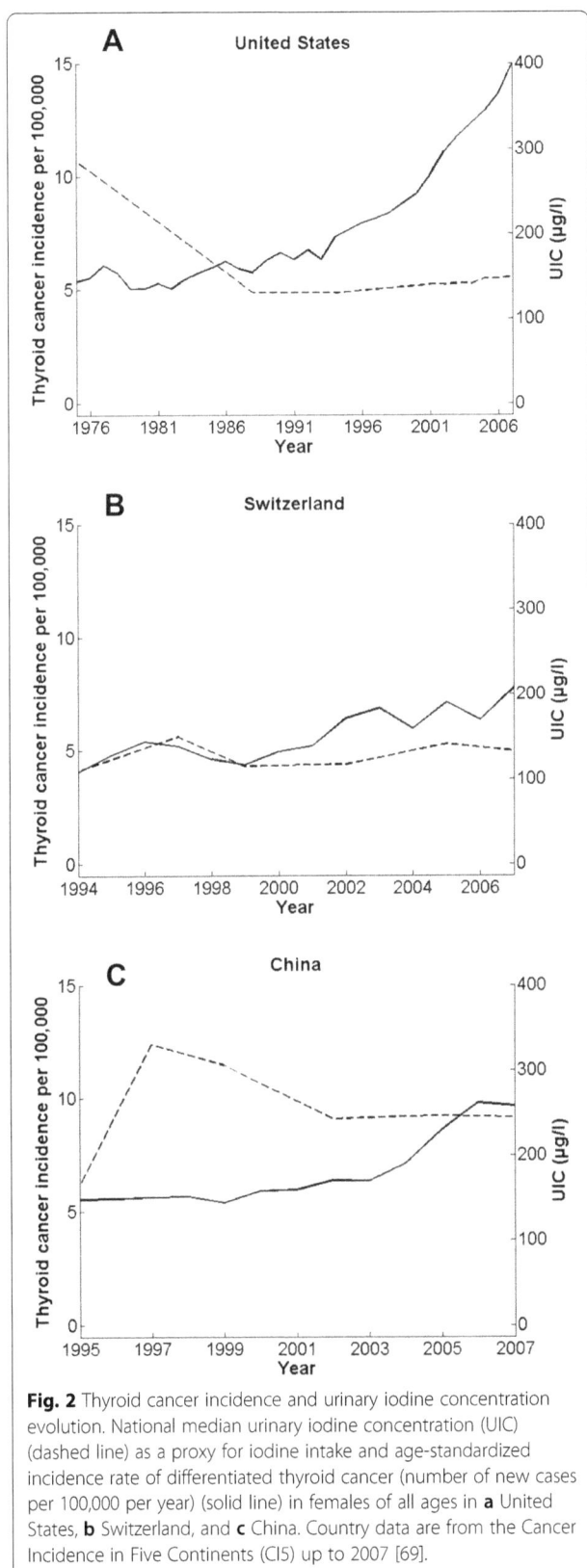

Fig. 2 Thyroid cancer incidence and urinary iodine concentration evolution. National median urinary iodine concentration (UIC) (dashed line) as a proxy for iodine intake and age-standardized incidence rate of differentiated thyroid cancer (number of new cases per 100,000 per year) (solid line) in females of all ages in a United States, b Switzerland, and c China. Country data are from the Cancer Incidence in Five Continents (CI5) up to 2007 [69].

the early 1970s (a median UIC of 320 μg/L), a more than 50 % decrease in iodine intakes to a median UIC of 145 μg/L in 1988 through 1994 [70], followed by sufficient and stable intakes during the period 2000–2010, with females having a median UIC of 142 μg/L and males a median UIC of 176 μg/L [71]. During this same period, incidence of thyroid cancer in the U.S. has been increasing by 6.6 % annually, and from 1973 to 2013, the annual incidence has increased by more than 500 % [72]. Thus, as shown in Fig. 2a, over past 4 decades in the U.S., while national iodine intakes have fallen from excess levels of intake to stabilize in the adequate range, there has been a steady increase in national incidence of differentiated thyroid cancer.

Northern Europe

Petersson et al. [73], using maps of goiter prevalence in Sweden from the 1930s to define iodine deficient versus iodine sufficient areas, found that during the period of 1958–1981, the relative risk of developing thyroid cancer was 0.92 in Swedish regions that were historically iodine deficient versus iodine sufficient. However, there was likely misclassification of exposure status as low-level iodine prophylaxis had been introduced in the formerly deficient areas before the study period. During the study period, the iodization level in salt was increased from 10 to 50 ppm and the iodine level in cattle feed supplements was increased, yet incidence rates of PTC increased similarly in both the iodine deficient and iodine sufficient regions, suggesting that the increasing rates were not related to original differences in iodine intakes.

Denmark introduced mandatory national fortification of salt used for bread making in 2000 and >90 % of Danish bread now contains iodized salt. This has improved iodine intakes but adults remain mildly iodine deficient with a median UIC of 83 μg/L because the fortification level is low, at 13 ppm [74]. The mean annual increase in the incidence of thyroid cancer in Denmark from 1943 to 2008 was 1.7 % in men and 1.8 % in women and was almost exclusively PTC [75]. The strongest increase in incidence began in the years before the iodization of salt, likely due to increased diagnostic activity. Because of differences in groundwater iodine content, before the introduction of iodized salt, the eastern part of Denmark was mildly iodine deficient (median UIC of 61 μg/L), while the western part was moderately deficient (median UIC of 45 μg/L). Although palpable goiter was found in 14.6 % in the area of moderate iodine deficiency versus 9.8 % in the area of mild deficiency [76], there were no regional differences in the overall incidence of thyroid cancer [77]. Also, the introduction of iodized salt did not result in a greater increase in the incidence of PTC in moderately iodine deficient western Denmark compared to eastern Denmark, suggesting that variations in iodine status are not a primary risk factor for thyroid cancer in the country [77].

In the Netherlands, the incidence of PTC has increased by only 2.1 % per year between 1989 and 2003, a less pronounced increase than in many other countries [78]. This might be partly explained by the stable and sufficient iodine intake of the Dutch population during the last 4 decades, together with the low level of radiation exposure and possibly the more conservative approach to incidentally discovered thyroid nodules [78].

The incidence of thyroid cancer is high in Iceland, a country with excess iodine intake from seafood and milk. In a study of surgical specimens for the period of 1944 to 1964 comparing Iceland and northern Scotland (where iodine intakes were presumed to be adequate), the PTC:FTC ratio was 6.5 in Iceland and 3.6 in Scotland [79]. The age-specific incidence rates for papillary carcinoma were approximately five times higher in Iceland than in Scotland in adults older than 35 years of age. It was hypothesized that high iodine intakes contribute to the high incidence of thyroid cancer in Iceland [79], but other authors have argued the high rates are due to the volcanic nature of the island [21]. Natural radiation is higher in volcanic areas, and radiation is known to increase risk for thyroid cancer, especially when the radiation occurs in childhood [21].

Central Europe

To correct severe endemic goiter and cretinism, iodized salt was introduced to northeastern Switzerland in 1923, and gradually spread to all Swiss cantons. In 1962, the iodine content in salt was increased from 5 to 10 ppm. A study analyzing more than 90'000 surgical specimens using the 1974 WHO classification reported a significant shift in the distribution of thyroid cancer subtypes comparing the period 1925 through 1941 to the period 1962 through 1973 [67]. In the former period, using age-adjusted data, 40 % of thyroid cancer was FTC, 38 % ATC and only 8 % was PTC. In the later period, 33 % were PTC, 30 % were FTC and 24 % were ATC. In a review of Swiss studies before 1973, the female:male ratio of thyroid cancer in areas of endemic goiter was 1.4 to 1.6, compared to those areas goiter-free or areas with iodized salt programs, where the female:male ratio was 2.1 to 3.0 [67]. In Geneva, between 1970–74 and 1995–98, when the iodine content and distribution of iodized salt did not change, the incidence of PTC increased from 0.7 to 1.8/100,000 for men and from 3.1 to 4.3/100,000 for women [64]. The authors suggested that the increasing incidence of PTC was mainly due to improved screening and diagnostic activity [64]. Figure 2b shows the relationship between Swiss national UIC data and national incidence of thyroid cancer for the period of 1994–2007; while iodine intakes in the population have remained stable, the prevalence of thyroid cancer has steadily increased.

In Germany, between 2003 and 2008, during which the country had sufficient iodine intakes from voluntary iodization of salt, the incidence rate of thyroid cancer rose from 2.7 to 3.4 (men) and from 6.5 to 8.9 (women) per 100,000 per year and was mainly PTC [80]. The incidence rate was higher in southern Germany, and the authors suggested this might be attributed in part to long-standing differences of iodine intake between different German regions, with the southern part of the country historically an area of iodine deficiency and endemic goiter.

Iodized salt was introduced into Austria in 1962 at a fortification level of 10 ppm. A study of thyroid cancer in surgical specimens in central Austria from 1952 to 1975 showed a significant increase in differentiated thyroid cancer and in the ratio of PTC:FTC, from 0.2 in 1952–1959 to 0.87 in 1970 to 1975 [66].

Southern Europe

Italy has one of the highest incidence rates for thyroid cancer; in 2007, the age-standardized (world population) incidence rate in women was nearly 20 per 100,000 women [1]. An Italian study analyzed thyroid cancer incidence from 25 cancer registries throughout the country between 1991 and 2005, before the national salt iodization program was introduced [81]. Populations located near the Alps and the Apennine Mountain Ranges, where iodine in soil and water is lowest, had low incidence rates for PTC compared to areas with higher iodine intake. However, the authors suggested this distribution of PTC was likely explained by local differences in medical surveillance, rather than iodine intake [81]. In a population-based study of ≈5600 subjects in Sicily in two regions with different iodine intakes during the period 1980 to 1990, surgery was performed in 792 patients on the basis of fine-needle biopsy of cold thyroid nodules. The frequency of thyroid cancer in patients with cold nodules was 5.3 % in the iodine sufficient area (mean UIC 114 μg/L) and 2.7 % in the iodine deficient area (mean UIC <50 μg/L) but was significantly different only in females [82].

A study in southern Greece examined patterns of thyroid cancer during the period from 1963 to 2000 [83]. The proportion of PTC was significantly higher in cases born in iodine sufficient areas (84 %, $n = 162/193$) than in cases born in previously iodine deficient areas (74 %, $n = 159/214$), while the iodine status of the current area of residence was not related to histological type [83].

In northwestern Spain, iodized salt was introduced in 1985. Rego-Iraeta et al. [84] studied rates of thyroid cancer during the period of 1978 to 2001 during the population's transition from mild iodine deficiency to iodine sufficiency. Comparing the years before and after salt iodization, the PTC:FTC ratio increased from 2.3 to 11.5, and the thyroid cancer incidence increased in females from 1.56/100,000 in the period from 1978 to 1985 to 8.23/100,000 in period from 1994 to 2001, with most of the new cases being papillary microcarcinomas [84].

China

Several Chinese studies have pointed out the temporal association between the introduction of the national program of mandatory salt iodization in 1996 and a subsequent increase in incidence of PTC [85, 86]. As shown in Fig. 2c, during the period from 1997 to 2002, the national median UIC has fallen and then remained stable, while the national incidence of thyroid cancer has steadily increased. In Shanghai, from 1983 to 2007, the annual percentage change in thyroid cancer incidence in women was 4.9 % from 1983 to 2003 and 19.9 % afterward [85]. Teng et al. [87] did a five-year follow-up study of thyroid disorders in three regions of China, one with highly excessive iodine intakes from iodine-rich drinking water (median UIC of 635 µg/L), one with mildly excessive intakes from iodized salt (median UIC of 350 µg/L) and one that was borderline iodine deficient (median UIC of 97 µg/L). No significant differences among cohorts were found in the cumulative incidence of either single or multiple thyroid nodules, but the region with highly excessive intakes had 13 new cases of thyroid cancer while none were diagnosed in the other two regions [87]. In contrast, a large cross-sectional study found no correlation between iodine status and the prevalence of thyroid cancer in a coastal region of China [88]. A large cross-sectional study in Hangzhou in 2010 found a higher risk of thyroid nodules in adults consuming non-iodized salt versus iodized salt (odds ratio (OR): 1.36; 95 % CI: 1.01, 1.83) and a higher risk of thyroid nodules in those with low iodine intakes, but not excess iodine intakes [89]. There have been changes in other suspected risk factors for thyroid cancer in China over recent decades, including increasing exposure to industrial pollution [90] and increasing adiposity [91]. Moreover, rapid improvements in health care during the same period have led to increasing diagnostic intensity for thyroid cancer, and this bias likely explains a major portion of the increasing thyroid cancer incidence in China.

Australia

Burgess et al. [92, 93] using data from Tasmania's and other regional cancer registries in Australia has reported regional and national thyroid cancer incidence and mortality trends, and related them to iodine status of the population. Tasmania and much of the Australian Eastern Seaboard were historically iodine deficient until about 1970, when a combination of iodization of bread (in Tasmania) and use of iodophors in the dairying industry

improved iodine intakes. Iodized bread was discontinued in 1974 and the use of iodophors in dairying decreased in the early 1980s, resulting in the return of mild-to-moderate iodine deficiency in the 1980s and 1990s. In 1996, the median UIC in Tasmania had fallen to 42 µg/L, and in 2004, median UICs in the eastern states of Australia were 74 to 89 µg/L, indicating mild iodine deficiency [94]. During this period of falling and then deficient iodine intakes, for the period 1978–1998 in Tasmania [92] and for the rest of Australia from 1982–1997 [93], thyroid cancer incidence rates increased steadily. In the latter study, the increase was 6.7 % per year for females and 4.4 % per year for males, primarily due to a rise in PTC incidence. The average annual increase in PTC incidence was most marked in moderately-iodine deficient Tasmania (24.7 % per annum) and mildly iodine deficient Victoria (13.2 %), New South Wales (10.1 %) and Queensland (14.1 %), compared to the presumed iodine sufficient western states (4.0–8.9 %) [93].

Argentina

In a study from northern Argentina of the period from 1958 to 2007, where iodized salt was introduced in 1963, the incidence rate for thyroid cancer showed a progressive increase from 1.6 per 100,000 in 1960 to 3.6 per 100,000 in 2001, and the ratio of PTC:FTC increased from 1.7 to 3.9 [95].

Iodine intake and undifferentiated thyroid cancer

Although ATC is a rare form of thyroid cancer, accounting for less than 5 % of thyroid cancer in most countries, patients with ATC have a poor prognosis, and thus mortality from ATC accounts for most of the mortality from thyroid cancer [96]. In contrast to differentiated thyroid cancer, which often has a subtle clinical presentation and may be difficult to detect, ATC is correctly diagnosed in nearly all cases in countries with adequate health care because of rapid tumor growth and clinical presentation. Also, its highly specific histological features are easy to recognize [97]. Thus, compared to differentiated thyroid cancer, varying diagnostic intensity or criteria are much less likely to bias changes in ATC incidence rates within countries over time. For these reasons, ecological studies that describe changes in ATC incidence before and after introduction of iodized salt may be more reliable than for differentiated thyroid cancer.

Before and after studies of the effect of iodine prophylaxis on ATC have mainly been done in areas of historic endemic goiter in Europe. Bacher-Stier et al. [98] reported on changes in ATC in the Tyrol region of Austria. In the early 1960s, this area was moderately iodine deficient (mean UIC was 36 µg iodine/g creatinine) and goiter was endemic. Iodized salt fortified at level of 10 ppm was introduced in 1963 and at 20 ppm in 1992, and this resulted in iodine sufficiency and a mean UIC of 145 μg iodine/g creatinine by the mid-1990s. Overall incidence of thyroid cancer did not change from 1952 to 1995, but there was a marked shift in the percentage of thyroid cancer that was ATC, from 28.6 % in 1952–1976 to 4.9 % in 1986–1995 [98].

In Slovenia, edible salt was fortified with 10 ppm iodine from 1972 to 1997 and the population was mildly iodine deficient with a mean UIC of 83 μg iodine/g creatinine [97]. Salt iodization was increased to 25 ppm from 1998 to 2008 and this resulted in adequate iodine intakes and a mean UIC of 148 μg iodine/g creatinine. The annual incidence of ATC in Slovenia before 1998 was 3.25 per million versus 1.9 per million afterward [97]. From 1981 to 1995 in southern Germany, iodine status improved from moderate iodine deficiency (median UIC of 40 μg/L) in 1986 to mild iodine deficiency (median UIC of 72 μg/L) in 1997, and the percentage of thyroid cancer that was ATC decreased from 11.3 % to 7.3 % [99]. Other studies have described similar decreases in ATC after correction of iodine deficiency through iodized salt in Switzerland, Austria, Italy and Sweden [66, 67, 73, 100]. Along with improved medical care, the significant decrease in the incidence of ATC after the introduction of iodized salt in Switzerland may have contributed to the marked decrease in mortality from thyroid cancer between 1921 and 1978 [101].

However, it should be noted that other European countries have reported similar reductions in ATC without changes in population iodine intake. In Scotland, there has been a decrease in the incidence of ATC without changes in iodination policy [102]. Similarly in the Netherlands, where iodine intakes have been stable and sufficient over the past few decades, the incidence of ATC decreased by 7.1 % per year between 1989 and 2003 [78].

Northern Argentina in 1960 was severely iodine deficient and mean UI excretion was 20 μg/day [103]. After iodized salt was introduced, mean UIC increased into the sufficient range, and was 152 μg iodine/g creatinine in 1975. Over this period, the percentage of thyroid cancer that was ATC decreased from 15.2 % before salt iodization to 2.6 % after salt iodination, and the annual incidence decreased from 1.4 per million to 0.1 per million [103]. A plausible explanation for why the percentage of thyroid cancer that is ATC is higher in areas of severe iodine deficiency is that when goiter is endemic in a population, individuals are less concerned by the occurrence of thyroid nodules or swelling, and this may delay diagnosis in many cases until serious symptoms occur. This delay in recognition may allow initially well-differentiated thyroid cancer to change into anaplastic cancer [104, 105].

Conclusions
Table 2 summarizes the before and after studies looking at either the effect of the introduction of salt iodization

or an increase in the salt iodization level on patterns of thyroid cancer. In three of eight studies that reported the gender ratio of thyroid cancer, the female: male ratio increased, while in two it decreased and in three it remained unchanged. The studies show a shift in the subtypes of thyroid cancer: all studies report an increase in the PTC:FTC ratio, and all but one show a decrease in the percentage of ATC. No studies have found an increase in incidence or frequency of ATC with increasing iodine intake. The findings in Table 2 are consistent with the earlier review of Williams [22], who reported that in countries with 'high' iodine intake (U.S., Iceland) the ratio of PTC:FTC ranged from 3.4 to 6.5, while in countries with 'moderate' iodine intake (the U.K. and northern Germany) the ratio was from 1.6 to 3.7, and in countries with 'low' iodide intake (Argentina, Columbia, Finland, southern Germany, Austria and Switzerland) the ratio was from 0.19 to 1.7.

Although the data in Table 2 suggest that populations in areas of sufficient iodine intake seem to have fewer of the more aggressive ATC and FTC, but more PTC, the comparisons may have been biased by other factors that may influence the presentation of thyroid cancer besides iodine intake. Interestingly, the increase in the PTC:FTC ratio and the decline in ATC is evident even in the study periods that preceded the introduction of increased diagnostic intensity for thyroid cancer. However, it should be remembered that increases in the incidence of differentiated thyroid cancer and the PTC:FTC ratio over the past two decades have occurred in countries with decreasing, stable and increasing iodine intakes. As shown in Fig. 2a-c, during the past several decades in the U.S., the incidence of thyroid cancer has been steadily increasing, but iodine intakes during the same period have decreased by about 50 %, and in Switzerland and China, two countries with well-established salt iodization programs, although iodine intakes have been stable, there have been steady increases in the incidence of thyroid cancer.

Iodine intake and mortality from thyroid cancer
In most areas of the world, while the incidence of thyroid cancer has been increasing over the past few decades, mortality has steadily declined [1]. Decreases in thyroid cancer mortality are due mainly to improved early diagnosis and surgery or ^{131}I therapy applied at an early tumor stage. However, because current or a history of goiter or thyroid nodules are strong risk factors for thyroid cancer [15], particularly the more aggressive subtypes (discussed below), it is possible that the substantial decline in iodine deficiency in many countries —particularly in low and middle-income areas that have introduced iodized salt— might also be contributing to the favorable trends in thyroid cancer mortality.

Table 2 Before-and-after studies on the effect of salt iodization on type of thyroid cancer. The effect of introduction of salt iodization or an increase in the salt iodization level on the sex ratio (female: male, F:M) of affected subjects and the subtypes of thyroid cancer, by country: changes in the papillary thyroid cancer to follicular thyroid cancer ratio (PTC:FTC), and the percentage of anaplastic thyroid cancer (% ATC).

Country (reference)	Years pre-iodized salt			Year and change in salt iodization	Years post-iodized salt		
	PTC:FTC	% ATC	F:M		PTC:FTC	% ATC	F:M
Basel, Switzerland [148]	1944–1953			1962	1964–1973		
	0.27	28.7	2.5	Increase from 5 to 10 ppm	0.74	27.7	2.5
Zurich, Switzerland [67]	1925–1941			1962	1962–1973		
	0.19	36.9	1.3	Increase from 5 to 10 ppm	1.1	23.8	2.1
Innsbruck, Austria [66]	1952–1959			1963	1970–1975		
	0.21	na	0.9	Introduction at 10 ppm	1.1	na	1.9
Tyrol, Austria [98]	1952–1975			1963; 1992	1986–1995		
	0.55	28.4	na	Introduction at 10 ppm; increase to 20 ppm	1.5	4.9	na
Klagenfurt, Austria [149]	1984–1989			1992	1990–1995		
	2.6	na	na	Increase from 10 to 20 ppm	4.0	na	na
Krakow and Nowy Sacz, Poland [150]	1986			1997	2001		
	1.0	na	na	Introduction at 30 ppm	5.9	na	na
Lower Franconia, Germany [99]	1981–1985			1993	1991–1995		
	1.5	11.3	3.0	Increased use by the food industry at 20 ppm	3.4	7.3	2.2
Salta, Argentina [95]	1958–1972			1963; 1970	1985–2007		
	1.7	16.9	2.9	Introduction at 40 ppm; decrease to 33 ppm	3.9	6.4	4.0
Galicia, Spain [84]	1978–1985			1985	1994–2001		
	2.3	na	4.3	Introduction at 60 ppm	11.5	na	3.4
Parma, Italy [100]	1998–2003			2005	2004–2009		
	13.0	2.3	3.1	Introduction at 30 ppm	13.6	1.0	3.2
Shenyang, China [86]	1992–1996			1995; 2000	1997–2009		
	2.3	7.1	3.2	Introduction at 20–60 ppm; decrease to 35 ppm	21.9	2.1	3.6

If population iodine status is a determinant of the pathogenesis of thyroid cancer, one might expect mortality rates in countries to be correlated with population iodine status. La Vecchia et al. [1], using data for thyroid cancer mortality and population size for countries in the period 1970–2012 from the WHO online database [106] estimated age-adjusted death rates from thyroid cancer at all ages in 2000 (1998–2002) and in 2010 (2008–2012) and percentage changes between these periods (Additional file 1: Table S1). Using these country data on thyroid cancer mortality, together with national or subnational median UIC data for same time periods, where available [18, 107], we calculated the change in age-adjusted death rates from thyroid cancer by gender between 2000 and 2010 versus the change in the population median UIC (μg/L) for the same time periods (Fig. 3). For women, there was a weak but significant indirect correlation ($r^2 = 0.135$; $p = 0.046$) that was not present for men. These country data suggest that, for women only, a greater increase in iodine intake over the

period 2000 to 2010 is associated with a greater decrease in thyroid cancer mortality.

Iodine intake and occult thyroid carcinoma at autopsy

Occult thyroid carcinomas (OTC) are often incidentally found at autopsy, and nearly all are papillary microcarcinomas. Unlike clinical PTC, differences in the occurrence of OTC at autopsy are not influenced by differences in screening and diagnostic intensity, but more likely reflect true differences due to genetic and/or environmental factors [108]. Although differences in autopsy methods used for thyroid sectioning and histological examination may bias comparisons, associations between iodine intake in populations and the occurrence of OTC at autopsy may be relatively free of ascertainment bias and therefore valuable.

Kovacs et al. [109] compared rates of OTC at autopsy in two ethnically and socioeconomically comparable populations in Hungary, one in an iodine deficient area (median UIC of 70 μg iodine/g creatinine) and one in an

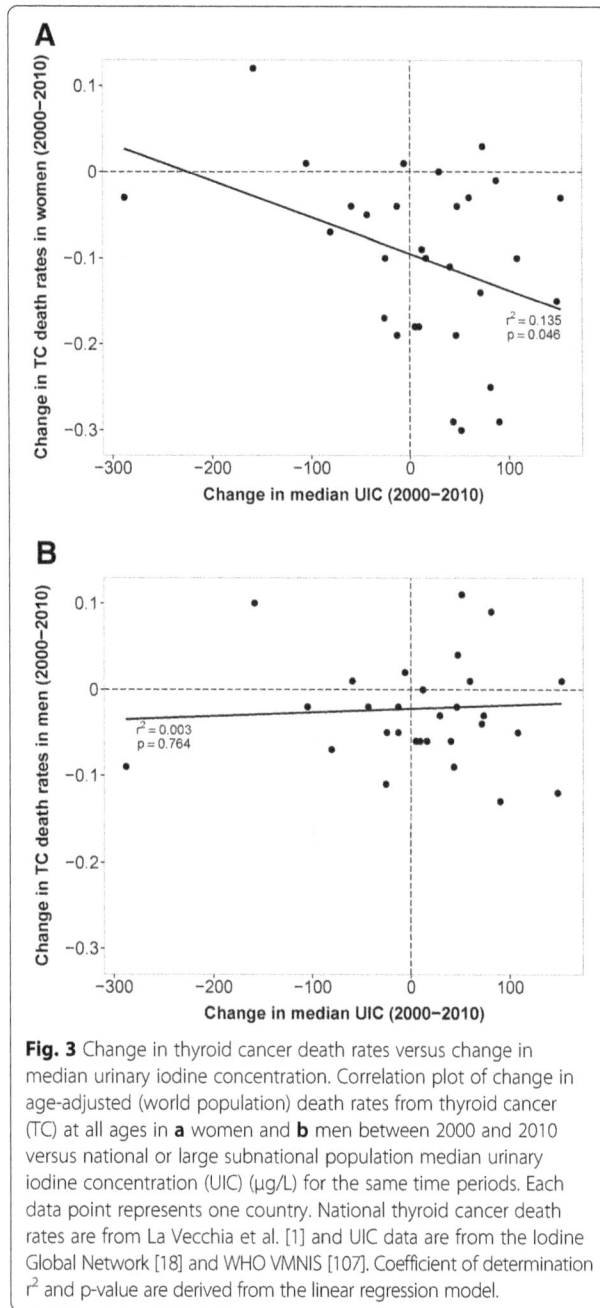

Fig. 3 Change in thyroid cancer death rates versus change in median urinary iodine concentration. Correlation plot of change in age-adjusted (world population) death rates from thyroid cancer (TC) at all ages in **a** women and **b** men between 2000 and 2010 versus national or large subnational population median urinary iodine concentration (UIC) (μg/L) for the same time periods. Each data point represents one country. National thyroid cancer death rates are from La Vecchia et al. [1] and UIC data are from the Iodine Global Network [18] and WHO VMNIS [107]. Coefficient of determination r^2 and p-value are derived from the linear regression model.

area of iodine excess due to iodine-rich drinking water (median UIC of 500 μg iodine/g creatinine). Goiter prevalence was 22.5 % in the iodine deficient area versus 2.3 % in the iodine excess area, and thyroid nodularity was more common in the iodine deficient area. However, the occurrence of OTC in the two areas was not different: 4.95 and 4.52 %, respectively, and OTC were not more common in glands with nodular goiter, consistent with findings from an earlier Austrian study [110]. In contrast, in autopsy studies performed in Japan [111] and Finland [112], OTC was more common in glands with nodular goiter.

Table 3 shows the occurrence of OTC in autopsy series, categorized by population iodine status based on the median UIC at the time of the study. Because migration studies suggest that Japanese ethnicity is a strong determinant of risk for OTC [108], we analyzed the data in Table 3 without the five Japanese autopsy studies shown at the bottom of the table. We also excluded as an outlier a Finnish study that reported a prevalence of OTC of 35.6 % [112]. In the remaining studies, that examined mainly Caucasian and Hispanic populations, in areas with deficient ($n = 11$), sufficient ($n = 10$), and excessive iodine intake ($n = 10$), the weighted mean prevalence of OPTC was 5.3, 6.0 and 3.3 %, respectively. Comparing the weighted means, the prevalence of OTC was significantly lower ($p < 0.01$) in areas of excess iodine intake versus areas of sufficient and deficient intakes, but there was no significant difference comparing rates between areas of deficient and sufficient intakes. These data differ from two previous reviews that suggested higher iodine intakes were associated with an increase in prevalence of OTC at autopsy [22, 109]. However, the first review may have been affected by misclassification bias as iodine status was only broadly defined as high, moderate and low and criteria for this classification were not given [22]. The conclusions of the second review are limited in that nearly all of the iodine deficient populations included were Caucasian, while nearly all the iodine excessive populations were Japanese [109].

Goiter, benign thyroid nodules and thyroid cancer

Iodine deficiency sharply increases risk of nodules and goiter in populations [19]. In nodular goiter, distinct clusters of follicular cells are proliferating independent of TSH control [113]. Iodine deficiency may trigger formation of nodules through chronic stimulation by TSH and/or the mutagenic effects of increased reactive oxygen species in the iodine deficient thyroid [114]. Franceschi et al. [15] did a pooled analysis of case–control studies of benign nodules and goiter and thyroid cancer, including 2519 cases (2008 were PTC) and 4176 controls from 11 studies of goiter and 8 studies of benign nodules/adenomas. The studies of goiter included populations from five regions with sufficient to excessive iodine intakes (four studies from the U.S. in the early 1980s, and one from Japan) and six populations with sufficient to mildly deficient intakes (one from coastal China before the introduction of iodized salt and five from Europe). For women, ORs for a history of goiter for all thyroid cancer were 5.9 (95 % CI: 4.2, 8.1), and for PTC and FTC were 5.5 (3.9, 7.8) and 6.9 (3.8, 12.4), respectively. For men, the OR for all thyroid cancer was 38.3 (95 % CI: 5.0, 291.2). In that review, with the exception of a Japanese study where the OR for thyroid cancer was very high for women (26.5), the individual ORs from the other ten studies did not vary

Table 3 Prevalence of occult thyroid cancer in adults at autopsy, by national iodine status. National population iodine status at the time of study as categorized according to WHO criteria for the median urinary iodine concentration (UIC) [23].[a]

Country (reference)	Year	No. autopsy cases	% with occult thyroid cancer
Probable deficient iodine intake (UIC < 100 µg/L) (n = 11)			
Italy [151]	1982	111	3.6
Chile [152]	1984	274	2.9
Poland [108]	1975	110	6.6
Portugal [153]	1979	600	1.0
Israel [154]	1981	260	4.2
Germany [155]	1987	1020	6.1
Spain [156]	1993	100	22.0
Belarus [157]	1993	215	8.8
Ukraine [158]	1996	162	10.8
Guatemala [159]	2005	150	2.0
Hungary [109]	2005	222	5.0
Mean			6.6
Weighted mean			5.3
Probable sufficient iodine intake (UIC = 100–299 µg/L) (n = 10)			
Canada [108]	1975	100	6.0
Sweden [160]	1981	500	6.4
USA [161]	1988	138	2.9
Brazil [162]	1989	300	1.0
Argentina [163]	1989	100	11.0
Iceland [164]	1992	199	6.0
Singapore [165]	1994	444	9.0
Austria [110]	2001	118	8.6
Greece [166]	2002	160	5.6
Turkey [167]	2011	108	3.7
Mean			6.0
Weighted mean			6.0
Probable excessive iodine intake (UIC ≥ 300 µg/L) (n = 10)			
USA [168]	1952	429	0.9
USA [169]	1955	1000	2.8
USA [170]	1955	221	1.4
USA [171]	1964	100	4.0
USA [172]	1966	300	2.7
USA [173]	1969	220	0.5
USA [174]	1974	157	5.7
Columbia [108]	1975	607	5.6
Hungary [109]	2005	221	4.5
Brazil [175]	2006	166	7.8
Mean			3.6
Weighted mean			3.3

Table 3 Prevalence of occult thyroid cancer in adults at autopsy, by national iodine status. National population iodine status at the time of study as categorized according to WHO criteria for the median urinary iodine concentration (UIC) [23].[a] (Continued)

Studies of Japanese populations in areas of excessive iodine intake (n = 5)			
USA, Japanese [176]	1971	100	24.0
Japan [174]	1974	1096	17.9
USA, Japanese [108]	1975	248	24.2
Japan [108]	1975	1167	28.4
Japan [111]	1990	408	15.7
Mean			22.0
Weighted mean			22.4

[a]Weighted means of iodine intake categories compared by using the Chi-squared test of independence: <100 µg/L vs. 100–299 µg/L (p = 0.244); ≥300 µg/L vs. <100 µg/L or 100–299 µg/L (both, p < 0.001)

widely. For women, OR for a history of benign nodules/adenomas for all thyroid cancer were 29.9 (95 % CI: 14.5, 62.0), and for PTC and FTC were 28.9 (13.6, 61.2) and 62.3 (18.9, 205.8), respectively. The excess risk for goiter and benign nodules/adenomas was greatest within 4 years prior to thyroid cancer diagnosis, but a significantly elevated OR was still present more than 10 years before diagnosis. Case–control and cohort studies published since this analysis [15] have supported a link between goiter and/or thyroid nodules and risk of thyroid cancer [115–117].

Because iodine deficiency increases risk for goiter and thyroid nodules, these data suggest risk for thyroid cancer might be increased by iodine deficiency. However, these associations might also be explained by an increased likelihood of thyroid cancer detection in iodine deficient populations because of more frequent thyroid surgery. Also, there are other causes of goiter (e.g., thyroiditis) than iodine deficiency. In contrast to the results of the pooled analysis [15], studies in the U.S. [118] and Australia [119] did not find that thyroid cancer mortality was higher in historically goitrous regions in those two countries.

A meta-analysis of 14 cross-sectional or retrospective cohort studies [120] found the risk of thyroid cancer was significantly lower in multinodular goiter than in single nodules (OR 0.8; 95 % CI: 0.67, 0.96). However, there was moderate inconsistency across studies (I^2 = 35 %): studies in iodine sufficient areas (U.S., Saudi Arabia, Nigeria, Croatia) found risk was lower in multinodular goiter than in single nodules (OR 0.77; 95 % CI: 0.65, 0.92), while studies in mildly iodine deficient areas (Italy, Turkey), where multinodular goiter would be expected to be more common, found no significant association (OR 0.88; 95 % CI: 0.68, 1.14).

Total iodine intake and thyroid cancer

Hawaii, U.S.

A case–control study in Hawaiian adults reported the association between dietary iodine intake and thyroid cancer in 191 cases (85 % PTC) and 442 controls [121]. A food frequency questionnaire was used to estimate iodine intake, but iodine content of local seafood was not available, so values were taken from other sources. Geometric mean daily iodine intake (μg/day) was higher in female cases than in controls (394 versus 326, $p = 0.01$). Iodine containing supplements contributed ≈7 % of iodine intake. When the highest iodine intake quartile was compared to the lowest, there was a no significant increase in risk for thyroid cancer in women (OR 1.6; 95 % CI: 0.8, 3.2) or in men (OR 1.3; 95 % CI: 0.4, 3.7). Selection bias was not likely in this study as cases were selected from a population-based registry and controls selected through random sample of that population. However, ORs were adjusted only for age and ethnicity but not for other confounding factors.

California, U.S.

A case–control study of 608 women with thyroid cancer and 558 controls between the ages of 20 and 74 in northern California (51 % Caucasian and 35 % Asian) examined dietary iodine intake via a food frequency questionnaire and iodine levels measured in toenail clippings [115]. The main iodine sources were rice and pasta dishes and pizza (30 % of mean daily intake); milk and other dairy products (13 %); bread products (12 %); multivitamin pills (11 %); and fish/shellfish (3 %). A significant reduction in the risk of PTC was seen in the highest iodine intake quintile (>537 μg/day) compared to the lowest (<273 μg/day) (OR 0.49; 95 % CI: 0.29, 0.84), with a similar OR for Caucasian and Asian women. Iodine intake from food alone was not associated with risk, but iodine intake from supplements was; thus, the protective effect for total dietary iodine was largely attributable to the higher consumption of multivitamin pills (most brands contain 150 μg of iodine) by controls. Of note, the highest quintile of dietary iodine was greater than three times the WHO RNI for iodine for this age group. There was no association between toenail iodine and PTC, but the usefulness of nail clippings as an exposure biomarker is uncertain. Although this study had a large sample size and controlled for confounding by many risk factors, there is also the possibility of selection bias as cases were found from a cancer registry but controls were obtained through random-digit dialing.

New Caledonia

Truong et al. [122] performed a countrywide case–control study of iodine intake and thyroid cancer in women on the Pacific island nation of New Caledonia. The country has a high incidence of thyroid cancer but was not exposed to iodizing radiation from past nuclear testing in the Pacific. The study included 293 cases and 354 population controls. An extensive food-frequency questionnaire was used to estimate iodine intake over the previous 5-year period. Iodine intake was computed using a French food composition table, which did not have data for some local seafood, so iodine intakes may have been underestimated. Overall, total iodine intakes were low, and tertiles of intake were: <75.0, 75.0–112.6 and ≥112.6 μg/day, compared to the WHO RNI of 150 μg/day. There was no significant association of iodine intake and thyroid cancer: comparing the upper tertile of intake versus the lower tertile, the OR was 1.13 (95 % CI: 0.68, 1.87). A high consumption of cruciferous vegetables was associated with thyroid cancer among women with iodine intakes less than 96 μg/day (OR 1.86; 95 % CI: 1.01, 3.43).

French Polynesia

French Polynesia has one of the world's highest incidence rates of thyroid cancer. A case–control study [123] included 229 cases of differentiated thyroid cancer (77 % PTC, 203 women, 26 men) matched with 371 controls. Daily dietary iodine intake was estimated from a food frequency questionnaire and was insufficient (<150 μg/day) in 60 % of both cases and controls. Dietary iodine intake (μg/day) was classified as: ≤74, severe or moderate deficiency; 75–149, mild deficiency, 150–299, optimal; and ≥300, excess. The ORs (95 % CI) for thyroid cancer at these intakes were: 2.57 (1.12, 5.93); 1.11 (0.63, 1.94); 1.00 (reference); 0.88 (0.38, 2.03) (p for trend = 0.04). These results did not change after adjustment with thyroid dose from prior exposure to radioactive fallout from nuclear testing in the area. A decreased risk of thyroid cancer was observed with a higher consumption of fish and shellfish, the main sources of iodine in the diet. More frequent iodized salt consumption was associated with an increased risk of thyroid cancer, but this result was likely biased because local doctors had advised patients who had a goiter or thyroid cancer to consume iodized salt.

Case–control studies: meta-analysis of total iodine intake and thyroid cancer

We examined the association between iodine intake and thyroid cancer by performing a meta-analysis of pooled measures of effect available from the four case–control studies described above [115, 121–123]. We report the size of the effect on thyroid cancer as adjusted OR for the highest iodine intake quantile compared to the lowest quantile (Fig. 4). For each study's subgroup, we algebraically derived the logarithmic estimate for OR (logOR) and its standard error (SE) from the available summary statistics. We calculated the overall pooled logOR and SE using random-effects model analysis with the DerSimonian and

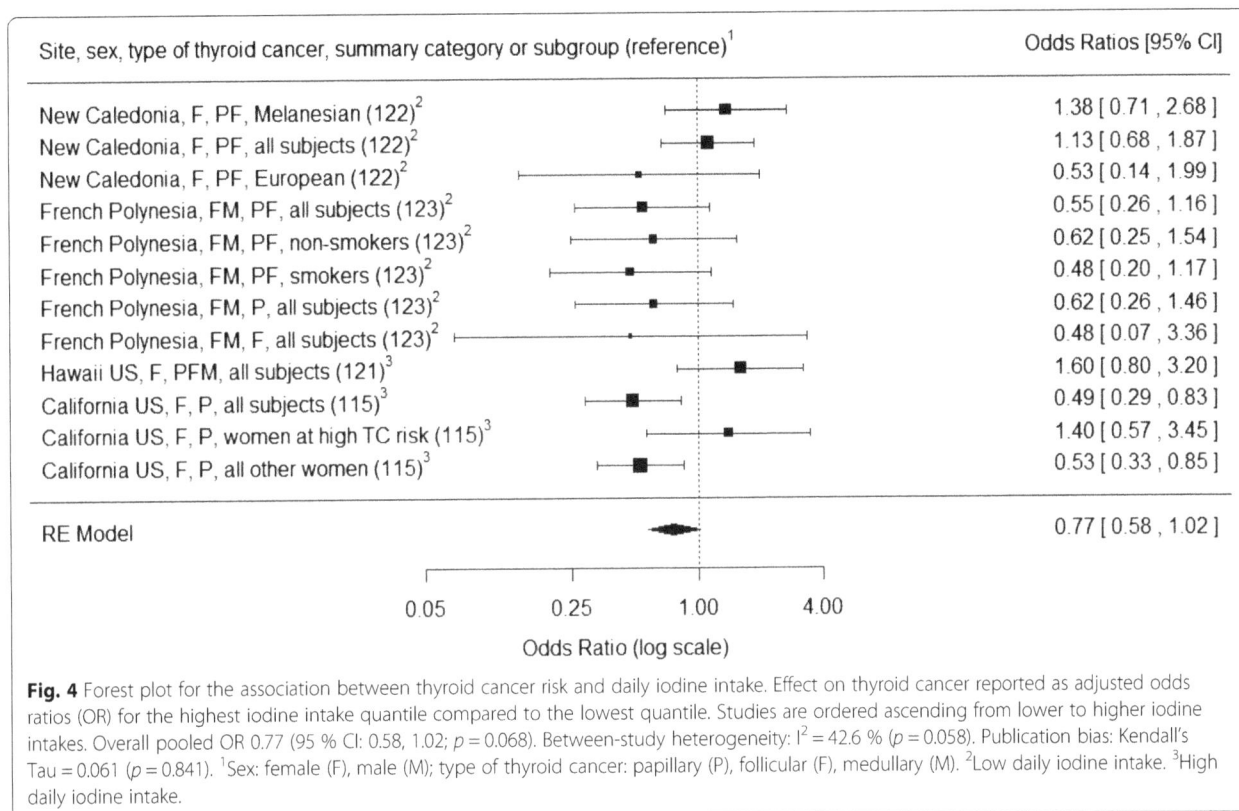

Fig. 4 Forest plot for the association between thyroid cancer risk and daily iodine intake. Effect on thyroid cancer reported as adjusted odds ratios (OR) for the highest iodine intake quantile compared to the lowest quantile. Studies are ordered ascending from lower to higher iodine intakes. Overall pooled OR 0.77 (95 % CI: 0.58, 1.02; $p = 0.068$). Between-study heterogeneity: $I^2 = 42.6$ % ($p = 0.058$). Publication bias: Kendall's Tau $= 0.061$ ($p = 0.841$). [1]Sex: female (F), male (M); type of thyroid cancer: papillary (P), follicular (F), medullary (M). [2]Low daily iodine intake. [3]High daily iodine intake.

Laird method to estimate the between-study variance [124], and evaluated residual heterogeneity between studies using the I^2 statistics. Publication bias was evaluated by visual inspection of the funnel plot of the random-effects model and by rank correlation test for funnel plot asymmetry. We performed data analysis with the R statistical programming environment (version 3.1.2) [125] using the metafor [126] and rmeta packages [127]. The meta-analysis indicates that the odds for thyroid cancer are 23 % less in the highest quantile of iodine intake versus the lowest, although this effect was only borderline significant (OR 0.77; 95 % CI: 0.58, 1.02; $p = 0.068$) (Fig. 4). There was moderate evidence for between-study heterogeneity ($I^2 = 42.6$ %; $p = 0.058$), but evaluation of iodine median intake as potential source of heterogeneity in a meta-regression model revealed no evidence of linearity between iodine intake and thyroid cancer ($p = 0.829$). There was no strong evidence of publication bias (Kendall's Tau $= 0.061$; $p = 0.841$).

Conclusions

In summary, two of the case–control studies (Hawaii and California) were done in areas of high iodine intakes, 2–3 fold higher than recommended intakes, while the other two were done in Pacific Island populations with mildly deficient intakes. The studies in California and French Polynesia suggest higher iodine intakes may

be protective against thyroid cancer, while the other two show no association. Our meta-analysis of these studies suggests a trend toward lower risk for thyroid cancer with higher iodine intake. However, in these case–control studies recall bias is always possible as cases may recall diet information differently than controls. Also, food composition data on iodine in local foods was limited and was often derived from foods from other geographic areas. Finally, the main weakness of these studies is that they did not measure UIC to assess total dietary iodine exposure and did not have data on iodine intake from iodized salt added in the household, likely an important source dietary iodine. Thus, there is a high possibility of misclassification of case of iodine exposure.

Case–control and cohort studies: seafood, milk and thyroid cancer
Seafood

Fish and shellfish are important sources of dietary iodine intake in populations that consume these products regularly. Liu and Lin [128] examined the relationship between fish consumption and risk of thyroid cancer in a meta-analysis of ten cohort or case–control studies. There was a 21 % decreased risk of thyroid cancer with high fish intake (OR 0.79; 95 % CI: 0.66, 0.94). Subgroup analysis was done comparing iodine sufficient populations in Norway and the U.S. to presumed iodine deficient populations in Italy, Sweden and French Caledonia. In the subgroup analysis, the summary OR was 0.74 (95 % CI: 0.59, 0.92) in the iodine deficient areas while no significant association was found in the iodine sufficient areas. Also, when the analysis was restricted to PTC, the authors found no significant association between fish intake and PTC risk. An earlier pooled analysis of case control studies published between 1980 and 1997 [129] from the United States, Japan, China and Europe found a borderline significant 12 % reduction in risk of thyroid cancer with high intakes of fish (OR 0.88: 95 % CI: 0.71, 1.1). There was a significant decrease in risk of thyroid cancer with high fish intake in regions with endemic goiter due to iodine deficiency (OR 0.65; 95 % CI: 0.48, 0.88) but not in iodine sufficient regions (OR 1.1; 95 % CI: 0.85, 1.5). The authors of these pooled analyses suggested that higher fish intakes exert a protective effect only in endemic goiter areas with suboptimal iodine intake.

Milk and milk products

In most European countries, the U.S. and Australia, population iodine intake from milk is typically greater than that from fish or seafood [130–132]. The native iodine content of milk is low, but the use of iodine-containing supplements for cows and iodophor disinfectants during dairying and transport result in high levels in milk and milk products [131]. Cross-sectional studies in iodine sufficient Chinese adults [89] and German university students [133] found no significant association between milk intake and the prevalence of thyroid nodules detected by ultrasound. A population-based case–control study in Sweden and Norway [134] reported a positive association of cheese (OR 1.5; 95 % CI: 1.0, 2.4) and butter (OR 1.6; 95 % CI: 1.1, 2.5) and thyroid cancer risk in adults, particularly in those who had lived in an endemic goiter area and had a high intake of all milk products. In a pooled analysis of four European case–control studies, high consumption of milk did not increase risk of thyroid cancer, but there was a significant increase in thyroid cancer risk for high intakes of cheese and butter (OR were 1.4 and 1.8 for the highest tertiles of intake) [135]. A later pooled analysis did not find a significant relationship of milk products and thyroid cancer [136] and case–control studies in iodine sufficient Poland [137] and New Caledonia [122] found no significant association between dairy consumption and risk of thyroid cancer. In a large U.S. cohort study of adults 50–71 years of age at baseline, during 7 years of follow-up there was no association between consumption of milk products (highest quintile had 1.4–1.6 dairy food servings per 1000 kcal) and risk of thyroid cancer in men (relative risk (RR) 0.78; 95 % CI: 0.45, 1.37) or women (RR 1.04; 95 % CI: 0.67, 1.62) [138].

Iodine status and risk of thyroid cancer after radiation exposure

External radiation to the thyroid increases risk for thyroid cancer, particularly when the radiation occurs in childhood [9, 10, 139, 140]. The Chernobyl nuclear accident in 1986 exposed populations of Belarus, Ukraine, and the Russian Federation to internal radiation from radioactive iodines deposited in the thyroid, resulting in sharp increase in pediatric and adolescent thyroid cancer, mainly PTC [141]. Historically, the areas exposed to Chernobyl fallout were affected by varying degrees of iodine deficiency [142]. Chronic iodine deficiency increases thyroidal clearance of plasma iodine, increases thyroid blood flow and increases thyroid size, all of which may increase thyroid uptake of ingested radioiodines [142]. Also, iodine deficiency increases thyroid activity and thyrocyte proliferation, thereby increasing vulnerability of the thyroid to the accumulated radioiodine [54]. In rat studies, combined with a single external radiation dose of 4 Gy, both iodine deficiency and iodine excess induced thyroid carcinomas (PTC and FTC) in 50–80 % of animals, while iodine sufficient animals did not develop thyroid carcinomas (Fig. 1b) [36].

Thus, many experts predicted the risk of radiation-related thyroid cancer after Chernobyl would be higher in more iodine deficient areas, and a number of studies have tested this hypothesis [143–146]. However, at the time of the accident, there had been no recent assessment of iodine status of the populations in the most exposed areas, so it is difficult to know with certainty which of the exposed populations were more iodine deficient when the accident occurred. Therefore, a variety of surrogates have been used to categorize iodine status at the time of exposure, such as soil iodine concentrations [144], residence in a rural versus urban area [144] or measures of iodine status more a decade after the accident [143, 145, 146].

Shakhtarin et al. [143] investigated a population-based sample of 3070 individuals (2590 aged 6–18 years, and 480 adults) from 75 villages in the most highly contaminated regions of the Bryansk Oblast of Russia, a region that was historically an area of endemic goiter. UIC was measured in the participants in 1996 (a decade after the accident) and the median UIC was determined for each village and used to divide the study area into four zones, as follows: median UIC ≥100; 75–99; 50–74; or <50 µg/L. Thirty four cases of thyroid cancer were identified in those born in 1968–1986 who lived in the study area at the time of the accident in 1986 (20 in females and 14 in males, median age 16 years). The excess relative risk (ERR) of thyroid cancer was directly associated with increasing thyroid radiation dose and indirectly associated with median UIC. There was a significant combined effect of radiation exposure and iodine deficiency: at 1 Gy of exposure, the

ERR in regions with a median UIC <50 µg/L (moderate iodine deficiency) was nearly two times that in areas of where the median UIC was ≥100 µg/L (iodine sufficiency).

Cardis et al. [144] performed a population-based case–control study of thyroid cancer in Belarus and Russia; cases were 276 thyroid cancers and controls were 1300 matched subjects below age 15 years at the time of the accident. Based on geologic maps of soil type in the affected areas, the authors estimated soil iodine concentration in rural settlements at the time of the Chernobyl accident and used these as a surrogate marker for iodine status, while classifying urban populations as iodine sufficient because it was assumed they were obtaining iodine sufficient foods from outside the local area. For subjects residing in areas with the lowest tertile of estimated soil iodine, the odds of developing thyroid cancer after a 1-Gy exposure were 3.2 (95 % CI: 1.9, 5.5) times higher than that for subjects living in areas of greater soil iodine. However, most of the areas studied had iodine deficient soils, so the comparison group (the higher two tertiles of soil iodine) was likely not iodine sufficient.

Tronko et al. [145] performed a prospective cohort study in 12 to 33 year-olds in the Ukraine who had been exposed to radiation from the Chernobyl accident during childhood. The authors assessed iodine status in subjects by goiter palpation and spot UICs more than a decade after the accident, in 1998–2000, when the median UIC was ≈50 µg/L. The study found no significant relationship between UIC and risk of thyroid cancer. A history of goiter was associated with a nonsignificant doubling in risk of thyroid cancer (OR 2.19; 95 % CI: 0.96, 5.03), but the study had limited statistical power due to a small number of cancer cases ($n = 45$). The later measurements of UIC and goiter may not reflect iodine status at the time of the accident because of changes in dietary habits and food distribution in the intervening period.

Zablotska et al. [146] screened nearly 12,000 individuals in Belarus aged 18 years or younger at the time of the Chernobyl accident. Past iodine deficiency was estimated by using self-reported history of diffuse and nodular goiter, as well as diffuse goiter and UICs measured during screening in 1996 through 2004. After adjustment for radiation dose, the prevalence rate for thyroid cancer was significantly higher for those with a self-reported history of nodular (OR 23.21) or diffuse goiter (OR 5.15), or with nodular or diffuse goiter diagnosed at screening (ORs 19.79 and 3.16). But UIC at screening was not associated with thyroid cancer; there was no significant increase in risk comparing those with moderate to severe iodine deficiency (UICs <50 µg/L) to those with higher UICs. However, Belarus began salt iodization in late 2000 and iodine status has generally been adequate in the population since then, so the later

UIC measurements in this study likely differ from those at the time of the accident in 1986 [147].

Conclusions

In these studies, the reliability of the proxy measures used to define iodine status at the time of the accident is uncertain, and therefore it is difficult to draw conclusions. However, an error in classification of iodine status in these studies would likely have been random and would have biased their estimates toward the null. Despite this, 3 out of 4 studies [143, 144, 146] found that poorer iodine status in children at the time of the accident was associated with a ≈2–3 fold increase in risk for developing thyroid cancer.

Conclusions

The incidence of thyroid cancer has been rising steadily over the past few decades in most countries [1]. Much of this increase is due to increased case finding because of improved screening and diagnosis methods, but there may also be a true increase, so it is important to clarify the role of suspected risk factors, including iodine intake. Population iodine intakes can vary up to 50 fold –from intakes less than 20 µg/d in areas of severe deficiency, to more than 1000 µg/d in areas with high iodine levels in drinking water or from intake of iodine-rich seaweed. Moreover, iodine intakes are shifting in many countries: they are increasing in some countries as iodized salt is introduced to correct iodine deficiency, while others report falling intakes, due to changes in dietary habits and patterns of iodine use by the food and dairy industry. It is well known that even small variations in population iodine intake are a determinant of benign thyroid disorders [16]. So why does the role of iodine intake in thyroid cancer remains uncertain, despite decades of study?

There are many reasons. Comparison studies of thyroid cancer epidemiology in populations and geographic areas are challenging because thyroid cancer is still a relatively rare and, in most cases, indolent cancer. Thus, long study periods in large populations are needed and this increases the likelihood of bias from changes in unmeasured risk factors other than iodine intake. There is the additional large uncertainty of the lag-time between changes in iodine exposure and changes in incidence of thyroid cancer; the lag-time between increasing iodine intake and the resolution of diffuse goiter and nodules in adult populations is several decades [67]. Accurate dietary assessment of iodine intake is notoriously difficult because discretionary use of household iodized salt and use of iodized salt in processed foods is difficult to quantify [24]. Finally, all of these difficulties are compounded by the current lack of an individual biomarker of iodine status: applying a population indicator such as the median

UIC to classify individual risk for thyroid cancer likely introduces substantial classification bias.

Animal studies indicate iodine deficiency is a weak initiator but a strong promoter of thyroid cancer, mainly of the follicular type. Less convincing evidence suggests iodine excess may be a weak promoter of thyroid cancer. The proposed mechanism for the effects of iodine deficiency –chronic elevation of TSH stimulates thyrocyte proliferation and increases the likelihood of mutagenesis– is plausible and supported by animal studies. However, TSH is not elevated in animals fed diets with excessive iodine, so the mechanism for the effects of excess iodine is unknown. Limited data from thyroid cell cultures suggest exposure to high amounts of iodine reduces RET/PTC3 and BRAF oncogene activation, but the relevance of these studies is uncertain because the iodine concentrations used were far above physiologic levels in the thyroid. A single human study found the RAS oncogene mutation rate was higher in FTC cases from an iodine deficient area, and in the two human studies investigating the BRAF mutation in PTC, one found no increased occurrence in cases from an iodine deficient area population while another found an increased occurrence in an iodine excess area. More well-controlled studies are needed to clarify the potential links between iodine intake and molecular alterations such as mutations of the BRAF and RAS genes and BRAF and RET rearrangements in thyroid cancer.

The overall incidence of thyroid cancer in populations does not appear to be influenced by the usual range of iodine intakes from dietary sources. The evidence is more convincing that increases in iodine intake may change the distribution of subtypes of thyroid cancer, particularly important are the data from countries before and after iodine prophylaxis done before the recent increases in diagnostic intensity (Table 3). These data are consistent in showing a higher percentage of the more-aggressive ATC and FTC in iodine deficient areas, whereas PTC seems to be more common in areas with high iodine intakes. Thus, by reducing FTC, and particularly ATC, iodized salt programs may be contributing to the decrease in thyroid cancer mortality seen in many countries; the data in Fig. 3 suggest this benefit may be strongest in women. However, firm conclusions cannot be made because of unmeasured covariates that may have changed over time along with iodine status, such as standards of medical care, environmental exposures, and histological classification.

Over the past 2 to 3 decades, there is clear temporal relationship in many countries between introduction of iodized salt and an increase in incidence of PTC. However, at the same time, several countries that have stable or decreasing iodine intakes, including Australia, the U.S. and Switzerland (Fig. 2), have also experienced an increase in PTC. Although a causal role of iodine intake in the etiology of PTC cannot be ruled out, a more likely explanation for the increasing incidence of PTC worldwide is the introduction and wider use of improved thyroid diagnostics. Compounding this, in areas without iodine deficiency and hence less goiter, individuals are more likely to notice a small change in their thyroid and go for medical examination. Thus, we may never have a clear answer to the question of whether changes in iodine intake contribute to PTC. Of note, autopsy studies of OTC are not confounded by changes in diagnostic and treatment, and they suggest that papillary microcarcinomas are actually less common in areas (outside of Japan) with high iodine intakes (Table 3).

The available data from case–control studies suggest higher iodine intakes and higher intakes of fish and seafood, particularly in iodine deficient populations, are linked to a small reduction in risk of thyroid cancer. However, the associations are weak and inconsistent and none of these studies were done in populations with clear iodine deficiency or excess. Future research should emphasize the collection of prospective data from large cohorts where total iodine exposure is assessed by measurement of repeated UICs, together with other iodine status biomarkers, such as serum thyroglobulin.

Overall, the available evidence suggests iodine deficiency is a risk factor for thyroid cancer, and that it particularly increases risk for FTC and possibly, ATC. This conclusion is based on: a) consistent data showing an increase in thyroid cancer (mainly follicular) in iodine deficient animals; b) a plausible mechanism (chronic TSH stimulation induced by iodine deficiency); c) consistent data from before and after studies of iodine prophylaxis showing a decrease in the percentage of thyroid cancer that is FTC and ATC; d) the indirect association between iodine intake and thyroid cancer mortality in the decade from 2000 to 2010; e) the autopsy studies of OTC showing microcarcinoma rates with lower iodine intakes; f) and the case control studies showing a trend toward lower risk for thyroid cancer with higher fish and total iodine intakes.

Abbreviations

ATC: Anaplastic thyroid cancer; BHP: N-nitrosobis(2-hydroxypropyl)amine; CI: Confidence intervals; TC: Thyroid cancer; DHPN: N-bis(2-hydroxypropyl)-nitrosamine; ERR: Excess relative risk; FTC: Follicular thyroid cancer; ICCIDD: International Council for the Control of Iodine Deficiency Disorders (now Iodine Global Network); MAPK: mitogen-activated protein kinase; NHANES: National Health and Nutrition Examination Surveys; NMU: N-nitrosomethylurea; OR: Odds ratio; OTC: Occult thyroid carcinomas; PTC: Papillary thyroid cancer; RNI: Recommended nutrient intake; RR: Relative risk; SE: Standard error; TSH: Thyroid-stimulating hormone; UIC: Urinary iodine concentration; UNICEF: United Nations Children's Fund; WHO: World Health Organization.

Competing interests
The authors declare that they have no competing interests.

Authors' contributions
MBZ wrote the draft of the manuscript. VG performed statistical analysis. Both authors read and approved the final manuscript.

Acknowledgements
The writing of this review was supported by a grant from the ETH Zürich, Switzerland.

Author details
[1]Laboratory of Human Nutrition, Department of Health Sciences and Technology, ETH Zürich, Schmelzbergstrasse 7, LFV D21, CH-8092 Zürich, Switzerland. [2]Laboratory of Human Nutrition, Department of Health Sciences and Technology, ETH Zürich, Schmelzbergstrasse 7, LFV E14, CH-8092 Zürich, Switzerland.

References
1. La Vecchia C, Malvezzi M, Bosetti C, Garavello W, Bertuccio P, Levi F, et al. Thyroid cancer mortality and incidence: a global overview. Int J Cancer. 2015;136:2187–95.
2. Rahib L, Smith BD, Aizenberg R, Rosenzweig AB, Fleshman JM, Matrisian LM. Projecting cancer incidence and deaths to 2030: the unexpected burden of thyroid, liver, and pancreas cancers in the United States. Cancer Res. 2014;74:2913–21.
3. Chen AY, Jemal A, Ward EM. Increasing incidence of differentiated thyroid cancer in the United States, 1988–2005. Cancer. 2009;115:3801–7.
4. Enewold L, Zhu K, Ron E, Marrogi AJ, Stojadinovic A, Peoples GE, et al. Rising thyroid cancer incidence in the United States by demographic and tumor characteristics, 1980–2005. Cancer Epidemiol Biomarkers Prev. 2009;18:784–91.
5. Morris LGT, Sikora AG, Tosteson TD, Davies L. The increasing incidence of thyroid cancer: the influence of access to care. Thyroid. 2013;23:886–92.
6. Udelsman R, Zhang Y. The epidemic of thyroid cancer in the United States: the role of endocrinologists and ultrasounds. Thyroid. 2014;24:472–9.
7. Ahn HS, Kim HJ, Welch HG. Korea's thyroid-cancer "epidemic" - screening and overdiagnosis. N Engl J Med. 2014;371:1765–7.
8. Bard D, Verger P, Hubert P. Chernobyl, 10 years after: health consequences. Epidemiol Rev. 1997;19:187–204.
9. Mazonakis M, Tzedakis A, Damilakis J, Gourtsoyiannis N. Thyroid dose from common head and neck CT examinations in children: is there an excess risk for thyroid cancer induction? Eur Radiol. 2007;17:1352–7.
10. Bounacer A, Wicker R, Caillou B, Cailleux AF, Sarasin A, Schlumberger M, et al. High prevalence of activating ret proto-oncogene rearrangements, in thyroid tumors from patients who had received external radiation. Oncogene. 1997;15:1263–73.
11. Renehan AG, Tyson M, Egger M, Heller RF, Zwahlen M. Body-mass index and incidence of cancer: a systematic review and meta-analysis of prospective observational studies. Lancet. 2008;371:569–78.
12. Rinaldi S, Lise M, Clavel-Chapelon F, Boutron-Ruault MC, Guillas G, Overvad K, et al. Body size and risk of differentiated thyroid carcinomas: findings from the EPIC study. Int J Cancer. 2012;131:E1004–14.
13. Hallgren S, Darnerud PO. Polybrominated diphenyl ethers (PBDEs), polychlorinated biphenyls (PCBs) and chlorinated paraffins (CPs) in rats - testing interactions and mechanisms for thyroid hormone effects. Toxicology. 2002;177:227–43.
14. Zhang Y, Guo GL, Han X, Zhu C, Kilfoy BA, Zhu Y, et al. Do Polybrominated Diphenyl Ethers (PBDEs) Increase the Risk of Thyroid Cancer? Biosci Hypotheses. 2008;1:195–9.
15. Franceschi S, Preston-Martin S, Dal Maso L, Negri E, La Vecchia C, Mack WJ, et al. A pooled analysis of case–control studies of thyroid cancer. IV. Benign thyroid diseases. Cancer Causes Control. 1999;10:583–95.
16. Zimmermann MB, Boelaert K. Iodine deficiency and thyroid disorders. Lancet Diabetes Endocrinol. 2015;3:286–95.
17. Wegelin C. Malignant disease of the thyroid gland and its relation to goitre in man and animals. Cancer Rev. 1928;3:297.
18. Global Iodine Nutrition Scorecard 2014. Available at: http://www.ign.org/cm_data/Scorecard_IGN_website_02_03_2015.pdf. Accessed 2 Mar 2015.
19. Carle A, Krejbjerg A, Laurberg P. Epidemiology of nodular goitre. Influence of iodine intake. Best Pract Res Clin Endocrinol Metab. 2014;28:465–79.
20. Cole WH, Majarakis JD, Slaughter DP. Incidence of carcinoma of the thyroid in nodular goiter. J Clin Endocrinol Metab. 1949;9:1007–11.
21. Feldt-Rasmussen U. Iodine and cancer. Thyroid. 2001;11:483–6.
22. Williams ED. Dietary iodide and thyroid cancer. In: Hall R, Köbberling J, editors. Thyroid disorders associated with iodine deficiency and excess. New York: Raven; 1985.
23. World Health Organization, United Nations Children's Fund, International Council for the Control of Iodine Deficiency Disorders. Assessment of iodine deficiency disorders and monitoring their elimination. A guide for programme managers. 3rd ed. Geneva: World Health Organization; 2007.
24. Zimmermann MB, Andersson M. Assessment of iodine nutrition in populations: past, present, and future. Nutr Rev. 2012;70:553–70.
25. Axelrad AA, Leblond CP. Induction of thyroid tumors in rats by a low iodine diet. Cancer. 1955;8:339–67.
26. Isler H, Leblond CP, Axelrad AA. Influence of age and of iodine intake on the production of thyroid tumors in the rat. J Natl Cancer Inst. 1958;21:1065–81.
27. Isler H. Effect of iodine on thyroid tumors induced in the rat by a low-iodine diet. J Natl Cancer Inst. 1959;23:675–93.
28. Schaller Jr RT, Stevenson JK. Development of carcinoma of the thyroid in iodine-deficient mice. Cancer. 1966;19:1063–80.
29. Fortner JG, George PA, Sternberg SS. The development of thyroid cancer and other abnormalities in Syrian hamsters maintained on an iodine deficient diet. Surg Forum. 1958;9:646–50.
30. Correa P, Welsh RA. The effect of excessive iodine intake on the thyroid gland of the rat. Arch Pathol. 1960;70:247–51.
31. Ohshima M, Ward JM. Promotion of N-Methyl-N-Nitrosourea-Induced Thyroid-Tumors by Iodine Deficiency in F344 Ncr Rats. J Natl Cancer I. 1984;73:289–96.
32. Ohshima M, Ward JM. Dietary iodine deficiency as a tumor promoter and carcinogen in male F344/Ncr rats. Cancer Res. 1986;46:877–83.
33. Kanno J, Onodera H, Furuta K, Maekawa A, Kasuga T, Hayashi Y. Tumor-promoting effects of both iodine deficiency and iodine excess in the rat-thyroid. Toxicol Pathol. 1992;20:226–35.
34. Yamashita H, Noguchi S, Murakami N, Kato R, Adachi M, Inoue S, et al. Effects of dietary iodine on chemical induction of thyroid-carcinoma. Acta Pathol Japon. 1990;40:705–12.
35. Cho YM, Imai T, Hasumura M, Hirose M. Lack of enhancement of susceptibility to mammary and thyroid carcinogenesis in rats exposed to DMBA and DHPN following prepubertal iodine deficiency. Cancer Sci. 2006;97:1031–6.
36. Boltze C, Brabant G, Dralle H, Gerlach R, Roessner A, Hoang-Vu C. Radiation-induced thyroid carcinogenesis as a function of time and dietary iodine supply: An in vivo model of tumorigenesis in the rat. Endocrinology. 2002;143:2584–92.
37. al-Saadi AA, Beierwaltes WH. Chromosomal changes in rat thyroid cells during iodine depletion and repletion. Cancer Res. 1966;26:676–88.
38. Riesco G, Taurog A, Larsen R, Krulich L. Acute and chronic responses to iodine deficiency in rats. Endocrinology. 1977;100:303–13.
39. Hill RN, Erdreich LS, Paynter OE, Roberts PA, Rosenthal SL, Wilkinson CF. Thyroid follicular cell carcinogenesis. Fundam Appl Toxicol. 1989;12:629–97.
40. Ward JM, Ohshima M. The role of iodine in carcinogenesis. Adv Exp Med Biol. 1986;206:529–42.
41. Kaplan MM. Progress in Thyroid-Cancer. Endocrin Metab Clin. 1990;19:469–78.
42. Doniach I, Williams ED. The development of thyroid and pituitary tumours in the rat two years after partial thyroidectomy. Br J Cancer. 1962;16:222–31.
43. Purves HD, Griesbach WE. Studies on experimental goitre; thyroid tumours in rats treated with thiourea. Br J Exp Pathol. 1947;28:46–53.
44. Wynford-Thomas D, Stringer BMJ, Williams ED. Desensitization of rat-thyroid to the growth-stimulating action of Tsh during prolonged goitrogen administration - persistence of refractoriness following withdrawal of stimulation. Acta Endocrinol (Copenh). 1982;101:562–9.
45. Uyttersprot N, Pelgrims N, Carrasco N, Gervy C, Maenhaut C, Dumont JE, et al. Moderate doses of iodide in vivo inhibit cell proliferation and the expression of thyroperoxidase and Na+/I- symporter mRNAs in dog thyroid. Mol Cell Endocrinol. 1997;131:195–203.
46. Eng PHK, Cardona GR, Fang SL, Previti M, Alex S, Carrasco N, et al. Escape from the acute Wolff-Chaikoff effect is associated with a decrease in thyroid

sodium/iodide symporter messenger ribonucleic acid and protein. Endocrinology. 1999;140:3404–10.

47. Krohn K, Maier J, Paschke R. Mechanisms of Disease: hydrogen peroxide, DNA damage and mutagenesis in the development of thyroid tumors. Nat Clin Pract Endoc. 2007;3:713–20.

48. Maier J, van Steeg H, van Oostrom C, Paschke R, Weiss RE, Krohn K. Iodine deficiency activates antioxidant genes and causes DNA damage in the thyroid gland of rats and mice. Biochim Biophys Acta. 2007;1773:990–9.

49. Vitale M, Di Matola T, D'Ascoli F, Salzano S, Bogazzi F, Fenzi G, et al. Iodide excess induces apoptosis in thyroid cells through a p53-independent mechanism involving oxidative stress. Endocrinology. 2000;141:598–605.

50. Cardoso LC, Martins DC, Figueiredo MD, Rosenthal D, Vaisman M, Violante AH, et al. Ca(2+)/nicotinamide adenine dinucleotide phosphate-dependent H(2)O(2) generation is inhibited by iodide in human thyroids. J Clin Endocrinol Metab. 2001;86:4339–43.

51. Langer R, Burzler C, Bechtner G, Gartner R. Influence of iodide and iodolactones on thyroid apoptosis. Evidence that apoptosis induced by iodide is mediated by iodolactones in intact porcine thyroid follicles. Exp Clin Endocr Diab. 2003;111:325–9.

52. Gartner R, Rank P, Ander B. The role of iodine and delta-iodolactone in growth and apoptosis of malignant thyroid epithelial cells and breast cancer cells. Hormones (Athens). 2010;9:60–6.

53. Kimura ET, Nikiforova MN, Zhu ZW, Knauf JA, Nikiforov YE, Fagin JA. High prevalence of BRAF mutations in thyroid cancer: genetic evidence for constitutive activation of the RET/PTC-RAS-BRAF signaling pathway in papillary thyroid carcinoma. Cancer Res. 2003;63:1454–7.

54. Liu XH, Chen GG, Vlantis AC, van Hasselt CA. Iodine mediated mechanisms and thyroid carcinoma. Crit Rev Cl Lab Sci. 2009;46:302–18.

55. Frasca F, Nucera C, Pellegriti G, Gangemi P, Attard M, Stella M, et al. BRAF(V600E) mutation and the biology of papillary thyroid cancer. Endocr Relat Cancer. 2008;15:191–205.

56. Guan H, Ji M, Bao R, Yu H, Wang Y, Hou P, et al. Association of high iodine intake with the T1799A BRAF mutation in papillary thyroid cancer. J Clin Endocrinol Metab. 2009;94:1612–7.

57. Fuziwara CS, Kimura ET. High iodine blocks a Notch/miR-19 loop activated by the BRAF(V600E) oncoprotein and restores the response to TGFbeta in thyroid follicular cells. Thyroid. 2014;24:453–62.

58. Shi YF, Zou MJ, Schmidt H, Juhasz F, Stensky V, Robb D, et al. High-rates of Ras Codon-61 mutation in thyroid-tumors in an iodide-deficient area. Cancer Res. 1991;51:2690–3.

59. Fiore AP, Fuziwara CS, Kimura ET. High iodine concentration attenuates RET/PTC3 oncogene activation in thyroid follicular cells. Thyroid. 2009;19:1249–56.

60. Xiang J, Wang XM, Wang ZY, Wu Y, Li DS, Shen Q, et al. Effect of different iodine concentrations on well-differentiated thyroid cancer cell behavior and its inner mechanism. Cell Biochem Biophys. 2015;71:299–305.

61. Langsteger W, Koltringer P, Wolf G, Dominik K, Buchinger W, Binter G, et al. The impact of geographical, clinical, dietary and radiation-induced features in epidemiology of thyroid cancer. Eur J Cancer. 1993;29A:1547–53.

62. Saxen E, Franssila K, Bjarnason O, Normann T, Ringertz N. Observer variation in histologic classification of thyroid cancer. Acta Pathol Microbiol Scand A. 1978;86A:483–6.

63. Hedinger CE, Sobin LH. Histological Typing of Thyroid Tumours. Geneva: World Health Organization (International Histological Classification of Tumours, No 11); 1974.

64. Verkooijen HM, Fioretta G, Pache JC, Franceschi S, Raymond L, Schubert H, et al. Diagnostic changes as a reason for the increase in papillary thyroid cancer incidence in Geneva, Switzerland. Cancer Causes Control. 2003;14:13–7.

65. Walthard B. Der Gestaltwandel Der Struma Maligna Mit Bezug Auf Die Jodprophylaxe Des Kropfes. Schweiz Med Wochenschr. 1963;93:809.

66. Hofstadter F. Frequency and morphology of malignant-tumors of the thyroid before and after the introduction of iodine-prophylaxis. Virchows Arch A Pathol Anat Histol. 1980;385:263–70.

67. Bubenhofer R, Hedinger C. [Thyroid neoplasms before and after the prophylactic supplementation of table salt with iodine]. Schweiz Med Wochenschr. 1977;107:733–41.

68. Leenhardt L, Bernier MO, Boin-Pineau MH, Conte Devolx B, Marechaud R, Niccoli-Sire P, et al. Advances in diagnostic practices affect thyroid cancer incidence in France. Eur J Endocrinol. 2004;150:133–9.

69. CI5plus: Cancer Incidence In Five Continents Time Trends. Available at: http://ci5.iarc.fr/CI5plus/Pages/online.aspx. Accessed 11 Dec 2014.

70. Hollowell JG, Staehling NW, Hannon WH, Flanders DW, Gunter EW, Maberly GF, et al. Iodine nutrition in the United States. Trends and public health implications: Iodine excretion data from National Health and Nutrition Examination Surveys I and III (1971–1974 and 1988–1994). J Clin Endocrinol Metab. 1998;83:3401–8.

71. Pan Y, Caldwell KL, Li Y, Caudill SP, Mortensen ME, Makhmudov A, et al. Smoothed urinary iodine percentiles for the US population and pregnant women: National Health and Nutrition examination survey, 2001–2010. Eur Thyroid J. 2013;2:127–34.

72. Lubitz CC, Kong CY, McMahon PM, Daniels GH, Chen YF, Economopoulos KP, et al. Annual financial impact of well-differentiated thyroid cancer care in the United States. Cancer. 2014;120:1345–52.

73. Pettersson B, Coleman MP, Ron E, Adami HO. Iodine supplementation in Sweden and regional trends in thyroid cancer incidence by histopathologic type. Int J Cancer. 1996;65:13–9.

74. Rasmussen LB, Jorgensen T, Perrild H, Knudsen N, Krejbjerg A, Laurberg P, et al. Mandatory iodine fortification of bread and salt increases iodine excretion in adults in Denmark - a 11-year follow-up study. Clin Nutr. 2014;33:1033–40.

75. Blomberg M, Feldt-Rasmussen U, Andersen KK, Kjaer SK. Thyroid cancer in Denmark 1943–2008, before and after iodine supplementation. Int J Cancer. 2012;131:2360–6.

76. Knudsen N, Bulow I, Jorgensen T, Laurberg P, Ovesen L, Perrild H. Goitre prevalence and thyroid abnormalities at ultrasonography: a comparative epidemiological study in two regions with slightly different iodine status. Clin Endocrinol (Oxf). 2000;53:479–85.

77. Sehestedt T, Knudsen N, Perrild H, Johansen C. Iodine intake and incidence of thyroid cancer in Denmark. Clin Endocrinol (Oxf). 2006;65:229–33.

78. Netea-Maier RT, Aben KKH, Casparie MK, den Heijer M, Grefte JMM, Slootweg P, et al. Trends in incidence and mortality of thyroid carcinoma in The Netherlands between 1989 and 2003: correlation with thyroid fine-needle aspiration cytology and thyroid surgery. Int J Cancer. 2008;123:1681–4.

79. Williams ED, Doniach I, Bjarnason O, Michie W. Thyroid Cancer in an Iodide Rich Area - Histopathological Study. Cancer. 1977;39:215–22.

80. Radespiel-Troger M, Batzler WU, Holleczek B, Luttmann S, Pritzkuleit R, Stabenow R, et al. Im Namen der Gesellschaft der epidemiologischen Krebsregister in Deutschland e V [Rising incidence of papillary thyroid carcinoma in Germany]. Bundesgesundheitsbl Gesundheitsforsch Gesundheitsschutz. 2014;57:84–92.

81. Lise M, Franceschi S, Buzzoni C, Zambon P, Falcini F, Crocetti E, et al. Changes in the incidence of thyroid cancer between 1991 and 2005 in Italy: a geographical analysis. Thyroid. 2012;22:27–34.

82. Belfiore A, La Rosa GL, La Porta GA, Giuffrida D, Milazzo G, Lupo L, et al. Cancer risk in patients with cold thyroid nodules: relevance of iodine intake, sex, age, and multinodularity. Am J Med. 1992;93:363–9.

83. Ilias I, Alevizaki M, Lakka-Papadodima E, Koutras DA. Differentiated thyroid cancer in Greece: 1963–2000. Relation to demographic and environmental factors. Hormones (Athens). 2002;1:174–8.

84. Rego-Iraeta A, Perez-Mendez LF, Mantinan B, Garcia-Mayor RV. Time trends for thyroid cancer in northwestern Spain: true rise in the incidence of micro and larger forms of papillary thyroid carcinoma. Thyroid. 2009;19:333–40.

85. Wang Y, Wang W. Increasing Incidence of Thyroid Cancer in Shanghai, China, 1983–2007. Asia Pac J Public Health. 2015;27:NP223–9.

86. Dong W, Zhang H, Zhang P, Li X, He L, Wang Z, et al. The changing incidence of thyroid carcinoma in Shenyang, China before and after universal salt iodization. Med Sci Monit. 2013;19:49–53.

87. Teng WP, Shan ZY, Teng XC, Guan HX, Li YH, Teng D, et al. Effect of iodine intake on thyroid diseases in China. New Eng J Med. 2006;354:2783–93.

88. Zhu W, Liu X, Hu X, Zhou S, Wang Y, Zhang Y. Investigation on the iodine nutritional status and the prevalence of thyroid carcinoma in Zhoushan Archipelago residents. Wei Sheng Yan Jiu. 2012;41:79–82.

89. Chen ZX, Xu WM, Huang YM, Jin X, Deng J, Zhu SJ, et al. Associations of noniodized salt and thyroid nodule among the Chinese population: a large cross-sectional study. Am J Clin Nutr. 2013;98:684–92.

90. Wong EY, Ray R, Gao DL, Wernli KJ, Li W, Fitzgibbons ED, et al. Reproductive history, occupational exposures, and thyroid cancer risk among women textile workers in Shanghai, China. Int Arch Occ Env Hea. 2006;79:251–8.

91. Yin JH, Wang CC, Shao Q, Qu DH, Song ZY, Shan PF, Zhang T, Xu J, Liang Q, Zhang SZ, Huang J. Relationship between the Prevalence of Thyroid Nodules and Metabolic Syndrome in the Iodine-Adequate Area of

Hangzhou, China: A Cross-Sectional and Cohort Study. Int J Endocrinol. 2014.

92. Burgess JR, Dwyer T, McArdle K, Tucker P, Shugg D. The changing incidence and spectrum of thyroid carcinoma in Tasmania (1978–1998) during a transition from iodine sufficiency to iodine deficiency. J Clin Endocrinol Metab. 2000;85:1513–7.

93. Burgess JR. Temporal trends for thyroid carcinoma in Australia: an increasing incidence of papillary thyroid carcinoma (1982–1997). Thyroid. 2002;12:141–9.

94. Li M, Eastman CJ, Waite KV, Ma G, Zacharin MR, Topliss DJ, et al. Are Australian children iodine deficient? Results of the Australian National Iodine Nutrition Study. Med J Aust. 2006;184:165–9.

95. Harach HR, Ceballos GA. Thyroid cancer, thyroiditis and dietary iodine: a review based on the Salta, Argentina Model. Endocr Pathol. 2008;19:209–20.

96. Chiacchio S, Lorenzoni A, Boni G, Rubello D, Elisei R, Mariani G. Anaplastic thyroid cancer: prevalence, diagnosis and treatment. Minerva Endocrinol. 2008;33:341–57.

97. Besic N, Hocevar M, Zgajnar J. Lower incidence of anaplastic carcinoma after higher iodination of salt in Slovenia. Thyroid. 2010;20:623–6.

98. Bacher-Stier C, Riccabona G, Totsch M, Kemmler G, Oberaigner W, Moncayo R. Incidence and clinical characteristics of thyroid carcinoma after iodine prophylaxis in an endemic goiter country. Thyroid. 1997;7:733–41.

99. Farahati J, Geling M, Mader U, Mortl M, Luster M, Muller JG, et al. Changing trends of incidence and prognosis of thyroid carcinoma in lower Franconia, Germany, from 1981–1995. Thyroid. 2004;14:141–7.

100. Ceresini G, Corcione L, Michiara M, Sgargi P, Teresi G, Gilli A, et al. Thyroid cancer incidence by histological type and related variants in a mildly iodine-deficient area of Northern Italy, 1998 to 2009. Cancer. 2012;118:5473–80.

101. Guberan E. [Mortality trends in Switzerland. 3. Tumors: 1921–1978]. Schweiz Med Wochenschr Suppl. 1980;Suppl 11:1–18.

102. Reynolds RM, Weir J, Stockton DL, Brewster DH, Sandeep TC, Strachan MW. Changing trends in incidence and mortality of thyroid cancer in Scotland. Clin Endocrinol (Oxf). 2005;62:156–62.

103. Harach HR, Galindez M, Campero M, Ceballos GA. Undifferentiated (Anaplastic) Thyroid Carcinoma and Iodine Intake in Salta, Argentina. Endocr Pathol. 2013;24:125–31.

104. Carcangiu ML, Steeper T, Zampi G, Rosai J. Anaplastic thyroid carcinoma. A study of 70 cases. Am J Clin Pathol. 1985;83:135–58.

105. Smallridge RC, Copland JA. Anaplastic thyroid carcinoma: pathogenesis and emerging therapies. Clin Oncol. 2010;22:486–97.

106. World Health Organization Statistical Information System (WHOSIS). WHO Mortality Database. Geneva: World Health Organization. Available at: http://apps.who.int/healthinfo/statistics/mortality/whodpms/.

107. WHO Vitamin and Mineral Nutrition Information System (VMNIS). Database on Iodine Deficiency. Available at: http://www.who.int/vmnis/database/iodine/en/. Accessed 11 Dec 2014.

108. Fukunaga FH, Yatani R. Geographic pathology of occult thyroid carcinomas. Cancer. 1975;36:1095–9.

109. Kovacs GL, Gonda G, Vadasz G, Ludmany E, Uhrin K, Gorombey Z, et al. Epidemiology of thyroid microcarcinoma found in autopsy series conducted in areas of different iodine intake. Thyroid. 2005;15:152–7.

110. Neuhold N, Kaiser H, Kaserer K. Latent carcinoma of the thyroid in Austria: a systematic autopsy study. Endocr Pathol. 2001;12:23–31.

111. Yamamoto Y, Maeda T, Izumi K, Otsuka H. Occult papillary carcinoma of the thyroid - a study of 408 autopsy cases. Cancer. 1990;65:1173–9.

112. Harach HR, Franssila KO, Wasenius VM. Occult papillary carcinoma of the thyroid - a normal finding in Finland - a systematic autopsy study. Cancer. 1985;56:531–8.

113. Derwahl M, Studer H. Nodular goiter and goiter nodules: Where iodine deficiency falls short of explaining the facts. Exp Clin Endocr Diab. 2001;109:250–60.

114. Krohn K, Fuhrer D, Bayer Y, Eszlinger M, Brauer V, Neumann S, et al. Molecular pathogenesis of euthyroid and toxic multinodular goiter. Endocr Rev. 2005;26:504–24.

115. Horn-Ross PL, Morris JS, Lee M, West DW, Whittemore AS, McDougall IR, et al. Iodine and thyroid cancer risk among women in a multiethnic population: the Bay Area Thyroid Cancer Study. Cancer Epidemiol Biomarkers Prev. 2001;10:979–85.

116. Memon A, Varghese A, Suresh A. Benign thyroid disease and dietary factors in thyroid cancer: a case–control study in Kuwait. Br J Cancer. 2002;86:1745–50.

117. Iribarren C, Haselkorn T, Tekawa IS, Friedman GD. Cohort study of thyroid cancer in a San Francisco Bay area population. Int J Cancer. 2001;93:745–50.

118. Pendergrast WJ, Milmore BK, Marcus SC. Thyroid cancer and thyrotoxicosis in the United States: their relation to endemic goiter. J Chronic Dis. 1961;13:22–38.

119. Clements FW. The relationship of thyrotoxicosis and carcinoma of the thyroid to endemic goitre. Med J Aust. 1954;2:894–7.

120. Brito JP, Yarur AJ, Prokop LJ, McIver B, Murad MH, Montori VM. Prevalence of thyroid cancer in multinodular goiter versus single nodule: a systematic review and meta-analysis. Thyroid. 2013;23:449–55.

121. Kolonel LN, Hankin JH, Wilkens LR, Fukunaga FH, Hinds MW. An epidemiologic study of thyroid cancer in Hawaii. Cancer Causes Control. 1990;1:223–34.

122. Truong T, Baron-Dubourdieu D, Rougier Y, Guenel P. Role of dietary iodine and cruciferous vegetables in thyroid cancer: a countrywide case–control study in New Caledonia. Cancer Causes Control. 2010;21:1183–92.

123. Clero E, Doyon F, Chungue V, Rachedi F, Boissin JL, Sebbag J, et al. Dietary iodine and thyroid cancer risk in French Polynesia: a case–control study. Thyroid. 2012;22:422–9.

124. Panityakul T, Bumrungsup C, Knapp G. On estimating residual heterogeneity in random-effects meta-regression: a comparative study. J Stat Theory Appl. 2013;12:253–65.

125. R Core Team. R: A language and environment for statistical computing. R Foundation for Statistical Computing, Vienna, Austria. Available at: http://www.R-project.org/. 2014.

126. Viechtbauer W. Conducting meta-analyses in R with the metafor package. J Stat Softw. 2010;36:1–48.

127. Lumley T. rmeta: Meta-analysis. R package version 2.16. Available at: http://CRAN.R-project.org/package=rmeta. 2012.

128. Liu ZT, Lin AH. Dietary factors and thyroid cancer risk: a meta-analysis of observational studies. Nutr Cancer. 2014;66:1165–78.

129. Bosetti C, Kolonel L, Negri E, Ron E, Franceschi S, Dal Maso L, et al. A pooled analysis of case–control studies of thyroid cancer. VI. Fish and shellfish consumption. Cancer Causes Control. 2001;12:375–82.

130. Perrine CG, Sullivan KM, Flores R, Caldwell KL, Grummer-Strawn LM. Intakes of dairy products and dietary supplements are positively associated with iodine status among US Children. J Nutr. 2013;143:1155–60.

131. Zimmermann MB. Symposium on 'Geographical and geological influences on nutrition': Iodine deficiency in industrialised countries. Proc Nutr Soc. 2010;69:133–43.

132. Haldimann M, Alt A, Blanc A, Blondeau K. Iodine content of food groups. J Food Compos Anal. 2005;18:461–71.

133. Brauer VF, Brauer WH, Fuhrer D, Paschke R. Iodine nutrition, nodular thyroid disease, and urinary iodine excretion in a German university study population. Thyroid. 2005;15:364–70.

134. Galanti MR, Hansson L, Bergstrom R, Wolk A, Hjartaker A, Lund E, et al. Diet and the risk of papillary and follicular thyroid carcinoma: a population-based case–control study in Sweden and Norway. Cancer Causes Control. 1997;8:205–14.

135. Franceschi S, Levi F, Negri E, Fassina A, La Vecchia C. Diet and thyroid cancer: a pooled analysis of four European case–control studies. Int J Cancer. 1991;48:395–8.

136. Mack WJ, Preston-Martin S, Dal Maso L, Galanti R, Xiang M, Franceschi S, et al. A pooled analysis of case–control studies of thyroid cancer: cigarette smoking and consumption of alcohol, coffee, and tea. Cancer Causes Control. 2003;14:773–85.

137. Bandurska-Stankiewicz E, Aksamit-Bialoszewska E, Rutkowska J, Stankiewicz A, Shafie D. The effect of nutritional habits and addictions on the incidence of thyroid carcinoma in the Olsztyn province of Poland. Endokrynol Pol. 2011;62:145–50.

138. Park Y, Leitzmann MF, Subar AF, Hollenbeck A, Schatzkin A. Dairy food, calcium, and risk of cancer in the NIH-AARP Diet and Health Study. Arch Intern Med. 2009;169:391–401.

139. Schneider AB, Shore-Freedman E, Weinstein RA. Radiation-induced thyroid and other head and neck tumors: occurrence of multiple tumors and analysis of risk factors. J Clin Endocrinol Metab. 1986;63:107–12.

140. Ron E, Lubin JH, Shore RE, Mabuchi K, Modan B, Pottern LM, et al. Thyroid cancer after exposure to external radiation: a pooled analysis of seven studies. Radiat Res. 1995;141:259–77.

141. Williams D. Twenty years' experience with post-Chernobyl thyroid cancer. Best Pract Res Clin Endocrinol Metab. 2008;22:1061–73.

142. Robbins J, Dunn JT, Bouville A, Kravchenko VI, Lubin J, Petrenko S, et al. Iodine nutrition and the risk from radioactive iodine: a workshop report in the chernobyl long-term follow-up study. Thyroid. 2001;11:487–91.

143. Shakhtarin VV, Tsyb AF, Stepanenko VF, Orlov MY, Kopecky KJ, Davis S. Iodine deficiency, radiation dose, and the risk of thyroid cancer among children and adolescents in the Bryansk region of Russia following the Chernobyl power station accident. Int J Epidemiol. 2003;32:584–91.

144. Cardis E, Kesminiene A, Ivanov V, Malakhova I, Shibata Y, Khrouch V, et al. Risk of thyroid cancer after exposure to 131I in childhood. J Natl Cancer Inst. 2005;97:724–32.

145. Tronko MD, Howe GR, Bogdanova TI, Bouville AC, Epstein OV, Brill AB, et al. A cohort study of thyroid cancer and other thyroid diseases after the chornobyl accident: Thyroid cancer in Ukraine detected during first screening. J Natl Cancer I. 2006;98:897–903.

146. Zablotska LB, Ron E, Rozhko AV, Hatch M, Polyanskaya ON, Brenner AV, et al. Thyroid cancer risk in Belarus among children and adolescents exposed to radioiodine after the Chornobyl accident. Br J Cancer. 2011;104:181–7.

147. Hatch M, Polyanskaya O, McConnell R, Gong ZH, Drozdovitch V, Rozhko A, et al. Urinary Iodine and goiter prevalence in Belarus: experience of the Belarus-American cohort study of thyroid cancer and other thyroid diseases following the Chornobyl nuclear accident. Thyroid. 2011;21:429–37.

148. Heitz P, Moser H, Staub JJ. Thyroid cancer: a study of 573 thyroid tumors and 161 autopsy cases observed over a thirty-year period. Cancer. 1976;37:2329–37.

149. Lind P, Langsteger W, Molnar M, Gallowitsch HJ, Mikosch P, Gomez I. Epidemiology of thyroid diseases in iodine sufficiency. Thyroid. 1998;8:1179–83.

150. Huszno B, Szybinski Z, Przybylik-Mazurek E, Stachura J, Trofimiuk M, Buziak-Bereza M, et al. Influence of iodine deficiency and iodine prophylaxis on thyroid cancer histotypes and incidence in endemic goiter area. J Endocrinol Invest. 2003;26:71–6.

151. Pingitore R. Rilievi morfologici autoptici su 111 tiroidi clinicamente normali in un'area italiana senza edemia gozzigena. Pathologica. 1982;74:545–52.

152. Arellano L, Ibarra A. Occult carcinoma of the thyroid gland. Pathol Res Pract. 1984;179:88–91.

153. Sobrinho-Simoes MA, Sambade MC, Goncalves V. Latent thyroid-carcinoma at autopsy - study from Oporto, Portugal. Cancer. 1979;43:1702–6.

154. Siegal A, Modan M. Latent Carcinoma of Thyroid in Israel - a Study of 260 Autopsies. Israel J Med Sci. 1981;17:249–53.

155. Lang W, Borrusch H, Bauer L. Occult carcinomas of the thyroid. Evaluation of 1,020 sequential autopsies. Am J Clin Pathol. 1988;90:72–6.

156. Martinez-Tello FJ, Martinez-Cabruja R, Fernandez-Martin J, Lasso-Oria C, Ballestin-Carcavilla C. Occult carcinoma of the thyroid. A systematic autopsy study from Spain of two series performed with two different methods. Cancer. 1993;71:4022–9.

157. Furmanchuk AW, Roussak N, Ruchti C. Occult thyroid carcinomas in the region of Minsk, Belarus. An autopsy study of 215 patients. Histopathology. 1993;23:319–25.

158. Avetisian IL, Petrova GV. Latent thyroid pathology in residents of Kiev, Ukraine. J Environ Pathol Toxicol Oncol. 1996;15:239–43.

159. Solares CA, Penalonzo MA, Xu M, Orellana E. Occult papillary thyroid carcinoma in postmortem species: prevalence at autopsy. Am J Otolaryng. 2005;26:87–90.

160. Bondeson L, Ljungberg O. Occult thyroid carcinoma at autopsy in Malmo, Sweden. Cancer. 1981;47:319–23.

161. Komorowski RA, Hanson GA. Occult thyroid pathology in the young-adult - an autopsy study of 138 patients without clinical thyroid-disease. Hum Pathol. 1988;19:689–96.

162. Bisi H, Fernandes VS, de Camargo RY, Koch L, Abdo AH, de Brito T. The prevalence of unsuspected thyroid pathology in 300 sequential autopsies, with special reference to the incidental carcinoma. Cancer. 1989;64:1888–93.

163. Ottino A, Pianzola HM, Castelletto RH. Occult papillary thyroid-carcinoma at autopsy in La-Plata, Argentina. Cancer. 1989;64:547–51.

164. Thorvaldsson SE, Tulinius H, Bjornsson J, Bjarnason O. Latent thyroid-carcinoma in Iceland at autopsy. Pathol Res Pract. 1992;188:747–50.

165. Chong PY. Thyroid carcinomas in Singapore autopsies. Pathology. 1994;26:20–2.

166. Mitselou A, Vougiouklakis T, Peschos D, Dallas P, Agnantis NJ. Occult thyroid carcinoma. A study of 160 autopsy cases. The first report for the region of Epirus-Greece. Anticancer Res. 2002;22:427–32.

167. Tanriover O, Comunoglu N, Eren B, Comunoglu C, Turkmen N, Dogan M, et al. Occult papillary thyroid carcinoma: prevalence at autopsy in Turkish people. Eur J Cancer Prev. 2011;20:308–12.

168. Hazard JB, Kaufman N. A survey of thyroid glands obtained at autopsy in a so-called goiter area. Am J Clin Pathol. 1952;22:860–5.

169. Mortensen JD, Woolner LB, Bennett WA. Gross and microscopic findings in clinically normal thyroid glands. J Clin Endocrinol Metab. 1955;15:1270–80.

170. Hull OH. Critical analysis of two hundred twenty-one thyroid glands; study of thyroid glands obtained at necropsy in Colorado. AMA Arch Pathol. 1955;59:291–311.

171. Brierre Jr JT, Dickson LG. Clinically unsuspected thyroid disease. GP. 1964;30:94–8.

172. Silverberg SG, Vidone RA. Carcinoma of thyroid in surgical and postmortem material - analysis of 300 cases at autopsy and literature review. Ann Surg. 1966;164:291–9.

173. Farooki MA. Epidemiology and pathology of cancer of the thyroid. I. Material, methods and results. Int Surg. 1969;51:232–43.

174. Sampson RJ, Woolner LB, Bahn RC, Kurland LT. Occult thyroid carcinoma in Olmsted County, Minnesota: prevalence at autopsy compared with that in Hiroshima and Nagasaki, Japan. Cancer. 1974;34:2072–6.

175. de Matos PS, Ferreira AP, Ward LS. Prevalence of papillary microcarcinoma of the thyroid in Brazilian autopsy and surgical series. Endocr Pathol. 2006;17:165–73.

176. Fukunaga FH, Lockett LJ. Thyroid carcinoma in the Japanese in Hawaii. Arch Pathol. 1971;92:6–13.

8

Reference interval of thyroid stimulating hormone and free thyroxine in a reference population over 60 years old and in very old subjects (over 80 years): comparison to young subjects

Rosita Fontes[1,2*], Claudia Regina Coeli[3], Fernanda Aguiar[3] and Mario Vaisman[1]

Abstract

Background: Studies based on laboratory data about thyroid stimulating hormone (TSH) and free thyroxine (FT4) reference interval (RI) show conflicting results regarding the importance of using specific values by age groups with advancing age. Retrospective laboratory data or non-specific criteria in the selection of subjects to be studied may be factors leading to no clear conclusions. The aim of this study is to test the hypothesis that TSH and FT4 have specific RI for subjects over 60 to 80 years.

Methods: We evaluated prospectively 1200 subjects of both sexes stratified by age groups, initially submitted to a questionnaire to do the first selection to exclude those with factors that could interfere in TSH or FT4 levels. Then, we excluded those subjects with goiter or other abnormalities on physical examination, positive thyroid peroxidase antibodies (TPOAb), thyroglobulin antibodies (TGAb), and other laboratory abnormalities.

Results: TSH increased with age in the whole group. There was no statistical difference in the analysis of these independent subgroups: 20–49 versus 50–59 years old (p > 0.05), and 60–69 versus 70–79 years old (p > 0.05). Consequently, we achieved different TSH RI for the three major age groups, 20 to 59 years old: 0.4 - 4.3 mU/L, 60 to 79 years old: 0.4 - 5.8 mU/L and 80 years or more: 0.4 - 6.7 mU/L. Conversely, FT4 progressively decreases = significantly with age, but the independent comparison test between the sub-groups showed that after age 60 the same RI was obtained (0.7 - 1.7 ng/dL) although the minimum value was smaller than that defined by manufacturer. In the comparison between TSH data obtained by this study and those defined by the manufacturer (without segmentation by age) 6.5% of subjects between 60 and 79 years and 12.5% with 80 years or more would have a misdiagnosis of elevated TSH.

Conclusions: TSH normal reference range increases with age, justifying the use of different RI in subjects 60 years old and over, while FT4 decreases with age. Using specific-age RI, a significant percentage of elderly will not be misdiagnosed as having subclinical hipothyroidism.

Introduction

In recent decades there has been increased life expectancy of the population and, consequently, of the aging process. Persons older than age 60 comprise 20 per cent of the world population in the more developed regions, and from 5 to 8 per cent in the less developed regions.

The oldest old, persons aged 80 years or older, is the fastest growing segment of the older population and by 2050 the number of this group is projected to be five times as large as at present [1].

Several aspects of the aging process affect the endocrine system and stimulate the use of screening programs for the detection of hormonal changes and drug interventions with hormone replacement therapies to provide better quality of life for the elderly. Evaluation of thyroid function in normal elderly is difficult, since the prevalence of non-thyroid disease and the use of medications that interfere with thyroid function is greater

* Correspondence: fontesrosita@hotmail.com
[1]Hospital Clementino Fraga Filho, Universidade Federal do Rio de Janeiro, Rua Prof. Rodolpho Paulo Rocco 255, Cidade Universitária, CEP 21941-913, Rio de Janeiro-RJ, Brazil
[2]Diagnósticos da América SA, Rio de Janeiro, Brazil
Full list of author information is available at the end of the article

than in young people. As a result, questions about the meaning of functional changes observed in the elderly are relatively common [2].

Data interpretation of thyroid function in the elderly has been changing over the past decades. In a study conducted in 1995 in a non-selected population, the authors considered that subjects of any age with some degree of TSH elevation had some grade of thyroid gland failure [3]. However, in 2002, the NHANES III study revisited this parameter data in a population excluding those with evidence of thyroid disease and, in this more uniform population, TSH still showed a progressive increase with age [4].

The International Federation of Clinical Chemistry and Laboratory Medicine (IFCC) Committee developed the theory of reference values for the "Reference Intervals and Decision Limits (CRIDL)" [5]. In 1995 the Clinical and Laboratory Standards Institute (CLSI) first published with IFCC the joint guideline "Defining, Establishing, and Verifying Reference Intervals in the Clinical Laboratory", reviewed in 2008 [6]. This document recommends application of prospective questionnaires and, if necessary, physical evaluation, of candidate subjects to be part of a control group. It also discourages the indirect approach in which database results are used to establish ranges, retroactively identifying acceptable reference populations. This has been a challenge since then, and many clinical laboratories do not have these procedures performed in accordance with the recommendations, due to the fact that they require time, additional costs, knowledge, and efforts to further clarify physicians and patients.

Recent studies have shown conflicting results regarding the decision to use reference intervals (RI) of TSH suitable for the elderly or not [7,8]. On studies with review of medical records, it is difficult to use strict inclusion and exclusion criteria in the selection of subjects representing a control group. Several bias may occur due to registration errors, and omission of information that were not actively taken from the patient. The consequent inclusion of a significant number of subjects with potential thyroid or general disease or use of interfering medications as belonging to the control group that may alter the final data obtained is a real possibility. Thus, the theme is still far from being exhausted, and this topic is relevant regarding the issue of not to hyper diagnose subclinical hypothyroidism in the elderly who actually could have higher TSH, but at appropriate levels for their age.

Likewise, as FT4 is the test of choice for the confirmation of thyroid disease, it is also relevant to assess whether there is a need for RI specific for subjects above 60 years and 80 years or older.

The aim of this study was to test the hypothesis that it is necessary to use specific RI for TSH and FT4 for subjects over 60 years old, and over 80 years old, compare the values with those of young subjects, and analyze the impact of using specific TSH RI for these age groups in the screening of thyroid dysfunction.

Materials and methods

Between March and December 2012, 1200 subjects of both sexes were evaluated prospectively distributed as follows: 120 males and 120 females in each of the following age ranges: 20–49, 50–59, 60–69, 70–79 and above 80 years, who attended a clinical laboratory to collect routine tests for which function evaluation and/ or thyroid autoimmunity had not been requested. They were invited to participate in order to arrive at the laboratory on pre-determined weekdays, according to availability of the researchers. A questionnaire was applied by one of the researchers, through direct interviews with participating candidates, which consisted of: 1) Identification data, address and phone number of the participants, as well as the name and telephone number of their physician for communication in case of abnormal results; characterization of their color or race according to themselves; if they consider themselves as healthy individuals; personal or familial thyroid disease in the present or past; current medications (among these, medications containing iodine in the last six months), smoking, hospitalization due to illness or accident in the last six months (and what the disease was), and pregnancy (for females who had not had menopause). Subjects were from the metropolitan area of Rio de Janeiro, belonging to middle and upper social class, as declared income, 77% white, 18% mulatto and 5% black. Subjects with negative thyroid peroxidase antibodies (TPOAb) and thyroglobulin antibodies (TGAb), normal lipid profile, ultrasensitive C-reactive protein level (CRP), blood count, renal function, and absence of goiter on palpation were in the inclusion criteria. The measurement of urinary iodine was not done since the salt iodization in Brazil is determined by federal law [9] and the authors have shown in previous study that the intake iodine in the Rio de Janeiro population is sufficient [10]. In addition, the National Health Surveillance Agency (ANVISA), which is the regulatory agency under the Ministry of Health, conducted a review of salt iodization in the samples used in Rio de Janeiro in the year before beginning of the study confirming that it was appropriate [11].

Exclusion criteria included past or present history of thyroid disease, previous thyroid surgery, family history of thyroid disease, TSH <0.1 mU/L or > 10.0 mU/L, as these results indicate a high probability of thyroid dysfunction [12], palpable goiter, smoking habit, use of medicines known as possible analytical or physiological interference on measurement of TSH or FT4 in the past three months (medicines and contrasts containing iodine in the past six months) mentioned in the list of medications and other drugs that may interfere with TSH and/or FT4 measurements [13-24], antidepressants, hospitalization in the past six months and pregnant females. As changes in thyroid morphology are significantly higher among the elderly, we assessed whether this was a factor in generating different results in the selection of subjects for the study. A thyroid ultrasonography (US) was performed on 687 subjects with exclusion of 24.1% who presented some thyroid change. More than 120 subjects still remained in each group. Comparing TSH and FT4 values between subjects who had normal US and those who did not perform US, there was no statistically significant difference (data not shown). Therefore, as this exam was not essential in the selection of subjects as controls, all of the initially selected subjects could be enrolled in the study, except those who were initially excluded and had been replaced by the same number of other subjects of the same age and sex in order of maintaining the initial number to be studied.

List of medications and other drugs that may interfere with TSH and/or FT4 measurements

2-3-dimercatopropanol, 2-4-dinitrophenol, 5-fluorouracil, 5-hydroxytryptophan
Acetazolamide, acetylsalicylic acid, alpha adrenergic blockers, aminoglutethimide, aminotriazole, amiodarone, androgens and other anabolic steroids, anphenona, anphetamines, antipyrine
Benserazide, beta adrenergic blockers, bexarotene, bromine, brompheniramine
Cadmium, carbamazepine, chromate, chromium picolinate, cimetidine, clofibrate, clomiphene, clomipramine, cobalt, complex anions, corticosteroids, cytostatics
Danazol, diphenylhydantoin, dinitrophenol, dobutamine, domperidone, dopamine and its agonists, other dopaminergic agents
Erythrosine, estrogens, ethionamide
Fenclofenac, fenoldopam, flunarizine, fluor, furosemide, fusaric acid
Growth hormone (GH), GH-Releasing hormone
Halofenate, heroin, heparin
Interleukins, iopanoic acid, other radiological contrasts, and other iodine-containing substances and drugs (potassium iodide and others), insulin-like Growth Factor-1, interferon
Ketoconazole
L-asparaginase, L-dopa inhibitors, levothyroxine, lithium, lovastatin,
Mefenamic acid, melatonin, metformin, methadone, methimazole, metoclopramide, mitotane
Nevirapine, niacin, nicotinic acid, nifedipine, NSAIDs, nitrate

O, p'-DDD, orphenadrine, opioids, oxcarbazepine
Para-aminobenzoic acid, perchlorate, perphenazine, phenidone, phenylbutazone, phenobarbital, pimozide, prazozin, primidone, propylthiouracil, pyridoxine
Quetiapine
Raloxifen, resorcinol, rifampicin, ritonavir, rubidium
Salsalate, serotonergics antagonists, somatostatin and its analogues, spironolactone, St. John's Wort, stavudine, sulfonamides, sulfonylureas, sulpiride, steroids hormones
Tamoxifen, thiocyanate, thyroid hormones and their analogs, troleandomycin, tyrosine kinase inhibitors
Valproic acid

Drugs are listed in alphabetical order and not in possible importance as interfering in TSH or thyroid hormone values.

The study was approved by the Research Ethics Committee of the Hospital Clementino Fraga Filho, Universidade Federal do Rio de Janeiro (HUCFF/UFRJ) and individuals agreed to participate by signing the informed consent form.

Collection of data and collection of samples

Serum was collected in the morning, in same species standard sampling tubes with separator gel. The measurements were done on the same day in primary tubes, after blood centrifugation at 3200 RPM for 15 min.

Biochemical data

Serum TSH, FT4, TPOAb and TGAb were measured by electrochemiluminescence immunoassays on the Roche Modular Analytics® E170 (Roche Diagnostics Australia Pty Ltd, Castle Hill, NSW, Australia).

Serum TSH concentrations were measured by an immunometric method, with an intra-assay percentage coefficient of variation (% CV) of 3.0% at concentrations of 0.040 ± 0.001 mU/L, 2.7% at 0.092 ± 0.002 mU/L and 1.1% at 9.4 ± 0.1 mU/L. The reference interval provided by the manufacturer is 0.3- 4.2 mU/L. Serum FT4, TPOAb and TGAb concentrations were measured by competitive assays. For FT4, the % CV was 1.4% at FT4 concentrations of 0.7 ± 0.01 ng/dL, 1.8% at 1.3 ± 0.02 and 2.0% at 2.7 ± 0.1 ng/dL. The reference interval provided by the manufacturer is 0.9 -1.7 ng/dL. For TPOAb the intra-assay % CV is 6.3% at TPO concentrations of 21.3 ± 1.34 IU/mL, 5.1% at 51.2 ± 2.6 IU/mL and 2.7% at 473 ± 12.7 IU/mL. According to the manufacturer, individuals without thyroid disease score lower than 34 IU/mL. For TGAb the intra-assay % CV is 4.9% at TG concentrations of 47.2 ± 2.3 IU/mL, 1.3% at 588 ± 7.4, and 1.3 at 3289 ± 42.0 IU/mL TGAb concentrations. According to the manufacturer, individuals without thyroid disease score lower than <115 IU/mL.

Statistical analysis

Data were analyzed using the program GraphPad Prism®, version 6.0 (GraphPad Software, Inc, California). In order to assess the Normal distribution of both data series (TSH and FT4) Kolmogorov-Smirnov tests were performed. Logarithmic 10 was used for analysis. TSH and FT4 were calculated for each subgroup and gender from 20 to 49 years, then, by 10-year age range until 80 years; all those aged older than 80 were grouped together. Descriptive analysis of serum TSH was reported as medians and 25% and 75% percentiles because it is not normally distributed. Two tailed Mann–Whitney test and Kruskal-Wallis test were used to compare the nonparametric TSH distributions in different subpopulations. Evaluation between two subgroups was made by independent test of Dunn multiple comparisons. Means and standard deviations were calculated for FT4, since it has showed a normal distribution. For comparing FT4 between all groups, two-way ANOVA tests were used when more than two data series were analyzed, and Student test in the case of two data series.

Outlying observations were calculated using the test proposed by Dixon. In all cases, the level of significance used was 0.05 [25]. For the RI, for both hormones 2.5% and 97.5% were taken. We used the method of Harris and Boyd [26] to decide whether it was necessary to separate the reference values for gender. According to this method, to calculate the statistical significance of the difference between the means of groups standard normal deviation (z), if the value z is less than 3 means there is no need to reference values separated by gender.

To calculate correlations between TSH and FT4 levels in all age groups, TSH data were transformed into logarithmic 10. With normal distribution the two-tailed

Pearson test was used; it was considered statistically significant if a p-value was less than 0.05. Pearson test was also used to analyze, individually, correlations between TSH and age and FT4 and age.

Results

TSH data

The reference group was comprised of 50% females and 50% males. The mean age by gender in each age subgroups are in Table 1. TSH data analysis by age or gender exhibited a non-Gaussian distribution. In each age group, there was no significant difference in serum TSH median between males and females (Table 1). Therefore, considering these factors, all individuals were eligible in each group for the establishment of reference intervals. Statistical parameters of TSH measurements are listed in Figure 1 and in Table 1. Analysis of median TSH as a whole group showed that there was a significant increase of this hormone with age (p < 0.001), but the analysis of independent subgroups, 20–49 years old *versus* 50–59 years old (p > 0.05), and 60–69 years old *versus* 70–79 years old (p > 0.05), showed no statistically significant difference. These data confirm that different RI for three major age groups should be used: 20 to 59 years, 60–79 years and 80 years or more. RI calculated for each sub-group are shown in Table 1.

FT4 data

FT4 exhibited a Gaussian distribution. Data of FT4 measurements are shown in Figure 2, and statistical parameters are listed in Table 2. Analysis of FT4 mean ± standard deviation (SD) shows that there is a significant reduction of the hormone with age as a whole group (p < 0.0001). However, despite a tendency to fall in FT4 with increasing

Table 1 Statistical data of TSH measurements

	Age groups				
	20-49	50-59	60-69	70-79	≥80
Mean age females (years old)	34.3	54.1	64.2	74.4	84.4
Mean age males (years old)	35.2	53.9	64.2	74.2	86.7
Median TSH in females	1.5		1.7		2.0
Median TSH in males	1.5		1.8		2.1
z values and p values between gender	z = −1.45 p = 0.30	z = −0.60 p = 0.69	z = −0.43 p = 0.54	z = −0.78 p = 0.40	z = −0.14 p = 0.99
Minimum TSH	0.3	0.4	0.2	0.3	0.2
Maximum TSH	5.8	5.9	8.4	9.5	9.3
25% TSH percentile	1.1	1.2	1.7	1.7	2.0
75% TSH percentile	2.2	2.6	2.8	3.0	3.5
Lower 95% CI	1.6	1.8	2.0	2.1	2.5
Upper 95% CI	1.9	2.1	2.4	2.5	2.9
Median TSH assumed	1.5		1.7		2.0
Minimum and maximum TSH RI assumed	0.4 – 4.3		0.4 – 5.8		0.4 – 6.7

RI: reference interval SD: standard deviation TSH in mU/L.

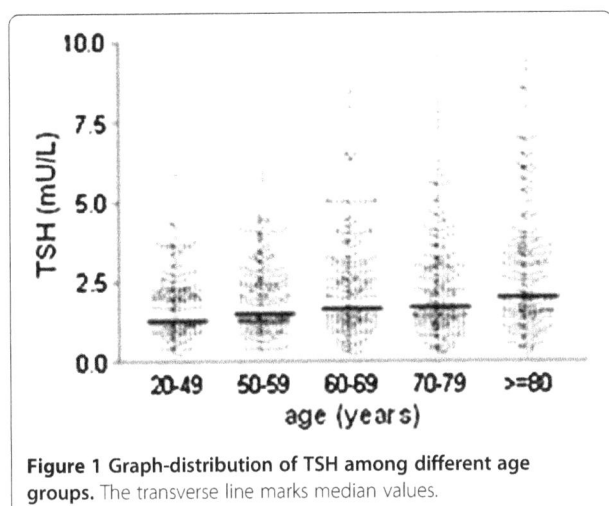

Figure 1 Graph-distribution of TSH among different age groups. The transverse line marks median values.

age, the independent comparison test between the sub-groups showed that there was no statistically significant difference between those over 60 years old. Reference intervals calculated for FT4 are shown in Table 2.

Regarding the correlation between TSH and FT4, a high level of significance was observed in all age sub-groups, independently analyzed (p < 0.0001), 20–49 years old: Pearson r = −0.4641, 95% confidence interval (CI) = −0.4961 to −0.2926, R squared = 0.1652; 50–59 years old: Pearson r = −0.3862, 95% CI = −0.4881 to −0.2739, R squared = 0.1492; 60–69 years old: Pearson r = −0.4653, 95% CI = −0.5583 to −0.3607, R squared = 0.2165; 70–79 years old: Pearson r = −0.4946, 95% CI = −0.5839 to −0.3934, R squared = 0.2446; 80 years old and over: Pearson r = −0.3951, 95% confidence interval = −0.4961 to −0.2835, R squared = 0.1561.

In order to assess whether the RI obtained in this study had clinical impact regarding the use of RI defined by the manufacturer in screening for thyroid disease, we compare the percentage of subjects who had TSH below

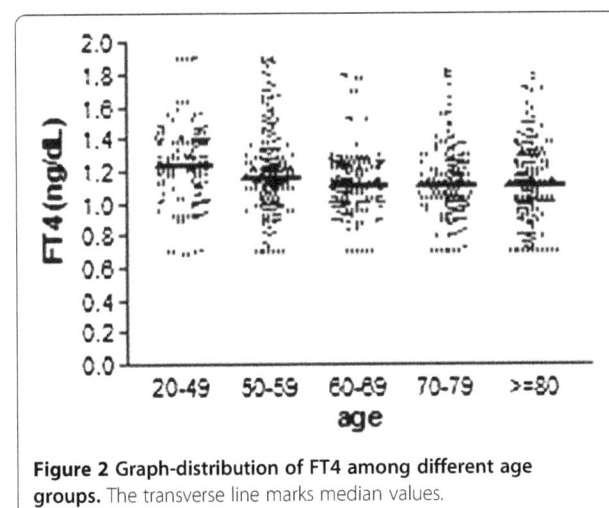

Figure 2 Graph-distribution of FT4 among different age groups. The transverse line marks median values.

or above the RI defined by age range obtained from this study with the values without segmentation by age. The results are showed in Table 3.

Discussion

Usually, for the interpretation of a laboratory test, clinical laboratories use RI provided by the manufacturer of lab kits. The result of a patient's test is then compared to this RI in order to diagnose whether it is normal or not. TSH concentration is the most sensitive test to reliably detect thyroid function abnormalities and is used as the screening test for studying thyroid function because of the inverse log-linear relationship between circulating TSH and FT4 concentrations [27,28].

This study, conducted prospectively with a reference population, showed that TSH increases progressively and significantly with age. The value of z less than 3.0 in all age groups indicates that the same RI should be adopted for both genders. On the other hand, FT4 tends to decrease with age. In the age groups above 60 years, FT4 values are equal between males and females. In subjects younger than 60, the value of z pointed that FT4 is lower in males than in females. A study of Kratzsch et al. also reports lower FT4 in males than in females [29]. However, as in our study, z result (3.0249) is very close to the cutoff point we consider that in the clinical routine, it is appropriate to use the same RI to both genders, the same way as in older subjects.

The lower TSH limit defined in this study of 0.4 mU/L is the same for all age groups over 60 years old, and does not differ from the lower limit of younger people. This value is in accordance with previous study using third generation immunometric TSH methodology, that refers to the lower TSH reference limit as approximately 0.3 to 0.4 mU/L, irrespective of the population studied or the method used [30]. The value found in this study, very slightly higher than that reported by the manufacturer, has no impact on an eventual reclassification of how many people have low TSH, as the difference between one and other is under 2%.

Association between TSH and age is highly significant. The median is 1.5 mU/L in people under 60 years old, increases to 1.7 mU/L from 60 to 79 years old, and to 2.0 mU/L for those aged 80 or more. Upper TSH limit increases from 4.3 mU/L under 60 years old, to 5.8 mU/L in the range of 60 to 79 years old and to 6.7 mU/L in those very old subjects, over 80. So, although the manufacturer's TSH kit is suitable for subjects less than 60 years of age, the same is not true for those 60 years or more, in which the limits are significantly higher.

Within the age ranges of 60–79 years and 80 years or over, a significant percentage of subjects are reclassified as having not elevated TSH if age-specific RI is adopted. The same does not occur in young subjects. According

Table 2 Statistical data of FT4 measurements

	Age groups				
	20-49	50-59	60-69	70-79	≥80
Mean FT4 ± SD in females	1.2 ± 0.03	1.2 ± 0.24	1.1 ± 0.22	1.2 ± 0.24	1.1 ± 0.24
Mean FT4 ± SD in males	1.3 ± 0.02	1.2 ± 0.25	1.1 ± 0.23	1.1 ± 0.22	1.1 ± 0.23
z values and p values between gender	$z = 3.02$ $p = -0.0001$	$z = 1.26$ $p = 0.28$	$z = 0.70$ $p = 0.31$	$z = -1.63$ $p = 0.08$	$z = 0.39$ $p = 0.31$
Minimum level FT4	0.7	0.7	0.7	0.7	0.7
Maximum level FT4	1.9	1.9	1.8	1.8	1.8
Lower FT4 95% CI	1.2	1.2	1.1	1.1	1.1
Upper FT4 95% CI	1.3	1.2	1.2	1.2	1.2
Mean FT4 ± SD assumed for both genders	1.2 ± 0.3	1.2 ± 0.3	1.1 ± 0.2	1.1 ± 0.2	1.1 ± 0.2
Minimum and maximum FT4 RI assumed for both genders	0.7 – 1.9			0.7 – 1.7	

RI: reference interval SD: standard deviation FT4 in ng/dL.

to the RI for each age group obtained in this study, 6.5% of subjects between 60 and 70 years and 12.5% of those with 80 years or more have less misdiagnosis of elevated TSH, leading to 19% reclassification from hypothyroidism to normal, using these criteria. With regard to the effects of age on serum TSH levels, other epidemiological studies indicate that the population's mean TSH levels increase with age [4,31,32]. The NHANES III was the best designed in selecting a control population, and data obtained were similar to the current study, indicating that increase in TSH is probably a physiological event for the elderly [33,34] or that this increase may be due to the presence of TSH isoforms with low bioactivity [35]. In each scenario one can avoid excessive diagnosis of subclinical hypothyroidism in the elderly adopting specific RI. And, to clarify the second hypothesis, the answer would be the development and clinical use of technologies to quantify only isoforms with normal TSH bioactivity.

Failure to find these differences in RI between the young and the elderly reported in other studies may be due to retrospective studies based, or selection choosing populations to be reference for which strict selection criteria were not applied through specific questionnaires and appropriate physical examination to exclude factors such as thyroid dysfunction in the subject or in the

family, interfering medications, other illnesses, recent hospitalizations, smoking habits and goiter.

Like TSH, FT4 has the same minimum reference value for all age groups. This value of 0.7 ng/dL however, is lower in relation to that defined by the manufacturer (0.9 ng/dL) in all groups. In relation to the maximum reference value, the level of 1.7 ng/dL is suitable to be used for subjects 60 years old and over. However, although this is not the scope of this study, the results obtained by us suggest that a higher reference superior value (1.9 ng/dL) should be used for young individuals.

Previous study demonstrated that FT4 remained relatively unchanged with age [36]. These data can be difficult to interpret because evaluation of thyroid function in the elderly is often complicated by the increased prevalence of chronic illness and the use of medication. In the present study, subjects with one or more of these factors were excluded. There is evidence that a low activity of thyroid hormone might be beneficial in the elderly. Low levels of FT4 have been associated with a better survival in elderly subjects [8,33,37,38]. On the other hand, even thyroid hormone levels within the normal range might be associated with thyroid hormone-related endpoints. As an example, in euthyroid subjects, especially the elderly, FT4, regardless of TSH levels is associated with atrial fibrillation, and

Table 3 Comparison of data of TSH (mU/L) obtained regarding RI defined by the manufacturer (without segmentation by age), with the results of this study that redefined RI specific for age range

Age ranges (y. old)	Results of TSH below RI (mU/L)			Results of TSH upper RI (mU/L)		
	Defined by the manufacturer	With segmentation by age in this study	Difference*	Defined by the manufacturer	With segmentation by age in this study	Difference*
< 60	0.4%	0.8%	+ 0.4%	1.7%	1.5%	- 0.2%
60-79	0.4%	2.1%	+ 1.7%	9.2%	2.7%	- 6.5%
≥ 80	0.4%	0.8%	+ 0.4%	14.5%	2.0%	- 12.5%

*Refers to percentage of subjects detected with TSH levels out of reference interval (RI) established by the manufacturer versus those where TSH was obtained in this study and RI was segmented by age.

lower physical performance [39,40]. One hypothesis is that these lower levels of thyroid hormone could possibly serve as an adaptive mechanism to prevent catabolism in the elderly [41].

We consider relevant the data obtained in this age-related prospective study, once it is very important to distinguish between normal and mildly elevated serum TSH concentrations in elderly subjects. Elevations of TSH in young individuals even light and without decreasing FT4 characterize subclinical hypothyroidism or minimal thyroid dysfunction and are related to comorbidities such as dyslipidemia, adverse obstetric events, impact on cognition, quality of life, cardiovascular events, and evolution to clinical hypothyroidism [42]. These effects have no correspondence in the elderly, since there is no evidence of these effects in this age group [43,44]. There is a consensus that subjects with TSH concentrations above 10.0 mU/L should be treated. However, according to Garber et al., in the Clinical Practice Guidelines for Hypothyroidism, very mild TSH elevations in older individuals, under this level, may not reflect subclinical thyroid dysfunction, but rather be a normal manifestation of aging. While the normal TSH reference may need to be narrowed range for some subpopulations [27,45], the normal RI may widen with aging [24]. This confirms that not all patients who have mild TSH elevations are hypothyroid and therefore would not require thyroid hormone therapy. These data are also relevant for the monitoring of subjects with hypothyroidism, since the target for TSH in levothyroxine treated subjects should be higher in elderly people. Pitfalls in the interpretation of TSH were carefully excluded in this study. Abnormal levels are observed in various non-thyroidal diseases and other conditions, but the effect of possible changes secondary to thyroid diseases were preventable excluding subjects who had used medication containing iodine during the previous 6 months, had had hospitalization, smokers, as well as those not using any medication that may alter minimally TSH or thyroid hormones.

Concluding, this data shows that prevalence of subclinical hypothyroidism is overestimated in the elderly, in almost 20% of subjects, unless age-specific RI is used. This might improve diagnostic accuracy and reduce the need of confirmatory unnecessary tests.

Competing interests
The author's declare that they have no competing interests.

Authors' contributions
RF did the study design, conducted the field study, made the final selection of study participants; computed the data and wrote the text. CRC made the initial guidance on the statistical requirements for the study, led and oversaw all statistical work. FA did the statistical field study under the supervision of CRC, being assisted during the course of the study also by the statistical mentioned in the acknowledgments. MV was the general supervisor of the study. He had discussions with the staff and the necessary modifications to the original design of the study; he revised, and made necessary adaptions

to the final text and made the final approval of the text submitted to the journal. All authors read and approved the final manuscript.

Acknowledgments
We appreciate the statistical assistance of Dr. Martha Mutis, MD, PhD, and the revision by Angelo Pereira, teacher and translator of English language.

Author details
[1]Hospital Clementino Fraga Filho, Universidade Federal do Rio de Janeiro, Rua Prof. Rodolpho Paulo Rocco 255, Cidade Universitária, CEP 21941-913, Rio de Janeiro-RJ, Brazil. [2]Diagnósticos da América SA, Rio de Janeiro, Brazil. [3]Núcleo de Estudos de Saúde Coletiva, Universidade Federal do Rio de Janeiro, Rio de Janeiro, Brazil.

References
1. United Nations publication: The Sex and Age distribution of the world populations. Sex and Age Popul Div, United Nations Secretariat, the 1998 Revis 1998, I:2–6. No. E.99.XIII.8.
2. Chiovato L, Mariotti S, Pinchera A: Thyroid diseases in the elderly. Baillieres Clin Endocrinol Metab 1997, 11:251–270.
3. Canaris GJ, Manowitz NR, Mayor G, Ridgway EC: The Colorado thyroid disease prevalence study. Arch Intern Med 2000, 160:526–534.
4. Hollowell JG, Staehling NW, Flanders WD, Hannon WH, Gunter EW, Spencer CA, Braverman LE: Serum TSH, T$_4$, and Thyroid Antibodies in the United States Population (1988 to 1994): National Health and Nutrition Examination Survey (NHANES III). J Clin Endocrinol Metab 2002, 87:489–499.
5. Ceriotti F: Prerequisites for use of common reference intervals. Clin Biochem Rev 2007, 28:115–121.
6. Horowitz GL, Altaie S, Boyd JC, Ceriotti F, Garg U, Horn P, Pesce A, Sine HE, Zakovski J: Defining, Establishing, and Verifying Reference Intervals in the Clinical Laboratory; Approved Guideline – Third Edition. Clin Lab Stand Inst 2008, 28:C28–A3.
7. Kahapola-Arachchige KM, Hadlow N, Wardrop R, Lim EM, Walsh JP: Age-specific TSH reference ranges have minimal impact on the diagnosis of thyroid dysfunction. Clin Endocrinol 2012, 77:773–779.
8. Vadiveloo T, Donnan PT, Murphy MJ, Leese GP: Age- and gender-specific TSH reference intervals in People with no obvious Thyroid disease in Tayside, Scotland: the Thyroid Epidemiology, Audit, and Research Study (TEARS). J Clin Endocrinol Metab 2013, 98:1147–1153.
9. Lei 1944/53 | Lei nº 1.944, de 14 de agosto de 1953 (Law 1944/53 | Law No. 1,944, of August 14, 1953) [http://presrepublica.jusbrasil.com.br/legislacao/128787/lei-1944-53]
10. Netto LS, Coeli CM, Micmacher E, Mamede SC, Nazar LO, Correa EK, Arrastia M, Galvão D, Buescu A, Vaisman M: Longitudinal study of pituitary-thyroid axis in pregnancy. Arq Bras Endocrinol Metab 2004, 48:493–498.
11. Resultado do Monitoramento do Teor de Iodo no Sal: Results of monitoring of iodine in salt. 2011 [http://portal.anvisa.gov.br/wps/wcm/connect/7d7bb4804be9dbf18c50ddbc0f9d5b29/Relat%C3%B3rio+Pro.Iodo+2011.pdf?MOD=AJPERES]
12. Surks MI, Ortiz E, Daniels GH, Sawin CT, Col NF, Cobin RH, Franklin JA, Hershman JM, Burman KD, Denke MA, Gorman C, Cooper RS, Weissman NJ: Subclinical thyroid disease: scientific review and guidelines for diagnosis and management. JAMA 2004, 291:228–238.
13. Oppenheimer JH, Schwartz HL, Dillman W, Surks MI: Effect of thyroid hormone analogues on the displacement of ^{125}I-L-triiodothyronine from hepatic and heart nuclei in vivo: possible relationship to hormonal activity. Bioch Bioph Res Commun 1973, 55:544–550.
14. Liewendahl K, Majuri H, Helenius T: Thyroid function tests in patients on long-term treatment with various anticonvulsivant drugs. Clin Endocrinol 1978, 8:185–191.
15. Smith PJ, Surks MI: Multiple effects of 5,5'-diphenylhydantoin on the thyroid hormone system. Endocr Rev 1984, 5:514–524.
16. Spencer C, Eigen A, Shen D, Duda M, Qualls S, Weiss S, Nicoloff J: Specificity of sensitive assays of thyrotropin (TSH) used to screen for thyroid disease in hospitalized patients. Clin Chem 1987, 33:1391–1396.
17. Larkin JG, Macphee GJA, Beastall GH, Brodie MJ: Thyroid hormone concentrations in epileptic patients. Eur J Clin Pharmacol 1989, 36:213–216.

18. Davies PH, Franklyn JA: The effects of drugs on tests of thyroid function. *Eur J Clin Pharmacol* 1991, **40**:439–451.

19. Stockigt JR: ree thyroid hormone measurement. *A Crit appraisal 2001 Endocrinol Metab Clin North Am* 2001, **30**:265–289.

20. Steele BW, Wang E, Klee GG, Thienpont LM, Soldin SJ, Sokoll LJ, Winter WE, Fuhrman SA, Elin RJ: Analytic bias of thyroid function tests: analysis of a college of American Pathologists fresh frozen serum pool by 3900 clinical laboratories. *Arch Pathol Lab Med* 2005, **129**:310–317.

21. Crofton KM: Thyroid disrupting chemicals: mechanisms and mixtures. *Int J Androl* 2008, **31**:209–223.

22. Stockigt JR, Lim CF: Medications that distort in vitro tests of thyroid function, with particular reference to estimates of serum free thyroxine. *Best Pract Clin Endocrinol Metab* 2009, **23**:753–767.

23. Beckett GJ: Mechanisms behind the non-thyroidal illness syndrome: an update. *J Endocrinol* 2010, **205**:1–13.

24. Garber JR, Cobin RH, Gharib H, Hennessey JV, Klein I, Mechanick JI, Pessah-Pollack R, Singer PA, Woeber KA: Clinical practice guidelines for hypothyroidism in adults: Cosponsored by the American Association of Clinical Endocrinologists and the American Thyroid Association. *Thyroid* 2012, **22**:1200–1235.

25. Dixon WJ: Processing data for outliers. *Biometrics* 1953, **9**:74–89.

26. Harris EK, Boyd JC: On dividing reference data into subgroups to produce reference ranges. *Clin Chem* 1990, **36**:265–270.

27. Baloch Z, Carayon P, Conte-Devolx B, Demers LM, Feldt-Rasmussen U, Henry JF, LiVosli VA, Niccoli-Sire P, John R, Ruf J, Smyth PP, Spencer CA, Stockigt JR: Laboratory medicine practice guidelines. Laboratory support for the diagnosis and monitoring of thyroid disease. *Thyroid* 2003, **13**:3–126.

28. Benhaldi N, Fliers E, Visser TJ, Reitsma JB, Wiersinga WM: Pilot study on the assessment of the setpoint on the hypothalamus-pituitary-tryroid axis in healthy volunteers. *Eur J Endocrinol* 2010, **162**:323–329.

29. Kratzsch J, Fiedler GM, Leichtle A, Brügel M, Buchbinder S, Otto L, Sabri O, Matthes G, Thiery J: New reference intervals for thyrotropin and thyroid hormones based on national academy of clinical biochemistry criteria and regular ultrasonography of the thyroid. *Clin Chem* 2005, **51**:1480–1486.

30. D'Herbomez M, Jarrige V, Darte C: Reference intervals for serum thyrotropin (TSH) and free thyroxine (FT4) in adults using the Access Immunoassay System. *Clin Chem Lab Med* 2005, **43**:102–105.

31. Brochmann H, Bjøro T, Gaarder PI, Hanson F, Frey HM: Prevalence of thyroid dysfunction in elderly subjects. A randomized study in a Norwegian rural community (Naerøy). *Acta Endocrinol (Copenh) 1988*, **117**:7–12.

32. Boucai L, Hollowell JG, Surks MI: An approach for development of age-, gender-, and ethnicity-specific thyrotropin reference limits. *Thyroid* 2011, **21**:5–11.

33. Atzmon G, Barzilai N, Hollowell JG, Surks MI, Gabriely I: Extreme longevity is associated with increased serum thyrotropin. *J Clin Endocrinol Metab* 2009, **94**:1251–1254.

34. Surks MI, Boucai L: Age- and race- based serum thyrotropin reference limits. *J Clin Endocrinol Metab* 2010, **95**:496–502.

35. Estrada JM, Soldin D, Buckey TM, Burman KD, Soldin OP: Thyrotropin isoforms – implications for TSH analysis and clinical practice. *Thyroid* 2013. in press.

36. Mariotti S, Franceschi C, Cossarizza A, Pinchera A: The aging thyroid. *Endocr Rev* 1995, **16**:686–715.

37. Gussekloo J, van Exel E, de Craen AJ, Meinders AE, Frölich M, Westendorp RG: Thyroid status, disability and cognitive function, and survival in old age. *JAMA* 2004, **292**:2591–2599.

38. Van Den Beld AW, Visser TJ, Feelders RA, Grobbee DE, Lamberts SWJ: Thyroid hormone concentrations, disease, physical function, and mortality in elderly Men. *J Clin Endocrinol Metab* 2005, **90**:6403–6409.

39. Gammage MD, Parle JV, Holder RL, Roberts LM, Hobbs FD, Wilson S, Sheppard MC, Franklyn JA: Association between serum free thyroxine concentration and atrial fibrillation. *Arch Intern Med* 2007, **167**:928–934.

40. Heeringa J, Hoogendoorn EH, von der Deure WM, Hofman A, Peeters RP, Hop WCJ, den Heijer M, Visser TJ, Witterman JCM: High-normal thyroid function and risk of atrial fibrillation. The rotterdam study. *Arch intern Med* 2008, **168**:2219–2224.

41. Peeters RP: Thyroid function and longevity: New insights into an Old dilemma. *J Clin Endocrinol Metab* 2009, **94**:4658–4660.

42. Biondi B, Cooper DS: The clinical significance of subclinical thyroid dysfunction. *Endocr Rev* 2008, **29**:76–131.

43. Laurberg P, Andersen S, Carle A, Karmisholt J, Knudsen N, Pedersen IB: The TSH upper reference limit: where are we at? *Nat Rev Endocrinol* 2011, **7**:232–239.

44. Tseng F-Y, Lin W-Y, Lin C-C, Lee L-T, Li T-C, Sung P-K, Huang K-C: Subclinical hypothyroidism is associated with increased risk for All-cause and cardiovascular mortality in adults. *J Am col Cardiol* 2012, **60**:730–737.

45. Wartofsky L, Dickey RA: The evidence for a narrower thyrotropin reference range is compelling 2005. *J Clin Endocrinol Metab* 2005, **90**:5483–5488.

9

The value of thyroperoxidase as a prognostic factor for differentiated thyroid cancer – a long-term follow-up study

Yurena Caballero[1*], Eudaldo M. López-Tomassetti[1], Julián Favre[1], José R. Santana[1], Juan J. Cabrera[2] and Juan R. Hernández[1]

Abstract

Background: Thyroperoxidase (TPO) is a membrane-bound protein essential for the production of thyroid hormones; because of this, TPO expression may be impaired in selected thyroid diseases. The goal of this study is to analyze TPO immune expression in differentiated thyroid cancer, and to determine whether TPO has any prognostic value.

Methods: A total of 139 patients who required surgery due to a thyroid nodule with signs or symptoms suspicious for malignancy during their physical, ultrasound and/or cytology examination were consecutively selected for the study. A study of TPO immunohistochemical expression was carried out on these patients using the MoAb47 monoclonal antibody. In addition, cell proliferation marker *Ki67* and tumor suppressor *p53* were also measured for comparison.

Results: A total of 139 cases, 43 benign tumors, 42 papillary carcinomas, 38 follicular carcinomas, 8 undifferentiated carcinomas, and 8 sporadic medullary carcinomas were analyzed. The relationship between TPO expression and disease was statistically significant ($p < 0.001$), and decreased with tumor dedifferentiation extent. Increased TPO expression in benign lesions as compared to decreased expression in papillary carcinomas and undifferentiated tumors is outstanding. Differences in TPO expression were observed in minimally invasive follicular carcinoma (MIFC) compared to widely invasive follicular carcinoma (WIFC). TPO expression decreases in undifferentiated malignancies in contrast with *p53* and *Ki67* expression, which increases in that setting. TPO, *p53* and *Ki67* expression was significantly related to TNM stage ($p < 0.001$). Survival rate was 72 % after a 20-year follow-up, and 100 % for subjects with higher TPO expression.

Conclusions: TPO may be useful in confirming or ruling out benign diseases from differentiated thyroid carcinoma, with the exception of low-risk carcinoma such as MIFC. It could be used as a prognostic factor for differentiated thyroid cancer and patient follow-up, together with other markers.

Keywords: Thyroid cancer, Thyroperoxidase, Ki67, p53

Background

Thyroperoxidase (TPO) is a membrane-bound protein essential for thyroid hormone production, characteristic of functional, normal thyroid cells. TPO expression is considered a thyroid differentiation marker. Qualitative and quantitative alterations in TPO activity, TPO messenger ribonucleic acid (mRNA), and protein expression can be related to thyroid changes and have been reported in pathological thyroid tissues [1]. TPO content has been shown to be significantly lower in thyroid malignancies as compared to benign conditions and normal tissue [2]; also, a reduction in TPO activity and TPO mRNA of 55–70 % is observed in differentiated thyroid carcinoma (DTC) [1, 3]. Moreover, anaplastic tumors have non-existent TPO expression. The biological meaning of this abnormal TPO expression is unclear; however, a deregulation of protein synthesis can be related. A progressive decrease in TPO levels, together with increased cell density, suggests an association with proliferation.

* Correspondence: yure_hop@hotmail.com
[1]General Surgery Department, Hospital Universitario Insular de Gran Canaria, Las Palmas de Gran Canaria, Las Palmas, Spain
Full list of author information is available at the end of the article

Molecular tests are emerging that measure different gene and protein combinations that may differentiate benign lesions from DTC [4–6]. Although these studies have shown good results and can be promising for the future, these techniques are not readily available in every hospital. On the other hand, immunohistochemistry techniques could be an easier option to differentiate between benign thyroid lesions and DTC.

Many studies have described immunohistochemical markers that improve the diagnosis of thyroid conditions such as TPO on their own or, alternatively, associated with other markers such as *galectine-3, CK19, HBME-1,* etc. De Micco determined that anti-TPO antibody MoAb47 recognized TPO expression in normal and benign thyroid tissues, but only in 3 % of malignant tumors [7]. TPO gene and protein expression in thyroid carcinoma have been analyzed, indicating low enzymatic activity [2], impaired solubility and suppressed TPO mRNA expression [8]. Savin et al. studied the value of TPO combined with *galectine-3* in DTC, observing that TPO had an intense expression in normal or hyperplasic thyroid tissue, and was down-regulated in thyroid pathologies. They reported an inverse correlation with known prognostic factors and TNM staging [9]. However, other reports have obtained the same TPO expression in both benign thyroid diseases and DTC [10].

This study analyzes the immunohistochemical expression of TPO (using MoAb-47) in both benign and malignant lesions to establish the relationship between TPO expression, histological type, differentiation degree, and tumor growth. In malignancies, including both differentiated and undifferentiated cancers; a comparative analysis of TPO with proliferation factor *Ki67* and cell-cycle suppressor protein *p53* was carried out [11–13].

Methods

Patients with thyroid nodules and signs or symptoms suspicious for malignancy during physical, ultrasound and/or cytology examination who required surgery during the period 1972 to 1995 were consecutively selected for this study. The ethical approval and informed consent of patients were obtained (The institutional review board was approved by the committe of the Hospital Universitario Insular de Gran Canaria and the University of Las Palmas of Gran Canaria). The institutional review board was approved by the committe of the Hospital Universitario Insular de Gran Canaria and the University of Las Palmas of Gran Canaria. Only 139 cases were included as we had a limited number of monoclonal antibodies available for the TPO immunohistochemical study. Data was prospectively collected and patients were divided into four groups according to their histological diagnosis: benign cases, papillary thyroid carcinoma (PTC), follicular thyroid carcinoma (FTC), and a fourth group called "others", which included undifferentiated thyroid carcinomas and sporadic medullary carcinomas. Specific variants were included in the study, such as the follicular variant of papillary carcinoma

and Hürthle cell carcinoma for the PTC group, clear cells and insular pattern for the FTC group. Even though sporadic medullary carcinomas are related to C-cells (and therefore to calcitonin levels) they were not excluded, as we wanted to evaluate TPO, *p53* and *ki67* expression.

Histological analysis

After gross examination, the specimens were fixed in 10 % formaldehyde and embedded in paraffin. Blocks were cut using a Leica microtome into 4–5 micron sections, and then studied with several staining techniques (Harris or Mayer hematoxylin, eosin, PAS).

Immunohistochemistry

The antibodies used for the immunohistochemical study included MoAb-47 for TPO, DO-7 for *p53*, and *Ki67* -MM1 against antigen *Ki67*.

Once obtained, histology blocks were placed in the heater for twelve hours at 37 °C and then soaked in xilol three times over 15 min, twice in absolute alcohol over 10 min, once over 5 min in 96 % alcohol, once in 70 % alcohol, and lastly once time during 5 min in distilled water. Afterwards, all slides were placed in a pressure cooker with citrate buffer solution as a recovery antigenic system. A process to inhibit endogenous peroxidase using 250 ml of 30 % hydrogen peroxide with 10 ml of methanol during 10 min followed this. Antibody solutions were prepared with the following dilutions: TPO 1:50, p53 1:50, and ki67 1:100; these were maintained at a temperature of 4 °C during the staining process. Then we started the incubation process without washing the slides with the primary antibody during 1 h, with the secondary antibody during another hour, and with the avidin-biotin-peroxidase complex during 30 min.

In the final stage, slides were washed in PBS for 15 min with agitation, and subsequently developed with chromogenic substrate for 3 to 6 min away from direct light (diaminobenzidine [DAB] solution); then they were washed with tap water for 5 min 3 times, and contrasted with Harris' or Mayer's hematoxylin for 1 min; finally they were dehydrated using a growing alcohol series (70 %, 96 %, and 100 % twice, and xylol clearing solution twice), and eventually mounted with coverslips using DPX).

Routine techniques such as Congo red under polarized light and calcitonin immunohistochemistry were used for sporadic medullary carcinomas.

Immunohistochemistry assessment

TPO expression was measured under a light microscope, in terms of percentage of stained cells and stain intensity, using different scores. For the percentage of stained cells an Arabic number was given: 0, 1–10 % stained cells = 1, 10–33 % = 2, 33–66 % = 3, >66 % = 4; and for stain intensity: negative = 0, mild = 1, moderate = 2, intense = 3. Intensity and proportion of stained cells were summed using the Vargas-Roig method [14] in order to obtain a single result. Thus, a tumor with a total result of 0–2 was classified as negative, one with 3–4 as mild positive, one with 4–5 as moderately positive, and one with 5–7 as intensely positive. One pathologist, who was blinded to cytology results, was in charge of the immunohistochemical expression measurement. Separately, another pathologist studied the surgical specimen and provided a final histological diagnosis. The scoring was performed with blinding to patient outcome.

Furthermore, mean, standard deviation, and 95 % confidence interval values were found for each area, both regarding percentage and intensity. The morphological aspects of immunostains were also described for the different pathologies. Overall survival was analyzed according to TPO level and TNM stage, as well as disease-free survival. Disease-free survival was considered for DTC when there was no clinical evidence of tumor, no imaging evidence of tumor, and undetectable serum thyroglobulin levels during TSH suppression and stimulation in the absence of interfering antibodies. For medullary thyroid carcinoma, calcitonin serum levels and carcinoembryonic antigen (CEA) levels were tested every 6 months during the first year, and then annually with an imaging procedure for control.

Statistical analysis

Data was analyzed using the SPSS v. 18.0 software. Statistical techniques included Pearson's squared chi test for the study of association between categorical variables; Student's t-test in the comparison of means for normally distributed numerical variables; Wilcoxon's non-parametric test in case of non-normality; a binary logistic regression model to find parameter profiles and TPO, $Ki67$, and $p53$ values; and a Cox proportional hazard analysis for assessing the effect of each prognostic factor on overall survival. A significance level of 5 % ($p < 0.05$) was established for all tests.

Results

This series includes a total of 139 cases, 43 benign and 96 malignant, classified in four groups. Table 1 summarizes the histological diagnoses by group. The surgical procedures performed included lobectomies, subtotal thyroidectomies (this type of procedure was carried out in patients from 1972 to 1995), and total thyroidectomies.

The immunohistochemical expression of TPO, $p53$ and $Ki67$ by disease is detailed in Figs. 1 and 2. TPO expression related to histological diagnosis was statistically significant ($p < 0.001$), with expression decreasing with cellular dedifferentiation. TPO staining patterns were also found in the different groups.

Table 1 Diagnosis by group

Group		Number (N)
Benign	Nodular hyperplasia	
	- Multinodular	10
	- Uninodular	9
	Chronic thyroiditis	
	- Hashimoto	7
	- Chronic nonspecific lymphocytic thyroiditis	3
	Adenoma	16
	Total	43
Papillary carcinoma	Papillary Carcinoma	38
	Follicular variant	4
	Total	42
Follicular carcinoma	Widely invasive	28
	- Clear cells	2
	- Hürthle cells	2
	- Insular pattern	5
	Minimally invasive	10
	Total	38
Other	Undifferentiated carcinoma	8
	Sporadic medullary carcinoma	8
	Total	16

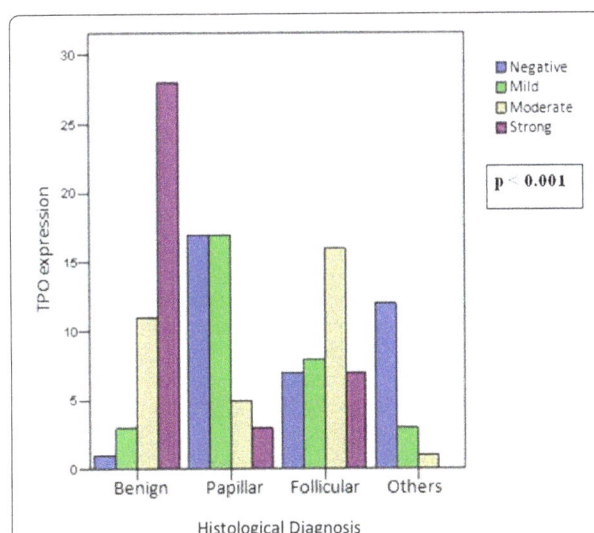

Fig. 1 TPO immunohistochemical expression according to tumor histology. TPO by groups showed an intense expression of TPO in benign cases when compared to the rest of groups, decreasing significantly in the papillary group, as well as in undifferentiated and sporadic medullary tumors (group "others"), where it was mainly negative. In the follicular group, TPO expression was variable, showing positive TPO expression but not as much as in the benign cases

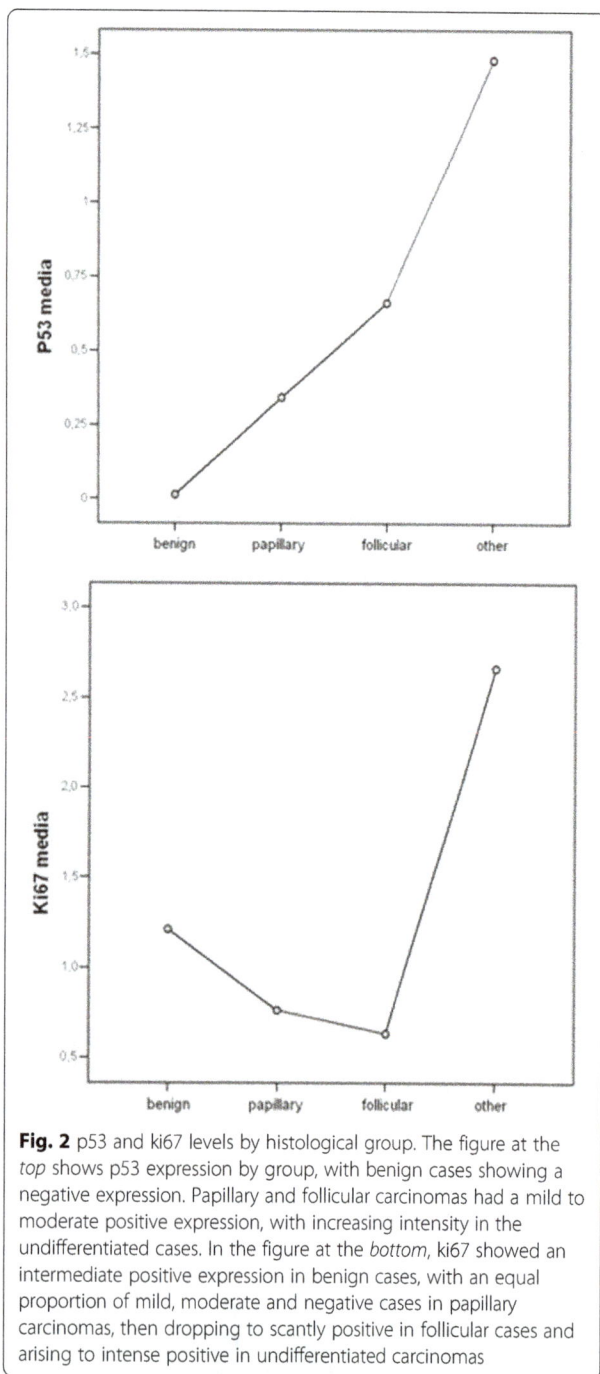

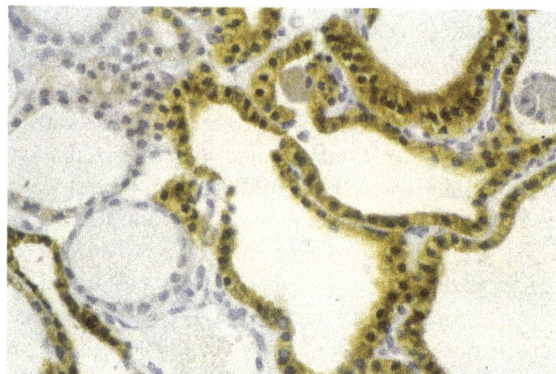

Fig. 3 Multinodular hyperplasia: Nodular hyperplasia showing cytoplasmic TPO expression (TPO x20) – highly intense in small follicles and apical areas

Fig. 2 p53 and ki67 levels by histological group. The figure at the *top* shows p53 expression by group, with benign cases showing a negative expression. Papillary and follicular carcinomas had a mild to moderate positive expression, with increasing intensity in the undifferentiated cases. In the figure at the *bottom*, ki67 showed an intermediate positive expression in benign cases, with an equal proportion of mild, moderate and negative cases in papillary carcinomas, then dropping to scantly positive in follicular cases and arising to intense positive in undifferentiated carcinomas

Benign pathology

In multinodular hyperplasia TPO was consistently positive in the cytoplasm (TPO staining scores: 2.7–5.5), with an irregular distribution highly intense in small follicles with apical TPO concentrations (Fig. 3). Uninodular cases showed moderate to high immunostaining (3.9 to 6.0) in the cytoplasm, particularly in microfollicular areas with cytoplasmic granules, as may be expected from a benign disease. A direct association between TPO intensity, presence of microfollicles, and localization in

areas near the capsule was found. In contrast, *p53* and *Ki67* expression was mostly negative.

TPO expression was moderate to high in all adenomas (mean 4.5), regularly distributed in the cytoplasm with a marked apical predominance. In Hürthle-cell adenomas low TPO positivity is characteristic both in central and subcapsular follicles; positivity is only outstanding for papillary growth patterns. The histological study of *p53* was negative in all but two cases – microfollicular and embryonic types. *Ki67* expression had intermediate positivity (1.2 to 2.4) in normal follicular, microfollicular and Hürthle-cell adenomas, with higher levels in a trabecular adenoma.

Papillary thyroid carcinoma

TPO staining was usually poor to moderate (<3) in 81 % of cases – higher TPO scores were only seen in four patients (3.6 and 6) – with positive expression in the apical pole of cells in the cystic epithelium and negative expression in Psammoma bodies (Fig. 4b). In follicular variants, negativity was seen in most fields except for focal areas with a regular and patchy distribution.

Protein *p53* had mild to moderate staining overall, and *Ki67* showed an equal distribution of mild, moderate and negative staining.

Follicular thyroid carcinoma

TPO results revealed positivity with irregular expression in most cases. Minimally invasive follicular cases (MIFC) (3.5 and 4.9) showed greater TPO immunostaining as compared to widely invasive follicular cases (WIFC) (1.4 and 2.9), with the presence of extensive, totally negative areas in contrast to their neighboring lesion zones (Fig. 4a). Five cases were totally negative. FTC showed decreased TPO immunostaining, both in intensity and percentage, when compared to hyperplasia and, to a lesser extent, thyroid adenoma. These lesions had an

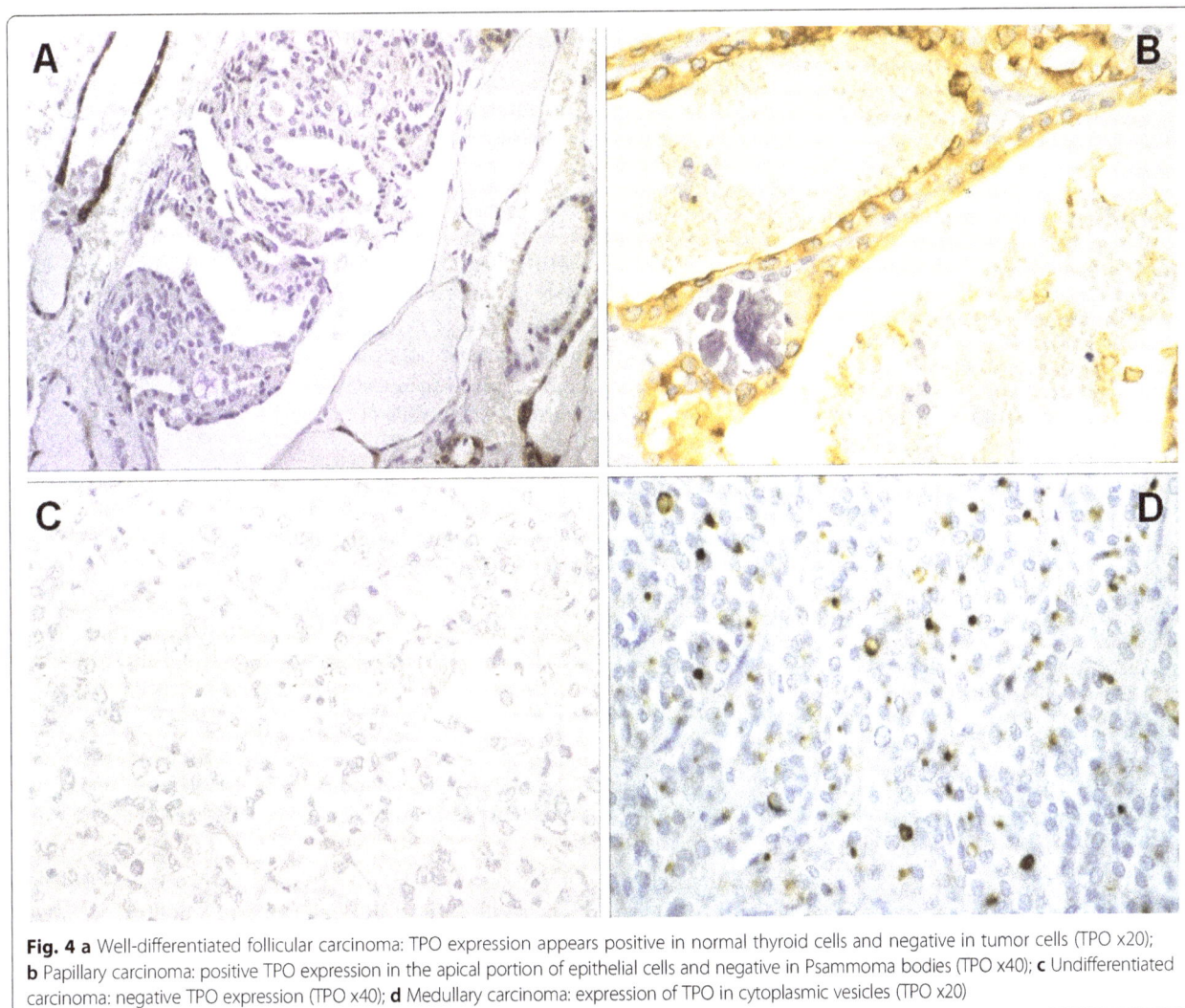

Fig. 4 a Well-differentiated follicular carcinoma: TPO expression appears positive in normal thyroid cells and negative in tumor cells (TPO x20); **b** Papillary carcinoma: positive TPO expression in the apical portion of epithelial cells and negative in Psammoma bodies (TPO x40); **c** Undifferentiated carcinoma: negative TPO expression (TPO x40); **d** Medullary carcinoma: expression of TPO in cytoplasmic vesicles (TPO x20)

irregular and cytoplasmic TPO stain, with mild and intense areas. In MIFCs TPO expression was moderate to intense in the cytoplasm and mild or negative in the nuclei; intracellular distribution was uniform from basal to apical areas. The presence of TPO in infiltrating follicles, including those protruding into the vascular lumen, is interesting. In WIFCs, expression was usually poorer.

P53 was negative for most MIFCs and positive in three Hürthle-cell carcinomas (1.5–3); WIFCs had scant positivity, and both clear-cell and insular-pattern lesions were negative. *Ki67* was scarcely positive in both MIFCs and WIFCs (0.4 and 1.3), with insular variants being moderately positive (1.4 and 3.7).

Others
Non-differentiated carcinoma
TPO was negative except in one case, which was considered follicular reclassified as anaplastic. *P53* positivity was generally intense (4 and 6.5), and *Ki67* was positive

in all cases with variable intensity (0.4 and 5.8), with anaplastic variants being more intensely positive (Fig. 4c).

Sporadic medullary carcinoma
TPO was negative in most cases and moderate in three; the presence of TPO in cytoplasmic vesicle-like deposits was noteworthy (Fig. 4d). *P53* immunostaining was negative except for two cases where it was markedly weak (0.2), and *Ki67* was negative in four cases and mild to moderate in the remaining four (2 y 4).

The cancer cohort was classified according to TNM stage. Figure 5 illustrates the association between TPO immunostaining and TNM stage, observing that TPO decreases as TNM increases.

Follow-up was carried out on an outpatient basis by the endocrinologist and the surgeon by way of physical examination, yearly thyroglobulin levels, and ultrasounds for suspected relapse. A maximum follow-up of 20 years was carried out. Minimum and median follow-up was 5

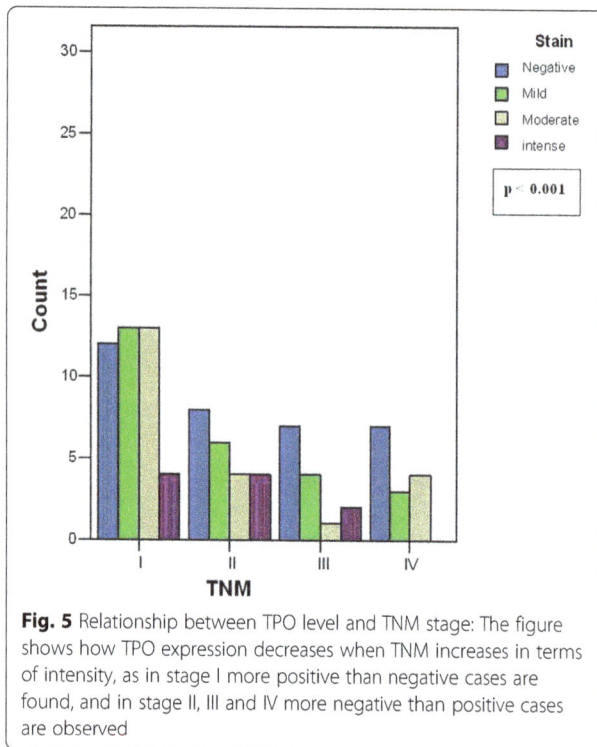

Fig. 5 Relationship between TPO level and TNM stage: The figure shows how TPO expression decreases when TNM increases in terms of intensity, as in stage I more positive than negative cases are found, and in stage II, III and IV more negative than positive cases are observed

and 15 years, respectively. A survival study was carried out, limited to patients with cancer, according to total TPO level (Fig. 6a) and TNM stage (Fig. 6b). Disease-free survival related to TPO expression (Fig. 6c) and TNM stage (Fig. 6d) was also analyzed.

According to TPO level, overall survival decreased in negative cases compared to positive cases without reaching statistical significance ($p = 0.34$). On the other hand, survival decreased with higher TNM stages ($p < 0.001$), as patients in stage IV had a 20-year survival of 52 % (SD 0.18) compared to patients in stage III and II, who had a 20-year survival of 83 % (SD 0.15) and 90 % (SD 0.09), respectively. We did not find any reason for the different survival rates in stages II and III, as they are differentiated by patient age and tumor size and localization.

Disease-free survival also decreased significantly in cases with higher TNM stages ($p < 0.001$). Patients in stage I had a 95 % disease-free survival after a 20-year follow-up. This rate dropped to 47 % for stage II, where patients under the age of 45 are included without taking into account tumor size or local or distant invasion. Stage III had a 29 % disease-free survival, whereas for stage IV all patients were ill at the end the observation period.

Discussion

TPO is a membrane-bound protein essential in the production of thyroid hormones. It catalyzes the iodination and coupling of tyrosyl residues to thyroglobulin to form

thyroid hormones T3 and T4. TPO expression pattern correlates with thyroid follicular cell function, both at the cytoplasm and apical membrane compartments. Quantitative and qualitative changes are related to hormone biosynthesis abnormalities usually due to thyroid disease. The biological meaning of abnormal TPO expression in thyroid tumors is unclear, but the progressive decrease of TPO levels together with an increase in cell density suggests it is correlated with proliferation [1–3].

Ki67 was used to study the proliferative activity of tumors, which determines their aggressiveness, progression, and metastatic potential. It is a monoclonal antibody that binds an antigen present in proliferating cells, but absent from quiescent cells [11]. On the other hand, gene *p53* is a suppressor gene that codes for a *p53* protein that plays a role in cell-cycle control, replication, and DNA repair. Mutated *p53* accumulates in the nucleus of tumor cells, and is promptly identifiable using immunohistochemical techniques [12, 13].

A huge variety of molecular tests are now available for the measurement of prognostic factors in thyroid carcinoma. Weber [4] identified a 3-gene combination to differentiate follicular adenomas from follicular carcinomas, with 100 % sensitivity and 97 % specificity. Rosen [5] compared gene expression in benign thyroid lesions versus papillary carcinoma, and described a set of 6 genes that predicted pathological diagnosis with 75 % sensitivity and 100 % specificity; Kroll [6] described fusion protein *PAX8/PPAR-γ* as a marker to distinguish benign from malignant follicular lesions. However, molecular techniques and gene studies are costly and time-consuming procedures that render their routine use difficult.

Our study's approach is different. Using simpler methods, such as immunohistochemistry, we analyzed TPO, *p53* and *Ki67* expression with the purpose of assessing whether TPO is useful as a prognostic marker by means of a long-term survival study. We have not found any literature describing a single study with such a long follow-up. The relationship between TPO expression and disease was statistically significant ($p < 0.001$) and decreased with tumor dedifferentiation extent. We do not know exactly why TPO is lost or increased according to tumor growth or development, albeit we suspect that differentiation criteria are involved. Increased TPO expression in benign lesions as compared to PTC and undifferentiated tumors is outstanding.

TPO increased in FTC to a lesser extent than in benign lesions, with differences in TPO expression between MIFC and WIFC being consistent with most reported studies [7, 15–17]. However, others such as Savin et al. among 47 cases of FTC observed an overall TPO expression of 78.7 % without correlation with degree of histopathological aggressiveness, as TPO expression in WIFC was not less reactive than in MIFC [9]. Microfollicular

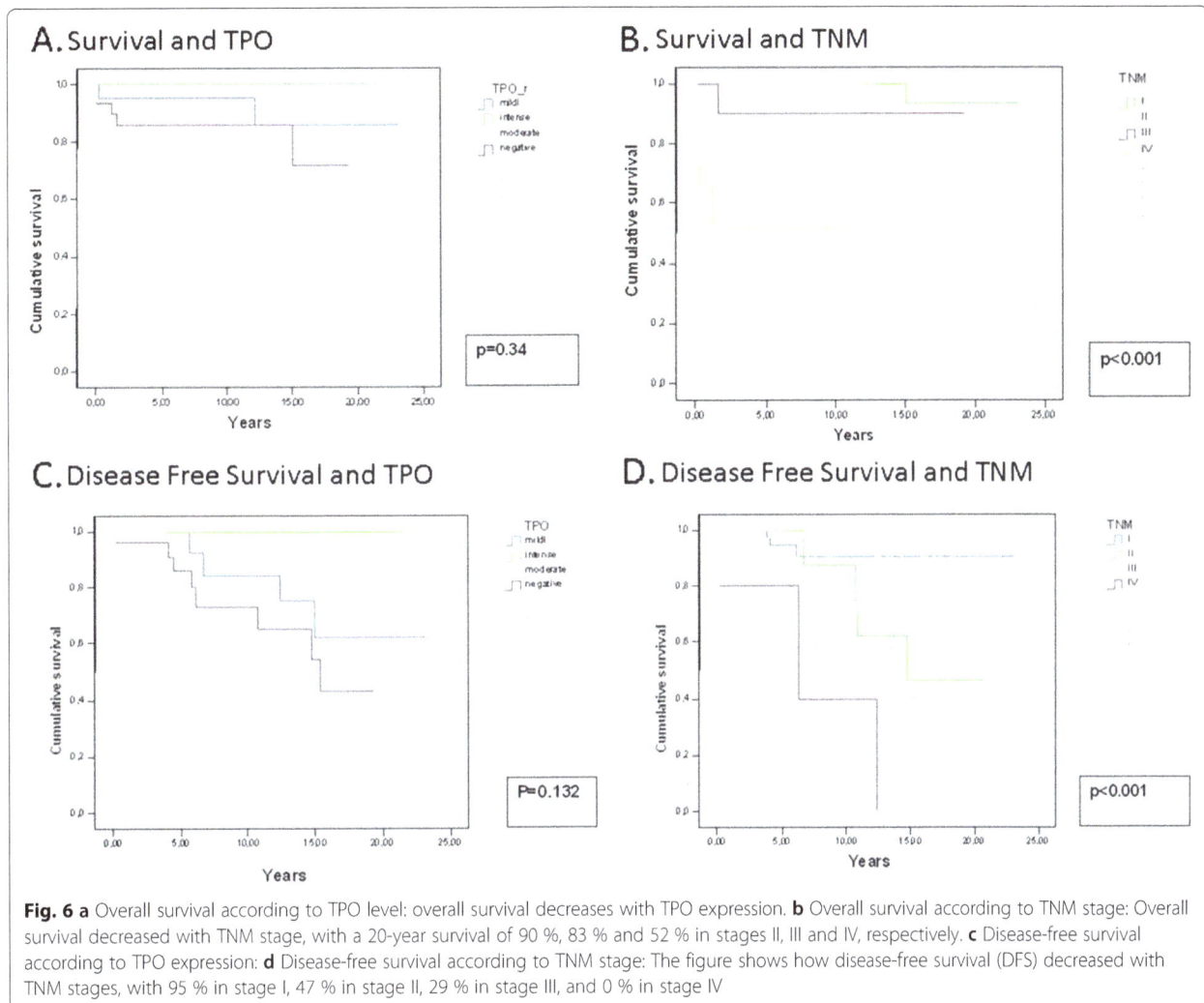

Fig. 6 a Overall survival according to TPO level: overall survival decreases with TPO expression. **b** Overall survival according to TNM stage: Overall survival decreased with TNM stage, with a 20-year survival of 90 %, 83 % and 52 % in stages II, III and IV, respectively. **c** Disease-free survival according to TPO expression: **d** Disease-free survival according to TNM stage: The figure shows how disease-free survival (DFS) decreased with TNM stages, with 95 % in stage I, 47 % in stage II, 29 % in stage III, and 0 % in stage IV

adenomas and MIFCs show increased TPO levels, which may reflect a failure of these invasive cells to lose function and differentiation despite their neoplastic course.

In contrast, De Micco [7, 15] observed that immunostaining was irregular in adenomas, moderate in 40 % of the remaining diseases, and negative in follicular carcinomas. This report does not include morphological criteria, immunostaining differences across areas, cytoplasmic localization, intensity assessment, or percentage per histological fields. Weber [4], in a series of 9 FTCs, found that only one was negative, thus reporting high positivity levels and a low sensitivity of TPO for this type of malignancy. In another study, Weber analyzed the use of TPO and galectine-3 separately for the diagnosis and prognosis of thyroid cancer — also combining both markers — and obtained with TPO staining a sensitivity of 39 % for any cancer, of 50 % for PTC, and of 11 % for FTC, which increased with galectine-3 immunostaining to 82 %, 96 % and 44 %, respectively [18]. Therefore, follicular cancer is associated with abnormal TPO expression in studies, with

a decrease in TPO immunostaining in 80–95 % of follicular carcinomas.

The scarce TPO staining of PTC in our series is consistent with other reports [15, 19, 20] that show strong TPO suppression in papillary carcinomas. The negative TPO expression found in undifferentiated carcinomas, where cells lack their endocrine function, supports an association between cell differentiation and TPO levels.

BRAF^{V600E} mutation is one of the most common genetic alterations in thyroid carcinogenesis. Its presence in papillary carcinomas has been reported to be associated with advanced stages [21] and poorer clinical outcome, although this remains controversial. Romei et al. analyzed the mRNA expression levels of TPO, among others, according to the presence of BRAF^{V600E} mutation [22]. They observed a higher prevalence of the mutation in classical PTC, rather than the follicular variant, and a significantly lower mRNA expression of TPO ($p < 0.0001$) in PTCs with BRAF^{V600E} mutation as compared to negative cases, suggesting that BRAF^{V600E}-mutated PTCs, although still well differentiated, are losing the typical features of follicular cells. Therefore, this mutation may be related to an early dedifferentiation process rather than advanced PTC stages. In this study we did not analyze TPO expression according to this mutation; however, we are looking forward to starting a new study in this respect.

TPO expression according to TNM stage shows that TPO substantially decreases when TNM increases. The comparison of mean TPO, *Ki67* and *p53* values was statistically significant ($p < 0.01$), which corroborates that the immunohistochemical study of TPO has prognostic value, as well as that of *Ki67* and *p53*. However, our results show that an initial analysis of TPO in cytology samples is not effective to distinguish benign from malignant lesions because of TPO expression variability in follicular tumors, consistent with other reports [23, 24]. Nevertheless, TPO may be useful, together with other markers, in confirming or ruling out benign diseases except for low-risk carcinomas such as MIFC.

The relationship between TPO expression and prognosis of thyroid disease has been determined in different studies. Weber, in his 1-year follow-up, observed that 100 % of patients with positive TPO and galectine-3 immunostaining were free of disease at the end of follow-up, compared to 57 % of patients with a negative TPO staining. It was suggested that the continued expression of TPO in cancer might predict clinical outcome, rather than the lack thereof [18]. Pulcrano et al. observed that detectable TPO expression was associated with a lower risk of metastasis in a 5-year follow-up, suggesting that persistent functional differentiation reflects a less aggressive behavior [25]. In the present study, overall survival according to TPO expression showed that patients with negative TPO had decreased survival rates, with a cumulative overall survival of 20 years, but the comparison between groups was not statistically significant ($p = 0.34$). In contrast, survival according to TNM stage was statistically significant ($p < 0.001$). Association between disease-free survival and TPO expression was not significant between groups; however, patients with negative or weak TPO levels had a survival of 72 % and 86 %, respectively, in contrast to the 20-year survival rate of 100 % seen with intense TPO expression.

Within the limitations of our study we must underscore the indolent nature of differentiated thyroid cancer and its low mortality rate. Therefore, assessing disease-free survival is challenging since relapses are usually asymptomatic. Nevertheless, this study has detected significant differences in overall survival according to TNM stage in association with TPO levels, and we believe this is due to our sample size and follow-up length, which reached a maximum of 20 years. Our results should be interpreted cautiously since the study may be influenced by a selection bias, as not all patients in the period referred were included in the study. Lastly, the number of thyroid malignancy samples analyzed is limited, especially when considering the subdivisions included in the classification of thyroid tumors, which may be considered an additional limitation.

Conclusions

In our study, TPO levels represent a useful prognostic factor for differentiated thyroid cancer. It may be highly useful for patient follow-up. A pronounced TPO fall requires assessment because of a high risk for local and/or distant relapse and decreased survival. The difference in TPO expression between MIFC and WIFC is an interesting finding in this study, and should be considered. In view of our results, TPO cannot be considered an effective diagnostic marker to separate benign from malignant disease following fine-needle aspiration in cases of follicular proliferation [18, 19]. Further prospective studies are needed.

Abbreviations
TPO: Thyroperoxidase; DTC: Differentiated thyroid carcinoma; MIFC: Minimally invasive follicular carcinoma; WIFC: Widely invasive follicular carcinoma; mRNA: Messenger ribonucleic acid; PTC: Papillary thyroid carcinoma; FTC: Follicular thyroid carcinoma.

Competing interests
All authors declare no financial competing interests, nor any other type of conflicts of interest.

Authors' contributions
CY helped in the acquisition of data and the statistical analysis, reviewed the literature about this topic, and drafted the manuscript. LE and FJ participated in the design of the study, was in charge of the recruitment of patients and data, and revised the manuscript critically. SJ designed the study with HJ, helped in the follow-up of patients, performed the statistical analysis, and took part in the immunohistochemical study of TPO. CJ carried out the immunohistochemical study, took part in the interpretation of data, and helped to draft the manuscript. HJ devised the study, helped to design it, was the main surgeon for patients, and was in charge of follow-up. All authors read and approved the final manuscript.

Author details
[1]General Surgery Department, Hospital Universitario Insular de Gran Canaria, Las Palmas de Gran Canaria, Las Palmas, Spain. [2]Pathology Department, Hospital Universitario Insular de Gran Canaria, Las Palmas de Gran Canaria, Las Palmas, Spain.

References
1. Valenta LJ, Valenta V, Wang CA, Vickery Jr AL, Caulfield J, Maloof F. Subcellular distribution of peroxidase activity in human thyroid tissue. J Clin Endocrinol Metab. 1973;37:560–9.
2. Mizukami Y, Matsubara F. Correlation between thyroid peroxidase activity and histopathological and ultrastructural changes in various thyroid diseases. Endocrinol Jpn. 1981;28:381–9.
3. Valenta LJ, Meichel-Bechet M. Ultrastructure and biochemistry of thyroid carcinoma. Cancer. 1977;40:284–300.
4. Weber F, Shen L, Aldred MA, Morrison CD, Frilling A, Saji M, et al. Genetic classification of benign and malignant thyroid follicular neoplasia based on a three-gene combination. J Clin Endocrinol Metab. 2005;90:2512–21.

5. Rosen J, He M, Umbricht C, Alexander HR, Dackiw AP, Zeiger MA, et al. A six-gene model for differentiating benign from malignant thyroid tumors on the basis of gene expression. Surgery. 2005;138:1050–6.

6. Kroll TG. Molecular events in follicular thyroid tumors. Cancer Treat Res. 2004;122:85–105.

7. De Micco C, Ruf J, Chrestian MA, Gros N, Henry JF, Carayon P. Immunohistochemical study of thyroid peroxidase in normal, hyperplastic, and neoplastic human thyroid tissues. Cancer. 1991;67:3036–41.

8. Masini-Repiso AM, Bonaterra M, Spitale L, Di Fulvio M, Bonino MI, Coleoni AH, et al. Ultrastructural localization of thyroid peroxidase, hydrogenperoxide-generating sites, and monoamine oxidase in benign and malignant thyroid diseases. Hum Pathol. 2004;35:436–46.

9. Savin S, Cvejic D, Isic T, Paunovic I, Tatic S, Havelka M. Thyroid peroxidase and galectin-3 immunostaining in differentiated thyroid carcinoma with clinicopathologic correlation. Hum Pathol. 2008;39:1656–63.

10. Ohta K, Endo T, Onaya T. The mRNA levels of thyrotropin receptor, thyroglobulin and thyroid peroxidase in neoplastic human thyroid tissues. Biochem Biophys Res Commun. 1991;14;174:1148–53.

11. Pisani T, Pentellini F, Centanni M, Vecchione A, Giovagnoli MR. Inmunocytochemical expression of Ki67 and laminin in Hürthle cell adenomas and carcinomas. Anticancer Res. 2003;23:3323–6.

12. Dobashi Y, Sakamoto A, Sugimura I, Machinemi R. Overexpression of p53 as possible prognostic factor in human thyroid carcinoma. Am J Surg Pathol. 1993;17:375–81.

13. Soares P, Cameselle-Teijeiro J, Sobrinho-Simões M. Immunohistochemical detection of p53 in differentiated, poorly differentiated and undifferentiated carcinomas of the thyroid. Histopathology. 1994;24:205–10.

14. Vargas-Roig LM, Gago FE, Aznar JC, Ciocca DR. Heat shock protein expression and drug resistance in breast cancer patients treated with induction chemotherapy. Int J Cancer. 1998;79:468–75.

15. De Micco C, Kopp F, Vassko V, Grino M. In situ hybridization and immunohistochemistry study of thyroid peroxidase expression in thyroid tumors. Thyroid. 2000;10:109–15.

16. Garcia S, Vassko V, Henry JF, De Micco C. Comparison of thyroid peroxidase expression with cellular proliferation in thyroid follicular tumors. Thyroid. 1998;8:745–9.

17. Franke WG, Zöphel K, Wunderlich GR, Mat R, Kühne A, Schimming C, et al. Thyroperoxidase: a tumor marker for post-therapeutic follow-up of differentiated thyroid carcinomas? Results of a time course study. Cancer Detect Prev. 2000;24:524–30.

18. Weber KB, Shroyer KR, Heinz DE, Nawaz S, Said MS, Haugen BR. The use of a combination of galectin-3 and thyroid peroxidise for the diagnosis and prognosis of thyroid cancer. Am J Clin Pathol. 2004;122:524–31.

19. Czarnocka B, Pastuszko D, Janota-Bzowski M, Weetman AP, Watson PF, Kemp EH, et al. Is there loss or qualitative changes in the expression of thyroid peroxidase protein in thyroid epithelial cancer? Br J Cancer. 2001;85:875–80.

20. Tanaka T, Umeki K, Yamamoto I, Sugiyama S, Noguchi S, Ohtaki S. Immunohistochemical loss of thyroid peroxidase in papillary thyroid carcinoma: strong suppression of peroxidase gene expression. J Pathol. 1996;179:89–94.

21. Namba H, Nakashima M, Hayashi T, Hayashida N, Maeda S, Rogounovitch Tim Ohtsuru A, et al. Clinical implication of hot spot BRAF mutation, V599E, in papillary thyroid cancers. J Clin Endocrinol Metab. 2003;88:4393–7.

22. Romei C, Ciampi R, Faviana P, Agate L, Molinaro E, Bottici V, et al. BRAFV600E mutation, but not RET/PTC rearrangements, is correlated with a lower expression of both thyroperoxidase and sodium iodide symporter genes in papillary thyroid cancer. Endocr Relat Cancer. 2008;15:511–20.

23. Paunovic I, Isic T, Havelka M, Tatic S, Cvejic D, Savin S. Combined immunohistochemistry for thyroid peroxidase, galectin-3, CK19 and HBME-1 in differential diagnosis of thyroid tumors. APMIS. 2012;120:368–79.

24. Savin S, Cvejic D, Isic T, Petrovic I, Paunovic I, Tatic S, et al. Thyroid peroxidase immunohistochemistry in differential diagnosis of thyroid tumors. Endocr Pathol. 2006;17:53–60.

25. Pulcrano M, Boukheris H, Talbot M, Caillou B, Dupuy C, Virion C, et al. Poorly differentiated follicular thyroid carcinoma: prognostic factors and relevance of the histological classification. Thyroid. 2007;17:639–46.

10

TSH receptor antibodies have predictive value for breast cancer

Paweł Szychta[1,4], Wojciech Szychta[1,5], Adam Gesing[1], Andrzej Lewiński[2,3] and Małgorzata Karbownik-Lewińska[1,3]*

Abstract

Background: Associations between breast cancer and thyroid disorders are reported in numerous studies. Relationships between thyroperoxidase antibodies (TPOAb), thyroglobulin antibodies (TgAb) and breast cancer have been previously demonstrated. However, no analysis has been performed concerning an association between thyrotropin (TSH) receptor antibodies (TSHRAb) and breast cancer. The aim of the study was to evaluate the prevalence of breast cancer or benign breast tumors in patients with Graves' disease and to analyze a possible relationship between Graves' disease and these two groups of breast diseases with emphasis to epidemiology and laboratory findings.

Patients and methods: Clinical and laboratory details of 2003 women hospitalized for endocrine disorders were retrospectively analyzed, using an unpaired Student's t-test, logistic regression analysis, χ^2 test of independence or the two-sided ratio comparison test.

Results: The coexistence of Graves' disease and breast cancer was statistically significant. We observed TSHRAb and TgAb more frequently in patients with breast cancer. We found that TSHRAb is the only variable possessing predictive value for breast cancer.

Conclusions: The strong relationship between Graves' disease and breast cancer is proposed. We suggest that TSHRAb could be described as a positive determinant of breast cancer. The present data call attention to the usefulness of screening for breast cancer in long-term follow-up of patients with autoimmune thyroid disorders, especially of those with Graves' disease. Similarly, screening for autoimmune thyroid disorders should be performed in patients with nodular breast disease. Additionally, the article draws ideas for further research in order to develop targeted treatment for more successful outcome in patients with breast cancer.

Keywords: Breast cancer, Thyroid, Autoimmune disease, Graves' disease, TSH receptor antibody, TSH, Thyroglobulin antibody, Thyroperoxidase antibody

Introduction

Breast cancer is a hormone dependent malignancy. Thyroid hormone receptors affect both the normal breast cell differentiation and breast cancer cell proliferation, with effects of thyroid hormones similar to those caused by estrogens [1,2]. Relationship between thyroid diseases, such as nodular hyperplasia, hyperthyroidism and thyroid cancer, with breast cancer was demonstrated in several studies [3-6]. However, ambiguous results concerning the

above association have been recently summarized [7]. In contrast, hypothyroidism due to Hashimoto's thyroiditis was documented as a protective factor against breast cancer [8-10], but also this observation was not confirmed in other sources [11].

Graves' disease, one of the thyroid autoimmune diseases, is characterized – in its typical form – by hyperthyroidism with laboratory results of decreased thyrotropin (TSH) level, increased free thyroxine (FT$_4$) and/or free triiodothyronine (FT$_3$) levels, detectable TSH receptor (TSHR) stimulating antibodies (TSHRAb), usually positive thyroid peroxidase antibodies (TPOAb) and thyroglobulin antibodies (TgAb) [12]. An exclusive diagnostic feature of Graves' disease is the presence of TSHRAb. The ligand

* Correspondence: MKarbownik@hotmail.com
[1]Department of Oncological Endocrinology, Medical University of Lodz, 7/9 Zeligowski St., 90-752, Lodz, Poland
[3]Department of Endocrinology and Metabolic Diseases, Polish Mother's Memorial Hospital, Research Institute, Lodz, Poland
Full list of author information is available at the end of the article

for TSHRAb, i.e. TSHR, is also present in breast cancer tissue [13].

Only limited aspects of potential association between Graves' disease and breast cancer have been postulated [14,15], whereas the exact mechanism has not been identified [16]. Genetic, environmental and molecular pathways of both female predominant diseases have been described, and integrated analysis of the above entities provides opportunity to identify the potential relevant common etiological mechanisms [17]. The potential relationship between antithyroid autoantibodies and breast cancer has not been clearly documented, as the elevated serum levels of TPOAb and TgAb in patients with breast cancer, detected in some studies [18-21], have not been confirmed elsewhere [22,23]. Moreover, no conclusive research has been undertaken concerning significance of TSHRAb in patients with breast cancer [24].

The aim of the study was to evaluate the prevalence of breast cancer or benign breast tumors in patients with Graves' disease and to analyze a possible relationship between Graves' disease and these two groups of breast diseases with emphasis to epidemiology and laboratory findings.

Patients and methods

Retrospective clinical details of 2003 women, who were hospitalized for endocrine disorders in the Department of Endocrinology and Metabolic Diseases at the Polish Mother's Memorial Hospital – Research Institute in Lodz within a 3-year period between 2002 and 2005, were retrieved from the hospital records following the internal audit approval. Inclusion criteria were female adults. Exclusion criteria were all oncological conditions other than breast neoplasia and thyroid disorders other than Graves' disease, such as nodular goiter, thyroid cancer, autoimmune thyroiditis (AIT), etc.

After exclusion, 1686 women aged 36.48 ± 15.95 years were enrolled to the study (Table 1). Two studied groups consisted of 47 patients with benign breast tumors (BBT), aged 46.27 ± 14.18 years and 9 patients with breast cancer (BC), aged 54.55 ± 9.60 years. Therefore, 1630 women hospitalized for several non-oncological diseases and without thyroid diseases other than Graves' disease (polycystic ovary syndrome, primary infertility,

osteopenia, osteoporosis, obesity, dwarfism, anorexia, atherosclerosis, cardiomyopathy, dyslipidemia, hirsutism, hypertension, ischemic heart disease, gastric ulcer, metabolic syndrome or diabetes of any type) were considered as a control group (C) with an average age of 36.10 ± 15.89 years.

Because of the relatively high age range of women with breast cancer and to analyze the cause-effect relation, age-matched groups of patients and healthy women could not be investigated in all stages of the analysis. Therefore, the predictors of breast cancer were analyzed in the age-matched group of 499 patients, including 9 patients with BC aged 54.55 ± 9.60 years and 490 control individuals (C) aged 53.86 ± 8.88 years (p > 0.05).

The following parameters were recorded with the use of the data analysis program, designed by one of co-authors of the study (P.S.): age and laboratory parameters, i.e. TSH, FT_4, FT_3, TSHRAb, TgAb and TPOAb. The following diagnoses were considered: Graves' disease, benign breast tumors (BBT) and breast cancer (BC). The normal ranges of the laboratory tests in our hospital are: TSH (0.27–4.2 mIU/L), FT_4 (0.93–1.7 ng/dL), FT_3 (1.8–4.6 pg/mL), TPOAb (<35 IU/mL), TgAb (<115 IU/mL) and TSHRAb (<1.8 IU/mL).

The data were statistically analyzed using an unpaired Student's t-test – for continuous variables. The two-sided ratio comparison test was used to evaluate the frequency of events. Univariate logistic regression analysis, followed by multivariate logistic regression analysis, was used to determine which continuous variable might have predicted breast cancer or benign breast tumors. The $\chi2$ test of independence was used to determine, which dichotomized variable might have predicted breast cancer or benign breast tumors. The results are presented as mean ± standard deviation (SD). Statistical significance was determined at the level of p < 0.05.

Results

Statistically significant differences were found in age distribution between patients with breast cancer (BC) and control group (C), as well as between women with benign breast tumors (BBT) and control group (C) (Table 1). However, there were no statistical differences

Table 1 Clinical characteristics of patients with breast cancer, benign breast tumors, Graves' disease and in controls

Parameter	Clinical characteristics				Statistical analysis		
	BC	BBT	C	All patients	p (BC vs. BBT)	p (BC vs. C)	p (BBT vs. C)
Patients – No (%)	9 (0.53%)	47 (2.78%)	1630 (96.6%)	1686 (100%)	ns	<0.0001	<0.0001
Age – yr (mean ± SD)	54.55 ± 9.60	46.27 ± 14.18	36.10 ± 15.89	36.48 ± 15.95	ns	0.0005	<0.0001
Graves' disease – No (%)	3 (33.3%)	6 (12.7%)	111 (6.8%)	120 (7.1%)	ns	0.0025	ns

Clinical characteristics of patients with breast cancer (BC), patients with benign breast tumors (BBT) and controls (C) and the occurrence of Graves' disease. Statistical evaluation was done by an unpaired Student's t-test (for age) or by the two-sided ratio comparison test (for no. of patients and for Graves' disease occurrence); ns, non-significant.

Table 2 Graves' disease as the dichotomized determinant of breast cancer or benign breast tumors

Dichotomized determinant	Association with BC (n = 9)		Association with BBT (n = 47)	
	χ^2	p	χ^2	p
Graves' disease (n = 120)	9.41	0.0021	2.33	ns

χ^2 test of independence analysis of the dichotomized determinant (i.e. Graves' disease occurrence) of breast cancer (BC) or of benign breast tumors (BBT), performed in all patients; ns, non-significant in all patients.

in age distribution between patients with benign breast tumors (BBT) and patients with breast cancer (BC).

Graves' disease was diagnosed on the basis of clinical findings and the presence of TSHRAb in 120 (7.11%) female patients aged 41.65 ± 15.19 years. Graves' disease coexisted more frequently with breast cancer (p = 0.0021), but not with benign breast tumors (p > 0.05) (Table 2).

In breast cancer patients, the mean values for TSH were 1.724 ± 3.629 mU/L and they did not differ significantly from those in controls (2.12 ± 5.41 mU/L) and from those in patients with benign breast tumors (1.35 ± 0.89 mU/L) (Figure 1). In turn, FT_4 was 1.283 ± 0.427 ng/dL in patients with breast cancer and did not differ significantly from levels found either in controls (1.34 ± 1.93 ng/dL) or in women with benign breast tumors (1.30 ± 0.67 ng/dL). In patients with breast cancer, FT_3 was 2.882 ± 1.617 pg/mL and was similar to controls (3.33 ± 1.91 pg/mL) and to patients with benign breast tumors (3.54 ± 1.65 pg/mL).

When levels of thyroid antibodies were compared among three groups of patients, the following differences were found. The mean values of serum TSHRAb were 25.65 ± 20.29 IU/ml in breast cancer patients, they were significantly lower in controls (4.83 ± 8.19 IU/ml, p = 0.0006), and were lower in patients with benign breast tumors (8.52 ± 14.04 IU/ml), but the differences between BC and BBT or between BBT and controls did not reach statistical significance (Figure 2). Serum concentrations

of TgAb in patients with breast cancer were 1120.8 ± 1914.9 IU/ml and were considerably higher than in controls (241.4 ± 565.0 IU/ml, p = 0.0100) and markedly higher than in patients with benign breast tumors (191.7 ± 267.1 IU/ml, p = 0.0443) (Figure 3). In turn, TPOAb in patients with breast cancer were at level of 157.8 ± 294.8 IU/ml and were similar to control group (135.7 ± 206.0 IU/ml, p > 0.05) and to benign breast tumors (178.9 ± 221.9, p > 0.05).

Several parameters, such as hormones and antibodies concentrations were submitted to a univariate and a multivariate logistic regression model. The purpose of the model was to determine which of those continuous variables might predict breast cancer or benign breast tumors either in the entire group of female patients or in age-matched groups. No predictive value for any of the examined hormones and for TPOAb was documented at univariate regression analysis in the entire group of patients (Table 3). In opposite, breast cancer predictive value for TSHRAb (OR = 1.10, 95% CI = 1.01-1.20, p = 0.0222) and TgAb (OR = 1.00, 95% CI = 1.00-1.01, p = 0.0377) was found at univariate regression analysis in the entire group of patients. Thus, TSHRAb and TgAb could be theoretically considered as positive risk factors for breast cancer. However, both above determinants lost their predictive value at multivariate analysis. In turn, meticulous logistic regression analysis, based on the age-matched

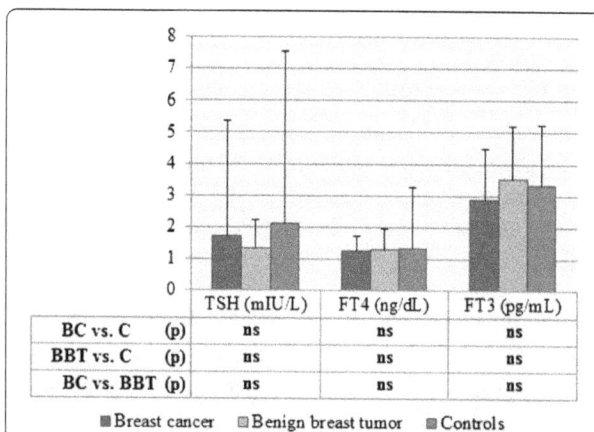

		TSH (mIU/L)	FT4 (ng/dL)	FT3 (pg/mL)
BC vs. C	(p)	ns	ns	ns
BBT vs. C	(p)	ns	ns	ns
BC vs. BBT	(p)	ns	ns	ns

■ Breast cancer ▨ Benign breast tumor ▨ Controls

Figure 1 Levels of hormones in patients with breast cancer, with benign breast tumors and in controls. Levels of hormones in: patients with breast cancer (BC), patients with benign breast tumors (BBT) or controls (C), expressed as mean ± SD; Statistical analysis with Student's unpaired t-test; ns, non-significant.

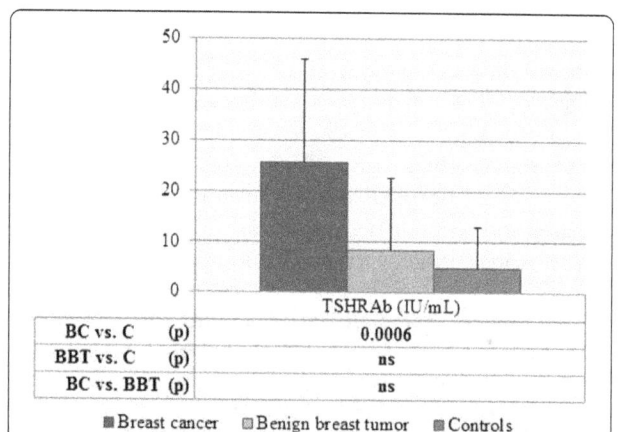

		TSHRAb (IU/mL)
BC vs. C	(p)	0.0006
BBT vs. C	(p)	ns
BC vs. BBT	(p)	ns

■ Breast cancer ▨ Benign breast tumor ▨ Controls

Figure 2 Levels of TSHRAb in patients with breast cancer, with benign breast tumors and in controls. Levels of TSHRAb in: patients with breast cancer (BC), patients with benign breast tumors (BBT) or controls (C), expressed as mean ± SD; Statistical analysis with Student's unpaired t-test; ns, non-significant.

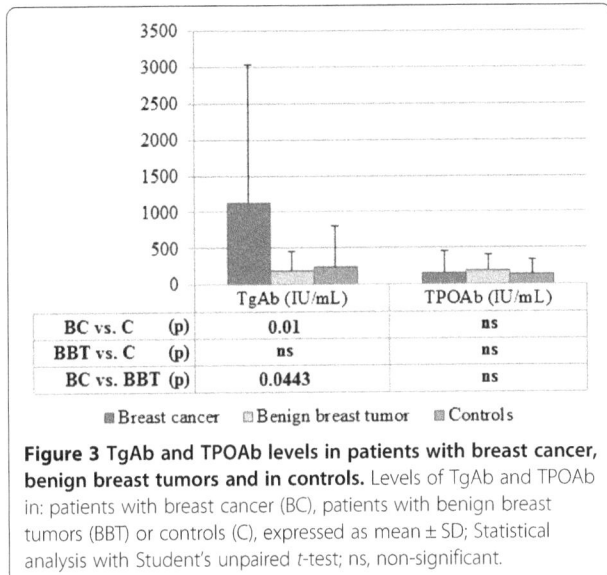

Figure 3 TgAb and TPOAb levels in patients with breast cancer, benign breast tumors and in controls. Levels of TgAb and TPOAb in: patients with breast cancer (BC), patients with benign breast tumors (BBT) or controls (C), expressed as mean ± SD; Statistical analysis with Student's unpaired t-test; ns, non-significant.

Discussion

Mammary gland is derived from iodide-concentrating ectoderm [17]. Breast functions are similar to the thyroid gland in relation to the absorption capacity of iodide for use as a milk ingredient during lactation [4,25]. Altered thyroid hormonal function due to abnormal iodine uptake has an impact on incidence of iodine deficiency disorders (IDD) [25], autoimmune diseases and could possibly affect cancer development. Increased intake of iodine is considered as a protective factor against the occurrence of breast cancer [26]. In conformity, low levels of iodine were described in the breast cancer tissues as compared to normal breast tissue or benign breast tumors [27].

Uptake of serum iodide into the breast alveolar and ductular cells happens in the mechanism of active transport via the glycoprotein – Na+/I-symporter (NIS) [28]. The expression of NIS occurs in 80% to 90% of breast cancer cases and, thus, symporter could be potentially used in the radio-isotope breast imaging with [125]I (alternatively [99]mTc) and in the breast cancer treatment with [131]I (alternatively [188]Re) [13], following administration of stimulants enhancing NIS expression [29,30].

groups of patients with breast cancer and controls, revealed that TSHRAb is the only variable possessing predictive value for breast cancer (OR = 1.09, 95% CI = 1.00-1.20, p = 0.0368) (Table 4). No other predictors of breast cancer or benign breast tumors were documented in our series.

Distribution of breast tumors in relation to age intervals and in comparison to Graves' disease is presented in Figure 4. A shift between diagnosis of Graves' disease and breast cancer was observed. Peak incidence of Graves' disease was seen in patients at age of about 35 years and the lowest frequency was observed at age of about 45 years, whereas peak level of breast cancer diagnosis were noted at about 65 years, and the lowest frequency at about 75 years. In contrast, we observed no similar distribution trends in relation to age intervals between benign breast tumors and breast cancers or between benign breast tumors and Graves' disease.

Assessment of hormonal thyroid function in breast cancer patients was assessed in our study with measurement of TSH, FT_4 and FT_3 levels and we found no differences among breast cancer patients, women with benign breast tumors and female controls. However, limited short-term hormone observations cannot be interpreted in relation to the long-term cancer development because of the changeable thyroid activity affected by several extrinsic and intrinsic factors. In turn, concerning the impact of autoimmune diseases on breast cancer incidence, we confirmed the high prevalence of breast cancer in patients with Graves' disease (Table 2).

Thyroid antibodies in the autoimmune thyroid disorders could interact with the receptors on breast tumors and thus they were previously designated as precursors for the coincidence of mammary and thyroid disorders [31]. Autoantigens, TPO in the thyroid and lactoperoxidases in

Table 3 Hormone and autoantibody concentrations as determinants of breast cancer or benign breast tumors

Parameter	Association with BC (n = 9)						Association with BBT (n = 47)		
	Univariate logistic regression			Multivariate logistic regression			Univariate logistic regression		
	OR	95% CI	p	OR	95% CI	p	OR	95% CI	p
TSH (mIU/L)	0.97	0.75-1.26	ns	-			1.20	0.92-1.55	ns
FT_4 (ng/dL)	0.96	0.42-2.21	ns				1.01	0.78-1.31	ns
FT_3 (pg/mL)	0.48	0.71-1.82	ns				0.95	0.81-1.11	ns
TSHRAb (IU/mL)	1.10	1.01-1.20	0.0222	0.92	0.66-1.28	ns	0.97	0.91-1.03	ns
TgAb (IU/mL)	1.00	1.00-1.01	0.0377	0.99	0.99-1.00	ns	1.00	0.99-1.00	ns
TPOAb (IU/mL)	1.00	0.99-1.01	ns	-			1.00	0.99-1.00	ns

Univariate and multivariate logistic regression analysis of the univariate determinants (such as hormone and autoantibody concentrations) of breast cancer (BC) or breast benign tumor (BBT), performed in all patients (n = 1686); OR, odds ratio; CI, confidence interval; ns, non-significant.

Table 4 Hormone and autoantibody concentrations as breast cancer or benign breast tumors determinants, in age-matched groups

Parameter	Association with BC (n = 9)		
	OR	95% CI	p
TSH (mIU/L)	0.96	0.77-1.21	ns
FT$_4$ (ng/dL)	0.92	0.32-2.67	ns
FT$_3$ (pg/mL)	0.69	0.29-1.62	ns
TSHRAb (IU/mL)	1.09	1.00-1.20	0.0368
TgAb (IU/mL)	1.00	0.99-1.00	ns
TPOAb (IU/mL)	0.99	0.99-1.00	ns

Univariate logistic regression analysis of the univariate determinants (such as hormone and autoantibody concentrations) of breast cancer (BC) or breast benign tumor (BBT), performed in the age-matched groups of patients (n = 499); OR, odds ratio; CI, confidence interval; ns, non-significant.

the breast, are required for organification of iodine to produce iodoproteins [32], as they catalyze H_2O_2 production to oxidize I⁻ [33]. Previously reported potential association between TPOAb or TgAb and breast cancer was arguable and the results were summarized in Table 5 [4,18,34-36]. The presence of TPOAb was previously described as a prognostic index of a more favorable outcome in patients with breast cancer, with similar importance to the tumor size and to the axillary nodal status [37]. In our study, TPOAb levels were similar among the three analyzed groups. In turn, TgAb levels were higher in our series in patients with breast cancer comparing to controls and to patients with benign breast tumors. However, the ligand for TgAb, thyroglobulin (Tg), has antigenicity affected by the iodine content within the protein [18,38], and thus TgAb are present non-specifically in different diseases coexisting with the altered iodine intake [39]. More importantly, TgAb can be also found in patients with chronic

disorders not involving thyroid [40] or even in healthy patients without any thyroid disease [41]. Thus, clinical impact of the elevated concentrations of TgAb is unreliable, as they were detected non-specifically to thyroid diseases or breast cancer.

Relationship between incidence of benign breast tumors and thyroid diseases with the increased levels of TgAb and TPOAb in serum has been also proposed [42]. Previous report documented the increased level of TPOAb in 28% of women with benign fibrocystic mastopathies and 80% had thyroid hypertrophy [21,43]. In contrary, we did not observe any association between Graves' disease, hormones or antibodies concentrations and occurrence of benign breast tumors.

Interaction between thyroid and breast cancer can occur in the mechanism involving TSHR, common in the adipose breast tissue [35]. Under physiological conditions, TSH via TSHR stimulates growth, differentiation and function of the thyroid cells [4,44]. This receptor is a target for THSRAb in Graves' disease. It should be stressed that TSHR expression is common in breast cancer, with higher prevalence in low-grade breast cancer [13]. The clinical significance of the serum TSHRAb in relation to breast cancer and Graves' disease was unresolved in the previous observations [6,15]. In our study, TSHRAb levels were significantly higher in breast cancer comparing to controls. They were positive determinants of breast cancer in the univariate logistic regression analysis, which did not reach statistical significance in multivariate logistic regression analysis. However, in the analysis of the age-matched groups of patients, TSHRAb was found to be the only positive determinant of breast cancer. Therefore, we suggest that TSHRAb can be called a positive predictor for the subsequent development of breast cancer. However,

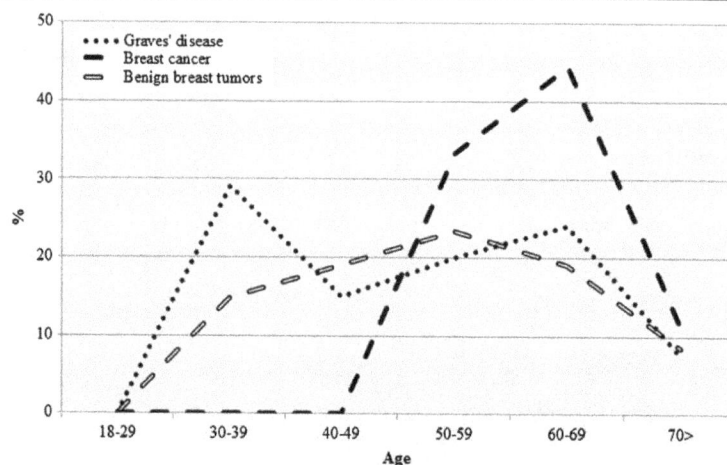

Figure 4 Trends in occurrence of breast cancer, benign breast tumors and Graves' disease. Distribution of breast cancer (BC) or benign breast tumors (BBT) in relation to age intervals and in comparison to Graves' disease, expressed as linear trends.

Table 5 Summarized previous reports concerning relationship between thyroid diseases and breast cancer or benign breast tumors

Parameter	[Previously reported data] (n = number of patients enrolled to study)														
	[3] (n = 150)			[18] (n = 115)			[34] (n = 61)			[35] (n = 175)			[36] (n = 48)		
	BC	C	p	BC	C	p	BC	C	p	BC	C	p	BC	C	p
n	150	100	-	66	49	-	36	100	-	100	75	-	26	22	-
Age-yr means ± SD (min-max)	63 (38–80)	age-matched	-	63.5 ± 11.8	68.4 ± 12.8	ns	52.8 ± 10.2	age-matched	-	63 (38–80)	-	-	(30–85)	age-matched	-
TSH	3.12 ± 1.40	1.46 ± 0.82	ns	1.77 (0.15–47.9)	1.52 (0.45–14.56)	ns	1.9 ± 0.7	1.8 ± 1.4	ns	4.12 ± 1.40	1.39 ± 0.79	0.030	1.36 ± 0.63	2.41 ± 0.35	<0.05
units	µIU/ml			mIU/dl			µIU/ml			µIU/ml			µIU/ml		
FT$_4$	2.64 ± 0.91	1.42 ± 0.31	ns	15.70 (7.38–22.63)	15.19 (10.5–21.5)	ns	9.76 ± 2.73	9.9 ± 2.4	ns	2.93 ± 0.57	1.39 ± 0.21	0.030	1.40 ± 1.64	1.10 ± 0.83	<0.05
units	ng/dl			pmol/dl			pg/ml			ng/dl			ng/dl		
FT$_3$	8.47 ± 0.75	4.48 ± 0.75	ns		-	ns	3.58 ± 0.7	3.2 ± 0.6	ns	7.25 ± 0.75	3.42 ± 0.91	0.030	3.56 ± 3.14	2.87 ± 3.12	<0.001
units	pmol/l						pg/ml			pmol/l			pmol/ml		
TgAb	140.92 ± 21.52	27.75 ± 7.60	ns	35.80 (26.1–6000.0)	27.70 (18.5–298.0)	<0.001	12/36	12/100	p < 0.01		-			-	
units	IU/ml			kIU/dl			Patients' ratio with positive TgAb								
TPOAb	105.82 ± 21.46	23.08 ± 4.16	0.030	6.10 (6.1–871.0)	6.10 (6.1–1621.6)	ns	12/36	8/100	p < 0.01	104.57 ± 19.39-	24.81 ± 5.16	0.030		-	
units	IU/ml			kIU/dl			Patients' ratio with positive TPOAb			IU/ml					
Diagnosis	BC	C	p	BC	C	p					-				
Graves' disease	-	-	-	0/66	0/49	-									
AITD	57/150	17/100	0.001	16/66	8/49	-									

Summary of the previously reported endocrine and immunological laboratory status in patients with breast cancer (BC) and controls (C); ns, non-significant.

further prospective research is required on a larger group of patients to determine unquestionably the significance of the above association.

Consequently, neutral TSHR antagonists (ligands inhibiting receptor activation by agonists), such as NIDDK-CEB-52, NCGC00242595 and NCGC00229600, could play a potential role in the breast cancer prophylaxis, acting as precursors of drugs preventing from TSHRAb activation in patients with Graves' disease [45]. Monoclonal antibodies, currently used in experimental studies on the medical therapeutic intervention in Graves' disease by vaccination with chemically altered autoantigens, could selectively deplete specific T lymphocytes subsets and block the T-cell receptor MHC interaction [46]. Additionally, no reports were found assessing the theoretical suppressive effect of blocking subtype of TSHRAb (causing hypothyroidism) on breast cancer and thus such clinical research would be advisable.

As discussed above, reduced iodide concentration, elevated levels of the thyroid hormones and antibodies contributed to an increased risk of breast cancer in previous reports and in our study. However, some authors suggested also the possible impact of breast cancer on the thyroid with the resulting increased level of thyroid hormones and the autoimmune response with the detectable thyroid antibodies [5]. In our series we found shift of about 15–20 years between the primary peak of the diagnosed Graves' disease and the secondary maximal incidence of breast cancer (Figure 4). However, the observed long shift is partially affected by the fact that participants in our study were younger than the general population of patients with Graves' disease, as they were hospitalized due to the more prominent symptoms. Older patients with usually more subtle clinical course of Graves' disease are treated as outpatients [47]. Despite some possible level of bias, we claim that it is the Graves' disease which could contribute to the subsequently observed development of breast cancer.

In conclusion, the strong relationship between Graves' disease and breast cancer is proposed. We suggest that TSHRAb could be described as a positive determinant of breast cancer. The present data call attention to the usefulness of screening for breast cancer in long-term follow-up of patients with autoimmune thyroid disorders, especially of those with Graves' disease. Similarly, screening for autoimmune thyroid disorders should be performed in patients with nodular breast disease. Additionally, the article draws ideas for further research in order to develop targeted treatment for more successful outcome in patients with breast cancer.

Competing interests
The authors declare that they have no competing interests.

Authors' contributions
PS, WS, AL & MKL have made substantial contributions to conception and design of the study. PS and WS were involved in the acquisition of data. PS designed the data analysis program. All authors (PS, WS, AG, AL & MKL) performed analysis and interpretation of data. PS was involved in drafting the manuscript. MKL revised the draft critically for important intellectual content. AL & MKL supervised and guided all the steps of preparing the manuscript and gave final approval of the version to be published. All authors read and approved the final manuscript.

Acknowledgements
The study was supported by the statutory funds No. 503/1-107-03/503-01 and No. 503/1-107-05/503-01 from the Medical University of Lodz.

Author details
[1]Department of Oncological Endocrinology, Medical University of Lodz, 7/9 Zeligowski St., 90-752, Lodz, Poland. [2]Department of Endocrinology and Metabolic Diseases, Medical University of Lodz, Lodz, Poland. [3]Department of Endocrinology and Metabolic Diseases, Polish Mother's Memorial Hospital, Research Institute, Lodz, Poland. [4]Current address: Department of Oncological Surgery and Breast Diseases, Polish Mother's Memorial Hospital, Research Institute, Lodz, Poland. [5]Current address: 1st Department of Cardiology, Medical University of Warsaw, Warsaw, Poland.

References
1. Dinda S, Sanchez A, Moudgil V: Estrogen-like effects of thyroid hormone on the regulation of tumor suppressor proteins, p53 and retinoblastoma, in breast cancer cells. *Oncogene* 2002, **21**:761–768.
2. Conde I, Paniagua R, Zamora J, Blanquez MJ, Fraile B, Ruiz A, Arenas MI: Influence of thyroid hormone receptors on breast cancer cell proliferation. *Ann Oncol* 2006, **17**:60–64.
3. Turken O, Narln Y, Demlrbas S, Onde ME, Sayan O, Kandemlr EG, Yaylacl M, Ozturk A: Breast cancer in association with thyroid disorders. *Breast Cancer Res* 2003, **5**:R110–R113.
4. Hellevik AI, Asvold BO, Bjøro T, Romundstad PR, Nilsen TI, Vatten LJ: Thyroid function and cancer risk: a prospective population study. *Cancer Epidemiol Biomarkers Prev* 2009, **18**:570–574.
5. Tosovic A, Bondeson AG, Bondeson L, Ericsson UB, Malm J, Manjer J: Prospectively measured triiodothyronine levels are positively associated with breast cancer risk in postmenopausal women. *Breast Cancer Res* 2010, **12**:R33.
6. Siegler JE, Li X, Jones SD, Kandil E: Early-onset breast cancer in a woman with Graves' disease. *Int J Clin Exp Med* 2012, **5**:358–362.
7. Angelousi AG, Anagnostou VK, Stamatakos MK, Georgiopoulos GA, Kontzoglou KC: Mechanisms in endocrinology: primary HT and risk for breast cancer: a systematic review and meta-analysis. *Eur J Endocrinol* 2012, **166**:373–381.
8. Ito K, Maruchi N: Breast cancer in patients with Hashimoto's thyroiditis. *Lancet* 1975, **2**:1119–1121.
9. Kapdi JJ, Wolfe JN: Breast cancer relationship to thyroid supplements for hypothyroidism. *JAMA* 1976, **236**:1124–1127.
10. Nelson M, Hercbergs A, Rybicki L, Strome M: Association between development of hypothyroidism and improved survival in patients with head and neck cancer. *Arch Otolaryngol Head Neck Surg* 2006, **132**:1041–1046.
11. Maruchi N, Annegers JF, Kurland LT: Hashimoto's thyroiditis and breast cancer. *Mayo Clin Proc* 1976, **51**:263–265.
12. Hamasaki H, Yoshimi T, Yanai H: A patient with Graves' disease showing only psychiatric symptoms and negativity for both TSH receptor autoantibody and thyroid stimulating antibody. *Thyroid Res* 2012, **5**:19.
13. Oh HJ, Chung JK, Kang JH, Kang WJ, Noh DY, Park IA, Jeong JM, Lee DS, Lee MC: The relationship between expression of the sodium/iodide symporter gene and the status of hormonal receptors in human breast cancer tissue. *Cancer Res Treat* 2005, **37**:247–250.
14. Munoz JM, Gorman CA, Elveback LR, Wentz JR: Incidence of malignant neoplasms of all types of patients with Graves' disease. *Arch Intern Med* 1978, **138**:944–947.

15. Chen YK, Lin CL, Chang YJ, Cheng FT, Peng CL, Sung FC, Cheng YH, Kao CH: Cancer risk in patients with Graves' disease: A nationwide cohort study. *Thyroid*. in press.

16. Hardefeldt PJ, Eslick GD, Edirimanne S: Benign thyroid disease is associated with breast cancer: a meta-analysis. *Breast Cancer Res Treat* 2012, **133**:1169–1177.

17. Venturi S: Is there a role for iodine in breast diseases? *Breast* 2001, **10**:379–382.

18. Jiskra J, Límanová Z, Barkmanová J, Smutek D, Friedmannová Z: Autoimmune thyroid diseases in women with breast cancer and colorectal cancer. *Physiol Res* 2004, **53**:693–702.

19. Smyth PP: The thyroid, iodine and breast cancer. *Breast Cancer Res* 2003, **5**:235–238.

20. Giani C, Fierabracci P, Bonacci R, Gigliotti A, Campani D, De Negri F, Cecchetti D, Martino E, Pinchera A: Relationship between breast cancer and thyroid disease: relevance of autoimmune thyroid disorders in breast malignancy. *J Clin Endocrinol Metab* 1996, **81**:990–994.

21. Smyth PPA, Shering S, Kilbane MT, Murray MJ, McDermott EWM, Smith DF, O'Higgins NJ: Serum thyroid peroxidase autoantibodies, thyroid volume and outcome in breast cancer. *J Clin Endocrinol Metab* 1998, **83**:2711–2716.

22. Kuijpens JL, Nyklíctek I, Louwman MW, Weetman TA, Pop VJ, Coebergh JW: Hypothyroidism might be related to breast cancer in post-menopausal women. *Thyroid* 2005, **15**:1253–1259.

23. Simon MS, Tang MT, Bernstein L, Norman SA, Weiss L, Burkman RT, Daling JR, Deapen D, Folger SG, Malone K, Marchbanks PA, McDonald JA, Strom BL, Wilson HG, Spirtas R: Do thyroid disorders increase the risk of breast cancer? *Cancer Epidemiol Biomarkers Prev* 2002, **11**:1574–1578.

24. Latif R, Morshed SA, Zaidi M, Davies TF: The thyroid-stimulating hormone receptor: impact of thyroid-stimulating hormone and thyroid-stimulating hormone receptor antibodies on multimerization, cleavage, and signaling. *Endocrinol Metab Clin North Am* 2009, **38**:319–341.

25. Zygmunt A, Adamczewski Z, Wojciechowska-Durczyńska K, Cyniak-Magierska A, Krawczyk-Rusiecka K, Zygmunt A, Karbownik-Lewińska M, Lewiński A: Evaluation of efficacy of iodine prophylaxis in Poland based on the examination of schoolchildren living in Opoczno Town (Lodz Voivodship). *Thyroid Res* 2012, **5**:23.

26. Mittra I, Perrin J, Kumaoka S: Thyroid and other autoantibodies in British and Japanese women: an epidemiological study of breast cancer. *BMJ* 1976, **1**:257–259.

27. Kilbane MT, Ajjan RA, Weetman AP, Dwyer R, McDermott EW, O'Higgins NJ, Smyth PP: Tissue iodine content and serum-mediated 125I uptake-blocking activity in breast cancer. *J Clin Endocrinol Metab* 2000, **85**:1245–1250.

28. Beyer SJ, Jimenez RE, Shapiro CL, Cho JY, Jhiang SM: Do cell surface trafficking impairments account for variable cell surface sodium iodide symporter levels in breast cancer? *Breast Cancer Res Treat* 2009, **115**:205–212.

29. Daniels GH, Haber DA: Will radioiodine be useful in treatment of breast cancer? *Nat Med* 2000, **6**:859–860.

30. Boelaert K, Franklyn JA: Sodium iodide symporter: a novel strategy to target breast, prostate, and other cancers? *Lancet* 2003, **361**:796–797.

31. Dumont JE, Maenhaut C: Growth factors controlling the thyroid gland. *Baillieres Clin Endocrinol Metabol* 1991, **5**:727–753.

32. Fernández-Soto ML, Jovanovic LG, González-Jiménez A, Lobón-Hernández JA, Escobar-Jiménez F, López-Cózar LN, Barredo-Acedo F, Campos-Pastor MM, López-Medina JA: Thyroid function during pregnancy and the postpartum period: iodine metabolism and disease states. *Endocr Pract* 1998, **4**:97–105.

33. Karbownik-Lewińska M, Kokoszko-Bilska A: Oxidative damage to macromolecules in the thyroid - experimental evidence. *Thyroid Res* 2012, **5**:25.

34. Giustarini E, Pinchera A, Fierabracci P, Roncella M, Fustaino L, Mammoli C, Giani C: Thyroid autoimmunity in patients with malignant and benign breast diseases before surgery. *Eur J Endocrinol* 2006, **154**:645–649.

35. Ali A, Mir MR, Bashir S, Hassan T, Bhat SA: Relationship between the levels of Serum Thyroid Hormones and the Risk of Breast Cancer. *J Biol Agr Healthc* 2011, **2**:56–60.

36. Saraiva PP, Figueiredo NB, Padovani CR, Brentani MM, Nogueira CR: Profile of thyroid hormones in breast cancer patients. *Braz J Med Biol Res* 2005, **38**:761–765.

37. Smyth PPA: Autoimmune thyroid disease and breast cancer: a chance association. *J Endocrinol Invest* 2000, **23**:42–43.

38. Belkadi A, Jacques C, Savagner F, Malthièry Y: Phylogenetic analysis of the human thyroglobulin regions. *Thyroid Res* 2012, **5**:3.

39. Cahoon EK, Rozhko A, Hatch M, Polyanskaya O, Ostroumova E, Tang M, Nadirov E, Yauseyenka V, Savasteeva I, McConnell RJ, Pfeiffer RM, Brenner AV: Factors associated with serum thyroglobulin levels in a population living in Belarus. *Clin Endocrinol (Oxf)* 2012. in press.

40. Molleston JP, Mellman W, Narkewicz MR, Balistreri WF, Gonzalez-Peralta RP, Jonas MM, Lobritto SJ, Mohan P, Murray KF, Njoku D, Rosenthal P, Barton BA, Talor MV, Cheng I, Schwarz KB, Haber BA, for the PEDS-C Clinical Research Network: Autoantibodies and Autoimmune Disease During Treatment of Children With Chronic Hepatitis C. *J Pediatr Gastroenterol Nutr* 2013, **56**:304–310.

41. Hill OW: Thyroglobulin antibodies in 1,297 patients without thyroid disease. *Br Med J* 1961, **5242**:1793–1796.

42. Tunbridge WM, Vanderpump MP: Population screening for autoimmune thyroid disease. *Endocrinol Metab Clin North Am* 2000, **29**:239–253.

43. Mizia-Stec K, Zych F, Widala E: Mastopathy and simple goiter–mutual relationships. *Przegl Lek* 1998, **55**:250–258.

44. Kopp P: The TSH receptor and its role in thyroid disease. *Cell Mol Life Sci* 2001, **58**:1301–1322.

45. Gershengorn MC, Neumann S: Update in TSH receptor agonists and antagonists. *J Clin Endocrinol Metab* 2012, **97**:4287–4292.

46. Swain M, Swain T, Mohanty BK: Autoimmune thyroid disorders-An update. *Indian J Clin Biochem* 2005, **20**:9–17.

47. Gesing A, Lewiński A, Karbownik-Lewińska M: The thyroid gland and the process of aging; what is new? *Thyroid Res* 2012, **5**:16.

11

Association between genetic mutations and the development of autoimmune thyroiditis in patients with chronic hepatitis C treated with interferon alpha

Janina Krupińska[1], Waldemar Urbanowicz[2^], Mariusz Kaczmarczyk[3], Grzegorz Kulig[1], Elżbieta Sowińska-Przepiera[1], Elżbieta Andrysiak-Mamos[1] and Anhelli Syrenicz[1*]

Abstract

Background: Considerable progress was made by the introduction of interferon to the treatment of chronic hepatitis C virus infection. This treatment, however, is associated with the risk of developing or exacerbating autoimmune diseases, with chronic autoimmune thyroiditis being one of them. The aim of our study was to evaluate the predisposition to autoimmune thyroiditis in patients with chronic hepatitis C virus during IFN-alpha therapy, depending on the presence of polymorphisms in the promoter region of CTLA-4C (−318)T gene and in exon 1 of A49G gene as well as C1858T transition of PTPN22 gene.

Methods: The study was conducted in 149 patients aged between 18 and 70 years (mean of 43.9 years), including 82 men and 67 women. Control group for the assessment of the distribution of analyzed polymorphism of genotypes consisted of 200 neonates, from whom umbilical blood was drawn for the tests. The patients were divided into three groups: group 1 consisted of 114 patients without thyroid impairment before and during IFN-alpha therapy, group 2 contained 9 patients with AT with the onset prior to IFN-alpha treatment, and group 3 comprised 26 patients with AT starting after the beginning of IFN-alpha therapy.

Results: The frequency of C1858Tand C(−318)T genotypes observed in the study group did not differ significantly from control group. A significant difference, however, was found for A49G polymorphism.

Conclusions: No association was demonstrated between the occurrence of autoimmune thyroiditis with the onset during IFN-alpha therapy and the presence of polymorphisms within CTLA-4 C(−318)T gene in the promoter region and A49G in exon 1, as well as C1858T transition of PTPN22 gene.

Keywords: Genetic mutations, Hepatitis C virus, Interferon alpha, Thyroiditis

Background

The development of autoimmune diseases is determined by the coexistence of autoimmune, environmental, and genetic factors. Genetic predisposition to autoimmune diseases depends on many genetic loci, of which three play a key role: alleles of major histocompatibility complex genes (human leukocyte antigen- HLA), mainly class II HLA-DR3; alleles of a gene coding cytotoxic T lymphocyte associated antigen-4 (CTLA-4), and alleles of PTPN22 gene coding for lymphoid-specific tyrosine phosphatase (LYP) [1].

CTLA-4 gene, located on chromosome 2q33, codes for membrane protein (cytotoxic lymphocyte antigen 4), which is important for the regulatory functions of T lymphocytes. Some variants of this gene predispose to autoimmune thyroiditis, including Graves' disease, as well as to type 1 diabetes, Addison's disease; also, such non-endocrine conditions as rheumatoid arthritis or coeliac disease [2-7]. In order for the autoimmune response to

* Correspondence: anhelli@asymed.ifg.pl
^Deceased
[1]Department of Endocrinology, Metabolic Diseases and Internal Diseases, Pomeranian Medical University, Szczecin, Poland
Full list of author information is available at the end of the article

take place, thyroid autoantigens must be presented to immunocompetent cells; class II HLA antigens participate in this process. Many proteins are involved in the activation of T cell dependent on antigen presentation, including CTLA-4, which inhibits this activation. Mutations of CTLA-4 occur spontaneously as a result of DNA copying error during replication or they may be induced by exposure to DNA-damaging chemical factors or viruses incorporated into the genome DNA during the life cycle. The mutation most likely to occur is the erroneous incorporation of a purine or pyrimidine (i.e. A↔G or T↔C substitution) [8]. Three CTLA-4-related polymorphisms have been described to date: substitution of adenine with guanine in exon 1 position 49 codon 17 (CTLA-4 A49G), substitution of thymine with cytosine at position 318 of CTLA-4(T318C) gene promoter, and elongation of AT sequence of microsatellite marker in 3' untranslated region (3'UTR(AT)n [6,7,9]. The majority of studies focus on the association between exon 1 CTLA-4 gene polymorphism (A49G) and the risk of developing diseases with autoimmune background [10,11].

The inhibition of T cell activation by CTLA-4 is governed by two mechanisms. In the first, activation is inhibited by the signal that constitutes a response to the activation of lymphocyte T receptor. It occurs at the early stage of immune response, when the expression of CTLA-4 and B7 receptor is restricted. Consequently, the inhibition of T cell proliferation and IL-2 secretion also take place. The second mechanism comprises surface competition between CTLA-4 and CD28 for B7 ligand on the antigen presenting cell. This mechanism depends on the expression of CTLA-4 on the surface of T lymphocyte and is known to join immune response at a later stage, when B7 and CTLA-4 expression increases. The consequence of B7 and CTLA-4 binding is the termination of response through restriction of signal from CD28, anergy of activated T lymphocytes, and their subsequent apoptosis. The impairment of CTLA-4 expression and/or function results in abnormal regulation of autoimmune response [12-14].

In 2004, Bottini et al. published the results of a study demonstrating that substitution of cytosine with thymidine at position 1858 of PTPN22 gene is associated with type 1 diabetes in patients from North America and Sardinia [15]. PTPN22 gene is located on chromosome 1p13.3-p13.1 [16]. A 1858T>C polymorphism leads to the substitution of arginine (R) with tryptophan (W) at position 620 (R620W), which makes it impossible for the PTPN22 gene-coded phosphatase to properly bind with Csk signaling molecules [16-18]. Under normal conditions, LYP-Csk complex causes the gradual inhibition of activation signal for T lymphocytes. Apart from polymorphisms within the major histocompatibility complex (MHC) and CTLA-4, a 1858 T>C polymorphism of

PTPN22 gene is currently a recognized risk factor for autoimmune diseases [17-20].

The aim of this study was to assess the predisposition to autoimmune thyroiditis in patients with chronic hepatitis C virus treated with IFN-α, depending on the presence of CTLA-4 C(–318)T polymorphism in gene promoter region and exon 1 CTLA-4 gene A49G polymorphism, as well as C1858T transition of PTPN22 gene.

Methods
Characteristics of study subjects
The study was approved by the Ethics Committee at Pomeranian Medical University in Szczecin (decision no. KB-0080/88/09).

The study group consisted of 149 patients aged between 18 and 70 years (mean of 43.9 years), including 82 men and 67 women. All subjects were HCV positive and remained under the care of Hepatology Outpatient Clinic at Regional Polyclinical State Hospital in Szczecin between 2003 and 2007. To assess genetic predisposition to autoimmune thyroiditis during IFN-α therapy, C (–318)T polymorphism in gene promoter region and exon 1 CTLA-4 gene A49G polymorphism, as well as C1858T transition of PTPN22 gene were analyzed. Molecular investigations were conducted at the Institute of Clinical Biochemistry and Molecular Diagnostics at Pomeranian Medical University in Szczecin.

The patients were divided into three groups: 1) Group 1 – 114 subjects without impairment of thyroid function before and during IFN-α therapy, 2) Group 2 – 9 subjects with the onset of autoimmune thyroiditis before IFN-α therapy, and 3) Group 3 – 26 patients with the onset of autoimmune thyroiditis after IFN-α therapy.

Detailed clinical characteristics of study subjects can be found in our earlier publication [21].

DNA isolation
To detect CTLA-4 polymorphisms and PTPN22 transition, 5 ml of venous blood was drawn into Vacutainer test tubes containing 0.1 ml 5% EDTA. The study material consisted of DNA isolated from peripheral blood leukocytes with the use of QIAMP® DNA Mini Kit (Qiagen).

The distribution of analyzed polymorphisms was also assessed in umbilical blood obtained from 200 neonates, who constituted the control group.

Sequence of starters
Selected polymorphisms of genes: CTLA-4 [rs 231775 A/G (A49G), rs5742909 C/T(C(–318)T)], and PTPN22 [rs2476601 C/T (C1858T)] were identified with PCR-RFLP (polymerase chain reaction-restriction fragment

length polymorphism) with the use of specific starter pairs (Table 1).

Amplification of CTLA-4 and PTPN22 sequences

Optimal PCR conditions for individual starter pairs were established in preliminary experiments (Table 2).

All amplifications were performed in Mastercycler Gradient thermal cycler (Eppendorf).

Amplifications of CTLA4 sequences were performed in 20 µl of reaction mixture containing the following ingredients: 40 ng of genome DNA, PCR buffer [10 mM of Tris–HCl, 50 mM of KCl, and 0.08% of Nonidet P40] (MBI Fermentas), dNTP [200 µM](MBI Fermentas), MgCl2 [1,5 mM](MBI Fermentas), upstream and downstream primer, 4 pmol each (synt. TIB MOLBIOL, Poznań), and 0.5 U of Taq polymerase (MBI Fermentas).

Amplifications of PTPN22 gene sequences were performed in 20 µl of reaction mixture containing: 40 ng of genome DNA, 1 x PCR buffer (QIAGEN), 1 x Q-Solution(QIAGEN), dNTP [200 µM] (MBI Fermentas), upstream and downstream primer, 4 pmol each (synt. TIB MOLBIOL, Poznań), and 1 U of Hot Star Taq polymerase (QIAGEN).

The following temperature-time profile was used in PCR: 1) phase I: preliminary denaturation 94°C – 5 min, 2) phase II (36–37 cycles; Table 2): denaturation: 94°C – 20 sec, annealing: 52-60°C (Table 2) – 40 sec, elongation: 72°C, 3) phase III: final elongation 72°C – 8 min.

Amplification products were subject to restriction analysis with appropriate enzymes (Table 3).

PCR products and restriction fragments were separated by electrophoresis in agarose gel of appropriate concentration and stained with ethidium bromide. The separation was conducted in 1 x TBE buffer (0.089 M of Tris, 0.089 M of boric acid, 2 mM of EDTA), at the temperature of 20°C and voltage of 80V. The length of restriction fragments was estimated on the basis of length marker DNA-pUC Mix Marker 8 (MBI Fermentas). The final stage consisted of photographing the obtained results with Polaroid camera (DS-34 Direct Screen Camera) under UV light (Transiluminator 4000, Stratagene). The photos were scanned and saved as jpeg files (Figures 1, 2, 3).

Table 1 Sequence of starters

Gene	Polymorphism	Sequence of starters
CTLA4	rs231775	5'-GCTCTACTTCTTGAAGACCT-3'
		5'-AGTCTCACTCACCTTTGCAG-3'
	rs5742909	5'-GGATGCCCAGAAGATTGA -3'
		5'-AAGGAAGCCGTGGGTTTA -3'
PTPN22	rs2476601	5'-ACCGCGCCCAGCCCTACTTTTG-3'
		5'-AGCCACCATGCCCATCCCACACT-3'

Table 2 Amplification conditions

Gene	Polymorphism	$T_{annealing}$ [°C]	No. of cycles	Amplicon [bp]
CTLA4	rs231775	58	37	162
	rs5742909	54	36	215
PTPN22	rs2476601	60	37	392

Statistical analysis

The conformity of genotype frequency with Hardy-Weinberg law was evaluated with an exact test using R "genetic" module (version 2.9.0; http://cran.r-project.org).

The analysis of polymorphisms was performed with χ2 test and logistic regression model for the calculation of odds ratio (OR) with 95% CI (confidence interval). Allele frequency was calculated on the basis of genotype frequency.

The compliance of genotype frequency with Hardy-Weinberg distribution was analyzed separately for the study group and in the control group, as well as for both of these groups together.

Results

Distribution of C1858T, A49G and C(–318)T genotypes in study and control groups

With the exception of A49G polymorphism, genotype frequency did not differ significantly from the theoretical distribution. In the case of A49G polymorphism, the deviations from Hardy-Weinberg equilibrium were found as following for each of the three groups analyzed groups: study group - p<0.0001, control group – p<0.05, study and control groups together - p<0.00001.

The distribution of genotypes of C1858T, A49G, and C(–318)T polymorphisms in the study group and in control group are presented in Table 4. The frequency of C1858T and C(–318)T genotypes in the study group did not differ significantly from that in the control group. A significant difference, however, was observed for A49G polymorphism; moreover, no GG homozygote was detected in the study group, while there were 14 GG

Table 3 Conditions of restriction analysis

Gene	Polymorphism	Restriction enzyme	Restriction fragments [bp]
CTLA4	rs 231775 A/G	Sat I [10 U, 37°C, 12 h]	allele A: 99 + 63
			allele G: 74 + 25 + 63
	rs5742909	Mse I [5 U, 65°C , 12 h]	allele C: 215
			allele T: 124 + 91
PTPN22	rs2476601 C/T	Rsa I [5 U, 37°C, 12 h]	allele C: 228 + 74 + 46 + 44
			allele T: 272 + 74 + 46

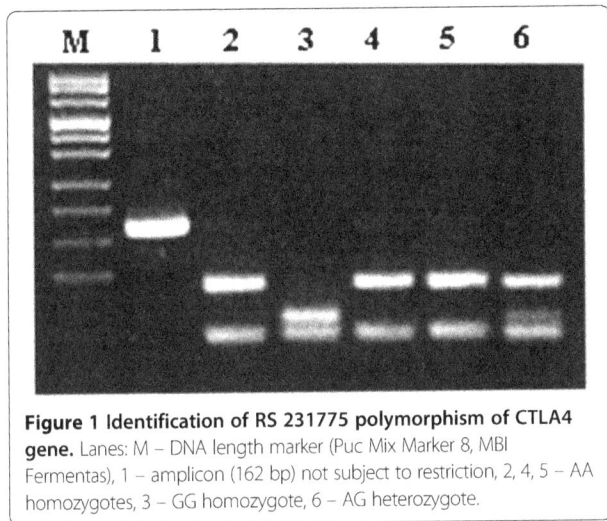

Figure 1 Identification of RS 231775 polymorphism of CTLA4 gene. Lanes: M – DNA length marker (Puc Mix Marker 8, MBI Fermentas), 1 – amplicon (162 bp) not subject to restriction, 2, 4, 5 – AA homozygotes, 3 – GG homozygote, 6 – AG heterozygote.

homozygotes in the control group, being equal to 7% of all genotypes in this group.

Predisposition to chronic viral hepatitis

The results of analysis in relations to different inheritance modes for minor alleles (dominant and recessive) of the mutated gene and to patient's gender are presented in Table 5. Dominant mode was defined as the presence of at least one minor allele in comparison to the absence of this allele, resulting in the following three sets of comparisons: TT+CT vs. CC (minor allele T), GG +AG vs. AA (minor allele G) and TT+CT vs. CC (minor allele T), for C1858T, A49G and C(−318)T polymorphisms, respectively. In the case of the recessive mode, homozygotes for minor alleles were compared with the carriers of major alleles, producing the following sets of comparisons: TT vs. CT+CC, GG vs. AG+AA and TT vs. CT+CC for C1858T, A49G, and C(−318)T, respectively.

Following gender adjustments, C1858T and C(−318)T polymorphisms, irrespective of the analyzed inheritance

mode and A49G polymorphism in the dominant mode (GG+AG vs. AA), did not demonstrate any relationship with the predisposition to chronic viral hepatitis. Odds ratio for A49G in the recessive mode (GG vs. AG+AA) could not be obtained due to the absence of GG homozygotes in the study group, but the observed difference in the frequency of GG homozygotes (0% of patients treated with interferon and 7% of the control group) and allele A carriers (100% of patients treated with interferon and 96% of the control group) was significant (p=0.00334, two-tailed Fisher's test).

Distribution of genotypes in patients with autoimmune thyroiditis and in patients without thyroid impairment

Table 6 presents the number and frequency of genotypes of C1858T, A49G, and C(−318)T polymorphisms in patients with autoimmune thyroiditis (AT, n=18) and in patients without impairment of thyroid function during treatment (n=62). The comparison of genotype frequencies in these two groups did not show any significant differences with regards to any of analyzed polymorphisms. It is worth noticing that there were no GG homozygotes of A49G polymorphism, both in AT group and in patients without thyroid impairment.

Predisposition to AT during IFN-α therapy

Our study attempted to assess the predisposition to AT depending on the possessed genotype in relation to two inheritance modes and the gender of the patient (Table 7). Since AT group lacked homozygotes of mutated TT C1858T, GG A49G, and TT C(−318)T alleles, the assessment of predisposition to AT in the carriers of these genotypes as compared to the carriers of wild-type (major) alleles (recessive mode) proved impossible. Additionally, A49G GG homozygotes were not detected in patients without thyroid impairment. Conversely, the carriers of mutated (minor) alleles (TT+CT C1858T, GG+AG A49G, and TT+CT C(−318)T) did not

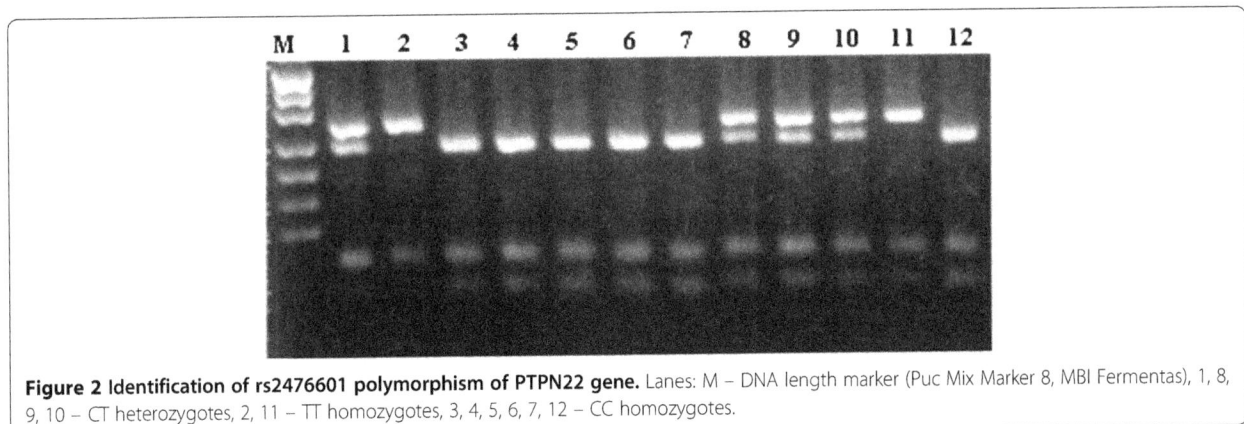

Figure 2 Identification of rs2476601 polymorphism of PTPN22 gene. Lanes: M – DNA length marker (Puc Mix Marker 8, MBI Fermentas), 1, 8, 9, 10 – CT heterozygotes, 2, 11 – TT homozygotes, 3, 4, 5, 6, 7, 12 – CC homozygotes.

show a greater predisposition to AT as compared to wild-type homozygotes (dominant mode).

OR was not obtained in three cases (recessive inheritance): C1858T – absence of TT homozygotes in the study group vs. one (1.6%) TT homozygote in the control group (p=1.0, two-tailed Fisher's test); A49G – no GG homozygotes in both groups; C(–318)T – no TT homozygotes in the study group as compared to 2 TT homozygotes (3.2%) in the control group (p=1.0, two-tailed Fisher's test).

Discussion

At present, genetic studies are being employed with increasing frequency for the assessment of predisposition to many diseases, especially those that are genetically determined (monogenic and polygenic) as well as those that involve the chromosomes. Diagnostic assessments have become markedly easier to carry out as a result of considerable progress in the investigational methods of molecular biology following the discovery of polymerase chain reaction (PCR) in early 1990s, allowing for the replication of selected DNA fragments in billions of copies. Approximately 80 monogenic diseases have a direct influence on body's endocrine function; although, polygenic factors are also known to play a role [2].

Genetic polymorphism is the consequence of two types of structural changes in gene sequence, i.e. single nucleotide polymorphism (SNP) and major structural changes such as simple sequence length polymorphism (SSLP), i.e. a variable number of tandem repeats-VNTR (147). According to current genetic research, a common genetic background of autoimmune diseases seems to comprise the following components: C1858T polymorphism of a single nucleotide of PTPN22 gene coding for lymphocyte-specific phosphatase and A/G polymorphism at position 49 of CTLA-4 gene, acting as a negative regulator of lymphocyte T activation, The first results in excessive activation of T lymphocytes, while the second modifies post-translation processes in endoplasmic reticulum through the substitution of threonine with alanine in a signal peptide and this, in turn, causes less effective glycosylation and reduced surface expression of CTLA-4 peptide [22-24]. In 2007, Lee et al. conducted a meta-analysis showing the association between C1858T polymorphism of PTPN22 gene and Graves' (G) disease, type 1 diabetes, rheumatoid arthritis, and lupus erythematosus [16,22]. Another study published in 2007 demonstrated a very strong causal relationship between 49A/G polymorphism of CTLA-4 gene and the development of Hashimoto Thyroiditis (HT) and the presence of anti-thyroid antibodies in Graves' disease and HT [25]. A solid correlation between autoimmune thyroid diseases and CTLA-4 polymorphism on chromosome 2q33 was proved by Bicek et al. in 2009, namely two A>G

polymorphisms of a single nucleotide of CTLA-4 gene at position +49 of exon 1 (49A/G) and +6230 (CT60) in 3'UTR [26]. We analyzed the distribution of genotypes of C1858T, A49G, and C(–318)T polymorphisms in the study subjects and in the control group. A significant difference was found for A49G polymorphism in the study group vs. control group, while the frequency of C1858T and C(–318)T genotypes did not differ significantly in both groups. The aim of our study was to assess the occurrence of C(–318)T polymorphism of CTLA-4 gene within the promoter region. Additionally, we aimed to evaluate A49G polymorphism in exon 1 and C1858T transition of PTPN22 gene in a group of patients with the onset of AT during INF-α therapy for HCV as compared to subjects without any impairment of thyroid function during treatment. The comparison of genotype frequency between these groups conducted in our study showed no significant differences for all polymorphisms. This result differs from that reported by Kula et al. in 2003, who found the strongest association between CTLA-4 polymorphism and the development and clinical picture of HT in a group of 89 Polish subjects [27]. 49A/G polymorphism associated with the activation of T lymphocytes influences the high level of anti-thyroid antibody production in G-B disease and HT [23,28]. Kula et al. [27] did not find any significant differences in mean TPOAb level for CTLA-4 gene in relation to the genotype with demonstrated association with the exacerbation of hypothyroidism and thyroid volume. Slovenian investigators examined 328 Caucasian patients with G-B disease and Postpartum Thyroiditis (PPT), and compared the results with those obtained in a control group of 117 healthy subjects. The distribution of genotypes of both polymorphisms was similar in these two groups. The frequency of GG genotype in G-B disease was 13.8% for 49A/G polymorphism as compared to 5.1% in the control group; the corresponding values for CT60 polymorphism were 40.7% in the study group and 25.6% in the control group. The frequencies of GG genotype for HT and PPT were comparable and were found to equal to 12.9% for 49AG polymorphism and 34.4% for CT60 polymorphism. A comparison of G allele vs. A allele for both polymorphisms within CTLA-4 gene was also performed and showed that the likelihood of developing G-B disease is 1.6 times greater for individuals with G allele in 49A/G or CT60 polymorphism of CTLA-4 gene. It was demonstrated that 49A/G and CT60 polymorphisms of CTLA-4 gene display strong causal relationship with autoimmune thyroid diseases (AITD) in Slovenian population [26]. Additionally, a correlation between the presence of GG genotype and the development of HT and PPT were also showed [11,26]. We evaluated the frequencies of genotypes in patients treated with INF-α and in the control group and, as mentioned before, a

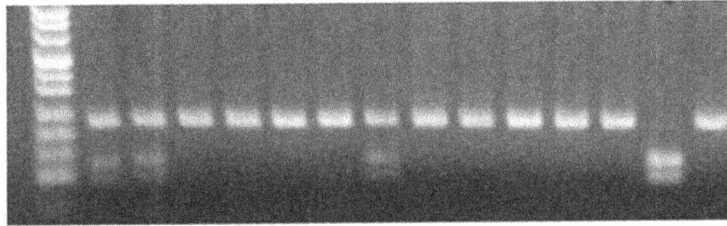

Figure 3 Identification of rs5742909 polymorphism of CTLA4 gene. Lanes: M – DNA length marker (pUC Mix Marker 8, MBI Fermentas), 1, 2, 7 – CT heterozygotes, 3, 4, 5, 6, 8, 9, 10, 11, 12, 14 – CC homozygotes, 13 – TT homozygote.

significant difference was observed for A49G polymorphism in both groups. Namely, no GG homozygotes were detected in the study group as compared to the control group with 14 GG homozygotes, constituting 7% of all genotypes in this group. Furthermore, A49G GG homozygotes were not found in patients without thyroid impairment. Conversely, in a meta-analysis published by Roycroft et al. in 2009, which examined C1858T polymorphism of PTPN22 gene in the population of Caucasian patients with Addison's disease living in Britain and in Poland [29], sixty-one out of 502 (12.2%) British patients were the carriers of T allele in PTPN22 C1858T(R620W)SNP. This allele was detected in 67 (7.8%) of 858 healthy subjects from the control group. In the Polish population of 174 patients, 1858T alleles were found in 34 (19.5%) subjects compared with 11.7% in the control group. The authors performed another comparison within this study, namely, they compared the frequency of 1858T allele in control groups originating from different parts of Europe and obtained the following results: Newcastle (England) – 7.8%, Sheffield (England) – 10.5%, and Norway – 10.8%. Therefore, it is our opinion that the correlation between the polymorphism of PTPN22 gene and the occurrence of Addison's disease in European population cannot be confirmed beyond a reasonable doubt as authors claim [29].

Ever since the relationship between CTLA-4 polymorphisms and G-B disease and type 1 diabetes in southern European countries was demonstrated for the first time, numerous studies have been conducted to link a given polymorphism with a specific disease. So far, many authors have stressed a strong association between G-B disease and the polymorphism of CTLA-4 gene; however, a considerable controversy has arisen as to the site of polymorphism. For example, Bicek et al., state that CT60 polymorphism shows the strongest correlation only with G-B disease and that its association with HT and PPT is weaker [26]. Petrone et al. demonstrated that in Italian population A49G polymorphism was correlated with G-B disease, especially when G allele was present [30]. Ban et al. observed a much greater frequency of G allele SNP CT60 associated with G-B disease in Japanese subjects than in Caucasian population: 72.6% vs. 52.3%, respectively [31]. In Japanese population, the presence of G allele CT60 was more common in patients with G-B disease than in the control group: 84.0% and 72.6%, respectively; just as it was in the whole group of patients with autoimmune thyroid diseases: 80.1% and 72.6%, respectively. A dominant genotype model among AITD patients was GG+GA vs. AA, while a recessive genotype model was found to be GG vs. AG+AA [32]. We tried to analyze the various modes of inheritance of mutated allele, i.e. dominant inheritance (a necessary condition was the presence of at least one mutated allele versus the absence of this allele), producing three sets of comparisons: TT+CT vs. CC (mutated T allele), GG +AG vs. AA

Table 4 Distribution of C1858T, A49G, and C(−318)T genotypes in the study group and control group

SNP	Genotypes	Study group (n=101)	Control group (n=200)
C1858T	CC	74 (73.2%)	147 (73.5%)
	CT	25 (24.8%)	50 (25.0%)
	TT	2 (2.0%)	3 (1.5%)
	p=0.95347		
A49G	AA	43 (42.6%)	81 (40.5%)
	AG	58 (57.4%)	105 (52.5%)
	GG	0 (0.0%)	14 (7.0%)
	p=0.02423		
C(−318)T	CC	79 (78.2%)	151 (75.5%)
	CT	20 (19.8%)	48 (24.0%)
	TT	2 (1.98%)	1 (0.5%)
	p=0.35636		

Table 5 Predisposition to chronic viral hepatitis

SNP	Variable	OR (95% CI)	p*
C1858T	TT+CT vs. CC	0.96 (0.56-1.67)	0.895
	TT vs. CT+CC	1.34 (0.22-8.26)	0.749
A49G	GG+AG vs. AA	0.94 (0.57-1.53)	0.799
	GG vs. AG+AA	—	—
C(−318)T	TT+CT vs. CC	0.87 (0.49-1.54)	0.630
	TT vs. CT+CC	3.82 (0.34-43.3)	0.278

*gender-adjusted p values.

Table 6 Distribution of genotypes in patients with AT and in patients without thyroid impairment

SNP	Genotypes	AT (n=18)	No thyroid impairment (n=62)
C1858T	CC	12 (66.7%)	49 (79.0%)
	CT	6 (33.3%)	12 (19.4%)
	TT	0 (0.0%)	1 (1.6%)
	p=0.41034		
A49G	AA	7 (38.9%)	26 (41.9%)
	AG	11 (61.1%)	36 (58.1%)
	GG	0 (0.0%)	0 (0.0%)
	p=0.81720		
C(−318)T	CC	14 (77.8%)	47 (75.8%)
	CT	4 (22.2%)	13 (21.0%)
	TT	0 (0.0%)	2 (3.2%)
	p=0.74153		

(mutated G allele), and TT+CT vs. CC (mutated T allele) for C1858T, A49Gm and C(−318)T polymorphisms, respectively. Recessive inheritance (the presence of both mutated alleles was necessary) resulting in the following genotypes: TT vs. CT+CC, GG vs. AG+AA, and TT vs. CT+CC for C1858T, A49G, and (C-318T) polymorphisms, respectively, was also analyzed. We found that the carriers of mutated alleles (TT+CT C1858T, GG +AG A49G, and TT+CT C(−318t)) did not have a higher predisposition to autoimmune thyroiditis (AT) as compared to homozygotes of dominant mode. We also tried to assess the predisposition to AT depending on the genotype possessed, taking into consideration two different modes of inheritance and patient's gender. However, since AT group lacked homozygotes of mutated alleles: TT C1858T, GG A49G, and TT C(−318)T, the evaluation of predisposition to AT in the carriers of these genotypes as compared to the carriers of wild-type alleles (recessive mode) was not feasible in our study. Kucharska et al. reports that among 68 HT patients, G allele and homozygotes with rare G/G allele were significantly more frequent. These authors found no significant difference in the occurrence of homozygotes with common A/A allele

Table 7 Predisposition to AT during IFN-α therapy

SNP	Variable	OR (95% CI)	p*
C1858T	TT+CT vs. CC	1.92 (0.57-6.44)	0.282
	TT vs. CT+CC	—	—
A49G	GG+AG vs. AA	1.26 (0.41-3.89)	0.678
	GG vs. AG+AA	—	—
C(−318)T	TT+CT vs. CC	1.02 (0.27-3.83)	0.971
	TT vs. CT+CC	—	—

*gender-adjusted p values.

and heterozygotes [9]. Kinjo et al. demonstrated that in a group of 144 patients with G-B disease, the frequency of AA, AG, and GG genotypes at position 49 of CTLA-4 gene was significantly higher than in the control group [28]. The frequency of GG genotype was significantly greater, while the frequency of AA genotype was significantly lower in patients with G-B disease as compared to the control. In 1997, Witas et al. analyzed the occurrence of polymorphic alleles of CTLA-4 gene in Polish population of 122 children and found C(−318)T polymorphism in 20.5% of analyzed subjects. Their data indicates that the frequency of T allele was 0.107 and estimated occurrence of heterozygotes 19.1% [33]. The study conducted in Germany by Deichmann et al. in a group of 239 patients with G-B disease demonstrated that C(−318)T polymorphism was found in 13.4% of patients, and heterozygotes were detected in 23.2% of cases [17]. The studies of genetic predisposition to autoimmune endocrine diseases, including autoimmune thyroiditis, focus on the search for polymorphisms within candidate genes responsible for autoimmune diseases. In Hashimoto's autoimmune thyroiditis, apart from known genetic liability related to the presence of histocompatibility antigens class II DR 3, 4 and 5, and the recognized effect of such environmental factors as the excess of iodine or medications (e.g. interferon), the presence of polymorphisms within CTLA-4 gene and PTPN22 gene must also be taken into account. The results of studies conducted to date are inconclusive; therefore, further research is necessary to explain the etiopathogenesis of autoimmune thyroid diseases.

Conclusions

No association was found between the occurrence of autoimmune thyroiditis during interferon therapy and the presence of polymorphisms within CTLA-4 C(−318) T gene in the promoter region and A49G in exon 1, as well as C1858T transition of PTPN22 gene.

Competing interests
The authors declare that they have no competing interests.

Authors' contributions
JK and AS conceived of the study, participated in its design and coordination, and helped to draft the manuscript. WU, GK, ESP and EAM conceived of the study and helped to draft the manuscript. MK carried out the molecular genetic studies and participated in the design and coordination of the study. All authors read and approved the final manuscript.

Author details
[1]Department of Endocrinology, Metabolic Diseases and Internal Diseases, Pomeranian Medical University, Szczecin, Poland. [2]Department of Infectious Diseases and Hepatology, Pomeranian Medical University, Szczecin, Poland. [3]Institute of Clinical Biochemistry and Molecular Diagnostics, Pomeranian Medical University, Szczecin, Poland.

Association between genetic mutations and the development of autoimmune thyroiditis in patients...

115

References

1. Syrenicz A, Syrenicz M: **Hyperthyroidism.** In *Endocrinology in clinical practice.* Edited by Syrenicz A. Szczecin: Pomeranian Medical University; 2011:170–181.

2. Ciechanowicz A, Kokot F: *Genetyka molekularna w chorobach wewnętrznych.* Warszawa: PZWL; 2009.

3. Dittmar M, Kahaly GJ: **Immunoregulatory and susceptibility genes in thyroid and polyglandular autoimmunity.** *Thyroid* 2005, **15:**239–250.

4. Donner H, Braun J, Seidl C, Rau H, Finke R, Ventz M, Walfish PG, Usadel KH, Badenhoop K: **Codon 17 polymorphism of the cytotoxic T lymphocyte antigen 4 gene in Hashimoto's thyroiditis and Addison's diseases.** *J Clin Endocrinol Metab* 1997, **82:**4130–4132.

5. Kavvoura FK, Akamizu T, Awata T, Ban Y, Chistiakov DA, Frydecka I, Ghaderi A, Gough SC, Hiromatsu Y, Ploski R, Wang PW, Ban Y, Bednarczuk T, Chistiakova EI, Chojm M, Heward JM, Hiratani H, Juo SH, Karabon L, Katayama S, Kurihara S, Liu RT, Miyake I, Omrani GH, Pawlak E, Taniyama M, Tozaki T, Ioannidis JP: **Cytotoxic T-lymphocyte associated antigen 4 gene polymorphism and autoimmune thyroid disease: a meta-analysis.** *J Clin Endocrinol Metab* 2007, **92:**3162–3170.

6. Vaidya B, Kendall-Taylor P, Pearce SHS: **The genetics of autoimmune thyroid disease.** *J Clin Endocrinol Metab* 2002, **87:**5385–5397.

7. Yeşilkaya E, Koç A, Bideci A, Camurdan O, Boyraz M, Erkal O, Ergun MA, Cinaz P: **CTLA-4 gene polymorphism in children and adolescents with autoimmune thyroid diseases.** *Genet Test* 2008, **12:**461–464.

8. Bradley JR, Johnson DR, Pober BR: *Genetyka medyczna.* Warszawa: PZWL; 2009.

9. Kucharska AM, Wiśniewska A, Rymkiewicz-Kluczyńska B: **Występowanie polimorfizmu w pozycji 49 eksonie 1 genu CTLA-4 u dzieci z chorobą Hashimoto.** *Endokrynol Diabetol Chor Przemiany Materii Wieku Rozw* 2006, **12:**163–166.

10. Suwalska K, Tutak A, Frydecka I: **Polimorfizm genu kodującego antygen supresorowy - ryzyko autoimmunizacji.** *Postępy Biologii Komórki* 2003, **30:**549–562.

11. Yang J, Qin Q, Yan N, Zhu YF, Li C, Yang XJ, Wang X, Pandey M, Hou P, Zhang JA: **CD40 C/T(−1) and CTLA-4 A/G(49) SNPs are associated with autoimmune thyroid diseases in the Chinese population.** *Endocrine* 2012, **41:**111–115.

12. Kosmaczewska A, Ciszak L, Boćko D, Frydecka I: **Expression and functional significance of CTLA-4, a negative regulator of T cell activation.** *Arch Immunol Ther Exp (Warsz)* 2001, **49:**39–46.

13. Benhatchi K, Jochmanová I, Habalová V, Wagnerová H, Lazúrová I: **CTLA-4 exon A49G polymorphism in Slovak patients with rheumatoid arthritis and Hashimoto thyroiditis - results and the review of the literature.** *Clin Rheumatol* 2011, **30:**1319–1324.

14. Kucharska AM, Górska E, Popka K, Wąsik M, Rymkiewicz-Kluczyńska B: **Ekspresja powierzchniowa CD 152(CTLA-4) na limfocytach krwi obwodowej u dzieci z chorobą Hashimoto.** *Endokrynol Diabetol Chor Przemiany Materii Wieku Rozw* 2006, **12:**167–170.

15. Bottini N, Musumeci L, Alonso A, Rahmouni S, Nika K, Rostamkhani M, MacMurray J, Meloni GF, Lucarelli P, Pellecchia M, Eisenbarth GS, Comings D, Mustelin T: **A functional variant of lymphoid tyrosine phosphatase is associated with type I diabetes.** *Nat Genet* 2004, **36:**337–338.

16. Lee YH, Rho YH, Choi SJ, Ji JD, Song GG, Nath SK, Harley JB: **The PTPN22 C1858T functional polymorphism and autoimmune diseases – a meta-analysis.** *Rheumatology (Oxford)* 2007, **46:**49–56.

17. Deichmann K, Heinzmann A, Brüggenolte E, Forster J, Kuehr J: **An Mse I RELP in the human CTLA-4 promotor.** *Biochem Biophys Res Commun* 1996, **225:**817–818.

18. Skórka A: **Cukrzyca typu 1 – aspekty genetyczne. Klinika Pediatryczna.** *Szkoła Pediatrii* 2009, **12:**5131–5134.

19. Eschler DC, Hasham A, Tomer Y: **Cutting edge: the etiology of autoimmune thyroid diseases.** *Clin Rev Allerg Immunol* 2011, **41:**190–197.

20. Yu X, Sun JP, He Y, Guo X, Liu S, Zhou B, Hudmon A, Zhang ZY: **Structure, inhibitor, and regulatory mechanism of Lyp, a lymphoid-specific tyrosine phosphatase implicated in autoimmune diseases.** *Proc Natl Acad Sci USA* 2007, **104:**19767–19772.

21. Krupińska J, Wawrzynowicz-Syczewska M, Urbanowicz W, Pobłocki J, Syrenicz A: **The influence of interferon alpha on the induction of autoimmune thyroiditis in patients treated for chronic viral hepatitis type C.** *Endokrynol Pol* 2011, **62:**517–522.

22. Wojewoda E: **Czynniki genetyczne w patogenezie i współwystępowaniu chorób autoimmunologicznych, ze szczególnym uwzględnieniem chorób reumatycznych wieku dziecięcego.** *Reumatologia* 2009, **47:**39–43.

23. Pastuszak-Lewandowska D, Sewerynek E, Domańska D, Gładyś A, Skrzypczak R, Brzezińska E: **Basic research CTLA-4 gene polymorphism and their influence on predisposition to autoimmune thyroid diseases (Graves' disease and Hashimoto's thyroiditis).** *Arch Med Sci* 2012, **3:**415–421.

24. Kucharska AM, Rogozińska I, Pyrżak B, Miszkurka G, Wiśniewska A: **Polimorfizm A/G w pozycji 49 eksonu 1 genu CTLA-4 u dzieci z cukrzycą typu 1 – doniesienie wstepne.** *Endokrynologia Pediatryczna* 2009, **8:**27–32.

25. Zalatel K: **Determinants of thyroid autoantibody production in Hashimoto's thyroiditis.** *Expert Rev Clin Immunol* 2007, **3:**217–222.

26. Bicek A, Zaletel K, Gaberscek S, Pirnat E, Krhin B, Stopar TG, Hojker S: **49A/G and CT60 polymorphisms of the cytotoxic T-lymphocyte-associated antigen 4 gene associated with autoimmune thyroid disease.** *Hum Immunol* 2009, **70:**820–824.

27. Kula D, Stęchły D, Jurecka-Lubieniecka B, Hasse-Lazar K, Krawczyk A, Szpak S, Jarząb M, Pawelczak A, Gubała E: **Predyspozycja genetyczna do choroby Hashimoto w populacji polskiej:związek z polimorfizmem genów TNF i CTLA-4.** *Endokrynol Pol* 2003, **54:**495–496.

28. Kinjo Y, Takasu N, Komiya I, Tomoyose T, Takara M, Kouki T, Shimajiri Y, Yabiku K, Yoshimura H: **Remission of Graves hyperthyroidism and A/G polymorphism at position 49 in exon 1 of cytotoxic T lymphocyte-associated molecule-4 gene.** *J Clin Endocrinol Metab* 2002, **87:**2593–2596.

29. Roycroft M, Fichna M, McDonald D, Owen K, Zurawek M, Gryczyńska M, Januszkiewicz-Lewandowska D, Fichna P, Cordell H, Donaldson P, Nowak J, Pearce S: **The tryptophan 620 allele of the lymphoid tyrosine phosphatase (PTPN22) gene predisposes to autoimmue Addison's disease.** *Clin Endocrinol (Oxf)* 2009, **70:**358–362.

30. Petrone A, Giorgi G, Galgani A, Alemanno I, Corsello SM, Signore A, Di Mario U, Nisticò L, Cascino I, Buzzetti R: **CT60 single nucleotide polymorphism of the cytotoxic T-lymphocyte-associated antigen-4 gene region is associated with Graves' disease in an Italian population.** *Thyroid* 2005, **15:**232–238.

31. Ban Y, Tozaki T, Taniyama M, Tomita M, Ban Y: **Association of a CTLA-4 3' untranslated region (CT60) single nucleotide polymorphism with autoimmune thyroid disease in the Japanese population.** *Autoimmunity* 2005, **38:**151–153.

32. Chopra IJ, Hershman JM, William M, Pardridge WM, Nicoloff JT: **Thyroid function in nonthyroidal illnesses.** *Ann Intern Med* 1983, **98:**946–957.

33. Witas HW, Różalski M, Młynarski W, Sychowski R, Bodalski J: **Polymorphism of CTLA-4 gene in Polish population.** *Przegl Pediatr* 1997, **27:**246–248.

12

Apoptosis induction by combination of drugs or a conjugated molecule associating non-steroidal anti-inflammatory and nitric oxide donor effects in medullary thyroid cancer models: implication of the tumor suppressor p73

Thierry Ragot[1,2,3], Claire Provost[4], Aurélie Prignon[4], Régis Cohen[5], Michel Lepoivre[6] and Sylvie Lausson[4*]

Abstract

Background: Medullary thyroid cancer (MTC) is a C-cell neoplasm. Surgery remains its main treatment. Promising therapies based on tyrosine kinase inhibitors demand careful patient selection. We previously observed that two non-steroidal anti-inflammatory drugs (NSAID), indomethacin, celecoxib, and nitric oxide (NO) prevented tumor growth in a model of human MTC cell line (TT) in *nude* mice.

Methods: In the present study, we tested the NO donor: glyceryl trinitrate (GTN), at pharmacological dose, alone and in combination with each of the two NSAIDs on TT cells. We also assessed the anti-proliferative potential of NO-indomethacin, an indomethacin molecule chemically conjugated with a NO moiety (NCX 530, Nicox SA) on TT cells and indomethacin/GTN association in rMTC 6–23 cells. The anti-tumoral action of the combined sc. injections of GTN with oral delivery of indomethacin was also studied on subcutaneous TT tumors in *nude* mice. Apoptosis mechanisms were assessed by expression of caspase-3, TAp73α, TAp73α inhibition by siRNA or Annexin V externalisation.

Results: The two NSAIDs and GTN reduced mitotic activity in TT cells versus control (cell number and PCNA protein expression). The combined treatments amplified the anti-tumor effect of single agents in the two tested cell lines and promoted cell death. Moreover, indomethacin/GTN association stopped the growth of established TT tumors in *nude* mice. We observed a significant cleavage of full length PARP, a caspase-3 substrate. The cell death appearance was correlated with a two-fold increase in TAp73α expression, with inhibition of apoptosis after TAp73α siRNA addition, demonstrating its crucial role in apoptosis.

Conclusion: Association of NO with NSAID exhibited amplified anti-tumoral effects on *in vitro* and *in vivo* MTC models by inducing p73-dependent apoptotic cell death.

Keywords: Medullary thyroid carcinoma, Non-steroidal anti-inflammatory drugs, NO-donors, Apoptosis, TT cells, rMTC 6–23 cells

* Correspondence: sylvielausson@aol.com
[4]Sorbonne Universités, UPMC University Paris 06, plateforme LIMP,
Laboratoire d'Imagerie Médicale Positonique, Hôpital Tenon, Paris 75020,
France
Full list of author information is available at the end of the article

Introduction

Medullary thyroid carcinoma (MTC) is a neuroendocrine neoplasm of C cells (for reviews see [1, 2]). This cancer releases large amounts of calcitonin (CT) correlated to tumor size [3]. MTC is sporadic in about 75 % of cases, and patients with sporadic carcinoma are usually diagnosed at late stage. Nowadays, surgical removal of the thyroid with lymph node dissection is the gold standard curative treatment of MTC. Prognostic remains poor since 40 to 60 % of patients are not cured. Current chemo- and radiotherapies are still ineffective. Hereditary germ-line mutations or somatic mutations of the RET proto-oncogene are involved in the carcinogenesis of familial and sporadic MTCs respectively. Several tyrosine kinase inhibitors (TKIs) that are notably RET receptor inhibitors are used and under evaluation for patients with advanced MTC with promising results [2, 4]. Thus TKIs vandetanib or cabozantinib can be used as single agent for first line systemic therapy in selected patients with advanced progressive MTC. But TKIs give only a significant increase of progression-free survival with no effect on death rate [5]. Thus, other or combined curative approaches are necessary to improve MTC treatments in the future.

The anti-tumor potential of non-steroidal anti-inflammatory drugs (NSAIDs) was recognized a few years ago [6–8]. The anti-proliferative effects of NSAIDs can result from the decrease of prostaglandin (PG) synthesis by inhibition of cyclooxygenase (COX) activity but also from anti-tumoral actions independent of PGs and COXs. We have previously demonstrated that the classical NSAID, indomethacin, reduced the development of xenografted TT tumors induced by injection of human MTC TT cells in *nude* mice [9]; indomethacin lowered PGE_2 secretion by TT cells. We also reported that a low dose of the selective COX-2 inhibitor, celecoxib (with less gastro-intestinal side effects than conventional drugs) significantly diminished the growth of TT tumors. This anti-tumor action was independent of PGE_2 and COX-2 [10].

Otherwise, we observed a very strong anti-tumor potential of nitric oxide (NO) on MTCs for two rat cell lines and TT cells [11]. More recently, authors reported that the chemical association of NO donors with a NSAID not only prevented side effects of the NSAID but also was able to amplify its anti-tumor action [12–14]. Elevation of the NO concentration can cause DNA damage, mutation and apoptosis [15]. The tumor suppressor protein p53 is a key player in the DNA damage response and the onset of apoptosis. NO has been shown to activate p53 which promotes pro-apoptotic effects [16]. Two *p53* related genes, *p63* and *p73*, have also been identified more than 15 years after the discovery of *p53* [17, 18]. The human *p73* gene generates two groups of isoforms,

some with a complete transactivation (TA) domain (TAp73) and others exhibiting a truncated TA domain (ΔNp73). Growth suppression or induction of apoptosis can be accomplished by the TAp73 isoforms. Studies have shown that p73 is required for apoptosis induction in response to DNA damage by chemotherapeutic drugs such as cis-platin [19]. Thus, p53 and p73 could be interesting targets to study in MTC chemotherapies: *p53* is not mutated in this cancer; in contrast, p73 was never studied in C cell but mutations in the *p73* gene are rare in cancer patients. p73 is not only involved in tumor suppression but has important functions in neural cells and it also could be well expressed in neuroendocrine C cells.

In the present study, we compared the anti-proliferative actions of a pharmacological dose of the NO-donor, glyceryl trinitrate (GTN) or Trinitrine, a drug used in cardiology, of two NSAID, indomethacin and celecoxib, of the combinations of one NSAID with GTN, and finally, of a chemically conjugated molecule, NO-indomethacin (NCX 530) from Nicox SA, an indomethacin molecule conjugated with a NO donor group. We also studied the implications of cell death mediators p53 and p73 in TT cells. The NSAID doses used in these cultures were those reproducing the anti-tumoral benefits with low side effects we have previously described *in vivo*. Moreover, we assessed the anti-proliferative effect of the indomethecin/GTN association in another MTC cell line, rMTC 6–23 and studied the anti-tumoral action of a combined administration of GTN in sc. injections with oral delivery of indomethacin on xenografted TT tumors.

Materials and methods

Materials

Celecoxib was a generous gift from Pfizer (USA). Indomethacin was purchased from Cayman Chemical (Ann Arbor, MI). The NO-donor glyceryl trinitrate (GTN) was obtained from Merck (Lyon, France). The conjugated molecule NO-indomethacin (NCX 530) was a gift from Nicox SA (Sophia Antipolis, France). The TT and rMTC 6–23 cell lines were from the American Type Culture Collection (Rockville, MD). Primary antibodies to p73 (IMG 313A, Imgenex, A300-126A, Bethyl Laboratories), p53 (sc 6243, Santa Cruz Biotechnology), PCNA (Santa Cruz Biotechnology), PARP-1 (c-2-10, Calbiochem) and α-tubulin (T9026, Sigma) were used for western blots. Detections were performed with fluorescent Alexa Fluor 680-conjugated anti-mouse (A 21057, Invitrogen/Molecular Probes) or IRDye 800CW-anti-rabbit (926–32211, LI-COR Biosciences) IgG. Rabbit anti-caspase-3 antibody (ab52293, Abcam), Starr Trek Universal detection kit (Biocare Medical/Eurobio) and AEC Peroxidase Substrate kit (Vector Laboratories/Eurobio) were used for the immunohistochemistry of TT tumor slides.

Cell culture

TT cells were cultured in RPMI 1640 medium (Invitrogen, Cergy-Pontoise, France) supplemented with 2 mM L-glutamine, 25 mM HEPES, 10 % heat-inactivated fetal calf serum (FCS), 100 U/mL penicillin and 100 µg/mL streptomycin (Invitrogen). RMTC 6–23 cells were cultured in Dulbecco's Modified Eagle's medium (DMEM) Gluta-MAX™ (Life Technologies, Cergy-Pontoise, France) supplemented with 1 % of Non-Essential Amino Acids (Life Technologies) and –5 % heat-inactivated FCS. To determine the anti-proliferative effects of the NSAID/GTN combinations or NCX 530, TT or rMTC 6–23 cells were seeded out in 6-well-plates at a density of 2 to 3×10^5 cells per well, respectively. Three days later, NSAIDs and/or GTN were added (or not, or vehicles only, for the controls) to cell culture medium. Medium was changed every two days (TT cells) or every 36 h (rMTC 6–23 cells). After various periods of treatment, cells were dissociated 5 min with trypsin-EDTA or TrypLE™ Express (Life Technologies) for TT or rMTC 6–23 cells, respectively. Cells were counted with an hemocytometer (Trypan Blue exclusion) and/or using counting slides with an automated cell counter (TC20™ Bio-Rad, Marnes-la-Coquette, France). NSAIDs were dissolved in DMSO and GTN in ethanol. The following doses were used: celecoxib 25 µM, indomethacin 100 or 200 µM, GTN 100 µM, and NCX 530, 100 and 200 µM for short term experiments, and 150 µM for long term experiments. Controls were performed in the presence of drug vehicles (DMSO and ethanol) at the same concentrations as in experimental wells (DMSO ≤ 0.4 % and ethanol = 0.2 %). For western blot analyses, cells were seeded out in 6-well plates at a density of 10^6 cells per well. Treatments began 3 days later. In proliferation and apoptosis detection experiments, triplicates were performed for each category; in experiments for immunoblotting analyses, duplicates were used.

Apoptosis detection

After cell counts, the cell suspensions were adjusted to 10^6 cells/ml in microfuge tubes. An Annexin V-FITC Apoptosis Detection kit (Calbiochem, Merck Millipore, Darmstadt, Germany), was used to quantify apoptosis/necrosis. The "Rapid Annexin V binding" protocol provided by the suppliers was followed. After incubation with Annexin V-FITC and addition of Propidium Iodide, fluorescence was immediately analyzed by flow cytometry (BD Accuri™ C6 Flow Cytometer, BD Biosciences) using 530/30 and 670 LP emission filters preventing spillover. Unlabeled samples were used to adjust the gates.

Immunoblotting analyses

Immunoblots were performed as described in Tebbi et al. [20]. After harvest, cells were washed twice in ice-cold phosphate buffered saline (PBS). Crude cell extracts were prepared in a 50 mM Tris–HCl lysis buffer, pH 7.4, supplemented with 150 mM NaCl, 1 % Triton X-100, 0.5 % sodium deoxycholate, 1 mM EDTA, 1 mM DTT and protease inhibitors including 1 mM Pefablock (Merck/Calbiochem). Soluble proteins (30 µg per lane) were separated by SDS-PAGE using a 10 %-acrylamide gel and transferred onto nitrocellulose membranes. These ones were blocked in 3 % skimmed milk. After overnight incubation at 4 °C with primary antibodies and four washes in PBS/Tween, membranes were incubated for 1 h with fluorescent dye-conjugated secondary antibodies. After washing, the infrared fluorescent signals at 680 and 800 nm were quantified with an Odyssey scanner (LI-COR Biosciences). Protein contents were standardized using α-tubulin band density.

Transfections with TAp73 siRNA

SiRNA sequences were reported and validated in Guittet et al. [21]. Cells were transfected with TAp73 Select siRNA (Ambion) or control siRNA (MWG) using Interferin transfection reagent (Polyplus Transfection). TT cells were plated in 6-well plates and grown to approximately 30-50 % confluency. Before transfection, culture medium was replaced by the same medium without antibiotics (4 mL per well). Interferin (corresponding to 15 µL per well) was incubated with siRNA for 10 min in antibiotic-free medium. Then, the mixture was added dropwise to wells, resulting in a siRNA concentration of 30 nM. We have previously verified that this method led to 80 % reduction of TAp73α expression, 3 days after mixture addition. Cells were maintained in the transfection medium for 16 h. They were then cultured in usual medium with GTN (100 µM) and celecoxib (25 µM) treatment or with DMSO and ethanol (control wells) during 2 days and 8 h.

In vivo experiment

5×10^6 TT cells were inoculated subcutaneously (sc) on the back of each *nude* mouse. When tumors became palpable, their diameters were regularly measured with a caliper and tumor volume (mm^3) was calculated using the following formula: (the shortest diameter)^2 × (the longest diameter) × 0.5. When the mean volume of tumors reached about 70 mm^3, animals were randomly divided into three groups: one control group (5) and two treated groups, one receiving sc injections of Nitronal each two days, (0.1 mg GTN/20 g of body weight during 6 days, then 0.15 mg, $n = 5$), the other group receiving the same doses of Nitronal with indomethacin (2 mg/day/kg of body weight in drinking water, $n = 4$). Animal manipulations were performed according to the recommendations of the French Ethical Committee and under the supervision of authorized investigators.

Mice were sacrificed at day 14 and tumors were removed and weighted. Tumors were divided in two parts. One part of the tumor was fixed in 4 % paraformaldehyde during 96 h and embedded in paraffin. Some tumor slides, chosen in three different levels (100 μm apart), were colored with hematotoxylin-phloxine-saffron (HPS) stain. The cavity area of colored slides was measured by ImageJ software at three levels in each tumor. For caspase-3 immunohistochemistry, we followed a method similar to that described in Bressenot et al. [22].

Statistical analyses

All results were analysed using ANOVA. Differences between two means were tested by the Fisher tests. Data are represented as means ± SEM. For each determination, two or three independent experiments were performed. The significance level was set at $P < 0.05$. For the proliferation experiments, we assessed the differences between treated cells and control cells at day 4 (D4). We also tested cell number reductions induced by NO-NSAID bi-therapies at D4 and D8 versus D0. For the immunoblotting analyses, we tested the differences between treated and control cells at D1 and D3. Moreover, for each NSAID/GTN combination (proliferation experiments at D4 and p73 expression at D3), we performed a two-factor variance analysis to assess the significance of NSAID or GTN effects individually and to test the presence of a NSAID/GTN interaction.

In the annexin V studies, a significant linear regression was obtained between apoptotic cell percentages and total number of cells, in controls: the apoptotic cell percentage increases when cell density grows. Thus, we compared the apoptotic cell percentage in each treated culture with a percentage (calculated with the regression) in a control containing the same total number of cells than the treated culture. For the *in vivo* experiment, we assessed the tumor volume growth and the mean differences between treatments by the two-factor analysis (time factor as repeated measures and treatment factor).

Results

Anti-proliferative effects of GTN, NSAID/GTN combinations and NO-indomethacin on TT cells

As previously reported, we observed that the NSAIDs celecoxib and indomethacin prevented the proliferation of TT cells: the cell number in treated samples was reduced by about 30 % at D2 and D4 versus controls (Fig. 1a and b). Moreover, we established that a NO-donor, GTN (100 μM), had a similar effect: the viable cell number was decreased by about 30 % versus controls (Fig. 1a and b). We revealed significant effects of each NSAID alone and GTN alone at D4. Interestingly, the combinations of one NSAID with GTN strongly

increased the anti-tumoral action seen for each individual molecule at D4 (cell number diminution of 50 to 60 % versus controls). Significant reductions were observed between D0 and D4, $P < 0.05$, after celecoxib/GTN incubation and $P < 0.01$, after indomethacin-GTN treatment. The two-factor analysis of variance did not reveal an interaction between each NSAID and GTN; this result suggests the presence of additive effects. NO-indomethacin, NCX530, had the same anti-tumor action than the GTN and indomethacin incubation. The reduction of cell population treated with NCX 530 versus control was dose-dependent (Fig. 1c).

Continuous anti-tumor action of NSAID/GTN combinations and NO-indomethacin after long-time administration on TT cells

When cells were treated with NO-NSAID combinations until D8, the cell number reduction was prolonged from D4 to D8: $P < 0.05$ for indomethacin/GTN, $P < 0.01$ for celecoxib/GTN and NO-indomethacin alone (Fig. 2a). In another experiment, TT cells were incubated with NSAID/GTN combinations or NO-indomethacin during 7 days then, cultured in drug-free medium until D12. Under these conditions, no growth rebound was observed between D7 to D12 (Fig. 2b). Thus, the anti-tumoral action was amplified when treatments were prolonged and this beneficial effect was maintained after treatment cessation.

NSAIDs, GTN and NSAID/GTN bi-therapies reduce mitotic proliferation of TT cells. NSAID/GTN combined treatments only lead to cell death

PCNA is a nuclear antigen expressed during cell mitotic division. The effects of drug exposition on PCNA expression were investigated by western blot analysis. Figure 3a shows a significant decrease in PCNA levels in all 3-day-treated cells versus controls: celecoxib alone, $P < 0.0001$, indomethacin alone, $P < 0.0001$, GTN alone, $P < 0.0001$, NSAID/GTN combinations, $P < 0.0001$ (NCX 530, $P < 0.01$). Thus, all these treatments reduced the levels of TT cell mitotic divisions.

PARP is a substrate of caspase-3, cleaved early during cell apoptosis. Western blot analyses revealed that PARP was cleaved in TT cells incubated with drug combinations (or NO-indomethacin alone, data not shown) during 3 days: the levels of PARP full-length polypeptide were significantly decreased ($P < 0.05$ versus control cells) for all bi-therapies, (Fig. 3b). No effect appeared after one day of treatment (data not shown). Thus, the reduction of viable cell numbers receiving bi-therapies after D2 also resulted from apoptotic cell death induction.

Increased expression of the tumor suppressors p53 and p73

We investigated the expression of the tumor suppressors p53 and p73 in TT cells at basal levels and in response

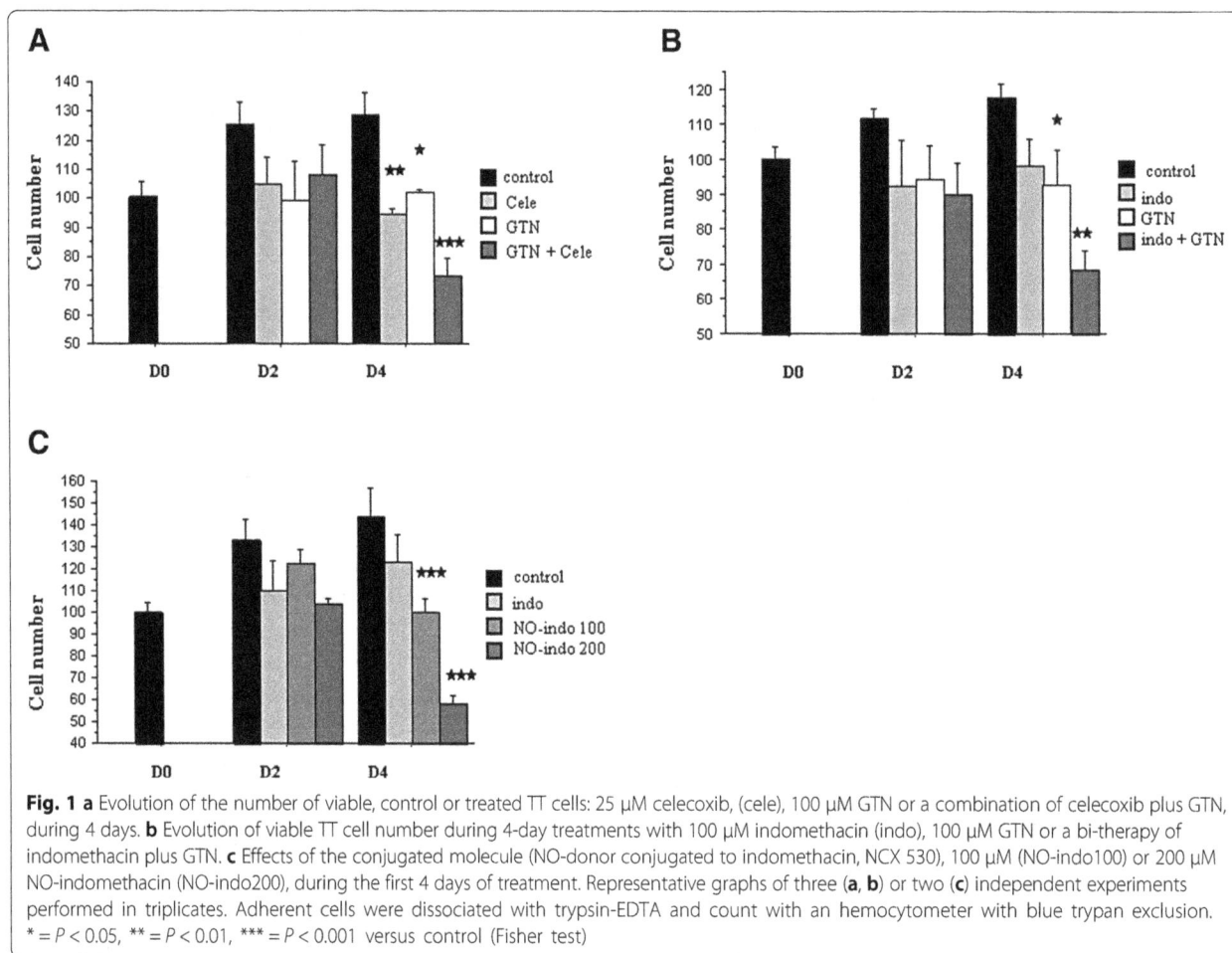

Fig. 1 a Evolution of the number of viable, control or treated TT cells: 25 µM celecoxib, (cele), 100 µM GTN or a combination of celecoxib plus GTN, during 4 days. **b** Evolution of viable TT cell number during 4-day treatments with 100 µM indomethacin (indo), 100 µM GTN or a bi-therapy of indomethacin plus GTN. **c** Effects of the conjugated molecule (NO-donor conjugated to indomethacin, NCX 530), 100 µM (NO-indo100) or 200 µM NO-indomethacin (NO-indo200), during the first 4 days of treatment. Representative graphs of three (**a**, **b**) or two (**c**) independent experiments performed in triplicates. Adherent cells were dissociated with trypsin-EDTA and count with an hemocytometer with blue trypan exclusion. * $= P < 0.05$, ** $= P < 0.01$, *** $= P < 0.001$ versus control (Fisher test)

to the different treatments by NSAIDs and NO. We found that this cell line expressed p53 and TAp73α at basal levels. ΔNp73 was not detected in control and treated TT cells. No change in p53 and p73 expressions was observed in 1-day treated cells (data not shown). Indomethacin, indomethacin plus GTN, and NO-indomethacin led to comparable increases in p53 levels at D3 while celecoxib and GTN had no effect (Fig. 3c).

In contrast, TAp73α expression increased by a factor two after 3-day NSAID/GTN combined treatments (Fig. 3d) or incubation with NO-indomethacin alone. These elevations were correlated with a reduction in PARP levels and TT cell number decrease between D2 and D4. The two-factor analysis of variance showed significant 50 %-increases of TAp73 level after 3-day treatments with NSAID alone or GTN alone: in the experiments with indomethacin plus GTN, $P = 0.05$ for indomethacin factor, $P = 0.01$ for GTN factor; in the experiment with celecoxib plus GTN, $P < 0.05$ for celecoxib and for GTN. No significant interaction between NSAIDs and GTN was revealed. Thus, additive effects lead to the strongest increases in TAp73 expression after 3-day combined treatments.

p73 siRNA transfection
Celecoxib/GTN combination induced a strong and significant increase of TAp73 expression in TT cells, after 2 days and 8 h of treatment ($P < 0.01$, Fig. 4a and b). Transfection of siRNA targeting TAp73 isoforms before this treatment, led to a significantly lower level of TAp73 (around minus 50 %, $P = 0.05$). We also observed a decrease of PARP heavy chain expression after the NSAID/GTN incubation ($P < 0.05$, Fig. 4a and c), while TAp73 siRNA suppressed this phenomenon. Thus, as suggested by the previously described correlation, the strong increase in p73 level must be responsible for PARP cleavage and cell apoptosis.

Confirmation of anti-proliferative effect of the indomethacin/GTN association on rMTC 6–23 cell cultures
Anti-proliferative actions of NO and indomethacin were also assessed by incubations with indomethacin alone (200 µM), GTN (100 µM) alone, or combinations of the two drugs in a second MTC cell line (Fig. 5). As observed in TT cells, indomethacine or GTN alone slowed the growth of rMTC 6–23 cell cultures; the combination amplified the anti-proliferative effect of each

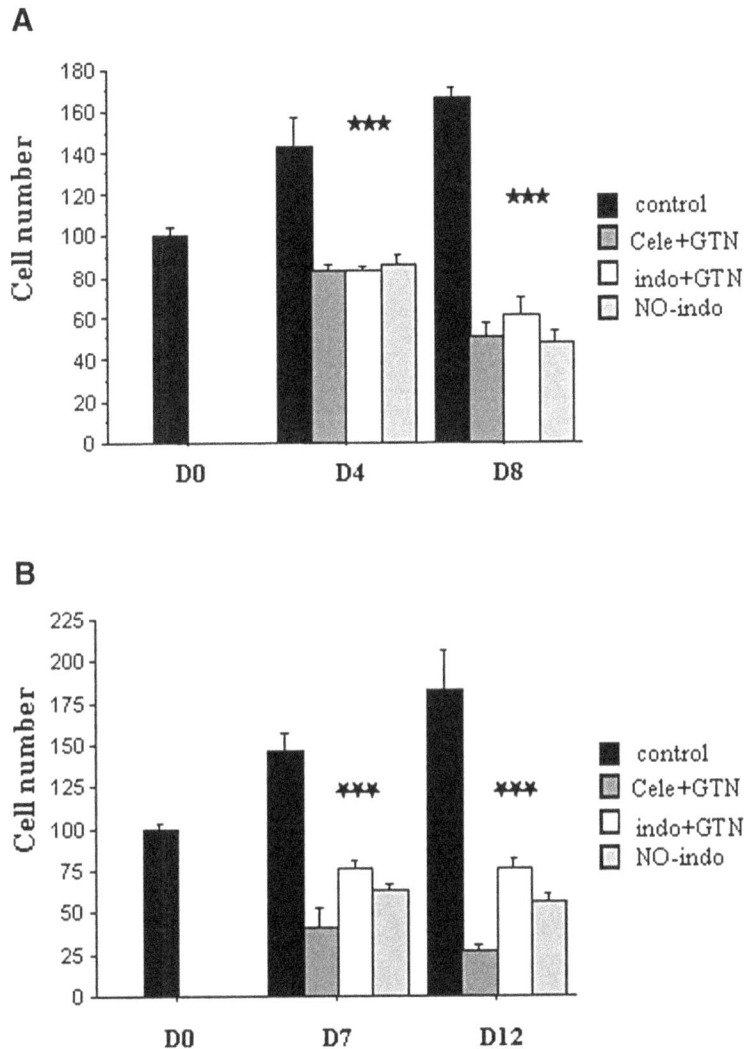

Fig. 2 a Evolution of viable TT cell number in control wells and in wells treated by NSAID/GTN combination: 25 µM celecoxib plus 100 µM GTN (cele + GTN), or 100 µM indomethacin plus 100 µM GTN (indo + GTN), or 150 µM NCX 530 (NO-indo), during 8 days. **b** Evolution of viable TT cell populations after cessation of treatments with NSAID/GTN bi-therapies or NCX 530 (25 µM celecoxib, 100 µM indomethacin, 100 µM GTN or 150 µM NCX 530). Representative graphs of two independent experiments performed in triplicates. Adherent cells were dissociated with trypsin-EDTA and count with a hemocytometer. *** = $P < 0.001$ versus control for each treatment (Fisher tests)

drug ($P < 0.01$ versus indomethacin alone, $P < 0.0001$ versus GTN alone, at D6) and even reduced the cell number at D6 versus D0 ($P < 0.05$). The apoptosis percentage was low, about 5 % in controls according to Annexin V staining and FACS analysis. Indomethacin did not produced significant change in apoptosis level versus control while GTN alone induced only a low elevation (145 %, $P < 0.05$) but the combination of both led to a stronger increase (308 %, $P < 0.001$), at D6. This ampification was significant ($P < 0.01$, combined treatment versus GTN incubation). Thus, also in this cell line, the strong anti-proliferative action of indomethacin/GTN association resulted from the promotion of apoptotic cell death.

Anti-tumoral action of combined administration of GTN plus indomethacin on established subcutaneous TT tumors in *nude* mice

Next, the *in vivo* activity of GTN alone or in combination with indomethacin was determined in *nude* mice. Figure 6 illustrated the effect of treatments on TT xenograft volumes. Subcutaneous injections of GTN did not significantly modified the growth of the subcutaneous tumors while the bi-therapy first slowed it down and then, stopped it from D7 to D12 (global analyses showed a significant effect of the bi-therapy versus control, $P < 0.0001$ and a significant effect of the combination versus GTN alone group, $P < 0.05$). Action on tumor weights at D14

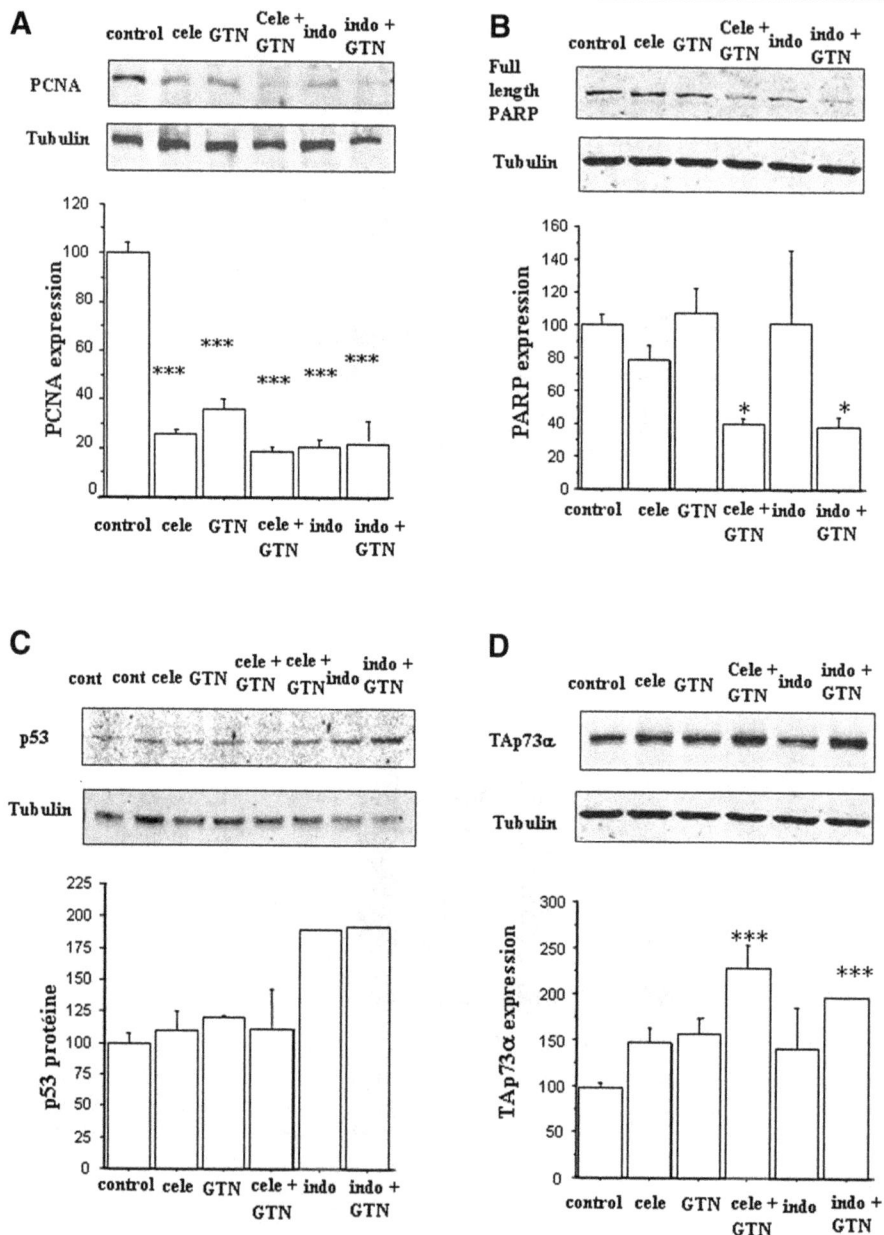

Figure 3 Expression of various proteins in TT cells after 3 days of exposition to 25 µM celecoxib (cele), 100 µM indomethacin (indo), 100 µM GTN or NSAID/GTN combinations. **a** PCNA protein. For each category, $n = 6$ to 3. **b** PARP heavy chain. For each category, $n = 4$ to 3. **c** Tumor suppressor p53. For each category, $n = 4$ to 2. **d** TAp73α. For each category, $n = 7$ to 4. Graphs obtained from associated results of two experiments on TT cells. Proteins from TT cell lysates were separated by SDS-PAGE using 10 % acrylamide gel and transferred onto nitro cellulose membranes. Immunoblots were probed with specific antibodies and a α-tubulin (internal control) antibody. $* = P < 0.05$, $*** = P < 0.001$ versus control (Fisher tests)

was strictly comparable to effect on tumor volumes at D12 (data not shown).

A HPS coloration of slides showed that control TT tumors were rather only composed of tumoral tissue. The GTN-treated tumors had the same appearance. On the contrary, numerous spaces empty of cancerous cells were visualized in tumors treated by the drug combination. The

cavity area represented 19 ± 2.8 % of the total tumor surface. In agreement with these observations, we found numerous cleaved caspase-3 stained cells in these tumors indicating that the combination led to cell death, probably by apoptosis. Such immunostaining observations were rare in the GTN-treated and control groups. The tumor growth arrest with formation of cavities and presence of

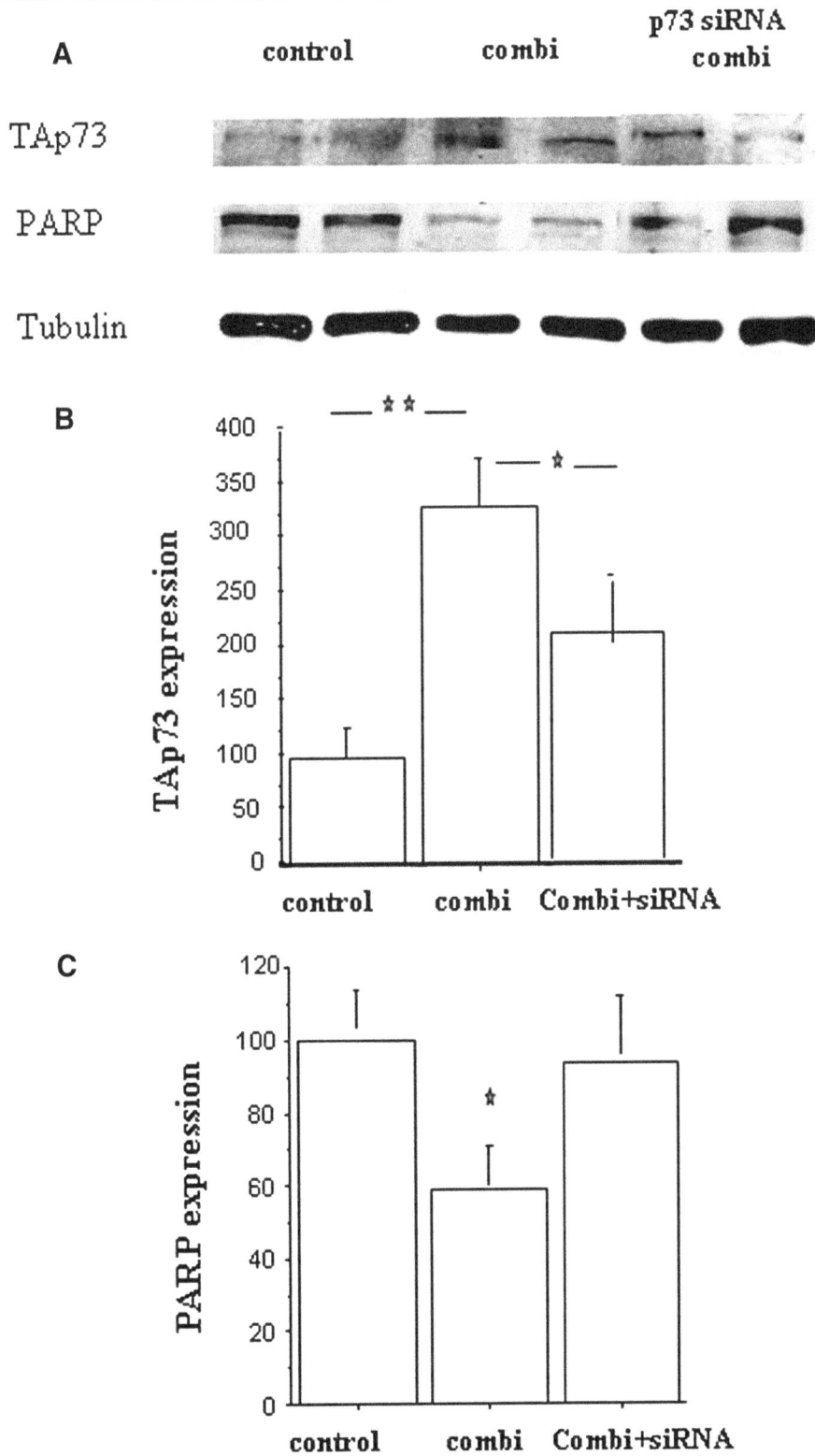

Fig. 4 a Effect of p73 siRNA pre-treatment on TAp73 and PARP expressions in TT cells receiving 25 µM celecoxib plus 100 µM GTN (combi) during 2 days and 8 h. **b** Effect of p73 siRNA pre-treatment on TAp73 expression in the same TT cells. **c** Effect of p73 siRNA pre-treatment on full length PARP expression in these cells. Graphs obtained from associated results of two experiments on TT cells. For each category, $n = 6$ to 4. Proteins from TT cell lysates were separated by SDS-PAGE using 10 % acrylamide gel and transferred onto nitro cellulose membranes. Immunoblots were probed with specific antibody and a α-tubulin (internal control) antibody. $* = P < 0.05$, $** = P < 0.01$ (Fisher tests)

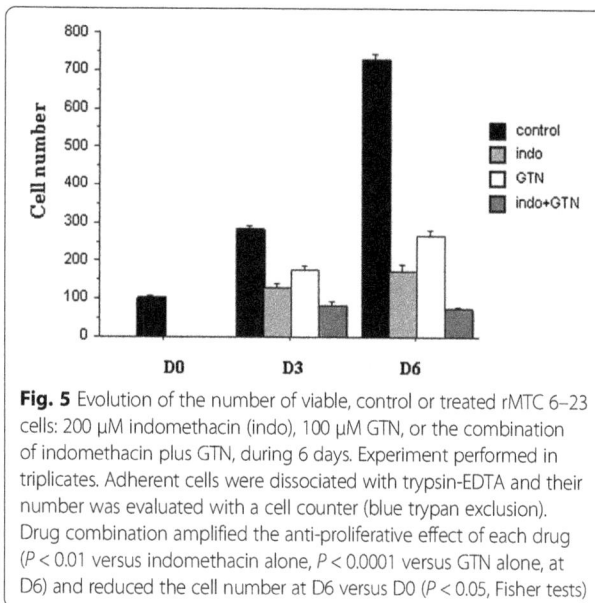

Fig. 5 Evolution of the number of viable, control or treated rMTC 6–23 cells: 200 µM indomethacin (indo), 100 µM GTN, or the combination of indomethacin plus GTN, during 6 days. Experiment performed in triplicates. Adherent cells were dissociated with trypsin-EDTA and their number was evaluated with a cell counter (blue trypan exclusion). Drug combination amplified the anti-proliferative effect of each drug ($P < 0.01$ versus indomethacin alone, $P < 0.0001$ versus GTN alone, at D6) and reduced the cell number at D6 versus D0 ($P < 0.05$, Fisher tests)

apoptotic cells suggested that the combined treatment reduced the cancer extension after D7 while GTN alone had no significant effect.

Discussion

In the present study we demonstrated the anti-proliferative value of NO donor plus NSAIDs on a human MTC cell line. The bi-therapies, celecoxib/GTN, indomethacin/GTN and NO-indomethacin amplified the anti-proliferative effects of each drug alone against TT cells. Indomethacin/GTN combination had the same action on the growth of rMTC 6–23 cells. Since the enhanced cytotoxicity of bi-therapies was correlated with increased expression of TAp73 in TT cells, we proposed that TAp73 might be implicated in the cytotoxic mechanism. In support of this hypothesis, knocking

down TAp73 reduced PARP cleavage, a marker of apoptotic cell death. Interestingly, the indomethacin/GTN combination also produced a reduction of tumoral tissue extension and induced cell death, in the *in vivo* model. We have previously reported that the administration of indomethacin alone at the same dose only reduced TT xenograft growth [9].

It has been widely shown that NSAIDs and aspirin prevented the growth of numerous cancers and notably human cancers. The anti-tumor and pro-apoptotic potentials of NO have often been reported. During the last few years, authors have tested various conjugated molecules associating a NO-donor with a non-selective COX inhibitor, *i.e.* classical NSAID (NO-NSAID). They described that NO-NSAID have better anti-proliferative activity than the parent NSAID, *in vitro* and *in vivo*, and in particular, in colon, bladder and prostate cancer [23–26, 13]. Moreover, the administration of NO reduces the side effects of NSAID. Recently, the anti-proliferative action of nitro-oxy derivatives of the COX-2 selective inhibitor, celecoxib, has been assessed in various cell lines. These interesting derivatives of celecoxib which have less toxicity than the parent NSAID, showed an anti-tumor activity comparable to that of celecoxib [27, 28].

With respect to MTCs, our group has found that celecoxib at a low dose and the classical NSAID, indomethacin, reduced the development of tumors arising -from human TT cell injection in *nude* mice [10, 9]. Tomoda et al. [29] also reported that indomethacin have a strong anti-proliferative action on TT cells and two other MTC lines, due to mitotic division reduction without amplification of cell death level. Moreover, we have observed that three MTC cell lines were very sensitive to the anti-proliferative effect of a NO-donor [11]. The present publication reports that a pharmacological dose of GTN, a NO pro-drug used in cardiology, reduced significantly TT cell proliferation *in vitro* via mitotic division decrease.

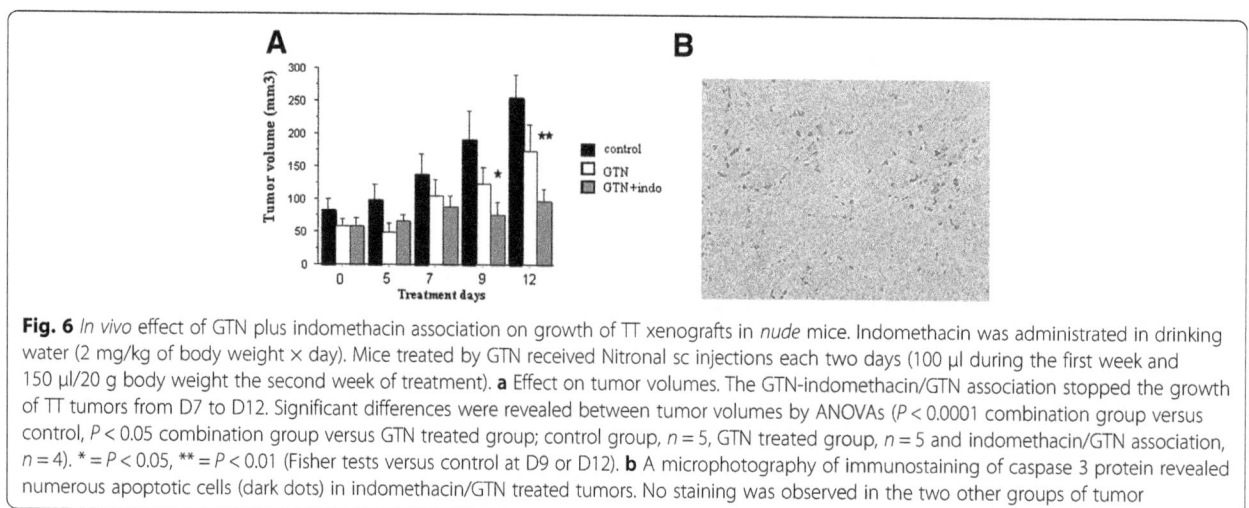

Fig. 6 *In vivo* effect of GTN plus indomethacin association on growth of TT xenografts in *nude* mice. Indomethacin was administrated in drinking water (2 mg/kg of body weight × day). Mice treated by GTN received Nitronal sc injections each two days (100 µl during the first week and 150 µl/20 g body weight the second week of treatment). **a** Effect on tumor volumes. The GTN-indomethacin/GTN association stopped the growth of TT tumors from D7 to D12. Significant differences were revealed between tumor volumes by ANOVAs ($P < 0.0001$ combination group versus control, $P < 0.05$ combination group versus GTN treated group; control group, $n = 5$, GTN treated group, $n = 5$ and indomethacin/GTN association, $n = 4$). * = $P < 0.05$, ** = $P < 0.01$ (Fisher tests versus control at D9 or D12). **b** A microphotography of immunostaining of caspase 3 protein revealed numerous apoptotic cells (dark dots) in indomethacin/GTN treated tumors. No staining was observed in the two other groups of tumor

As previously described for other cancer cells, incubation with NO and indomethacin strongly amplified the anti-tumoral effect of treatments alone in TT cell cultures. NO-indomethacin (NCX 530) had a stronger action than the individual NSAID. Interestingly, in our model, the association of GTN with celecoxib also increased the anti-proliferative activity of the drugs used as single agents. After analyses of the mitotic division and apoptosis markers, PCNA and PARP, we found that this phenomenon resulted from the induction of TT apoptotic cell death by combinations of a NO donor with each NSAID, while each molecule alone only acted on mitotic division.

In cancer biology, both positive and negative actions of NO have been reported. Low doses could promote cancer proliferation. Elevation of NO concentration can cause cell damage and apoptosis [15] and the tumor suppressor protein p53 have been implicated in the onset of cell death [16]. Recently, Tebbi et al. [20] described that NO induced the overexpression of the tumor suppressor isoform TAp73α in leukemia cells. In our model, the NO donor GTN, at low dose, did not increase p53 expression and only induced mitotic division reduction without apoptosis induction. This treatment moderately elevated TAp73α expression in TT cells but only after three days of exposition. The pathway leading to in vitro proliferation reduction remains unknown. Anyway, only a moderate, not significant growth reduction was obtained in vivo. This result could come from the difficulties to reveal a significant effect in vivo compared to in vitro experiment, from lower NO doses in tissues but also from the promotion of tumor angiogenesis which favors tumor cell proliferation.

The mechanisms of NSAID action are not completely elucidated. The anti-tumor effect of these drugs can result from the decrease of PG by inhibition of synthesis enzymes, COX 1 and/or 2. However, various mechanisms, independent of PG and COX have been also described [30, 31]. Increase of p53 expression was frequently observed after NSAID treatments of various models. In particular, Lau et al. [32] found that COX inhibitors induce apoptosis by increasing p53 stability and nuclear accumulation. Targeting p53 in MTCs may represent an attractive strategy since this protein is not mutated in these tumors [33]. In the present study, we found that only indomethacin increased p53 expression, in TT cells. Indomethacin alone acts on mitotic division [9]. However, p53 level elevation did not seem to intervene in the cell division reduction as this phenomenon appeared before p53 level increase.

Recently for the first time, Lau et al. [34] demonstrated the implication of p73 in the anti-tumor effect of a NSAID: the apoptotic response to celecoxib resulted from the increase of the TAp73β:ΔNp73 ratio in neuroblastoma cells. In our hand, both celecoxib and indomethacin increased the expression of the TAp73α isoform in TT cells. It is noteworthy that ΔNp73 and TAp73β were not detected in this cell line. The moderate elevation of TAp73α expression by a 1.5 factor did not promote the anti-mitotic action of the NSAIDs since this anti-tumor effect appeared during the first day of treatment while the variations in protein expression was only observed after more than two days. However we have not investigated post-translational modifications of TAp73α, such as phosphorylation that might be implicated in the anti-mitotic effects of these NSAIDs. Moreover, in our model, the increase of TAp73α after incubation with NSAIDs alone did not induce cell apoptosis. In fact, TAp73α would be a less potent apoptosis inducer than TAp73β [35].

Combinations of NO with one of the NSAIDs did not reinforce the cell division reduction as PCNA level in cells treated with only one simple drug was comparable to the protein expression in cells which have received combined treatment. But interestingly and for the first time, we observed the addition of NO and NSAID effects on TAp73α expression. Thus combinations led to a stronger elevation of this isoform level. Bi-therapies only promoted apoptosis resulting from the TAp73α expression increase as demonstrated by full length PARP western blot after TAp73α siRNA adjunction in TT cell cultures.

In the in vitro experiments, we used celecoxib and indomethacin doses that reproduced anti-tumor effects obtained for long term in vivo treatments; the NO-donor GTN was used at a pharmacological dose. Thus, the in vitro observations described here allow to study a phenomenon that can be also induced in vivo as demonstrated in our in vivo experiments. More in vivo validation has to be done but the bases are set to expect similar results. The expression of p73 must also be verified in human MTCs.

It could be of interest for many reasons to consider clinical studies with NSAID and/or NO-donor therapies. First, these drugs have a low cost and are currently used with many years of experience in healthy subjects. Second, these drugs could be used for a long period at all stage of the disease (advanced or not). Third, combined anti-proliferative actions of NO donor and NSAIDs demonstrated in this study seem independent of known actions of TKI and synergic actions with them could be of value [36]. Unfortunately, clinical experience with use of indomethacin in patients with recurrent or metastatic MTC has been limited to three cases. In only two out of three patients, indomethacin therapy for 3 or 4 months caused marked reduction in tumor mass as well as calcitonin levels [37]. The efficacy of these drugs remains to be determined by clinical trials.

Competing interests

The authors declare that they have no competing interests.

Authors' contribution
TR carried out rMTC 6.23 cell studies and FACS analyses, and participated to the redaction of the manuscript. CP and AP carried out the work on nude mice. RC gave medical advice. ML carried out his knowledge on p73, western blots, and siRNAs. SL conceived the global study, carried out works on TT cells and on histological and statistical analyses. SL wrote the manuscript with TR. All authors read and approved the final manuscript.

Acknowledgements
We thank Nicox SA for a gift of NCX 530 and Pfizer that gave us celecoxib. We also thank S. Dumont and F. Merabtene (plateforme d'histomorphologie, IFR 65, UPMC, Paris, France) and A. Rodenas (service d'anatomopathologie, Hôpital Tenon, Paris, France) for technical assistance in immunohistochemistry.

Author details
[1]UMR 8203, Gustave Roussy, Laboratoire de Vectorologie et de Thérapeutiques Anticancéreuses, Villejuif 94805, France. [2]UMR 8203, CNRS, Laboratoire de Vectorologie et Thérapeutiques Anticancéreuses, Villejuif 94805, France. [3]UMR 8203, Univ Paris-Sud, Laboratoire de Vectorologie et Thérapeutiques Anticancéreuses, Villejuif 94805, France. [4]Sorbonne Universités, UPMC University Paris 06, plateforme LIMP, Laboratoire d'Imagerie Médicale Positonique, Hôpital Tenon, Paris 75020, France. [5]Hopital Delafontaine, Endocrinology Unit, Saint Denis, France. [6]IBBMC, CNRS 8619, bat 430, Université Paris Sud XI, Orsay, Paris 91405, France.

References

1. Vitale G, Caraglia M, Ciccarelli A, Lupoli G, Abbruzzese A, Tagliaferri P, et al. Current approaches and perspectives in the therapy of medullary thyroid carcinoma. Cancer. 2001;91:1797–808.
2. Pacini F, Castagna MG, Cipri C, Schlumberger M. Medullary thyroid carcinoma. Clin Oncol. 2010;22(6):475–85.
3. Cohen R, Campos J, Salaün C, Heshmati H, Kraimps J, Proye C, et al. Preoperative calcitonin levels are predictive of tumor size and postoperative calcitonin normalization in medullary thyroid carcinoma. J Clin Endocrinol Metab. 2000;85:919–22.
4. Schlumberger M, Carlomagno F, Baudin E, Bidart J, Santoro M. New therapeutic approaches to treat medullary thyroid carcinoma. Nat Clin Pract Endocrinol Metab. 2008;4:22–32.
5. Wells Jr SA, Asa SL, Dralle H, Elisei R, Evans DB, Gagel RF, et al. Revised american thyroid association guidelines for the management of medullary thyroid carcinoma. Thyroid. 2015;25:567–610.
6. DuBois RN, Giardiello FM, Smalley WE. Nonsteroidal anti-inflammatory drugs, and colorectal cancer prevention. Gastroenterol Clin North Am. 1996;25:773–91.
7. Langman MJ, Cheng KK, Gilman EA, Lancashire RJ. Effect of anti-inflammatory drugs on overall risk of common cancer: case–control study in general practice research database. BMJ. 2000;320:1642–6.
8. Rothwell PM, Price JF, Fowkes FG, Zanchetti A, Tognoni G, Lee R, et al. Short-term effects of daily aspirin on cancer incidence, mortality, and non-cardiovascular death: analysis of the time course of risks and benefits in51 randomised controlled trials. Lancet. 2012;379:1602–12.
9. Quidville V, Segond N, Pidoux E, Cohen R, Jullienne A, Lausson S. Tumor growth inhibition by indomethacin in a mouse model of human medullary thyroid cancer: implication of cyclooxygenases and 15-hydroxyprostaglandin dehydrogenase. Endocrinology. 2004;145:2561–71.
10. Quidville V, Segond N, Tebbi A, Cohen R, Jullienne A, Lepoivre M, et al. Anti-tumoral effect of a celecoxib low dose on a model of human medullary thyroid cancer in nude mice. Thyroid. 2009;19:613–21.
11. Soler MN, Bobe P, Benihoud K, Lemaire G, Roos BA, Lausson S. Gene therapy of rat medullary thyroid cancer by naked nitric oxide synthase II DNA injection. J Gene Med. 2000;2:344–52.
12. Wallace JL, Del Soldato P. The therapeutical potential of NO-NSAIDs. Fundam Clin Pharmacol. 2003;17:11–20.
13. Rao CV, Reddy BS, Steele VE, Wang CX, Liu X, Ouyang N, et al. Nitric oxide-releasing aspirin and indomethacin are potent inhibitors against colon cancer in azoxymethane-treated rats: effects on molecular targets. Mol Cancer Ther. 2006;5:1530–8.
14. Ouyang N, Williams JL, Tsioulias GJ, Gao JJ, Iatropoulos MJ, Kopelovich L, et al. Nitric oxide-donating aspirin prevents pancreatic cancer in a hamster tumor model. Cancer Res. 2006;66:4503–11.
15. Akaike T, Fujii S, Kato A, Yoshitake J, Miyamoto Y, Sawa T, et al. Viral mutation accelerated by nitric oxide production during infection in vivo. Faseb J. 2000;14:1447–54.
16. Messmer UK, Ankarcrona M, Nicotera P, Brune B. p53 expression in nitric oxide-induced apoptosis. FEBS Lett. 1994;355:23–6.
17. Kaghad M, Bonnet H, Yang A, Creancier L, Biscan JC, Valent A, et al. Monoallelically expressed gene related to p53 at 1p36, a region frequently deleted in neuroblastoma and other human cancers. Cell. 1997;90:809–19.
18. Yang A, Kaghad M, Wang Y, Gillett E, Fleming MD, Dotsch V, et al. p63, a p53 homolog at 3q27-29, encodes multiple products with transactivating, death-inducing, and dominant-negative activities. Mol Cell. 1998;2:305–16.
19. Muller M, Schleithoff ES, Stremmel W, Melino G, Krammer PH, Schilling T. One, two, three–p53, p63, p73 and chemosensitivity. Drug Resist Updat. 2006;9:288–306.
20. Tebbi A, Guittet O, Cottet MH, Vésin F, Lepoivre M. TAp73 induction by nitric oxide. JBC. 2011;286:7873–84.
21. Guittet O, Tebbi A, Cottet MH, Vesin F, Lepoivre M. Upregulation of the p53R2 ribonucleotide reductase subunit by nitric oxide. Nitric Oxide. 2008;19:84–94.
22. Bressenot A, Marchal S, Bezdetnaya L, Garrier J, Guillemin F, Plénat F. Assessment of apoptosis by immunohistochemistry to active caspase-3, active caspase-7, or cleaved PARP in monolayer cells and spheroid and subcutaneous xenografts of human carcinoma. J Histochem Cytochem. 2009;57:289–300.
23. Kashfi K, Ryan Y, Qiao LL, Williams JL, Chen J, Del Soldato P, et al. Nitric oxide-donating non-steroidal anti-inflammatory drugs inhibit the growth of various cultured human cancer cells: evidence of a tissue type-independent effect. J Pharmacol Exp Ther. 2002;303:1273–82.
24. Huguenin S, Fleury-Feith J, Kheuang L, Jaurand MC, Bolla M, Riffaud JP, et al. Nitrosulindac (NCX 1102): a new nitric oxide- donating non steroidal anti-inflammatory drug (NO-NSAID), inhibits proliferation and induces apoptosis in human prostatic epithelial cell lines. Prostate. 2004;61:132–41.
25. Huguenin S, Vacherot F, Kheuang L, Fleury-Feith J, Jaurand MC, Bolla M, et al. Antiproliferative effect of nitrosulindac (NCX 1102), a new nitric oxide- donating non steroidal anti-inflammatory drug, on human bladder carcinoma cell lines. Mol Cancer Ther. 2004;3:291–8.
26. Fabbri F, Brigliadori G, Ulivi P, Tesei A, Vannini I, Rosetti M, et al. Pro-apototic effect of nitric oxide- donating NSAID, NCX 4040, on bladder carcinoma cells. Apoptosis. 2005;10:1095–103.
27. Bozzo F, Bassignana A, Lazzarato L, Boschi D, Gasco A, Bocca C, et al. Novel nitro-oxy derivatives of celecoxib for the regulation of colon cancer cell growth. Chem Biol Interact. 2009;182(2–3):183–90.
28. Bocca C, Bozzo F, Bassignana A, Miglietta A. Antiproliferative effects of COX-2 inhibitor celecoxib on human breast cancer cell lines. Mol Cell Biochem. 2011;350:59–70.
29. Tomoda C, Moatamed F, Naeim F, Hershman JM, Sugawara M. Indomethacin inhibits cell growth of medullary thyroid carcinoma by reducing cell cycle progression into S phase. Exp Biol Med. 2008;233:1433–40.
30. Kashfi K, Rigas B. Non-COX-2 targets and cancer: expanding the molecular target repertoire of chemoprevention. Biochem Pharmacol. 2005;70:969–86.
31. Grösch S, Maier T, Schiffmann S, Geisslinger G. Cyclooxygenase-2 (COX-2)-independent anticarcinogenic effects of selective COX-2 inhibitors. J Natl Cancer Inst. 2006;98:736–47.
32. Lau L, Hansford LM, Cheng LS, Hang M, Baruchel S, Kaplan DR. Cyclooxygenase inhibition modulate the p53/HDM2 pathway and enhance chemotherapy-induced apoptosis in neuroblastoma. Oncogene. 2007;26:1920–31.
33. Herfarth KKF, Wick MR, Marshall HN, Gartner E, Lum S, Moley JF. Absence of TP53 alterations in pheochromocytomas and medullary thyroid carcinomas. Genes Chromosom Cancer. 1997;20:24–9.
34. Lau LMS, Wolter JK, Lau JTML, Cheng LS, Smith KM, Hansford LM, et al. Cyclooxygenase inhibitors differentially modulate p73 isoforms in neuroblastoma. Oncogene. 2009;28:2024–33.
35. Gonzalez S, Perez-Perez MM, Hernando E, Serrano M, Cordon-Cardo C. P73beta-mediated apoptosis requires p57kip2 induction and IEX-1 inhibition. Cancer Res. 2005;65:2186–92.

Apoptosis induction by combination of drugs or a conjugated molecule associating non-steroidal...

127

36. Broutin S, Commo F, De Koning L, Marty-Prouvost B, Lacroix L, Talbot M, et al. Changes in signaling pathways induced by vandetanib in a human medullary thyroid carcinoma model, as analyzed by reverse phase protein array. Thyroid. 2014;24:43–51.

37. Sugawara M, Ly T, Hershman JM. Medullary Thyroid cancer current treatment strategy, novel therapies and perspectives for the Future. Horm Cancer. 2012;3:218–26.

13

Potassium iodide, but not potassium iodate, as a potential protective agent against oxidative damage to membrane lipids in porcine thyroid

Magdalena Milczarek[1], Jan Stępniak[1], Andrzej Lewiński[2,3] and Małgorzata Karbownik-Lewińska[1,3]*

Abstract

Background: Fenton reaction ($Fe^{2+}+H_2O_2 \rightarrow Fe^{3+}+{}^{\cdot}OH+OH^-$) is of special significance in the thyroid gland, as both its substrates, i.e. H_2O_2 and Fe^{2+}, are required for thyroid hormone synthesis. Also iodine, an essential element supplied by the diet, is indispensable for thyroid hormone synthesis. It is well known that iodine affects red-ox balance. One of the most frequently examined oxidative processes is lipid peroxidation (LPO), which results from oxidative damage to membrane lipids. Fenton reaction is used to experimentally induce lipid peroxidation. The aim of the study was to evaluate effects of iodine, used as potassium iodide (KI) or potassium iodate (KIO_3), on lipid peroxidation in porcine thyroid homogenates under basal conditions and in the presence of Fenton reaction substrates.

Methods: Porcine thyroid homogenates were incubated in the presence of either KI (0.00005 – 500 mM) or KIO_3 (0.00005 – 200 mM), without or with addition of $FeSO_4$ (30 μM) + H_2O_2 (0.5 mM). Concentration of malondialdehyde + 4-hydroxyalkenals (MDA + 4-HDA) was measured spectrophotometrically, as an index of lipid peroxidation.

Results: Potassium iodide, only when used in the highest concentrations (≥50 mM), increased lipid peroxidation in concentration-dependent manner. In the middle range of concentrations (5.0; 10; 25; 50 and 100 mM) KI reduced Fenton reaction-induced lipid peroxidation, with the strongest protective effect observed for the concentration of 25 mM. Potassium iodate increased lipid peroxidation in concentrations ≥2.5 mM. The damaging effect of KIO_3 increased gradually from the concentration of 2.5 mM to 10 mM. The strongest damaging effect was observed at the KIO_3 concentration of 10 mM, corresponding to physiological iodine concentration in the thyroid. Potassium iodate in concentrations of 5–200 mM enhanced Fenton reaction-induced lipid peroxidation with the strongest damaging effect found again for the concentration of 10 mM.

Conclusions: Potassium iodide, used in doses generally recommended in iodide prophylaxis, may prevent oxidative damage to membrane lipids in this gland. Toxic effects of iodide overload may result from its prooxidative action. Potassium iodate does not possess any direct beneficial effects on oxidative damage to membrane lipids in the thyroid, which constitutes an additional argument against its utility in iodine prophylaxis.

Keywords: Potassium iodide, Potassium iodate, Thyroid, Lipid peroxidation, Ferrous ion, Hydrogen peroxide

* Correspondence: MKarbownik@hotmail.com
[1]Department of Oncological Endocrinology, Medical University of Łódź, 7/9 Żeligowski Street, Łódź 90-752, Poland
[3]Polish Mother's Memorial Hospital – Research Institute, 281/289, Rzgowska Street, Łódź 93-338, Poland
Full list of author information is available at the end of the article

Background

Iodine, an essential trace element, is indispensable for thyroid hormone synthesis in humans and animals [1]. The only natural source of iodine is the diet. However, in numerous areas in the world iodine supply from natural sources is inadequate, resulting in iodine deficiency disorders (IDD) [2,3]. Precisely elaborated programs of iodine prophylaxis were introduced in different countries to prevent IDD [4]. These programs are mainly based on salt iodization with the use of either potassium iodide (KI) or potassium iodate (KIO_3).

These two compounds are characterised by different chemical properties and some differencies in potential toxicity/safety. Iodate is more stable, as iodide is readily oxidized to iodine and lost by evaporation [5]. Whereas reliable methods are validated for quantifying KIO_3 salt content, further validation is required for countries that use KI in salt iodization programs [6]. All other differences between KIO_3 and KI suggest the superiority of the latter over the former. First, human iodine bioavailability from KI is higher than from KIO_3 [7,8]. Second, in biofortification of vegetables with iodine, KI was found to be much more effective than KIO_3 [9,10].

In turn, according to some health authorities, the safety of KIO_3 to humans and animals is not completely documented and in 2002 the French Agency for Food Safety [11] did even question the use of KIO_3 instead of KI in iodine prophylaxis. Therefore, several experimental studies have been performed to clarify this issue. For example, it has been shown in experimental studies that KIO_3 does not reveal genotoxic effects [12]. Also comparative studies of the oxidative properties of iodate and other halogenate salts, such as bromate and chlorate, have shown that iodate would be of low, if any, genotoxic potential [13]. It is worth mentioning that both, KI and KIO_3, reveal similar effectiveness as blockers of radioiodine uptake by the thyroid in rats [14].

Nevertheless, according to similar effectiveness in iodine prophylaxis, both KI and KIO_3 were initially proved to be used for fortifying salt by the Joint WHO/FAO Expert Committee on Food Additives and Contaminants [15] and they are, along with other iodine salts, still admitted to be added to foods, including food supplements [16].

It is well known that iodine affects red-ox balance [17]. It is especially known for its excellent antioxidative properties in physiological conditions [18,19]. However, prooxidative effects of iodine were also demonstrated in experimental models. For example, in studies in vivo, iodine – given as iodide – expectedly increased MDA level in the rat thyroid and liver [20], or it increased Schiff's bases in rat lung and liver [21] and – when given as KIO_3 – in mice liver [22]. The latter change was accompanied by the increased activities of antioxidative enzymes, such as glutathione peroxidase and superoxide dismutase, but only after longer time

(3 months) of iodine exposure [22]. Thus, the balance between anti- and prooxidative effects of iodine depends on different factors, such as iodine dose/concentration or the time of action.

However, anti- or prooxidative effects of iodine on the thyroid gland with relation to iodine source, i.e. a chemical compound containing iodine, have never been examined in vitro, thus under conditions reflecting direct effects of these compounds on thyroid follicular cells.

Fenton reaction ($Fe^{2+}+H_2O_2 \rightarrow Fe^{3+}+^{\cdot}OH+OH^-$), being the basic reaction of oxidative stress, is of special significance in the thyroid gland, as both its substrates, i.e. H_2O_2 and Fe^{2+}, are required for thyroid hormone synthesis [23]. One of the most frequently examined oxidative processes is lipid peroxidation (LPO), which results from oxidative damage to membrane lipids. Bivalent iron (Fe^{2+}) and H_2O_2, which initiate Fenton reaction, have been frequently used to experimentally induce lipid peroxidation in different tissues [24-29], the thyroid gland included [30,31]. Also oxidative damage to nuclear and mitochondrial DNA has been induced by Fenton reaction substrates [32].

The aim of the study was to evaluate effects of iodine, used as potassium iodide (KI) or potassium iodate (KIO_3), on lipid peroxidation in porcine thyroid homogenates under basal conditions and in the presence of Fenton reaction substrates.

Preliminary results of the study were presented (as a poster presentation) during International and European Congress of Endocrinology in 2012 [33].

Methods

Ethical approval

The procedures, used in the study, were approved by the Ethics Committee of the Medical University of Lodz, Poland.

Chemicals

Potassium iodide (KI), potassium iodate (KIO_3), ferrous sulfate ($FeSO_4$) and hydrogen peroxide (H_2O_2) were purchased from Sigma (St. Louis, MO). The ALDetect Lipid Peroxidation Assay Kit was obtained from Enzo Life Sciences, Inc. (Zandhoven, Belgium). MilliQ-purified H_2O was used for preparing all solutions. All the used chemicals were of analytical grade and came from commercial sources.

Animals

Porcine thyroids were collected from forty five (45) animals at a slaughter-house, frozen on solid CO_2, and stored at -80°C until assay. Each experiment was repeated three to five times. Therefore, three to five tissue pools were prepared, with nine (9) thyroid glands used for each homogenate pool.

Assay of lipid peroxidation

Thyroid tissue was homogenized in ice cold 20 mM Tris-HCl buffer (pH = 7.4) (10%, w/v), and then incubated for 30 min at 37°C in the presence of examined substances. Porcine thyroid homogenates were incubated in the presence of either KI (500; 250; 100; 50; 25; 10; 5.0; 2.5; 1.0; 0.5; 0.25; 0.1; 0.05; 0.025; 0.01; 0.005; 0.0025; 0.001; 0.0005; 0.00025; 0.0001; 0.00005 mM) or KIO$_3$ (200; 150; 100; 50; 25; 10; 5.0; 2.5; 1.0; 0.5; 0.25; 0.1; 0.05; 0.025; 0.01; 0.005; 0.0025; 0.001; 0.0005; 0.00025; 0.0001; 0.00005 mM) without or with addition of Fenton reaction substrates, i.e. FeSO$_4$ (30 μM) + H$_2$O$_2$ (0.5 mM), or with addition of FeSO$_4$ (30 μM) only. According to different solubility of KI and KIO$_3$, different highest concentrations of these compounds were used in the study. Eight (8) separate experiments were performed, as it is specified in the Results section. The reactions were stopped by cooling the samples on ice. Each experiment was run in duplicate and repeated three to five times.

Measurement of lipid peroxidation products

The concentrations of malondialdehyde + 4-hydroxyalkenals (MDA + 4-HDA), as an index of lipid peroxidation, were measured in thyroid homogenates, with the ALDetect Lipid Peroxidation Assay Kit. The homogenates were centrifuged at 3,000 x g for 10 min at 4°C. After obtaining supernatant, each experiment was carried out in duplicate. The supernatant (200 μl) was mixed with 650 μl of a methanol: acetonitrile (1:3, v/v) solution, containing a chromogenic reagent, N-methyl-2-phenylindole, and vortexed. Following the addition of 150 μl of methanesulfonic acid (15.4 M), the incubation was carried out at 45°C for 40 min. The reaction between MDA + 4-HDA and N-methyl-2-phenylindole yields a chromophore, which is spectrophotometrically measured at the absorbance of 586 nm, using a solution of 10 mM 4-hydroxynonenal as the standard. The level of lipid peroxidation is expressed as the amount of MDA + 4-HDA (nmol) per mg protein. Protein was measured, using Bradford's method [34], with bovine albumin as the standard.

Statistical analyses

Results are expressed as means ± SE. The data were statistically analyzed, using a one-way analysis of variance (ANOVA), followed by the Student-Neuman-Keuls' test. The level of $p < 0.05$ was accepted as statistically significant.

Results

Two examined substances, i.e. KI and KIO$_3$, did not reveal the same effects on oxidative damage to membrane lipids in porcine thyroid homogenates, both under basal conditions and in the presence of Fenton reaction substrates.

Potassium iodide, when used in the highest concentrations (≥50 mM), did increase lipid peroxidation in concentration-dependent manner. In turn, KI in concentrations ≤25 mM did not affect lipid peroxidation (Figure 1).

When KI was used together with Fe^{2+}+H$_2$O$_2$, the following results were obtained. Potassium iodide used in the middle range of concentrations (5.0; 10; 25; 50 and 100 mM) reduced Fenton reaction-induced lipid peroxidation, with the strongest protective effect observed for the concentration of 25 mM, which completely prevented experimentally-induced lipid peroxidation (Figure 2). Interestingly, KI either in higher (≥250 mM) or lower (≤2.5 mM) concentrations did not affect significantly Fenton reaction-induced lipid peroxidation, which means that the level of lipid peroxidation in the presence of KI (≥250 mM or ≤2.5 mM) plus Fe^{2+}+H$_2$O$_2$ was the same as in the presence of Fe^{2+}+H$_2$O$_2$ only (Figure 2).

Subsequently, to compare prooxidative effects of KI alone to prooxidative effects of KI plus Fenton reaction substrates, the separate experiment was performed, in which thyroid homogenates were incubated in the presence of KI (in concentrations of 0.25-500 mM) alone or together with Fe^{2+}+H$_2$O$_2$ (Figure 3). The level of lipid peroxidation was significantly higher when KI (in concentrations ≤100 mM) was used together with Fe^{2+}+H$_2$O$_2$. However, KI did not enhanced Fenton reaction-induced lipid peroxidation (Figure 3), which is in agreement with results shown in Figure 2.

In our earlier study [31], Fe^{2+} used alone (i.e. as only one of Fenton reaction substrates), in opposite to H$_2$O$_2$,

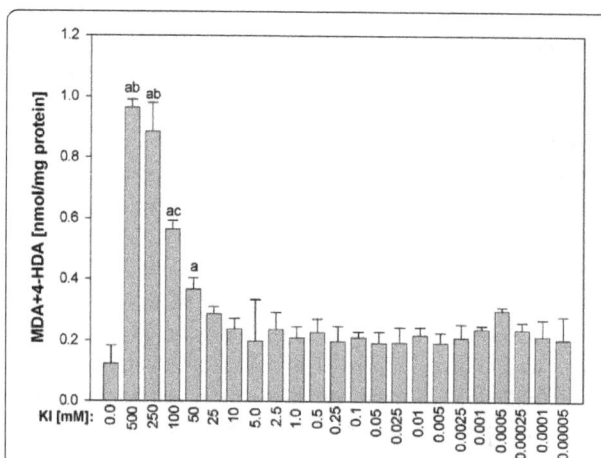

Figure 1 Lipid peroxidation, measured as MDA + 4-HDA level, in porcine thyroid homogenates. Homogenates were incubated in the presence of KI alone [500; 250; 100; 50; 25; 10; 5.0; 2.5; 1.0; 0.5; 0.25; 0.1; 0.05; 0.025; 0.01; 0.005; 0.0025; 0.001; 0.0005; 0.00025; 0.0001; 0.00005 mM]. Data are expressed as nmol/mg protein. Data are from four independent experiments. Values are expressed as mean ± SE (error bars). ^{a}p < 0.05 vs. control (in the absence of KI); ^{b}p < 0.05 vs. KI concentrations ≤100 mM; ^{c}p < 0.05 vs. any other KI concentration.

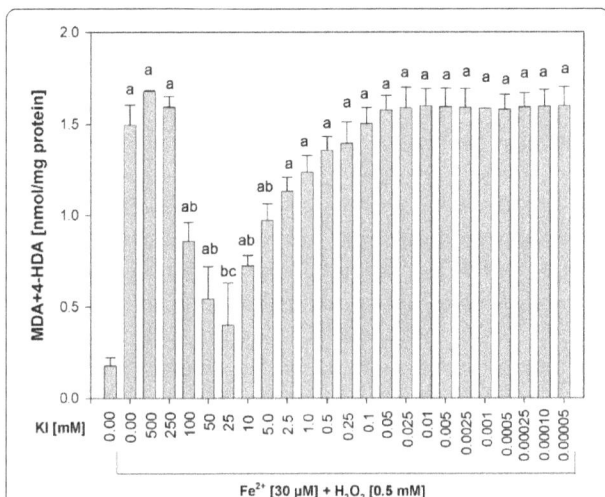

Figure 2 Lipid peroxidation, measured as MDA + 4-HDA level, in porcine thyroid homogenates. Homogenates were incubated in the presence of KI [500; 250; 100; 50; 25; 10; 5.0; 2.5; 1.0; 0.5; 0.25; 0.1; 0.05; 0.025; 0.01; 0.005; 0.0025; 0.001; 0.0005; 0.00025; 0.0001; 0.00005 mM] and, additionally, in the presence of both Fenton reaction substrates, namely in the presence of $FeSO_4$ [30 μM] plus H_2O_2 [0.5 mM]. Data are expressed as nmol/mg protein. Data are from three independent experiments. Values are expressed as mean ± SE (error bars). [a]$p < 0.05$ vs. control (in the absence of KI or $Fe^{2+}+H_2O_2$); [b]$p < 0.05$ vs. $Fe^{2+}+H_2O_2$, vs. KI [500 mM] + $Fe^{2+}+H_2O_2$, vs. KI [250 mM] + $Fe^{2+}+H_2O_2$; [c]$p < 0.05$ vs. KI [100 mM] + $Fe^{2+}+H_2O_2$.

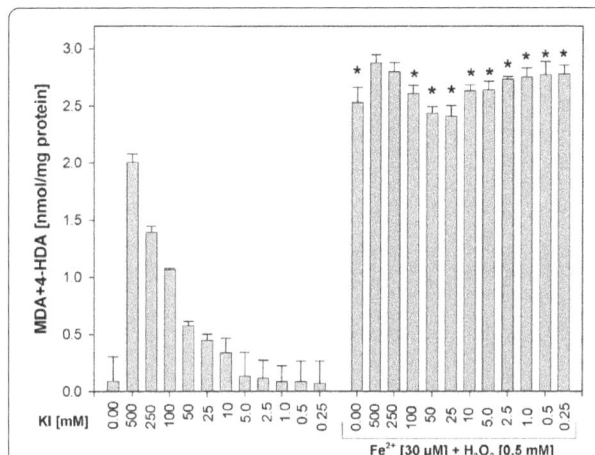

Figure 3 Lipid peroxidation, measured as MDA + 4-HDA level, in porcine thyroid homogenates. Homogenates were incubated in the presence of KI alone [500; 250; 100; 50; 25; 10; 5.0; 2.5; 1.0; 0.5; 0.25 mM] or in the presence of KI [500; 250; 100; 50; 25; 10; 5.0; 2.5; 1.0; 0.5; 0.25 mM] together with both substrates of Fenton reaction, namely in the presence of $FeSO_4$ [30 μM] plus H_2O_2 [0.5 mM]. Data are expressed as nmol/mg protein. Data are from three independent experiments. Values are expressed as mean ± SE (error bars). *$p < 0.05$ vs. respective concentration of KI alone (i.e. in the absence of $Fe^{2+}+H_2O_2$).

induced lipid peroxidation in thyroid homogenates. Therefore, in the present study we have performed the additional experiment with use of KI (in concentrations of 0.25-500 mM) alone or together with Fe^{2+} (Figure 4). No significant differences in lipid peroxidation were found for respective concentrations of KI in the presence or in the absence of Fe^{2+} (Figure 4).

In the opposite to KI, KIO_3 revealed, depending on the concentration or the presence/absence of $Fe^{2+}+H_2O_2$, either no protective effect at all or even strong pro-oxidative action (Figures 5 and 6). When KIO_3 was used alone, it did increase lipid peroxidation in concentrations ≥2.5 mM (Figure 5). The damaging effect of KIO_3 increased gradually from the concentration of 2.5 mM to 10 mM and, then, it decreased again gradually, however still being significantly stronger at the highest used KIO_3 concentration (200 mM) than in control (Figure 5). The strongest damaging effect to membrane lipids was observed at the KIO_3 concentration of 10 mM (Figure 5).

When KIO_3 was used together with $Fe^{2+}+H_2O_2$, the following results were obtained. Potassium iodate enhanced Fenton reaction-induced lipid peroxidation, when it was used in concentrations of 5 mM to 200 mM, with the strongest damaging effect of KIO_3 found again for the concentration of 10 mM (Figure 6). Concentration-dependent effects of KIO_3 used together with Fenton

reaction substrates were similar to those caused by KIO_3 alone (compare Figures 5 and 6).

In comparative experiment (i.e. in the presence and in the absence of Fenton reaction substrates), the addition of $Fe^{2+}+H_2O_2$ enhanced KIO_3-induced lipid peroxidation, but only for KIO_3 concentration ≤10 mM) (Figure 7). Strong

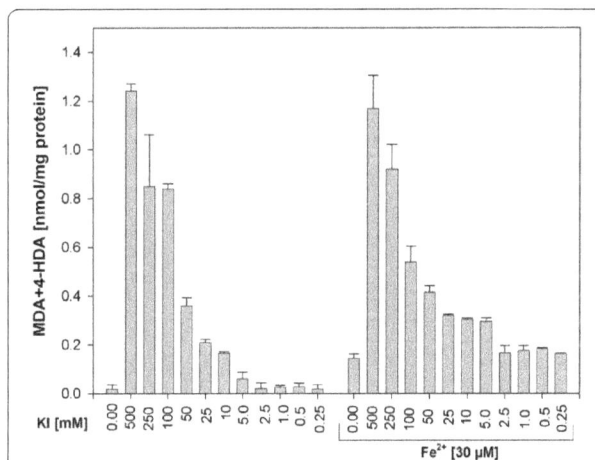

Figure 4 Lipid peroxidation, measured as MDA + 4-HDA level, in porcine thyroid homogenates. Homogenates were incubated in the presence of KI alone [500; 250; 100; 50; 25; 10; 5.0; 2.5; 1.0; 0.5; 0.25 mM] or in the presence of KI [500; 250; 100; 50; 25; 10; 5.0; 2.5; 1.0; 0.5; 0.25 mM] together with one substrate of Fenton reaction, namely in the presence of $FeSO_4$ [30 μM]. Data are expressed as nmol/mg protein. Data are from three independent experiments. Values are expressed as mean ± SE (error bars). No statistical differences between respective concentrations of KI (i.e. in the presence and in the absence of Fe^{2+}) were found.

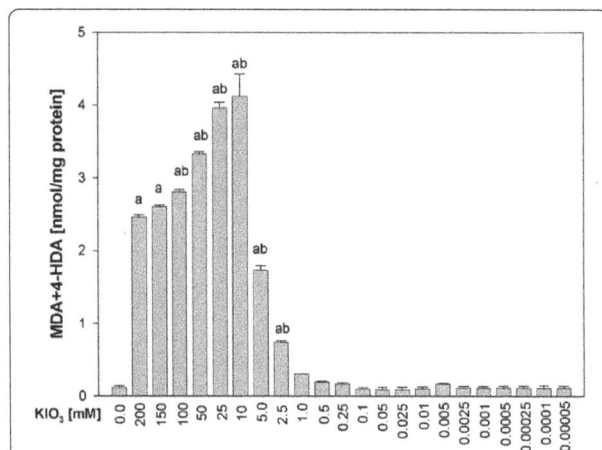

Figure 5 Lipid peroxidation, measured as MDA + 4-HDA level, in porcine thyroid homogenates. Homogenates were incubated in the presence of KIO_3 alone [200; 150; 100; 50; 25; 10; 5.0; 2.5; 1.0; 0.5; 0.25; 0.1; 0.05; 0.025; 0.01; 0.005; 0.0025; 0.001; 0.0005; 0.00025; 0.0001; 0.00005 mM]. Data are expressed as nmol/mg protein. Data are from five independent experiments. Values are expressed as mean ± SE (error bars). [a]$p < 0.05$ vs. control (in the absence of KIO_3); [b]$p < 0.05$ vs. any other KIO_3 concentration.

prooxidative effects of KIO_3 in concentrations ≥ 25 mM was not enhanced by Fenton reaction substrates (Figure 7).

In turn, no significant differences were found for respective concentrations of KIO_3 in the presence or in the absence of Fe^{2+} (Figure 8).

Discussion

Molar concentrations of KI and KIO_3 were calculated in the present study with regard to whole compounds. Among chemical elements forming either KI or KIO_3, iodine is characterized by the highest molecular mass – much higher than potassium (K) and oxygen (O), thus it constitutes the crucial part of both compounds concerning their molecular masses, i.e. iodine constitutes 76.45% of molecular mass of KI, and in case of KIO_3 it constitutes 59.30% of the molecular mass of this compound. In turn, the molecular mass of KI constitutes 77.57% of that one of KIO_3, so the molecular masses of these two compounds are of the same order of magnitude. Therefore, concentrations of KI and of KIO_3, calculated in the present study, may be used in comparative analyses either of effects of iodide ions (I^-) formed from both KI and KIO_3, or of effects of the whole compounds, i.e. KI and KIO_3.

It is worth mentioning that in vitro KI treatment of the thyroid cell line $PCCl_3$ resulted in the increased reactive oxygen species production [35]. Similar effect has not been evaluated after KIO_3 treatment.

Only few studies have been performed till now to compare effects of iodine present in two different sources, namely in KI and KIO_3. No differences were found between tissue (the thyroid gland, liver, kidney, muscle, abdominal fat tissue and skin) iodine content or blood thyroid hormone concentrations after in vivo treatment with high doses of either KI or KIO_3 [8]. In similar in vivo model the same group of authors evaluated some parameters of oxidative stress [36]. Different compounds of iodine, i.e. KI or KIO_3, have

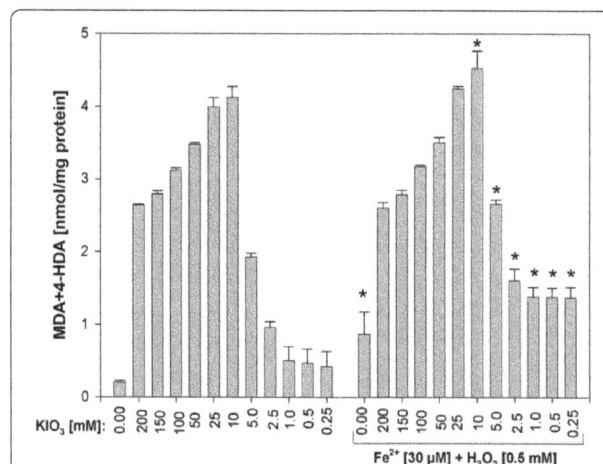

Figure 6 Lipid peroxidation, measured as MDA + 4-HDA level, in porcine thyroid homogenates. Homogenates were incubated in the presence of KIO_3 [200; 150; 100; 50; 25; 10; 5.0; 2.5; 1.0; 0.5; 0.25; 0.1; 0.05; 0.025; 0.01; 0.005; 0.0025; 0.001; 0.0005; 0.00025; 0.0001; 0.00005 mM] and, additionally, in the presence of both Fenton reaction substrates, namely in the presence of $FeSO_4$ [30 μM] plus H_2O_2 [0.5 mM]. Data are expressed as nmol/mg protein. Data are from five independent experiments. Values are expressed as mean ± SE (error bars). [a]$p < 0.05$ vs. control (in the absence of KIO_3 or $Fe^{2+}+H_2O_2$); [b]$p < 0.05$ vs. $Fe^{2+}+H_2O_2$ (in the absence of KIO_3); [c]$p < 0.05$ vs. any other concentration of KIO_3.

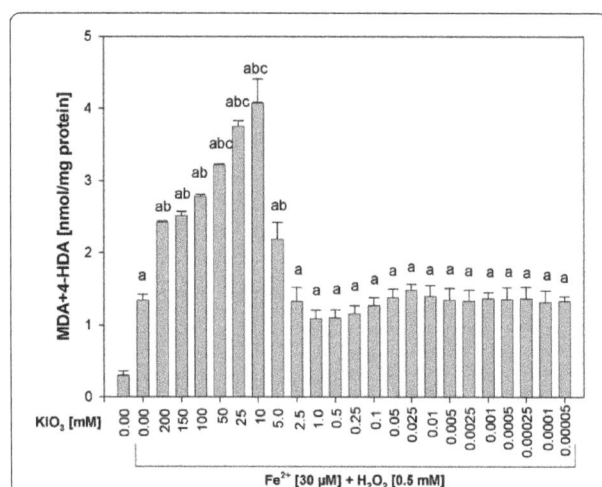

Figure 7 Lipid peroxidation, measured as MDA + 4-HDA level, in porcine thyroid homogenates. Homogenates were incubated in the presence of KIO_3 alone [200; 150; 100; 50; 25; 10; 5.0; 2.5; 1.0; 0.5; 0.25 mM] or in the presence of KIO_3 [200; 150; 100; 50; 25; 10; 5.0; 2.5; 1.0; 0.5; 0.25 mM] together with both substrates of Fenton reaction, namely in the presence of $FeSO_4$ [30 μM] plus H_2O_2 [0.5 mM]. Data are expressed as nmol/mg protein. Data are from three independent experiments. Values are expressed as mean ± SE (error bars). *$p < 0.05$ vs. respective concentration of KIO_3 alone (i.e. in the absence of $Fe^{2+}+H_2O_2$).

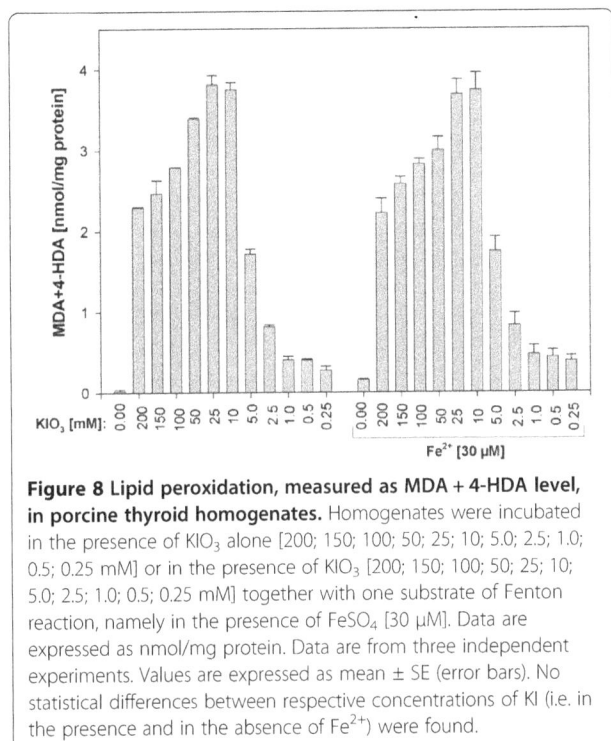

Figure 8 Lipid peroxidation, measured as MDA + 4-HDA level, in porcine thyroid homogenates. Homogenates were incubated in the presence of KIO_3 alone [200; 150; 100; 50; 25; 10; 5.0; 2.5; 1.0; 0.5; 0.25 mM] or in the presence of KIO_3 [200; 150; 100; 50; 25; 10; 5.0; 2.5; 1.0; 0.5; 0.25 mM] together with one substrate of Fenton reaction, namely in the presence of $FeSO_4$ [30 μM]. Data are expressed as nmol/mg protein. Data are from three independent experiments. Values are expressed as mean ± SE (error bars). No statistical differences between respective concentrations of KI (i.e. in the presence and in the absence of Fe^{2+}) were found.

similar effects on lipid peroxidation level (measured as MDA concentration) in the liver and the muscle, however certain differences were observed concerning mRNA expressions or the activities of antioxidative enzymes in different tissues [36]. However, such comparative studies have not been performed under in vitro conditions. The present study is the first one in which KI was found to be superior to KIO_3 in the thyroid gland concerning oxidative damage to macromolecules.

More favourable effects of KI comparing to KIO_3 were observed both, when each of these compounds was used separately or together with Fenton reaction substrates. Concerning the first situation, both KI and KIO_3 revealed – when used in high concentrations – damaging effects to membrane lipids in the thyroid. However, the difference between these unfavourable actions of KI and KIO_3 was crucial. Namely, the damaging effect of KI decreased gradually with decreasing concentrations of this compound and these undesired effects were not observed for concentrations below 50 mM, thus concentrations corresponding to inorganic iodine level normally present in the thyroid under physiological conditions. On the basis of experimental findings [37-39] the concentration of inorganic iodine in the human or rat thyroid was calculated by the authors of the present work to be approx. 9 mM. Taking into account close similarity between human and porcine thyroid in terms of thyroid volume and of thyroid hormone synthesis with all elements and all steps of this process [40], it may be estimated that iodine concentration in porcine thyroid

(used in the present study) is at similar level. Thus, the concentrations of KI resulting in thyroid level of inorganic iodine close to that observed under physiological conditions do not reveal prooxidative effects, at least in terms of oxidative damage to membrane lipids.

In opposite, when KIO_3 was used alone, the highest lipid peroxidation was found for its concentration of 10 mM, thus corresponding to the physiological concentration in the thyroid, which was calculated to be 9 mM. It should be recalled that the same concentration of KI did not increase the level of lipid peroxidation (compare Figures 1 and 2).

When KI or KIO_3 were added to the incubation medium together with Fenton reaction substrates, KI appeared to be also superior to KIO_3 concerning their influence on lipid peroxidation in the thyroid gland. Whereas KI in concentrations of 5–100 mM (Figure 2), i.e. corresponding to physiological concentrations of inorganic iodine, diminished experimentally-induced lipid peroxidation, KIO_3 did not reveal any protective action (Figure 5). Additionally, KI in concentration of 25 mM, thus being one order of magnitude higher than physiological iodine concentration, completely prevented Fenton reaction-induced lipid peroxidation. In turn, KIO_3 enhanced Fenton reaction-induced lipid peroxidation, when it was used in concentrations of 5 mM to 200 mM, with the strongest damaging effect of KIO_3 found again for the concentration of 10 mM (Figure 6).

Additionally it is clearly visible that prooxidative effects of KI was enhanced by Fenton reaction substrates. At the same time the damaging effects of KIO_3 were so strong that they were only weakly enhanced by Fenton reaction substrates (compare Figures 1 and 2, Figures 5 and 6, Figures 3 and 7). These comparative analyses reveal additionally the superiority of KI over KIO_3.

Ferrous ion (Fe^{2+}), which was in our earlier study [31] documented to induce lipid peroxidation in the thyroid gland, when it was used as only one of Fenton reaction substrates, did not modify significantly in the present study the effect of either KI or of KIO_3. This is probably due to the fact that prooxidative effects of Fe^{2+} alone is clearly weaker than those ones caused by both Fenton reaction substrates [31]. Potential mechanisms of differences between KI and KIO_3 effects on lipid peroxidation in thyroid homogenates, observed in the present study, should be discussed. Thus, the following explanation is proposed.

The reduction of IO_3, the process occurring when the tissue is exposed to KIO_3, requires the time and energy and possibly it is associated with unfavorable oxidative reactions and the damaging effects.

In turn, KIO_3 belongs to halogenate salts, which are known for their potentially toxic effects [5,13,41]. In our earlier studies, one of halogenate salts, namely potassium bromate ($KBrO_3$), being classified as carcinogen (group 2B according to IARC 1986 [42]), was shown to exert damaging effect to membrane lipids in porcine thyroid under in vitro (5 mM) and in vivo conditions [43]. Thus, $KBrO_3$ and KIO_3 increased lipid peroxidation in porcine thyroid homogenates when used in the same range of concentrations. At the same time, iodine used as KI (in concentrations ≤ 25 mM) did not reveal in the present study any toxic effects to membrane lipids and even it prevented experimentally induced lipid peroxidation, when used in the same range of concentrations (5–100 mM).

However, from among three halogenate salts, i.e. iodate, bromate and chlorate, the first one is characterized by the lowest redox potential. Therefore, KIO_3 seems to be potentially less toxic than bromate and chlorate, at least when oxidative mechanisms are considered.

Our study was performed under in vitro conditions and, therefore, it cannot be extrapolated directly into in vivo conditions, especially that IO_3^- is reduced to I^- before approaching the thyroid cell. However, our study is the first one which supports the statement that the use of KI in iodine prophylaxis is more safe than of KIO_3, in terms of their influence on oxidative damage to macromolecules. Additionally, not only the thyroid gland should be considered in the aspect of prooxidative effects of KIO_3 but, more importantly, other tissues, in particular digestive system, which is approached by KIO_3 earlier, i.e. immediately after exposure to this salt.

Conclusions

Potassium iodide, used in doses generally recommended in iodide prophylaxis, thus resulting in physiological iodine concentration in the thyroid, may prevent oxidative damage to membrane lipids in this gland. Toxic effects of iodide overload may result from its prooxidative action. Potassium iodate does not possess any direct beneficial effects on oxidative damage to membrane lipids in the thyroid, which constitutes an additional argument against its utility in iodine prophylaxis.

Competing interests
Authors declare that they have no competing interests.

Authors' contributions
MM carried out the experiments, performed the statistical evaluation and prepared the draft of the manuscript. JS accompanied the steps of the study related to lipid peroxidation measurement. AL revised the final version of the manuscript. MK-L designed the study, supervised its conducting and prepared the final version of the manuscript. All authors read and approved the final manuscript.

Acknowledgement
The research was supported by a grant from the National Science Centre (polish abbr. NCN) to the Medical University of Lodz (Project No. N N401 539540). This study constitutes a part of Ph.D. thesis of the first author of the paper (MM).

Author details
[1]Department of Oncological Endocrinology, Medical University of Łódź, 7/9 Żeligowski Street, Łódź 90-752, Poland. [2]Department of Endocrinology and Metabolic Diseases, Medical University of Łódź, 281/289 Rzgowska Street, Łódź 93-338, Poland. [3]Polish Mother's Memorial Hospital – Research Institute, 281/289, Rzgowska Street, Łódź 93-338, Poland.

References
1. Thilly CH, Vanderpas JB, Bebe N, Ntambue K, Contempre B, Swennen B, Moreno-Reyes R, Bourdoux P, Delange F: Iodine deficiency, other trace elements, and goitrogenic factors in the etiopathogeny of iodine deficiency disorders (IDD). Biol Trace Elem Res 1992, 32:229–243.
2. Zimmermann MB, Andersson M: Assessment of iodine nutrition in populations: past, present, and future. Nutr Rev 2012, 70:553–570.
3. Pearce EN, Andersson M, Zimmermann MB: Global iodine nutrition: where do we stand in 2013? Thyroid 2013, 23:523–528.
4. World Health Organization, United Nations Children's Fund, and the International Council for the Control of Iodine Deficiency Disorders: Indicators for Assessment of Iodine Deficiency Disorders and Their Control Programmes, Report of a Joint WHO/UNICEF/ICCIDD Consultation, 3–5 November 1992. Geneva: World Health Organization; 1993. Document WHO/NUT/93.1.
5. Bürgi H, Schaffner TH, Seiler JP: The toxicology of iodate: a review of the literature. Thyroid 2001, 11:449–456.
6. Rohner F, Garrett GS, Laillou A, Frey SK, Mothes R, Schweigert FJ, Locatelli-Rossi L: Validation of a user-friendly and rapid method for quantifying iodine content of salt. Food Nutr Bull 2012, 33(Suppl 4):330–335.
7. Murray MM, Pochin EE: Thyroid uptake of iodine from ingested iodate in man. J Physiol 1951, 114(Suppl):1–14.
8. Li Q, Mair C, Schedle K, Hammerl S, Schodl K, Windisch W: Effect of iodine source and dose on growth and iodine content in tissue and plasma thyroid hormones in fattening pigs. Eur J Nutr 2012, 51:685–691.
9. Zhu YG, Huang YZ, Hu Y, Liu YX: Iodine uptake by spinach (Spinaciaoleracea L.) plants grown in solution culture: effects of iodine species and solution concentrations. Environ Int 2003, 29:33–37.
10. Voogt W, Holwerda HT, Khodabaks R: Biofortification of lettuce (Lactuca sativa L.) with iodine: the effect of iodine form and concentration in the nutrient solution on growth, development and iodine uptake of lettuce grown in water culture. J Sci Food Agric 2010, 90:906–913.
11. AFSSA: Avis de l'Agence franc̜aise de se'curite' sanitaire des aliments relatif a' la modification de l'arre te' du 28 mai 1997 portant sur le sel alimentaire et aux substances d'apport nutritionnel pouvant e tre utilise'es pour sa supple'mentation; 2002. available: www.afssa.fr.
12. Poul JM, Huet S, Godard T, Sanders P: Lack of genotoxicity of potassium iodate in the alkaline comet assay and in the cytokinesis-block micronucleus test. Comparison to potassium bromate. Food Chem Toxicol 2004, 42:203–209.
13. Parsons JL, Chipman JK: The role of glutathione in DNA damage by potassium bromate in vitro. Mutagenesis 2000, 15:311–316.
14. Pahuja DN, Rajan MG, Borkar AV, Samuel AM: Potassium iodate and its comparison to potassium iodide as a blocker of 131I uptake by the thyroid in rats. Health Phys 1993, 65:545–549.
15. Joint WHO/FAO Expert Committee on Food Additives: Matters of interest arising from the forty-third World Health Assembly. In Evaluation of Certain Food Additives and Contaminants. Geneva: World Health Organization (WHO technical report series No. 806, Annex5; 1991.
16. European Commission: Commission Regulation (EC) No 1170/2009 of 30 November 2009 amending Directive 2002/46/EC of the European Parliament and of Council and Regulation (EC) No 1925/2006 of the European Parliament and of the Council as regards the lists of vitamin and minerals and their forms that can be added to foods, including food supplements. Official Journal of the European Union 2009, L 314:36.
17. Aceves C, Anguiano B, Delgado G: The extrathyronine actions of iodine. Antioxidant, apoptotic and differentiator factor in iodine-uptake tissues. Thyroid. in press.
18. Venturi S, Venturi M: Iodide, thyroid and stomach carcinogenesis: evolutionary story of a primitive antioxidant? Eur J Endocrinol 1999, 140:371–372.
19. Küpper FC, Carpenter LJ, McFiggans GB, Palmer CJ, Waite TJ, Boneberg EM, Woitsch S, Weiller M, Abela R, Grolimund D, Potin P, Butler A, Luther GW 3rd, Kroneck PM, Meyer-Klaucke W, Feiters MC: Iodide accumulation provides kelp with an inorganic antioxidant impacting atmospheric chemistry. Proc Natl Acad Sci U S A 2008, 105:6954–6958.
20. Joanta AE, Filip A, Clichici S, Andrei S, Daicoviciu D: Iodide excess exerts oxidative stress in some target tissues of the thyroid hormones. Acta Physiol Hung 2006, 93:347–359.
21. Sewerynek E, Swierczyńska-Machura D, Lewiński A: Effect of propylthiouracil on the level of Schiff's bases in tissues of rats on diet with different doses of potassium iodide. Neuro Endocrinol Lett 2006, 27:595–599.

22. Xia Y, Qu W, Zhao LN, Han H, Yang XF, Sun XF, Hao LP, Xu J: Iodine excess induces hepatic steatosis through disturbance of thyroid hormone metabolism involving oxidative stress in BALB/c mice. *Biol Trace Elem Res* 2013, **154**:103–110.

23. Karbownik M, Lewiński A: The role of oxidative stress in physiological and pathological processes in the thyroid gland; possible involvement in pineal-thyroid interactions. *Neuroendocrinol Lett* 2003, **24**:293–303.

24. Karbownik M, Reiter RJ, Garcia JJ, Tan D: Melatonin reduces phenylhydrazine-induced oxidative damage to cellular membranes: evidence for the involvement of iron. *Int J Biochem Cell Biol* 2000, **32**:1045–1054.

25. Karbownik M, Gitto E, Lewiński A, Reiter RJ: Relative efficacies of indole antioxidants in reducing autoxidation and iron-induced lipid peroxidation in hamster testes. *J Cell Biochem* 2001, **81**:693–699.

26. Karbownik M, Lewiński A, Reiter RJ: Anticarcinogenic actions of melatonin which involve antioxidative processes: Comparison with other antioxidants. *Int J Biochem Cell Biol* 2001, **33**:735–753.

27. Cabrera J, Burkhardt S, Tan DX, Manchester LC, Karbownik M, Reiter RJ: Autoxidation and toxicant-induced oxidation of lipid and DNA in monkey liver: reduction of molecular damage by melatonin. *Pharmacol Toxicol* 2001, **89**:225–230.

28. Gitto E, Tan DX, Reiter RJ, Karbownik M, Manchester LC, Cuzzocrea S, Fulia F, Barberi I: Individual and synergistic antioxidative actions of melatonin: studies with vitamin E, vitamin C, glutathione and desferrioxamine (desferoxamine) in rat liver homogenates. *J Pharm Pharmacol* 2001, **53**:1393–1401.

29. Karbownik-Lewińska M, Kokoszko-Bilska A: Oxidative damage to macromolecules in the thyroid - experimental evidence. *Thyroid Res* 2012, **5**:

30. Karbownik M, Lewiński A: Melatonin reduces Fenton-induced lipid peroxidation in porcine thyroid tissue. *J Cell Biochem* 2003, **90**:806–811.

31. Stępniak J, Lewiński A, Karbownik-Lewińska M: Membrane lipids and nuclear DNA are differently susceptive to Fenton reaction substrates in porcine thyroid. *Toxicol In Vitro* 2013, **27**:71–78.

32. Karbownik-Lewińska M, Stępniak J, Lewiński A: High level of oxidized nucleosides in thyroid mitochondrial DNA; damaging effects of Fenton reaction substrates. *Thyroid Res* 2012, **5**:24–32.

33. Milczarek M, Stępniak J, Lewiński A, Karbownik-Lewińska M: Potassium iodide, but not potassium iodate, as a potential protective agent against oxidative damage to membrane lipids in porcine thyroid. In *Proceedings of the 15th International & 14th European Congress of Endocrinology: 05–09 May 2012; Florence, European Society of Endocrinology*. Edited by KB Bioscientifica. Euro House, Bristol; 2012.

34. Bradford MM: A rapid and sensitive method for the quantitation of microgram quantities of protein utilizing the principle of protein-dye binding. *Anal Biochem* 1976, **72**:248–254.

35. Leoni SG, Kimura ET, Santisteban P, De la-Vieja A: Regulation of thyroid oxidative state by thioredoxin reductase has a crucial role in thyroid responses to iodide excess. *Mol Endocrinol* 2011, **25**:1924–1935.

36. Li Q, Mair C, Schedle K, Hellmayr I, Windisch W: Effects of varying dietary iodine supplementation levels as iodide or iodate on thyroid status as well as mRNA expression and enzyme activity of antioxidative enzymes in tissues of grower/finisher pigs. *Eur J Nutr* 2013, **52**:161–168.

37. Taurog A, Chaikoff IL, Feller DD: The mechanism of iodineconcentration by the thyroid gland: its non-organic iodine-binding capacity in the normal and propylthiouracil-treated rat. *J Biol Chem* 1947, **171**:189–201.

38. Taurog A, Tong W, Chaikoff IL: Non-thyroglobulin iodine of the thyroid gland II. Inorganic iodide. *J Biol Chem* 1951, **191**:677–682.

39. Tiran B, Karpf E, Tiran A, Lax S, Langsteger W, Eber O, Lorenz O: Iodine content of thyroid tissue in the Styrian population. *Acta Med Austriaca* 1993, **20**:6–8.

40. Kuzmuk KN, Schook LB: Pigs as a Model for Biomedical Sciences. In *The Genetics of the Pig. 2nd edition*. Edited by Rothschild MF, Ruvinsky A. Wallingford: CAB International; 2011:426–444.

41. National Toxicology Program (NTP): Toxicology and carcinogenesis studies of sodium chlorate (CAS No. 7775-09-9) in F344/N rats and B6C3F1 mice (drinking water studies), Technical Report Series no. 517. NIH Publication No. 06–4457. Research Triangle Park, NC: National Institutes of Health, Public Health Service, U.S. Department of Health and Human Services; 2005.

42. WHO/IARC: IARC Monographs on the Evaluation of the Carcinogenic Risk of Chemicals to Humans, Vol. 40, Some Naturally Occurring and Synthetic Food Components, Furocoumarins and Ultraviolet Radiation. Lyon: WHO/IARC; 1986:207–220.

43. Karbownik M, Stasiak M, Zasada K, Zygmunt A, Lewinski A: Comparison of potential protective effects of melatonin, indole-3-propionic acid, and propylthiouracil against lipid peroxidation caused by potassium bromate in the thyroid gland. *J Cell Biochem* 2005, **95**:131–138.

14

Role of metallothioneins in benign and malignant thyroid lesions

Bartosz Pula[1], Pawel Domoslawski[2], Marzena Podhorska-Okolow[1] and Piotr Dziegiel[1,3]*

Abstract

Recent findings in the past two decades have brought many insights into the biology of thyroid benign and malignant lesions, in particular the papillary and follicular thyroid cancers. Although, much progress have been made, thyroid cancers still pose diagnostic problems regarding differentiation of follicular lesions in relation to their aggressiveness and the treatment of advanced and undifferentiated thyroid cancers. Metallothioneins (MTs) were shown to induce cancer cells proliferation, mediate resistance to apoptosis, certain chemotherapeutics and radiotherapy. Therefore, MTs may be of utility in diagnosis and management of patients with benign and malignant lesions of the thyroid.

Keywords: Metallothionein, Thyroid, Nodular goiter, Cancer

Introduction

Thyroid cancer is regarded as the most common cancer of the endocrine organs and among all cancers it accounts approximately up to 2.5% of all malignancies [1,2]. Although, the death rates remain relatively low, there is a growing trend towards higher incidence of thyroid cancer which might not be explained by progress in detection of even relatively small thyroid cancers [1,3,4]. The majority of cancers of this organ develop from follicular epithelial cells and due to their morphology and biology are divided grossly into two groups. The first group, the well differentiated thyroid cancers, which include the papillary thyroid carcinoma (PTC) and the follicular thyroid carcinoma (FTC) are usually slow growing, characterized by iodine intake and susceptible to TSH-suppressive therapy [5-7]. The PTC accounts for approximately up to 80% of thyroid tumours, whereas the FTC accounts for 5-15% of diagnosed thyroid malignancies [8]. These cancers are usually curable utilizing combined surgical and radioiodine therapy in contrast to the anaplastic thyroid cancer (ATC), which represents the poorly differentiated thyroid cancers [7]. ATC comprises only 1-2% of all diagnosed thyroid malignancies, but is characterized by

rapid and invasive growth resulting in fulminant disease course and poor outcome [7,9]. In thyroid, approximately 5% of thyroid malignancies are diagnosed as medullary carcinoma, which in turn originates from the parafollicular C cells [7].

All the above mentioned histological variants of thyroid carcinomas may be easily distinguished upon histopathological examination, however in case of FTC problems may occur in distinguishing these tumors from benign follicular adenomas (FA) and follicular variants of PTC (FVPTC) [6]. In case of FTC and FA the differential diagnosis is made by identification of signs of invasiveness into the tumour capsule in numerous serial hematoxyline and eosine stained slides. This renders the fine-needle aspirates (FNA) of thyroid follicular nodules useless for diagnostic purposes and biopsies not allowing for determination of the lesions malignant potential are determined as of indeterminate significance [5]. Up to 40% of FNA are regarded as indeterminate and subsequently the majority of the patients undergo surgery, but only the minority of the resected thyroid nodules are classified as malignant [10-14]. Moreover, no immunohistochemical markers of invasiveness in FNA have been so far discovered [5,15]. Molecular testing of FNA and resected thyroid specimens may be of value, but none of the recently discovered mutations in thyroid tissue is widely used in the clinical practice [7,16].

* Correspondence: piotr.dziegiel@am.wroc.pl
[1]Department of Histology and Embryology, Medical University in Wroclaw, Wroclaw, Poland
[3]Department of Physiotherapy, Wroclaw University School of Physical Education in Wroclaw, Wroclaw, Poland
Full list of author information is available at the end of the article

Recent progress in molecular methods resulted in better understanding of the biology of thyroid tumours. It seems that metallothioneins (MTs), due to their characteristic properties may help in the differential diagnosis of thyroid tumours and patients management. This review presents the current knowledge regarding their expression in benign, as well as malignant thyroid lesions.

Metallothionein structure, synthesis and biological functions

MTs are low molecular weight proteins (6-7kDa), which are expressed in almost all types of organisms [17-19]. MTs were first isolated in 1957 from horse renal cortex and since then our knowledge concerning these highly conserved proteins have evolved [18,20]. All MTs posses a highly conserved amino acid sequence and MTs isolated from different animal species show little structural changes. A single MT molecule consists of 61-68 amino acids, depending on the isoform, where up to one third of proteins sequence is composed of cysteine (Cys) residues [17,21]. Interestingly, this residues are organized in typical tandem sequences, with up to two other amino acids occurring between two cysteins [21]. Due to such high cysteine content, MT possess the ability to bind up to seven bivalent metal ions, such as zinc, copper, mercury, lead [19], Moreover, MTs may bind up to twelve univalent metal ions [19,22].

In the overall structure of MTs two domains have been recognized, the domain α and β [23]. The domain α comprises amino acids 31-68 and is located on the C-terminal edge, whereas the N-terminal domain β comprises amino acids 1-30 [20]. The latter due to its highest antigencity is used for production of antibodies, but due to high homology of particular MT isoforms, the utility of such obtained antibodies in distinguishing particular MT isoforms is therefore highly limited [20,24,25]. Although, MTs form a homogenous group of proteins (according to their amino acid sequence and overall structure leading to charge differences), four principal isoforms could be distinguished: MT-1, MT-2, MT-3 and MT-4 [26]. Most of our knowledge concerning MTs biology stems from research directed on examination of the MT-1 and MT-2 isoforms (MT-1/2), which are ubiquitously expressed in almost all cells of the organism [27]. Expression of MT-3 at first seemed to be more specific and restricted only to neurons and was first isolated from rat brain extracts suffering to experimental Alzheimer disease [28-30]. MT-3 is also known under the synonym growth inhibitory factor (GIF) as it experimentally blocked the regeneration of neurons in injured nervous tissue [30]. Recent studies have brought more insights into the biology of this protein, as it was also found to be expressed in some normal tissues as well as in different tumour types [31-37]. The expression of MT-4 seems to be restricted only to

squamous epithelium of the skin and upper parts of the alimentary tract [38].

MTs are encoded by 17 genes located within the 16q13 region, from which 13 code for MT-1, two for MT-2 and one gene each coding for MT-3 and MT-4 [26,38,39]. However, at least 10 genes code for functional MT proteins: MT-1A, MT-1B, MT-1E, MT-1F, MT-1G, MT-1H, MT-1X, MT-2A, MT-3 and MT-4 [24,26]. Beside the functional isoforms, there were also seven non-functional isoforms identified: MT-1C, MT-1D, MT-1I, MT-1J, MT-1K, MT-1L and MT-2B [26,40]. MTs were found to be localized in cells cytoplasm, as well as in cell nucleus [20,41]. Isoforms of the MT-1 and MT-2 family were shown to be induced by several substances and agents e.g. heavy metals, steroids, cytokines, growth factors and free radicals [42-46]. Zinc ion seems to represent the natural biological compound responsible for the induction of MTs expression. Zinc ions bind to the metal response element-binding transcription factor (MTF-1), which interacts *via* its zinc finger domains with a particular DNA region - the so called metal response element (MRE). Binding of MTF-1 to MRE results in initiation of MT-1/2 gene transcription [47-49]. Metal ions, other than zinc, induce MT-1/2 expression independently of the binding to the MTF-1 transcription factor as they may not activate this protein. However, these metal ions possess higher affinity to MT-1/2 proteins as compared to zinc ions, what results with the release of the latter to the cytoplasm. As result, free zinc ions bind to the MTF-1, what activates the transcription of MT-1/2 genes [50-52]. Similar mechanism is observed during oxidative stress, in which MTs oxidation by hydrogen peroxide (H_2O_2) leads to release of zinc ions from these proteins [53,54]. Regulation of MTs expression by glucocorticoid hormones is regulated independently of the above mentioned mechanism, as glucocorticoid receptors bind to the specific regulatory sequence (GRE; glucocorticoid response element) in the promoter region of MTs genes activating their transcription [27,55]. MTs expression may be also induced during stress conditions *via* the antioxidant response element (ARE) [17,56,57].

Although, MT-3 shows approximately 70% sequence similarity to other MTs, however there are some differences in its structure, what might reflect its functional diversity in comparison to other MTs. MT-3 posses a glutamate-rich hexapeptide near the C-terminus and contains a CPCP (Cys-Pro-Cys-Pro) motif (amino acids 6-9), which is absent in other MTs [29,58]. This might be reflected by the unique growth inhibitory role of MT-3, not apparent in other MTs [28-30,58].

Metallothioneins in neoplasia

Lines of evidence point to significant role of MTs of the MT-1 and MT-2 isoforms in development and progression of numerous neoplastic diseases [18,41,59,60]. Due to the metal binding properties of MTs, these proteins may act as possible zinc ions donors for zinc-dependent enzymes and transcription factors, which play crucial role in processes such as replication, transcription and translation [18,61]. It was shown, that in inactive cells (G0 phase) MTs can be detected in the cytoplasm, whereas in cells undergoing division MTs are shifted to the nucleus. In addition, the high cytoplasmic expression of MTs is noted at the end of G1 phase and at the G1/S threshold, while the highest MTs concentration in cell nucleus was noted in the S and G2 phases [62,63]. The translocation of MTs into the nucleus during G1/S phase in tumour cells suggests that MTs facilitates cell proliferation by donating zinc ions to various transcription factors. Moreover, numerous reports based on immunohistochemical methods seemed to confirm the results obtained *in vitro* suggesting the role o MTs in cell cycle regulation, as MTs expression was detected in the cell cytoplasm and nucleus in organs undergoing growth or regeneration (e.g. liver, kidney and parabasal cells of stratified epithelium) [64-67]. In addition, MTs overexpression is frequently observed in various malignancies (epithelial as well as mesenchymal tumours) and in some cases increased with growing malignancy grade of those tumours [20,24,66-75]. Lines of evidence suggest, that MTs may diminish the suppressor function of the p53 protein leading to uncontrolled growth and proliferation [61,76]. Numerous experimental data have, shown a positive correlation of MT expression and Ki-67 or PCNA (proliferating cell nuclear antigen) antigens in human tumour tissues, supporting the pro-proliferative role of MTs [24,25,59,68,69,77,78].

Higher expression of MTs in human tumours was also linked to increased chemoresistance of some tumour types (e.g. gastric, ovarian, breast cancer), as it levels increased after chemotherapy with agents such as cisplatin, bleomycin, irinotecan or cyclophosphamide [41,79-81]. Due to the structure of MTs, they may diminish the effects of agents inducing the oxidative stress (daunorubicin, doxorubicin), in mechanism involving inactivation of free radicals [20,82]. Thanks to the high affinity of MTs to metal ions, these proteins may also inactivate alkylating drugs, characterized by cytotoxic effects dependent on heavy metal compounds (e.g. cisplatin, carboplatin) [83]. Several studies have shown that MTs may mediate cancer cells chemoresistance in human malignant tumours characterized by MTs overexpression [79,81,84-86]. Moreover, free radicals scavenging properties MTs may also take part in cancer cells resistance to radiotherapy [87].

Most of the studies have revealed, that MT-1/2 overexpression in malignant cells is associated with poor survival of patients with e.g. non-small cell lung cancer, intrahepatic cholangiocarcinoma, synovial sarcoma, renal cancer or melanoma [24,70,71,88-90]. However, some of the studies have showed that MTs in some tumour types do not yield any prognostic significance, or - in some case - were even associated with patients better prognosis [72,91]. Interestingly, in some studies MT-1G (hepatocellular and papillary thyroid cancer), MT-1F (colorectal cancer) and MT-3 (gastric and esophageal cancer) isoform were regarded as potent tumour suppressors [92-97]. In spite of many efforts, the role of MT-3 in neoplastic disease remains ambiguous and the results of the studies were frequently inconsistent [31,32,36,37,98,99]. Therefore it seems, that the role of particular metallothionein isoforms differ significantly and the utilization of MTs as potent prognostic factors in human cancers requires further research.

Metallothionein expression in thyroid tissues

First study regarding MTs expression in human thyroid tissue was performed by Nartney *et al.* in 1987, who used a polyclonal rabbit anti-MT antibody to examine the expression levels of MTs in surgically resected tumour samples and normal thyroid tissue biopsied from autopsy cases [100]. This pilot study revealed that in paraffin embedded tissues of normal thyroid, only 20% of analyzed cases expressed MTs in the nucleus of follicular thyroid cells, whereas a nuclear-cytoplasmic expression pattern of MT was noted in majority of the surgically resected tumour samples (91%) [100]. The results obtained by Nartney *et al.* regarding MTs expression in normal thyroid tissues were not in accordance with the results obtained by other studies, which showed that MTs expression is mostly downregulated in thyroid cancers when compared to normal thyroid follicular cells or benign lesions of the thyroid e.g. nodular goiter (Figure 1) [15,92,101,102]. These studies were performed either on paraffin-embedded tissues using immunohistochemistry or on fresh frozen material utilizing expression microarrays or real-time PCR. The latter allowed to distinguish the expression of particular functional MTs isoforms - data not possible to obtain with currently available antibodies due to the homogenous structure of MTs isoforms [92,101,102].

The microarray studies identified MT-1G gene expression as downregulated in PTC and FTC, supporting recent reports of MT-1G suppressor role in human colon and hepatocellular carcinoma [91-93,101,102]. Lines of evidence suggest that hypermethylation of gene promoters occurs frequently in thyroid cancers and may be responsible for altered expression of sodium-iodide symporter (NIS), proteins associated with adhesion or cell cycle [103-105]. Moreover, treatment of thyroid cancer cell lines with demethylating agents could restore the dedifferentiation of thyroid cancer cell lines and their ability to iodide uptake [105]. The decreased expression of

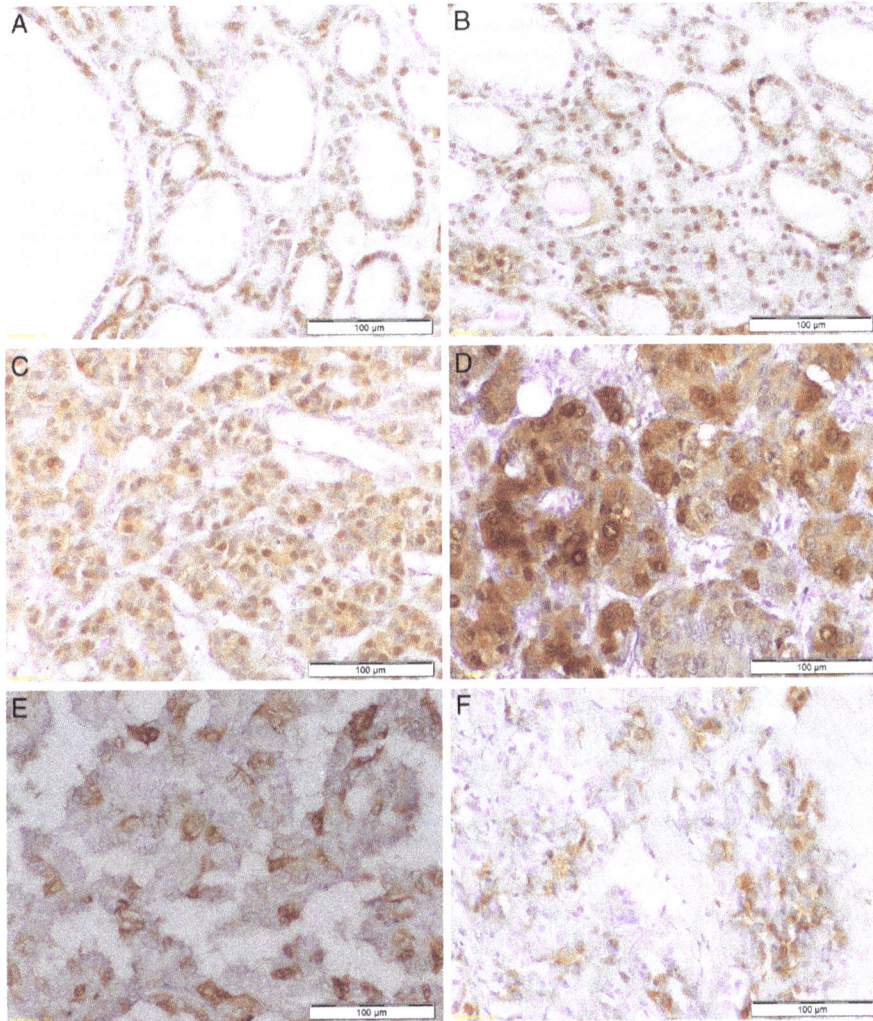

Figure 1 Differentiated nyclear cytoplasmic MT-1/2 expression in normal thyroid cells (A), nodular goiter (B), follicular adenoma (C), follicular carcinoma (D), papillary carcinoma (E) and medullary carcinoma (F). Magnification ×200.

MT-1G in PTC was caused by the hypermethylation of the CpG islands, but not the loss of heterozygosity (LOH) [103]. This observations were also confirmed on cell lines derived from human PTCs: NPA-87 (poorly differentiated), K1 and K2 (well-differentiated) [103,106,107]. The treatment of K2 cell line, which showed the highest level of methylation, with demethylating agent 5-aza-2'-deoxycytidene and/or trichostatin A (a histone deacetylase inhibitor) induced the higher expression level of MT-1G [103]. Similar results were described with the K1 cell line [92].

Beside the MT-1G, also MT-1H and MT-1X were shown to be downregulated in human PTC and FTC [92]. Also in the study of Finn *et al.*, it was demonstrated that in PTCs with classic morphology, as well as in the FVPTCs, MTs expression was downregulated what points to a potential application of MTs as markers of thyroid malignancy [101]. Nevertheless, also in this aspect

the biological significance of the above mentioned findings requires further research.

Biological significance of MTs expression in thyroid cancers

The biological importance of MTs expression was only assessed in relation to the MT-1G isoform in the study of Ferrario *et al.*, in which the expression of this isoform was restored in the K1 thyroid papillary cancer cell line with use of a MT-1G-myc expression plasmid [92]. MT-1G introduction into the K1 cell line resulted in reduced growth rate in respect to control cells subsequently leading to formation of smaller colonies. The suppressory role of MT-1G was additionally confirmed *in vivo* in athymic nude mice, as K1 cells with MT-1G expression yielded reduced tumour growth as compared to control cells [92]. Downregulation of MTs in PTC may be also partly responsible for decreased inactivation of reactive oxygen species observed in this tumour type, what might contribute to the carcinogenesis process [108,109].

Impact of MTs expression on carcinogenesis of thyroid cancer was also analysed in both studies of Liu *et al.* with regard to papillary (KAT5 cells) and anaplastic thyroid cancer (ARO cell line) [110,111]. In both studies the cell lines were subjected to treatment with cadmium ions (a potent inductor of MTs expression), in order to examine the impact of MTs isoforms on carcinogenesis. Cadmium treatment led to the induction of MT-1 and MT-2 isoforms in both cell lines, although differences in MT profile were observed [110,111]. In the KAT5 cells, the MT-1G and MT-2A levels were identified as being the most abundant isoforms upon cadmium treatment, whereas in the ARO cell line additionally the MT-1A, MT-1F, MT-1H, MT-1X were identified as the main functional isoforms [110,111]. Both studies have shown that induction of those isoforms was accompanied by alteration in the cell cycle leading to increase of proportion of cells in the S and G2-M phase and decrease in the proportion of cells in the G0/G1 phase [110,111]. Moreover, cadmium treatment resulted also in rise of calcium ions influx and led to a moderate rise in the phoshorylated ERK1/2 (extracellular signal-regulated kinase), both processes capable of stimulating cells proliferation [112]. Although, it was shown that the expression of MT-1G may alter proliferative response of KAT5 cells, the results of both studies should be taken with caution, because the study design did not allow clear assessment of MTs role in the observed cell cycle alterations [92,110,111]. Moreover, in our own study we did not observe any significant correlation between the expression of the MT-1/2 and the proliferation antigen Ki-67 in the series of PTC and FTC cases [15].

Clinical significance of MTs in thyroid

Although, the prognostic significance of MTs expression in thyroid cancer remains to be clarified, some of the obtained results may have potential to be to applied in clinical practice. Recent advance in molecular testing of thyroid carcinomas led to the identification of genes altered in particular type of the thyroid cancer [3,5,9,16]. It has become apparent that PTC and FTC harbour different mutations. PTC is characterized by the mutations in the RAS and BRAF genes as well as by rearrangements of the RET/PTC genes capable of activating the mitogen activated kinase (MAPK) pathway. In FTC alterations in the RAS gene and PAX8/PPARγ rearrangements were identified in majority of the cases [16]. However, these mutations were also shown to occur in benign thyroid lesions. This fact, on one hand confirms the multistep carcinogenesis process in the thyroid, but on the other may render difficulties in introducing these new findings

into clinical practice [7]. MTs expression shown as downregulated in majority of the thyroid cancer studies, could be used as an ancillary marker helping in differential diagnosis of indeterminate FNA or surgical specimens of thyroid lesions [15,92,101-103]. We have recently shown that immunohistochemical examination of MT-1/2 expression may be of use in differentiating FA from FTC, which are impossible to distinguish in FNA examination [6,8]. The higher expression of MT-1/2 observed in FTC as compared to FA may be of clinical importance, although this finding must be confirmed on a larger patients cohort with establishing proper cut-off points for the diagnosis [15]. Moreover, the pronounced expression of MT-1/2 in FTC may be linked to resistance to radiotherapy.

Conclusions

MTs due to their wide functional properties, potentially associated with progression of majority of human cancers may pose an interesting point of research in relation to human malignant thyroid lesions.

Competing interests

The authors declare that no competing financial interests exist.

Authors' contributions

All the authors drafted the manuscript. All the authors read and approved the final manuscript.

Acknowledgements

This work was supported by the scientific grant of Wroclaw Medical University, No. ST-442.

Author details

[1]Department of Histology and Embryology, Medical University in Wroclaw, Wroclaw, Poland. [2]Department of General, Gastroenterological and Endocrinological Surgery, Medical University in Wroclaw, Wroclaw, Poland. [3]Department of Physiotherapy, Wroclaw University School of Physical Education in Wroclaw, Wroclaw, Poland.

References

1. Patel KN, Shaha AR: **Poorly differentiated and anaplastic thyroid cancer.** *Cancer Control* 2006, **13**:119–128.
2. Siegel R, Naishadham D, Jemal A: **Cancer statistics, 2012.** *CA Cancer J Clin* 2012, **62**:10–29.
3. Smallridge RC, Marlow LA, Copland JA: **Anaplastic thyroid cancer: molecular pathogenesis and emerging therapies.** *Endocr Relat Cancer* 2009, **16**:17–44.
4. Davies L, Welch HG: **Increasing incidence of thyroid cancer in the United States, 1973-2002.** *JAMA* 2006, **295**:2164–2167.
5. LiVolsi VA: **Papillary thyroid carcinoma: an update.** *Mod Pathol* 2011, **24**(Suppl 2):S1–9.
6. Sobrinho-Simoes M, Eloy C, Magalhaes J, Lobo C, Amaro T: **Follicular thyroid carcinoma.** *Mod Pathol* 2011, **24**(Suppl 2):S10–18.
7. Catalano MG, Poli R, Pugliese M, Fortunati N, Boccuzzi G: **Emerging molecular therapies of advanced thyroid cancer.** *Mol Aspects Med* 2010, **31**:215–226.
8. Mazzaferri EL: **Thyroid cancer in thyroid nodules: finding a needle in the haystack.** *Am J Med* 1992, **93**:359–362.
9. Smallridge RC, Copland JA: **Anaplastic thyroid carcinoma: pathogenesis and emerging therapies.** *Clin Oncol (R Coll Radiol)* 2010, **22**:486–497.
10. Cooper DS, Doherty GM, Haugen BR, Kloos RT, Lee SL, Mandel SJ, Mazzaferri EL, McIver B, Pacini F, Schlumberger M, Sherman SI, Steward DL, Tuttle RM:

Revised American Thyroid Association management guidelines for patients with thyroid nodules and differentiated thyroid cancer. *Thyroid* 2009, 19:1167–1214.

11. Cooper DS, Doherty GM, Haugen BR, Kloos RT, Lee SL, Mandel SJ, Mazzaferri EL, McIver B, Sherman SI, Tuttle RM: **Management guidelines for patients with thyroid nodules and differentiated thyroid cancer.** *Thyroid* 2006, 16:109–142.

12. Sclabas GM, Staerkel GA, Shapiro SE, Fornage BD, Sherman SI, Vassillopoulou-Sellin R, Lee JE, Evans DB: **Fine-needle aspiration of the thyroid and correlation with histopathology in a contemporary series of 240 patients.** *Am J Surg* 2003, 186:702–709. discussion 709-710.

13. Greaves TS, Olvera M, Florentine BD, Raza AS, Cobb CJ, Tsao-Wei DD, Groshen S, Singer P, Lopresti J, Martin SE: **Follicular lesions of thyroid: a 5-year fine-needle aspiration experience.** *Cancer* 2000, 90:335–341.

14. Alexander EK, Kennedy GC, Baloch ZW, Cibas ES, Chudova D, Diggans J, Friedman L, Kloos RT, LiVolsi VA, Mandel SJ, Raab SS, Rosai J, Steward DL, Walsh PS, Wilde JI, Zeiger MA, Lanman RB, Haugen BR: **Preoperative diagnosis of benign thyroid nodules with indeterminate cytology.** *N Engl J Med* 2012, 367:705–715.

15. Krolicka A, Kobierzycki C, Pula B, Podhorska-Okolow M, Piotrowska A, Rzeszutko M, Rzeszutko W, Rabczynski J, Domoslawski P, Wojtczak B, Dawiskiba J, Dziegiel P: **Comparison of metallothionein (MT) and Ki-67 antigen expression in benign and malignant thyroid tumours.** *Anticancer Res* 2010, 30:4945–4949.

16. Nikiforov YE: **Molecular analysis of thyroid tumors.** *Mod Pathol* 2011, 24(Suppl 2):S34–43.

17. Vasak M, Meloni G: **Chemistry and biology of mammalian metallothioneins.** *J Biol Inorg Chem* 2011, 16:1067–1078.

18. Pedersen MO, Larsen A, Stoltenberg M, Penkowa M: **The role of metallothionein in oncogenesis and cancer prognosis.** *Prog Histochem Cytochem* 2009, 44:29–64.

19. Coyle P, Philcox JC, Carey LC, Rofe AM: **Metallothionein: the multipurpose protein.** *Cell Mol Life Sci* 2002, 59:627–647.

20. Dziegiel P: **Expression of metallothioneins in tumor cells.** *Pol J Pathol* 2004, 55:3–12.

21. Vasak M: **Advances in metallothionein structure and functions.** *J Trace Elem Med Biol* 2005, 19:13–17.

22. Palmiter RD: **The elusive function of metallothioneins.** *Proc Natl Acad Sci USA* 1998, 95:8428–8430.

23. Zangger K, Shen G, Oz G, Otvos JD, Armitage IM: **Oxidative dimerization in metallothionein is a result of intermolecular disulphide bonds between cysteines in the alpha-domain.** *Biochem J* 2001, 359:353–360.

24. Werynska B, Pula B, Muszczynska-Bernhard B, Gomulkiewicz A, Piotrowska A, Prus R, Podhorska-Okolow M, Jankowska R, Dziegiel P: **Metallothionein 1F and 2A overexpression predicts poor outcome of non-small cell lung cancer patients.** *Exp Mol Pathol* 2012, doi:pii: S0014-4800(12)00153-0. 10.1016/j.yexmp.2012.10.006. [Epub ahead of print].

25. Werynska B, Pula B, Muszczynska-Bernhard B, Piotrowska A, Jethon A, Podhorska-Okolow M, Dziegiel P, Jankowska R: **Correlation between expression of metallothionein and expression of Ki-67 and MCM-2 proliferation markers in non-small cell lung cancer.** *Anticancer Res* 2011, 31:2833–2839.

26. Mididoddi S, McGuirt JP, Sens MA, Todd JH, Sens DA: **Isoform-specific expression of metallothionein mRNA in the developing and adult human kidney.** *Toxicol Lett* 1996, 85:17–27.

27. Davis SR, Cousins RJ: **Metallothionein expression in animals: a physiological perspective on function.** *J Nutr* 2000, 130:1085–1088.

28. Uchida Y: **Growth-inhibitory factor, metallothionein-like protein, and neurodegenerative diseases.** *Biol Signals* 1994, 3:211–215.

29. Uchida Y, Takio K, Titani K, Ihara Y, Tomonaga M: **The growth inhibitory factor that is deficient in the Alzheimer's disease brain is a 68 amino acid metallothionein-like protein.** *Neuron* 1991, 7:337–347.

30. Uchida Y, Tomonaga M: **Neurotrophic action of Alzheimer's disease brain extract is due to the loss of inhibitory factors for survival and neurite formation of cerebral cortical neurons.** *Brain Res* 1989, 481:190–193.

31. Garrett SH, Park S, Sens MA, Somji S, Singh RK, Namburi VB, Sens DA: **Expression of metallothioein isoform 3 is restricted at the post-transcriptional level in human bladder epithelial cells.** *Toxicol Sci* 2005, 87:66–74.

32. Garrett SH, Sens MA, Shukla D, Nestor S, Somji S, Todd JH, Sens DA: **Metallothionein isoform 3 expression in the human prostate and cancer-derived cell lines.** *Prostate* 1999, 41:196–202.

33. Garrett SH, Sens MA, Todd JH, Somji S, Sens DA: **Expression of MT-3 protein in the human kidney.** *Toxicol Lett* 1999, 105:207–214.

34. Hoey JG, Garrett SH, Sens MA, Todd JH, Sens DA: **Expression of MT-3 mRNA in human kidney, proximal tubule cell cultures, and renal cell carcinoma.** *Toxicol Lett* 1997, 92:149–160.

35. Kim D, Garrett SH, Sens MA, Somji S, Sens DA: **Metallothionein isoform 3 and proximal tubule vectorial active transport.** *Kidney Int* 2002, 61:464–472.

36. Sens MA, Somji S, Garrett SH, Beall CL, Sens DA: **Metallothionein isoform 3 overexpression is associated with breast cancers having a poor prognosis.** *Am J Pathol* 2001, 159:21–26.

37. Sens MA, Somji S, Lamm DL, Garrett SH, Slovinsky F, Todd JH, Sens DA: **Metallothionein isoform 3 as a potential biomarker for human bladder cancer.** *Environ Health Perspect* 2000, 108:413–418.

38. Quaife CJ, Findley SD, Erickson JC, Froelick GJ, Kelly EJ, Zambrowicz BP, Palmiter RD: **Induction of a new metallothionein isoform (MT-IV) occurs during differentiation of stratified squamous epithelia.** *Biochemistry* 1994, 33:7250–7259.

39. Palmiter RD, Findley SD, Whitmore TE, Durnam DM: **MT-III, a brain-specific member of the metallothionein gene family.** *Proc Natl Acad Sci USA* 1992, 89:6333–6337.

40. Stennard FA, Holloway AF, Hamilton J, West AK: **Characterisation of six additional human metallothionein genes.** *Biochim Biophys Acta* 1994, 1218:357–365.

41. Cherian MG, Jayasurya A, Bay BH: **Metallothioneins in human tumors and potential roles in carcinogenesis.** *Mutat Res* 2003, 533:201–209.

42. Haq F, Mahoney M, Koropatnick J: **Signaling events for metallothionein induction.** *Mutat Res* 2003, 533:211–226.

43. Ghoshal K, Jacob ST: **Regulation of metallothionein gene expression.** *Prog Nucleic Acid Res Mol Biol* 2001, 66:357–384.

44. Ghoshal K, Majumder S, Li Z, Bray TM, Jacob ST: **Transcriptional induction of metallothionein-I and -II genes in the livers of Cu, Zn-superoxide dismutase knockout mice.** *Biochem Biophys Res Commun* 1999, 264:735–742.

45. Ghoshal K, Wang Y, Sheridan JF, Jacob ST: **Metallothionein induction in response to restraint stress. Transcriptional control, adaptation to stress, and role of glucocorticoid.** *J Biol Chem* 1998, 273:27904–27910.

46. Jacob ST, Ghoshal K, Sheridan JF: **Induction of metallothionein by stress and its molecular mechanisms.** *Gene Expr* 1999, 7:301–310.

47. Saydam N, Adams TK, Steiner F, Schaffner W, Freedman JH: **Regulation of metallothionein transcription by the metal-responsive transcription factor MTF-1: identification of signal transduction cascades that control metal-inducible transcription.** *J Biol Chem* 2002, 277:20438–20445.

48. Otsuka F, Okugaito I, Ohsawa M, Iwamatsu A, Suzuki K, Koizumi S: **Novel responses of ZRF, a variant of human MTF-1, to in vivo treatment with heavy metals.** *Biochim Biophys Acta* 2000, 1492:330–340.

49. Langmade SJ, Ravindra R, Daniels PJ, Andrews GK: **The transcription factor MTF-1 mediates metal regulation of the mouse ZnT1 gene.** *J Biol Chem* 2000, 275:34803–34809.

50. Murata M, Gong P, Suzuki K, Koizumi S: **Differential metal response and regulation of human heavy metal-inducible genes.** *J Cell Physiol* 1999, 180:105–113.

51. Koizumi S, Suzuki K, Ogra Y, Yamada H, Otsuka F: **Transcriptional activity and regulatory protein binding of metal-responsive elements of the human metallothionein-IIA gene.** *Eur J Biochem* 1999, 259:635–642.

52. Lichtlen P, Schaffner W: **The "metal transcription factor" MTF-1: biological facts and medical implications.** *Swiss Med Wkly* 2001, 131:647–652.

53. Nguyen T, Sherratt PJ, Pickett CB: **Regulatory mechanisms controlling gene expression mediated by the antioxidant response element.** *Annu Rev Pharmacol Toxicol* 2003, 43:233–260.

54. Andrews GK: **Regulation of metallothionein gene expression by oxidative stress and metal ions.** *Biochem Pharmacol* 2000, 59:95–104.

55. Hernandez J, Carrasco J, Belloso E, Giralt M, Bluethmann H, Kee Lee D, Andrews GK, Hidalgo J: **Metallothionein induction by restraint stress: role of glucocorticoids and IL-6.** *Cytokine* 2000, 12:791–796.

56. Bi Y, Palmiter RD, Wood KM, Ma Q: **Induction of metallothionein I by phenolic antioxidants requires metal-activated transcription factor 1 (MTF-1) and zinc.** *Biochem J* 2004, 380:695–703.

57. Campagne MV, Thibodeaux H, van Bruggen N, Cairns B, Lowe DG: **Increased binding activity at an antioxidant-responsive element in the metallothionein-1 promoter and rapid induction of metallothionein-1**

and -2 in response to cerebral ischemia and reperfusion. *J Neurosci* 2000, **20**:5200–5207.

58. Ding ZC, Ni FY, Huang ZX: Neuronal growth-inhibitory factor (metallothionein-3): structure-function relationships. *FEBS J* 2010, **277**:2912–2920.

59. Dziegiel P, Dumanska M, Forgacz J, Wojna A, Zabel M: Intensity of apoptosis as related to the expression of metallothionein (MT), caspase-3 (cas-3) and Ki-67 antigen and the survival time of patients with primary colorectal adenocarcinomas. *Rocz Akad Med Bialymst* 2004, **49**(Suppl 1):5–7.

60. Nielsen AE, Bohr A, Penkowa M: The balance between life and death of cells: roles of metallothioneins. *Biomark Insights* 2007, **1**:99–111.

61. Ostrakhovitch EA, Olsson PE, von Hofsten J, Cherian MG: P53 mediated regulation of metallothionein transcription in breast cancer cells. *J Cell Biochem* 2007, **102**:1571–1583.

62. Cherian MG, Apostolova MD: Nuclear localization of metallothionein during cell proliferation and differentiation. *Cell Mol Biol (Noisy-le-Grand)* 2000, **46**:347–356.

63. Levadoux-Martin M, Hesketh JE, Beattie JH, Wallace HM: Influence of metallothionein-1 localization on its function. *Biochem J* 2001, **355**:473–479.

64. Zalups RK, Fraser J, Koropatnick J: Enhanced transcription of metallothionein genes in rat kidney: effect of uninephrectomy and compensatory renal growth. *Am J Physiol* 1995, **268**:F643–650.

65. Cherian MG, Kang YJ: Metallothionein and liver cell regeneration. *Exp Biol Med (Maywood)* 2006, **231**:138–144.

66. Zamirska A, Matusiak L, Dziegiel P, Szybejko-Machaj G, Szepietowski JC: Expression of metallothioneins in cutaneous squamous cell carcinoma and actinic keratosis. *Pathol Oncol Res* 2012, **18**:849–855.

67. Bieniek A, Pula B, Piotrowska A, Podhorska-Okolow M, Salwa A, Koziol M, Dziegiel P: Expression of metallothionein I/II and Ki-67 antigen in various histological types of basal cell carcinoma. *Folia Histochem Cytobiol* 2012, **50**:352–357.

68. Gomulkiewicz A, Podhorska-Okolow M, Szulc R, Smorag Z, Wojnar A, Zabel M, Dziegiel P: Correlation between metallothionein (MT) expression and selected prognostic factors in ductal breast cancers. *Folia Histochem Cytobiol* 2010, **48**:242–248.

69. Wojnar A, Pula B, Piotrowska A, Jethon A, Kujawa K, Kobierzycki C, Rys J, Podhorska-Okolow M, Dziegiel P: Correlation of intensity of MT-I/II expression with Ki-67 and MCM-2 proteins in invasive ductal breast carcinoma. *Anticancer Res* 2011, **31**:3027–3033.

70. Dziegiel P, Jelen M, Muszczynska B, Maciejczyk A, Szulc A, Podhorska-Okolow M, Cegielski M, Zabel M: Role of metallothionein expression in non-small cell lung carcinomas. *Rocz Akad Med Bialymst* 2004, **49**(Suppl 1):43–45.

71. Dziegiel P, Suder E, Surowiak P, Kornafel J, Zabel M: Expression of metallothionein in synovial sarcoma cells. *Appl Immunohistochem Mol Morphol* 2002, **10**:357–362.

72. Pastuszewski W, Dziegiel P, Krecicki T, Podhorska-Okolow M, Ciesielska U, Gorzynska E, Zabel M: Prognostic significance of metallothionein, p53 protein and Ki-67 antigen expression in laryngeal cancer. *Anticancer Res* 2007, **27**:335–342.

73. Surowiak P, Matkowski R, Materna V, Gyorffy B, Wojnar A, Pudelko M, Dziegiel P, Kornafel J, Zabel M: Elevated metallothionein (MT) expression in invasive ductal breast cancers predicts tamoxifen resistance. *Histol Histopathol* 2005, **20**:1037–1044.

74. Szelachowska J, Dziegiel P, Jelen-Krzeszewska J, Jelen M, Tarkowski R, Spytkowska B, Matkowski R, Kornafel J: Correlation of metallothionein expression with clinical progression of cancer in the oral cavity. *Anticancer Res* 2009, **29**:589–595.

75. Szelachowska J, Dziegiel P, Jelen-Krzeszewska J, Jelen M, Tarkowski R, Wlodarska I, Spytkowska B, Gisterek I, Matkowski R, Kornafel J: Prognostic significance of nuclear and cytoplasmic expression of metallothioneins as related to proliferative activity in squamous cell carcinomas of oral cavity. *Histol Histopathol* 2008, **23**:843–851.

76. Fan LZ, Cherian MG: Potential role of p53 on metallothionein induction in human epithelial breast cancer cells. *Br J Cancer* 2002, **87**:1019–1026.

77. Hengstler JG, Pilch H, Schmidt M, Dahlenburg H, Sagemuller J, Schiffer I, Oesch F, Knapstein PG, Kaina B, Tanner B: Metallothionein expression in ovarian cancer in relation to histopathological parameters and molecular markers of prognosis. *Int J Cancer* 2001, **95**:121–127.

78. Dziegiel P, Salwa-Zurawska W, Zurawski J, Wojnar A, Zabel M: Prognostic significance of augmented metallothionein (MT) expression correlated

79. Chun JH, Kim HK, Kim E, Kim IH, Kim JH, Chang HJ, Choi IJ, Lim HS, Kim IJ, Kang HC, Park JH, Bae JM, Park JG: Increased expression of metallothionein is associated with irinotecan resistance in gastric cancer. *Cancer Res* 2004, **64**:4703–4706.

80. Dutta R, Sens DA, Somji S, Sens MA, Garrett SH: Metallothionein isoform 3 expression inhibits cell growth and increases drug resistance of PC-3 prostate cancer cells. *Prostate* 2002, **52**:89–97.

81. Surowiak P, Materna V, Maciejczyk A, Pudelko M, Markwitz E, Spaczynski M, Dietel M, Zabel M, Lage H: Nuclear metallothionein expression correlates with cisplatin resistance of ovarian cancer cells and poor clinical outcome. *Virchows Arch* 2007, **450**:279–285.

82. Cai L, Cherian MG: Zinc-metallothionein protects from DNA damage induced by radiation better than glutathione and copper- or cadmium-metallothioneins. *Toxicol Lett* 2003, **136**:193–198.

83. Shimoda R, Achanzar WE, Qu W, Nagamine T, Takagi H, Mori M, Waalkes MP: Metallothionein is a potential negative regulator of apoptosis. *Toxicol Sci* 2003, **73**:294–300.

84. Surowiak P, Materna V, Kaplenko I, Spaczynski M, Dietel M, Lage H, Zabel M: Augmented expression of metallothionein and glutathione S-transferase pi as unfavourable prognostic factors in cisplatin-treated ovarian cancer patients. *Virchows Arch* 2005, **447**:626–633.

85. Yap X, Tan HY, Huang J, Lai Y, Yip GW, Tan PH, Bay BH: Over-expression of metallothionein predicts chemoresistance in breast cancer. *J Pathol* 2009, **217**:563–570.

86. Smith DJ, Jaggi M, Zhang W, Galich A, Du C, Sterrett SP, Smith LM, Balaji KC: Metallothioneins and resistance to cisplatin and radiation in prostate cancer. *Urology* 2006, **67**:1341–1347.

87. Cai L, Satoh M, Tohyama C, Cherian MG: Metallothionein in radiation exposure: its induction and protective role. *Toxicology* 1999, **132**:85–98.

88. Schmitz KJ, Lang H, Kaiser G, Wohlschlaeger J, Sotiropoulos GC, Baba HA, Jasani B, Schmid KW: Metallothionein overexpression and its prognostic relevance in intrahepatic cholangiocarcinoma and extrahepatic hilar cholangiocarcinoma (Klatskin tumors). *Hum Pathol* 2009, **40**:1706–1714.

89. Weinlich G, Zelger B: Metallothionein overexpression, a highly significant prognostic factor in thin melanoma. *Histopathology* 2007, **51**:280–283.

90. Tuzel E, Kirkali Z, Yorukoglu K, Mungan MU, Sade M: Metallothionein expression in renal cell carcinoma: subcellular localization and prognostic significance. *J Urol* 2001, **165**:1710–1713.

91. Arriaga JM, Levy EM, Bravo AI, Bayo SM, Amat M, Aris M, Hannois A, Bruno L, Roberti MP, Loria FS, Pairola A, Huertas E, Mordoh J, Bianchini M: Metallothionein expression in colorectal cancer: relevance of different isoforms for tumor progression and patient survival. *Hum Pathol* 2012, **43**:197–208.

92. Ferrario C, Lavagni P, Gariboldi M, Miranda C, Losa M, Cleris L, Formelli F, Pilotti S, Pierotti MA, Greco A: Metallothionein 1G acts as an oncosupressor in papillary thyroid carcinoma. *Lab Invest* 2008, **88**:474–481.

93. Kanda M, Nomoto S, Okamura Y, Nishikawa Y, Sugimoto H, Kanazumi N, Takeda S, Nakao A: Detection of metallothionein 1G as a methylated tumor suppressor gene in human hepatocellular carcinoma using a novel method of double combination array analysis. *Int J Oncol* 2009, **35**:477–483.

94. Smith E, Drew PA, Tian ZQ, De Young NJ, Liu JF, Mayne GC, Ruszkiewicz AR, Watson DI, Jamieson GG: Metallothionien 3 expression is frequently down-regulated in oesophageal squamous cell carcinoma by DNA methylation. *Mol Cancer* 2005, **4**:42.

95. Deng D, El-Rifai W, Ji J, Zhu B, Trampont P, Li J, Smith MF, Powel SM: Hypermethylation of metallothionein-3 CpG island in gastric carcinoma. *Carcinogenesis* 2003, **24**:25–29.

96. Yan DW, Fan JW, Yu ZH, Li MX, Wen YG, Li DW, Zhou CZ, Wang XL, Wang Q, Tang HM, Peng ZH: Downregulation of metallothionein 1F, a putative oncosuppressor, by loss of heterozygosity in colon cancer tissue. *Biochim Biophys Acta* 2012, **1822**:918–926.

97. Peng D, Hu TL, Jiang A, Washington MK, Moskaluk CA, Schneider-Stock R, El-Rifai W: Location-specific epigenetic regulation of the metallothionein 3 gene in esophageal adenocarcinomas. *PLoS One* 2011, **6**:e22009.

98. Gurel V, Sens DA, Somji S, Garrett SH, Nath J, Sens MA: Stable transfection and overexpression of metallothionein isoform 3 inhibits the growth of MCF-7 and Hs578T cells but not that of T-47D or MDA-MB-231 cells. *Breast Cancer Res Treat* 2003, **80**:181–191.

99. Somji S, Garrett SH, Sens MA, Gurel V, Sens DA: Expression of metallothionein isoform 3 (MT-3) determines the choice between apoptotic or necrotic cell death in Cd+2-exposed human proximal tubule cells. *Toxicol Sci* 2004, **80**:358–366.

100. Nartey N, Cherian MG, Banerjee D: Immunohistochemical localization of metallothionein in human thyroid tumors. *Am J Pathol* 1987, **129**:177–182.

101. Finn SP, Smyth P, Cahill S, Streck C, O'Regan EM, Flavin R, Sherlock J, Howells D, Henfrey R, Cullen M, Toner M, Timon C, O'Leary JJ, Sheils OM: Expression microarray analysis of papillary thyroid carcinoma and benign thyroid tissue: emphasis on the follicular variant and potential markers of malignancy. *Virchows Arch* 2007, **450**:249–260.

102. Huang Y, Prasad M, Lemon WJ, Hampel H, Wright FA, Kornacker K, LiVolsi V, Frankel W, Kloos RT, Eng C, Pellegata NS, de la Chapelle A: Gene expression in papillary thyroid carcinoma reveals highly consistent profiles. *Proc Natl Acad Sci USA* 2001, **98**:15044–15049.

103. Huang Y, de la Chapelle A, Pellegata NS: Hypermethylation, but not LOH, is associated with the low expression of MT1G and CRABP1 in papillary thyroid carcinoma. *Int J Cancer* 2003, **104**:735–744.

104. Stephen JK, Chitale D, Narra V, Chen KM, Sawhney R, Worsham MJ: DNA methylation in thyroid tumorigenesis. *Cancers (Basel)* 2011, **3**:1732–1743.

105. Venkataraman GM, Yatin M, Marcinek R, Ain KB: Restoration of iodide uptake in dedifferentiated thyroid carcinoma: relationship to human Na+/I-symporter gene methylation status. *J Clin Endocrinol Metab* 1999, **84**:2449–2457.

106. Fagin JA, Matsuo K, Karmakar A, Chen DL, Tang SH, Koeffler HP: High prevalence of mutations of the p53 gene in poorly differentiated human thyroid carcinomas. *J Clin Invest* 1993, **91**:179–184.

107. Jones CJ, Shaw JJ, Wyllie FS, Gaillard N, Schlumberger M, Wynford-Thomas D: High frequency deletion of the tumour suppressor gene P16INK4a (MTS1) in human thyroid cancer cell lines. *Mol Cell Endocrinol* 1996, **116**:115–119.

108. Durak I, Bayram F, Kavutcu M, Canholat O, Ozturk HS: Impaired enzymatic antioxidant defense mechanism in cancerous human thyroid tissues. *J Endocrinol Invest* 1996, **19**:312–315.

109. Mano T, Shinohara R, Iwase K, Kotake M, Hamada M, Uchimuro K, Hayakawa N, Hayashi R, Nakai A, Ishizuki Y, Nagasaka A: Changes in free radical scavengers and lipid peroxide in thyroid glands of various thyroid disorders. *Horm Metab Res* 1997, **29**:351–354.

110. Liu ZM, Hasselt CA, Song FZ, Vlantis AC, Cherian MG, Koropatnick J, Chen GG: Expression of functional metallothionein isoforms in papillary thyroid cancer. *Mol Cell Endocrinol* 2009, **302**:92–98.

111. Liu ZM, Chen GG, Shum CK, Vlantis AC, Cherian MG, Koropatnick J, van Hasselt CA: Induction of functional MT1 and MT2 isoforms by calcium in anaplastic thyroid carcinoma cells. *FEBS Lett* 2007, **581**:2465–2472.

112. Dumaz N, Marais R: Integrating signals between cAMP and the RAS/RAF/MEK/ERK signalling pathways. Based on the anniversary prize of the Gesellschaft fur Biochemie und Molekularbiologie Lecture delivered on 5 July 2003 at the Special FEBS Meeting in Brussels. *FEBS J* 2005, **272**:3491–3504.

15

Metastatic carcinoma to the thyroid gland from renal cell carcinoma: role of ultrasonography in preoperative diagnosis

Kaoru Kobayashi[*], Mitsuyoshi Hirokawa, Tomonori Yabuta, Mitsuhiro Fukushima, Hiroo Masuoka, Takuya Higashiyama, Minoru Kihara, Yasuhiro Ito, Akihiro Miya, Nobuyuki Amino and Akira Miyauchi

Abstract

Background: Patients with metastases to the thyroid from renal cell carcinoma (RCC) that need surgical management are not many and unfamiliar to clinicians and thyroid endocrinologists. Therefore, little information is available on ultrasonographic features of metastatic carcinoma in the thyroid. The strategic value of ultrasound in preoperative surgical planning for patients with thyroid nodules has become increasingly appreciated. The purposes of this article are to clarify the ultrasound characteristics of metastatic carcinoma to the thyroid from RCC by evaluating many patients in one institute, and to investigate the role of ultrasonography in preoperative diagnosis.

Methods: Ten patients with these carcinomas who had undergone surgical management were investigated clinically and ultrasonographically. Ultrasonographic features to be evaluated were the form of involvement in the thyroid, size, shape, pattern, calcifications, vascularity, and tumor thrombus. Clinical features were previous history of RCC, serum thyroglobulin levels, cytology, preoperative diagnosis, and surgery.

Results: Ultrasonographic features of these carcinomas were more likely to involve a solitary, irregular, and solid without calcifications, and prominent intra-tumoral vascularity and tumor thrombus in the vein. These patients tended to be older, and to have relatively late recurrence in the thyroid, RCC in the right kidney as the primary site, and relatively low serum thyroglobulin levels.

Conclusions: Metastatic carcinomas to the thyroid from RCC presented highly characteristic features on ultrasonography. These ultrasonographic features combined with cytological findings and previous medical history of RCC can provide the optimal process for the preoperative diagnosis of such patients.

Keywords: Thyroid, Ultrasonography, Metastatic carcinoma, Renal cell carcinoma, Diagnosis, Tumor thrombus

Background

Metastases of renal cell carcinoma to multiple sites occur in the course of the disease and are generally regarded as the result of spread by a hematogenous route [1]. The thyroid gland is one of the metastatic sites from the primary lesion [1-3], but metastases to the thyroid that need surgical management are infrequent. It is reported that a surgical approach for such patients is associating with a favorable prognosis, when metastatic tumors are confined within the thyroid [1,3-6]. Therefore, preoperative diagnosis has clinical significance. Needless to say, previous medical history of renal cell carcinoma

and fine-needle aspiration cytology of thyroid tumors of such patients are important for preoperative diagnosis.

The strategic value of ultrasound in preoperative surgical planning of patients with thyroid nodules has become increasingly appreciated [7,8]. The ultrasonogaphic features of a metastatic tumor to the thyroid from renal cell carcinoma are unfamiliar to clinicians and thyroid endocrinologists because of the rarity of such patients. It is unclear whether the ultrasonogaphic features can be helpful in the preoperative diagnosis, in addition to characteristic findings of cytology and previous medical history of renal cell carcinoma.

In this article, we focus on the ultrasonographic features of metastatic carcinomas to the thyroid from renal

* Correspondence: kobayashi@kuma-h.or.jp
Kuma Hospital, 8-2-35 Shimoyamate-dori, Chuo-ku, Kobe-City 650-0011, Japan

cell carcinoma, and discuss the significance of ultrasound for the preoperative diagnosis of such patients.

Methods

We retrospectively reviewed the medical database of patients with thyroid malignancies who underwent surgery between January 1998 and December 2013 in Kuma Hospital. A total of 10 patients with metastatic carcinoma to the thyroid from renal cell carcinoma undergoing thyroid surgery were included in this study. Preoperative ultrasonography was performed in all patients who had thyroid surgery during this time period. The ultrasound readings that were used in this study were made as part of the care of the patients. Surgical samples of the thyroid, tumor thrombi, and lymph nodes were cut before fixation. Specimens were fixed in buffered formalin and embedded in paraffin, and HE and immunohistochemical staining was performed. All related pathological specimens were reviewed (by M.H.), and the histopathological diagnosis was included in this study. The preoperative ultrasound readings were confirmed visually by surgeons at surgery and histopathological examination postoperatively. The surgical findings and histopathological diagnosis were recorded in the medical database of the hospital. The ethics committee of Kuma Hspital approved the study protocol (US-RCC meta), which was in adherence to the Declaration of Helsinki.

Ultrasonographic examination was performed by well-trained, registered ultrasonographers, using a TOSHIBA Aplio SSA-770A ultrasound system with PLT-1204AX (7–14 MHz) and PLT-805AT (5–12 MHz) linear probes. We used both grayscale and power Doppler ultrasonography. Power Doppler ultrasonography was used predominantly to assess the vascularity of the thyroid tumor and to identify the presence or absence of tumor thrombus in the vein.

Age at thyroid surgery, sex, previous history of renal cell carcinoma, serum thyroglobulin level, anti-thyroglobulin autoantibody, and ultrasonographic findings of the thyroid tumor, fine-needle aspiration cytology, preoperative diagnosis, and surgery were investigated.

The ultrasonographic features of metastatic carcinomas to the thyroid from renal cell carcinoma to be estimated were as follows:

(1) Form of involvement in the thyroid
Tumor formation or diffuse involvement in the thyroid gland was estimated.

(2) Location in the thyroid gland and size of tumors
In terms of the right or left lobe, or the isthmus of the thyroid gland, the site where the tumor was located was estimated. The size of the tumor was recorded in mm.

(3) Shape of tumor, tumor pattern, and strong echoes (calcifications)
The shape of the tumor was classified into regular or irregular. The tumor pattern was classified into solid, mixed, or cystic. The presence or absence of strong echoes with acoustic shadowing (calcifications) was estimated within the tumor lesion.

(4) Vascularity and distribution of blood signals
The intensity of blood signals in the tumor was estimated by Doppler ultrasonography, and classified into -, ±, +, or ++. The distribution of blood signals was classified into intra-tumoral or peripheral dominant.

(5) Extrathyroidal spread (swollen lymph node and tumor thrombus)
The presence or absence of swollen lymph nodes in the neck and tumor thrombus in the thyroid veins and the internal jugular vein adjacent to the thyroid tumor was estimated.

Results

Clinical findings

There were 10 surgical patients with metastatic carcinoma to the thyroid from renal cell carcinoma in this period (Table 1). The histopathological diagnosis of the thyroid tumors was the clear cell variant of renal cell carcinoma in all of the 10 patients. One patient (Patient 7) revealed metastatic carcinoma in benign adenomatous nodule. The patients were 4 men and 6 women, and the age at thyroid surgery was 67.8 ± 7.3 years old (range, 57–79 years old; median, 68.5 years old). Eight patients presented with a previous medical history of nephrectomy for renal cell carcinoma 13.4 ± 8.4 years earlier (range, 2–30 years; median, 12.5 years). In two patients (Patients 9 and 10), renal cell carcinoma in the right kidney was discovered as a primary carcinoma after the thyroid surgery and the histopathological diagnosis of metastatic carcinoma to the thyroid gland. The side of renal cell carcinoma was the right in nine patients (Patients 1–6, and 8–10) and the left in one patient (Patient 7). One patient (Patient 5) revealed positivity for anti-thyroglobulin auto-antibody. Serum thyroglobulin (normal range, < 40 ng/ml) was 136. 9 ± 285.2 ng/ml (range, 9.3-894.6 ng/ml; median, 30.2 ng/ml) in the other 9 patients without autoantibody.

Ultrasonographic features

Form of involvement in the thyroid

Metastatic carcinomas showed tumor formation in the thyroid in all 10 of the patients (Figures 1, 2 and 3), and did not show diffuse involvement in the thyroid.

Table 1 Patients with metastatic carcinoma to the thyroid from renal cell carcinoma and ultrasonographic features

Patient No	Age, Sex	History, Side of RCC	Serum Tg, TgAb	Ultrasonographic features of metastatic carcinoma				FNAC	Pre-op. DX	Surgery
				Location, Size (mm)	Shape, Pattern, Calc.	Intra-tumoral vascularity	Tumor thrombus			
1	70F	8 yr, Right	81.3 (-)	Rt, 36x19x36	irregular solid, (-)	++	(-)	malignant, meta/RCC	meta/RCC	LO
2	77M	9 yr, Right	9.3 (-)	Rt, 56x35x48	irregular solid, (-)	++	(-)	indeterminate	meta/RCC	LO
3	72M	30 yr, Right	27.4 (-)	Lt, 31x19x24	irregular solid, (-)	++	(-)	benign, AN	meta/RCC	LO
4	58F	10 yr, Right	68.2 (-)	Rt, 39x23x36	irregular solid, (-)	++	(+) TV-IJV	indeterminate	meta/RCC	LO+RTV+RIJV
5	67F	18 yr, Right	128.5 (+)	Rt, 81x41x70 / Lt, 27x16x18	irregular solid, (-)	++ / ++	(+) TV-IJV	malignant, meta/RCC	meta/RCC	TT+RTV+RIJV
6	63F	2 yr, Right	894.6 (-)	Rt, 48x29x30 +LNS	irregular solid, (-)	++	(-)	malignant, meta/RCC	meta/RCC	LO+MND
7*	57M	15 yr, Left	26.1 (-)	Rt, 48x40x43	irregular solid, (-)	+	(+) TV	malignant, meta/RCC	meta/RCC	LO+RTV
8	79F	15 yr, Right	24.5 (-)	Rt, 45x33x34	irregular solid, (-)	++	(-)	benign, AN	AN	LO
9	65F	(-)** Right	70.7 (-)	Rt, 23x20x21	regular solid, (-)	+	(-)	fol. tumor, FT	FT	LO
10	70M	(-)** Right	30.2 (-)	Rt, 25x19x19 / Lt, 12x5x10	irregular solid, (-)	++	(+) TV	benign, AG	AG or PC?	TT+CND+RTV

A previous history of renal cell carcinoma was recognized in 7 patients (Patients 1-7) before surgery, and in 3 patients (Patients 8-10) it was not. Age: age at thyroid surgery, F: female, M: male, Rt: right, Lt: left, History: previous history of nephrectomy for renal cell carcinoma, RCC: renal cell carcinoma, Tg: thyroglobulin (normal range: < 40 ng/ml), TgAb: anti-thyroglobulin autoantibody. Shape of the tumor was classified into regular or irregular. Pattern of the tumor was classified into solid, mixed, or cystic. Calc.: intra-tumoral calcification; (+) or (-). Intra-tumoral vascularity was classified into -, +, or ++ according to the intensity of blood signals by Doppler ultrasonography. FNAC: fine-needle aspiration cytology, Pre-op. DX: preoperative diagnosis, meta/RCC: metastatic carcinoma to the thyroid from renal cell carcinoma, LO: lobectomy of the thyroid, TT: total thyroidectomy, MND: modified neck dissection, CND: central node dissection, TV: thyroid vein, IJV: internal jugular vein RIJV: partial resection of internal jugular vein, RTV: resection of thyroid vein, LNS: lymph node swelling in the neck, FT: follicular tumor, AN: adenomatous nodule, AG: adenomatous goiter, PC: papillary carcinoma. Patient 7*: Metastatic renal cell carcinoma in benign adenomatous nodule. The benign part of the tumor could not be detected on ultrasonography because of small size. (-)**: Existence of renal cell carcinoma was recognized after the thyroid surgery and the histopathological diagnosis of thyroid tumor.

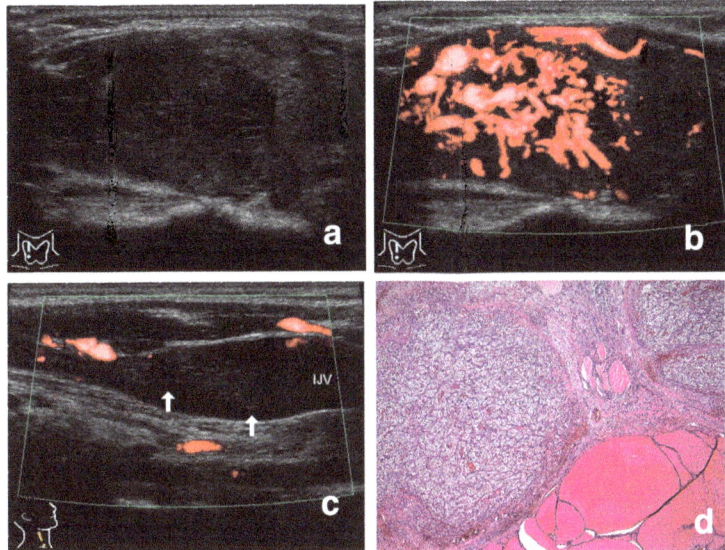

Figure 1 (Patient 4). a. Ultrasonography of the right lobe. A solid tumor. The margins are well demarcated and irregular, and the internal echo is predominantly hypoechoic and partially anechoic. Strong echoes with acoustic shadowing (calcifications) are not present. **b**. Power Doppler ultrasonography of the same section as in Figure 1a. Marked chaotic vascularity is predominantly shown in the intra-tumoral lesions. **c**. Power Doppler ultrasonography of the right internal jugular vein. A solid mass (arrows), that is, tumor thrombus, is shown as an "echogenic tongue" in the lumen. **d** Hematoxylin & eosin staining. Metastatic carcinoma of the clear cell variant of renal cell carcinoma and normal thyroid tissue are shown. Tissue of the tumor histopathogically demonstrates a pseudo-alveolar or pseudo-follicular structure and no calcifications.

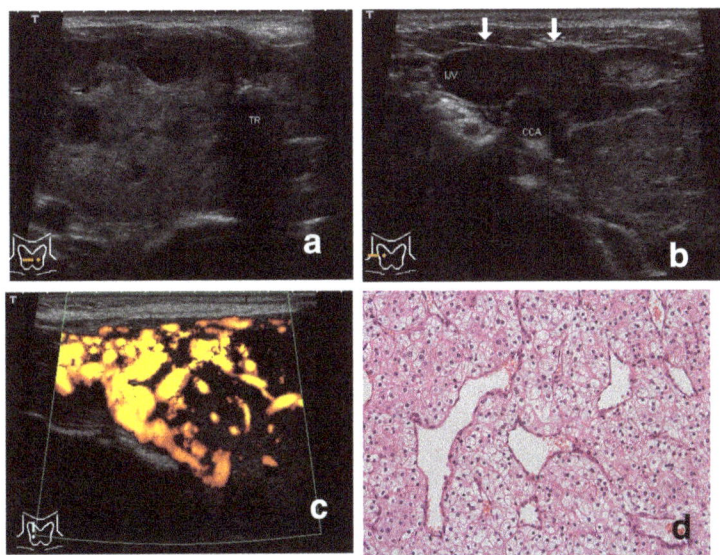

Figure 2 (Patient 5). a. Ultrasonography of the right lobe. A predominantly solid tumor. Internal echo shows homogenity in the solid area and interspersed cystic-like areas. (Power Doppler showed intense blood signals in these cystic-like areas). **b** Ultrasonography of the right lobe and the jugular vein. A solid mass (arrow on the left), that is, tumor thrombus, is shown in the lumen of the jugular vein. The lumen of the middle thyroid vein is completely occupied with tumor thrombus (arrow on the right). **c**. Power Doppler ultrasonography. Marked chaotic vascularity. **d** Hematoxylin & eosin staining. A rich vascular network.

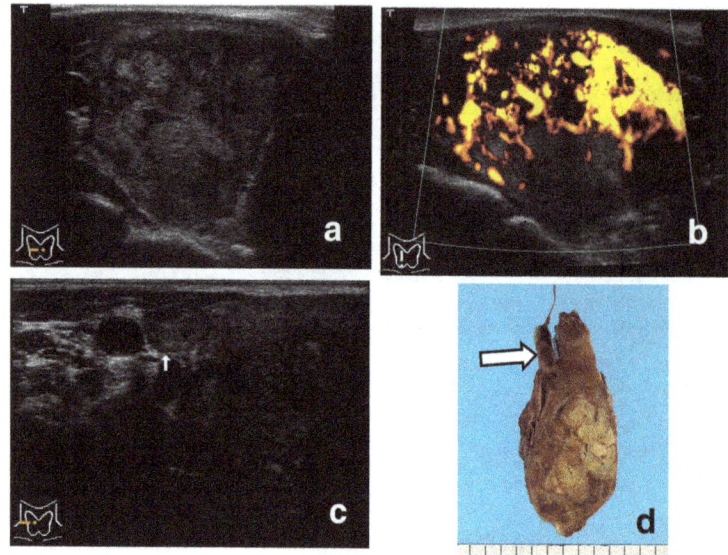

Figure 3 (Patient 7). a. Ultrasonography of the right lobe. A solid tumor. The internal echo is iso- to hypo-echoic and heterogeneous, and appears to show multiple small masses in the tumor. **b**. Power Doppler ultrasonography. **c**. Ultrasonography of the right lobe. Tumor thrombus (arrows) is observed in the superior thyroid vein. **d**. Gross resected specimen. Solid tumor in the right lobe of the thyroid and bulbous intravascular component, tumor thrombus (arrow), are shown.

Location and size of thyroid tumor

The location of metastatic tumors was the right lobe of the thyroid gland in 9 patients, and the left lobe in 3 patients (Patients 3, 5, and 10). Two patients (Patients 5 and10) presented two tumors in the right and left lobes of the thyroid gland. The maximum size of the tumors was 39.3 ± 18.2 mm (range, 12–81 mm; median, 37.5 mm).

Shape of tumor, tumor pattern, and calcifications

The shapes of the tumors were irregular and well demarcated, and the tumor pattern showed a solid and hypoechoic level without a capsule-like structure and direct contact to the normal thyroid tissue in all 10 of the patients. None of the tumors demonstrated strong echoes with acoustic shadowing (calcifications) within them.

Vascularity and distribution of blood signals

The intensity of vascularity in the tumors by Doppler ultrasonography was ++ in 8 patients (Figures 1b, 2c, 3b) and + in 2 patients. Blood signals were more dominant in intra-tumoral lesions than in peripheral lesions of the tumors in all of the patients.

Extrathyroidal spread (swollen lymph node and tumor thrombus)

One patient (Patient 6) showed swollen lymph nodes in the neck in addition to the thyroid tumor. Direct tumor extension into the adjacent veins, that is, tumor thrombi, was detected in 4 patients preoperatively. Tumor thrombi within the internal jugular vein via the thyroid vein ("echogenic tongue") were demonstrated in two patients (Patients 4 and 5) (Figures 1c, 2b), and those within the thyroid veins in two patients (Patienta 7 and 10) (Figure 3c). Intravascular components of the lesions appeared as a solid and hypoechoic mass without calcifications (Figures 1c, 2b, 3c).

Fine-needle aspiration cytology (FNAC)

FNAC showed metastatic carcinoma to the thyroid from renal cell carcinoma in 4 patients, indeterminate in 2 patients (Patients 2 and 4), benign in 3 patients (Patients 3, 8, and 10), and follicular neoplasm in one patient (Patient 9).

Preoperative diagnosis

Among the eight patients who had a previous history of nephrectomy for renal cell carcinoma, seven patients were accurately diagnosed with metastatic carcinoma to the thyroid from renal carcinoma preoperatively, and one patient (Patient 8) was diagnosed with a benign thyroid tumor. Two patients (Patients 9 and 10) who did not have a previous history of nephrectomy for renal cell carcinoma were misdiagnosed with follicular tumor and benign tumor, or papillary carcinoma preoperatively as the primary tumors.

Surgery

Total thyroidectomy was performed in 2 patients and lobectomy in 8 patients. Resection of thyroid veins or partial resection of internal jugular veins was performed in 4 patients because of tumor thrombi in the veins (Patients 4, 5, 7, and 10). Central and modified neck lymph node dissections in addition to thyroid lobectomy were performed in two patients (Patients 6 and 10).

Discussion

Table 1 reveals that these patients tend to be older, and to have relatively late recurrence in the thyroid, renal cell carcinoma in the "right" kidney as a primary site, and relatively low serum thyroglobulin levels. Three patients (Patients 8–10) could not be correctly diagnosed preoperatively, although 7 patients (Patients 1–7) were identified to have metastatic carcinoma. The previous history of renal cell carcinoma could not be obtained preoperatively in one patient (Patient 8). In 2 patients (Patients 9 and 10), thyroid metastasis was the initial presentation of the renal cell carcinoma. It is of interest that ultrasonography played an important role in preoperative diagnosis.

Thyroid ultrasound is particularly useful for estimating the location of a nodule, its size, and its solid or cystic nature, and also for guiding the performance of fine-needle aspiration biopsies. Therefore, it has already become established as the diagnostic procedure of choice in guidelines [7,8] for the management of thyroid nodules by every professional organization of endocrinologists. Papillary thyroid carcinoma is the most common and primary malignancy, and ultrasound features of such patients, for example, a predominantly solid, hypoechoic, ill-circumscribed nodule and lymph node swelling in the neck [9], have already become familiar. On the other hand, patients with metastases to the thyroid from renal cell carcinoma that need surgical management are not many and unfamiliar to clinicians and endocrinologists. It is reported that a surgical procedure for thyroid metastasis from renal cell carcinoma has benefits for the prognosis of such patients [1,3-6]. Little information is available on the ultrasonographic features of metastatic tumor to the thyroid from renal cell carcinoma [2,10-13]. For the reasons mentioned above, ultrasound features of metastatic carcinoma to the thyroid from renal cell carcinoma should be clarified by the evaluation of many patients. A full understanding of ultrasound features is clinically important and essential for such patients' care.

The most common primary site from which metastasis to the thyroid gland occurs is reported to be the kidney in a clinical series [1,2]. Renal cell carcinoma arises from the renal tubular epithelial cells, and the clear cell type is the most common variant [14]. Histopathologically, clear cell carcinoma shows polygonal cells with clear cytoplasm, distinct cell membranes, and small compact eccentric nuclei, and a rich vascular network [14]. The propensity of primary renal cell carcinoma in the kidney

to spread to regional lymph nodes and virtually every organ site is well recognized [14]. Furthermore, this carcinoma often invades regional veins and forms tumor thrombus in the lumen of the renal veins or the inferior vena cava. In addition, this carcinoma behaves unpredictably and its recurrence after nephrectomy is highly variable, presenting as late metastases several years after the initial surgery [1-3,5,10,12,13]. In this situation, metastatic carcinomas in the thyroid occur as a result of hematogenous spread from renal cell carcinoma [14].

A pseudo-alveolar or pseudo-follicular pattern of clear cell carcinoma may resemble the clear cell variant of thyroid carcinoma and adenoma histopathologically. Recently, it has been described that metastatic tumor in the thyroid should be diagnosed based on rich vascularity, abundant extravasated erythrocytes, pseudofollicular spaces filled with blood, negativity for thyroglobulin, and positivity for CD10 and positivity for the renal cell carcinoma marker carbonic anhydrase IX [15]. Histopathological features of the thyroid tumors inevitably reflect ultrasound images of these tumors. Sonographers and endocrinologists must be aware that the ultrasound images of thyroid tumors should be read and understood on the basis of the histopathological features of the tumors.

According to our series (Table 1), metastatic carcinomas to the thyroid from renal cell carcinoma formed one or two nodules within any portion of the thyroid glands in all 10 of the patients. No patients revealed diffuse involvement in the thyroid such as diffuse sclerosing variant of papillary thyroid carcinoma or diffuse swelling of Hashimoto's thyroiditis on histopathology. Furthermore, these tumors did not form a distinct capsule of the tumor histopathologically, and neoplastic cells of these tumors were directly exposed to the normal thyroid tissue and showed invasiveness to adjacent tissue (Figure 1d). For that reason, these tumors showed an irregular margin without a capsule-like structure and directly contacted the normal thyroid region on ultrasonography (Figures 1, 2 and 3).

The tissue of these tumors histopathologically demonstrated a pseudo-alveolar or pseudo-follicular structure (Figures 1d, 2d), and cystic degeneration did not occur within the tumor. Additionally, calcifications did not form within these tumors, and there was a very rich vascular network in the tumor parenchyma (Figure 2d). In terms of the echogenicity of the internal echo of these tumors, they were hypoechoic compared with normal thyroid tissue, which reflected the homogenity of the tissue of these tumors on histopathology. These tumors did not demonstrate cystic anechoic lesions with posterior acoustic enhancement, or any type of echogenic foci with acoustic shadowing, that is, calcifications, on ultrasonography. Doppler ultrasonography showed intensive blood signals or prominent chaotic vascularity in the intra-tumoral area, but did not show prominent vascularity in the peri-tumoral area (Figures 1b, 2c, 3b).

Neoplastic cells of these tumors directly invaded intra-tumoral vessels and formed tumor thrombi in the lumen of the vessels. Grayscale and Doppler ultrasonography showed an "echogenic tongue", that is, tumor thrombus, in the lumen of the thyroid vein or the internal jugular vein (Figures 1c, 2b, 3c) in 4 of the 10 patients. We previously reported on tumor thrombus in surgical patients with thyroid malignancies [16]. Of the 5507 patients with thyroid malignancies, there were 9 patients with tumor thrombi. (Two of these previously reported patients are Patients 4 and 5 in Table 1 of this article.) It can be said that metastases to the thyroid from renal cell carcinoma have a high frequency of tumor thrombus as extrathyroidal spread on ultrasonography. In the literature, tumor thrombi were also reported in a small number of patients with metastatic carcinoma from renal cell carcinoma [4,10,17]. Tumor thrombi in veins adjacent to the thyroid gland can be described as a noteworthy ultrasonographic feature because they are highly suggestive of malignancy. We believe that the detection of tumor thrombus by ultrasonography is useful for preoperative determination of the surgical procedure for such patients [4,10,17] as well as for the diagnosis of metastasis from renal cell carcinoma.

In one patient (Patient 7), small nest of benign adenomatous nodule were demonstrated in the peripheral tissue of the tumor histopathologically, although the majority of the tumor was occupied with clear cell carcinoma. This tumor revealed metastatic renal cell carcinoma in benign adenomatous nodule. The benign part of the tumor could not be detected on ultrasonography preoperatively because of small size. It is reported that renal cell carcinoma rarely metastasized to primary thyroid tumors [18].

There are some ultrasonographic classification systems for thyroid nodules. Among them, Kuma Hospital's ultrasound classification system (Kuma's USC, USC 1–5) [19,20] and the Thyroid imaging reporting and date system (TIRADS, TIRADS 1–6) [21] are popular and useful for clinical management at present. These ultrasound classification systems represent the risk of malignancy of thyroid nodules. When these two ultrasound classification systems are applied to the tumors in these 10 patients, they are classified in USC 4 (probably malignant) and 5 (malignant) on Kuma's USC, and TIRADS 5 (probably malignant) and 6 (malignant) on the TIRADS classification. In particular, tumors with tumor thrombi (Patients 4, 5, 7, and 10) can be easily classified into USC 5 and TIRADS 6.

Quasi-static and shear-wave elastography now become available for diagnostic ultrasonic procedures in addition to conventional grayscale and Doppler ultrasonography. Quasi-static elastography is a relatively new technology that maps the relatively elastic properties of soft tissues, and shear-wave elastography is a new technology that shows quantitative stiffness value of tissues by measuring the velocity of wave propagation. Currently, Adamczewski et al. reported the findings of these two different elastography techniques in a patient with metastases of renal clear-cell carcinoma to the thyroid [22]. Both techniques revealed differences in relative stiffness (strain ratio) between the normal tissue and metastases. However, the absolute stiffness values for metastases in shear-wave elastography were within the range characteristic benign lesions. The data accumulation of these new techniques will add to the interpretation of conventional ultrasound images, and be helpful for ultrasonic diagnosis.

Thyroid metastasis from renal cell carcinoma has some characteristic ultrasonographic findings, such as prominent chaotic intra-tumoral vascularity and tumor thrombus as mentioned above; however, these findings are not specific to this disease. It is thus necessary to perform ultrasonography and fine-needle aspiration biopsy and to obtain information on the previous history of renal cell carcinoma in order to make a correct diagnosis preoperatively. It is reported that fine-needle aspiration cytology can suggest the possibility of metastatic tumor from renal cell carcinoma, and is essential for preoperative diagnosis [1,3,23]. Cytological findings of thyroid metastasis from renal cell carcinoma tend to be bloody, a lack of colloid, and striped nuclei with only occasional cells showing clear cytoplasm [23]. When clear cells are identified within the thyroid gland, primary tumors with clear cell features including papillary, follicular, and medullary thyroid carcinoma, and secondary tumor such as those from lung and salivary gland also need to be considered.

When a previous history of nephrectomy for renal cell carcinoma is recognized in such a patient, ultrasound examination as well as cytology is effective and helpful in order to diagnose it preoperatively. Actually, three patients (Patients 2, 3, and 4) showed an "indeterminate" or "benign" status because of too many blood cells and no neoplastic cells in cytology. However, these patients had a previous history of nephrectomy for renal cell carcinoma and demonstrated characteristic ultrasonographic findings for metastatic carcinoma from renal cell carcinoma. Therefore, we could make the correct preoperative diagnosis. In contrast, when we do not recognize a previous history of renal cell carcinoma, or thyroid metastasis is the first symptom as renal cell carcinoma in a patient, it seems to be difficult to diagnose it preoperatively because of the rarity of the disease. Unfortunately, two patients (Patients 9 and 10) who had no previous history of renal cell carcinoma were not correctly diagnosed preoperatively in spite of the existence of characteristic features on ultrasonography. Preoperative recognition of a previous history of renal cell carcinoma in a patient must be the most important clue for the correct diagnosis of the disease, which many articles in the literature have emphasized [1,2,6].

Cytology was falsely negative in four patients with previous history of renal cell carcinoma (Patients 2, 3, 4, and 8). We should have measured thyroglobulin in the washout of fine-needle aspiration cytology. When thyroglobulin was low or detectable, clinical suspicion of metastatic nodule would become more definitely.

Conclusions

Comprehensive judgment of ultrasonographic findings of thyroid tumor, cytological findings, and previous medical history of renal cell carcinoma are suggested to lead to the correct diagnosis of patients with metastases to the thyroid from renal cell carcinoma. In this situation, ultrasound is the initial examination and such characteristic features on ultrasonography mentioned above can be clues to the correct diagnosis.

Consent

Written informed consent was obtained from the patient's guardian/parent/next of kin for the publication of this report and any accompanying images.

Competing interests
The authors declare that they have no competing interests.

Authors' contributions
All authors read and approved the final manuscript.

References

1. Chung AY, Tran TB, Brumund KT, Weisman RA, Bouvet M. Metastases to the thyroid: a review of the literature from the last decade. Thyroid. 2012;22:258–68.
2. Sindoni A, Rizzo M, Tuccari G, Ieni A, Barresi V, Calbo L, et al. Thyroid metastases from renal cell carcinoma: review of the literature. Scientific World Journal. 2010;10:590–602.
3. Hegerova L, Griebeler ML, Reynolds JP, Henry MR, Gharib H: Metastasis to the thyroid gland: Report of a large series from the Mayo Clinic. Am J Clin Oncol doi: [10.1097/COC.0b013e31829d1d09]
4. De Stefano, Carluccioo R, Zanni E, Marchiori D, Cicchetti G, Bertaccini A, et al. Management of thyroid nodules as secondary involvement of renal cell carcinoma: case report and literature review. Anticancer Res. 2009;29:473–6.
5. Assouad J, Banu E, Brian E, Pham DN, Dujon A, Foucault C, et al. Strategies and outcomes in pulmonary and extrapulmonary metastases from renal cell cancer. Eur J Cardiothorac Surg. 2008;33:794–8.
6. Duggal NM, Horattas MC. Metastatic renal cell carcinoma to the thyroid gland. Endocr Pract. 2008;4:1040–6.
7. Gharib H, Papini E, Paschke R, Duick DS, Valcavi R, Hegedues L, et al. AACE/AME/ETA Task Force on Thyroid Nodules: American Association of Clinical Endocrinologists and Associazione Medici Endocrinologi for clinical practice for the diagnosis an management of thyroid nodules. Endocrine Pract. 2006;12:63–102.
8. American Thyroid Taskforce on Thyroid Nodules and Differentiated Thyroid Cancer, Cooper DS, Doherty GM, Haugen BR, Kloos RT, Lee SL, et al. Revised American Thyroid Association management guideline for patients with and differentiated thyroid cancer. Thyroid. 2009;19:1167–214.
9. Ahuja AT: Head and Neck. Differentiated thyroid carcinoma; In *Diagnostic Imaging: Ultrasound*, ed 1, Salt Lake City, Utah. AMIRSYS: 2007; 6–11.
10. Pickhardt PJ, Pickard RH. Sonography of delayed thyroid metastasis from renal cell carcinoma with jugular vein extension. Am J Roentgenol. 2003;81:272–4.
11. Kim AY, Park SB, Choi HS, Hwang JC. Isolated thyroid metastasis from renal cell carcinoma. J Ultrasound Med. 2007;26:1799–802.
12. Kihara M, Yokomise H, Yamauchi. Metastasis of renal cell carcinoma to the thyroid gland 19 years after nephrectomy: a case report. Auris Nasus Larynx. 2004;31:95–100.
13. Wada N, Hirakawa S, Rino Y, Hasuo K, Kawachi K, Nakatani Y, et al. Solitary metachronous metastasis to the thyroid from renal clear cell carcinoma 19 years after nephrectomy: report of a case. Surg Today. 2005;35:483–7.
14. Russo P. Renal cell carcinoma: presentation, staging, and surgical treatment. Semin Oncol. 2000;27:160–76.
15. Cimino-Mathew A, Sharma R, Netto GJ. Diagnostic use of PAX8, CAIX, TTF-1, and TGB in metastatic renal cell carcinoma of the thyroid. Am J Surg Pathol. 2011;35:757–61.
16. Kobayashi K, Hirokawa M, Yabuta T, Fukushima M, Kihara M, Higashiyama T, et al. Tumor thrombus of thyroid malignancies in veins: Importance of detection by ultrasonography. Thyroid. 2011;21:527–31.
17. Matei DV, Brescia A, Nordio A, Spinelli MG, Melegari S, Cozzi G, et al. Renal cell carcinoma and synchronous thyroid metastasis with neoplastic thrombosis of the internal jugular vein: report of a case. Arch Ital Urol Androl. 2001;3:203–6.
18. Bohn OL, De las Casas LE, Leon ME. Tumor-to-tumor metastasis: Renal cell carcinoma metastatic to papillary carcinoma of thyroid-report of a case and review of the literature. Head Neck Pathol. 2009;3:327–30.
19. Yokozawa T, Miyauchi A, Kuma K, Sugawara M. Accurate and simple method of diagnosing nodules the modified technique of ultrasound-guided fine needle aspiration biopsy. Thyroid. 1995;5:141–5.
20. Ito Y, Amino N, Yokozawa T, Ota H, Ohshita M, Murata N, et al. Ultrasonographic evaluation of thyroid nodules in 900 patients: comparison among ultrasonographic, cytological, and histological findings. Thyroid. 2007;17:1269–76.
21. Horvath E, Majlis S, Rossi R, Franco C, Niedmann JP, Castro A, et al. An ultrasonogram reporting system for thyroid nodules stratifying cancer risk for clinical management. J Clin Endoccrinol Metab. 2009;94:1748–4751.
22. Adamczewski Z, Dedecjus M, Skowronska-Jozwiak E, Lewinski A. Metastases of renal clear-cell carcinoma to the thyroid: a comparison of shear-wave and quasi-static elastograhy. Pol Arch Med Wewn. 2014;124:485–6.
23. Bhalla R, Popp A, Nassar A. Case report: metastatic renal carcinoid to the thyroid diagnosed by fine needle aspiration biopsy. Diagn Cytopathol. 2007;35:597–600.

16

Proposed algorithm for management of patients with thyroid nodules/focal lesions, based on ultrasound (US) and fine-needle aspiration biopsy (FNAB); our own experience

Zbigniew Adamczewski and Andrzej Lewiński[*]

Abstract

Background: The standard management in patients with thyroid nodules is to assess the risk of malignancy, based on cytological examination. On the other hand, there are thyroid patterns of ultrasound (US) image, associated with an increased risk of malignancy.

The aim of our study was to create a diagnostic algorithm that would employ both data from US examination (expressed by a total score, according to our scoring system) and FNAB results, classified according to Bethesda system (The Bethesda System for Reporting Thyroid Cytopathology - TBSRTC categories).

Material and methods: 100 thyroid cancer foci (94 papillary carcinomas, 4 medullary carcinomas, 2 undifferentiated carcinomas) and 100 benign focal lesions were selected during postoperative histopathological examination of thyroid glands excised during surgery from 111 patients. The corresponding US images of each lesion – performed in the course of preoperative diagnostics – were evaluated for the presence of seven (7) different features in US image, suggesting a malignant character of lesion, viz. vascularity, i.e., the increased central intranodular blood flows, microcalcifications, "taller-than-wide" orientation, solid composition, hypoechogenicity, irregular margin and either absence of peripheral halo or the presence of outer shell of uneven thickness, surrounding the lesion. The sensitivity, specificity, positive predictive values, negative predictive values and odds ratios for each US feature were calculated.

Results: In US image of the analyzed cancer foci, we obtained the following values of odds ratio for each of the above mentioned features suggesting malignancy: "taller-than-wide" orientation - odds ratio - 301.0, microcalcifications - 24.67, increased intranodular vascularity - 20.44, hypoechogenicity - 18.61, irregular margins - 7.81, absence of halo - 5.88, and solid composition - 4.16.

Taking into account our own experience and the present data, in juxtaposition with the opinions of other authors, we propose a division of US features into 3 groups of different prognostic importance, expressed by a total score calculated based on our scoring system. Accordingly, microcalcifications, "taller-than-wide" orientation, the increased intranodular vascularity, and hypoechogenicity constitute one group - each of the features in this group is awarded 1 point. In turn, the characteristics of minor prognostic importance, such as irregular margin, absence of halo, solid composition, and large size (a diameter longer than 3.0 cm) - are associated with the granting 0.5 points each. The most important prognostic features – a rapid growth (enlargement) of nodules/focal lesions and a presence of pathologically altered lymph nodes are associated with the granting 3 points for each.

(Continued on next page)

---

[*] Correspondence: alewin@csk.umed.lodz.pl
Department of Endocrinology and Metabolic Diseases, Medical University of Lodz, Polish Mother's Memorial Hospital – Research Institute, Rzgowska 281/289, 93-338, Lodz, Poland

(Continued from previous page)

Our scoring system can be applied in order to better assessment of thyroid US patterns in whole. In patients with a total score ranging from $0 < 4$ points there is US pattern of a low risk of malignancy, with $\geq 4 < 7$ points - intermediate risk, and in patients with a score ≥ 7 points – a high risk in question.

Conclusion: Complementary use of our scoring system and FNAB TBSRTC categories can help to make optimal clinical decisions as regards the selection of treatment strategy.

Background

Common use of ultrasonography (US) in the diagnostics of thyroid diseases and of other diseases in the neck region caused rapid increase of the number of detected impalpable, asymptomatic lesions in the gland. According to some authors, it allows to visualize 10 times more US lesions than the number of palpable nodules detected during the physical examination [1-3]. It creates diagnostic and therapeutic dilemmas, dominated by the question: what is the most proper medical management – observation and careful monitoring of existing nodule, or – the opposite - referring the patients for surgery. While follow up, the most frequent way to proceed are the repeated US examination and a fine needle aspiration biopsy (FNAB). Even though the biopsy is considered by many doctors as a basis for further monitoring, performing FNAB of any identified lesions may not be prudent [4,5]. It happens that FNAB confirms the benign nature of the lesion and, nevertheless, it is quite frequently repeated (often many times) in spite of the fact that US image pattern does not change during a long-term observation. On the other hand, the surgical treatment in patients with obvious clinical signs and symptoms of malignant neoplastic disease is sometimes delayed because of unnecessary diagnostic procedures (e.g., due to awaiting for recommended time after which FNAB should be performed again). Thus, the endocrinologist - while diagnosing the thyroid nodule - cannot forget a question of fundamental importance – what is a bigger threat to the patients – observation, i.e., monitoring of lesion and live with the existing thyroid nodule or subjecting the patient to surgical treatment of his/her thyroid.

The aim of our study was to create an algorithm that would employ both data from US examination and FNAB results, classified according to Bethesda recommendations (The Bethesda System for Reporting Thyroid Cytopathology - TBSRTC categories), in order to optimise diagnostic and therapeutic management in case of nodules/US focal lesions in the thyroid [6].

Methods

The algorithm was developed on the basis of prospective diagnostics in patients with nodules/US focal lesions of the thyroid, hospitalized in the Department of Endocrinology and Metabolic Diseases, in the time period from January 2008 to June 2012, who – then - were referred for surgery. At the same time, data of other authors on assessing the risk of thyroid malignancy, based on US characteristics, FNAB results, family medical history, and - above all - clinical signs and symptoms were considered.

100 thyroid cancer foci (94 papillary carcinomas, 4 medullary carcinomas, 2 undifferentiated carcinomas) and 100 benign focal lesions were selected during postoperative histopathological examination of thyroid glands excised during surgery carried out in 111 patients, aged 23 to 79 years (mean age – 57.0 years). The corresponding US images of each lesion – obtained in the course of preoperative diagnostics – were evaluated in order to assess seven (7) US characteristics, the most useful in differentiating benign and malignant lesions [7-10]. All examinations were performed by the same diagnostician, with extensive experience in thyroid US, using Toshiba Aplio XG US device with a linear probe PLT 1204 BT 12–18 MHz. An evaluation of focal lesions was carried out in the grey scale (B-mode), also with use of Power-Doppler method.

The following US features were subjected to analysis (for each characteristics - an appearance suggesting a malignant character of lesion is specified, followed by the respective image of the same feature, speaking for its benign nature):

1. Vascularity - defined as the presence of irregular chaotic intranodular hypervascularity; also images of a total absence of blood flow in hypoechogenic, solid lesions were included into that group; in contrast to the peripheral, subcapsular blood flows, suggesting benign lesions [11,12].
2. Calcifications - assessed as the presence of microcalcifications, also their coexistence with other forms of calcifications (e.g., dystrophic); in contrast to the absence of calcifications, the latter suggesting benign nature of lesions.
3. Orientation - "taller than wide" shape of lesion in transverse and/or longitudinal planes; in contrast to all other lesion shapes.
4. Composition - solid lesions, also mixed lesions with cystic component not exceeding 10% of the volume; in contrast to lesions with cystic parts greater than 10% of total volume and/or to solely cystic lesions.

Table 1 Distribution of US characteristics in malignant and benign thyroid lesions; p values indicating a statistical significance are marked by bold

Parameter	No. of cases (%)	Malignant lesions No. of cases (%)	Benign lesions No. of cases (%)	p value
Vascularity				
Intranodular and increased or completely absent	150 (75.0)	96 (64.0)	54 (46.0)	**<0.0001**
Peripheral, subcapsular	50 (25.0)	4 (8.0)	46 (92.0)	
Microcalcifications				
Positive	128 (64.0)	93 (72.7)	35 (27.3)	**<0.0001**
Negative	72 (36.0)	7 (9.7)	65 (90.2)	
Orientation				
Taller-than-wide	88 (44.0)	86 (97.7)	2 (2.3)	**<0.0001**
Wider-than-tall or of other shape	112 (56.0)	14 (12.5)	98 (87.5)	
Composition				
Solid	173 (86.5)	94 (54.3)	79 (65.7)	**0.0032**
Mixed	27 (23.5)	6 (22.2)	21 (77.8)	
Echogenicity				
Hypoechogenic	106 (53.0)	84 (79.2)	22 (20.1)	**<0.0001**
Isoechogenic	94 (47.0)	16 (17.0)	78 (83.0)	
Margins				
Irregular	107 (53.5)	77 (71.9)	30 (28.1)	**<0.0001**
Well circumscribed	93 (46.5)	23 (24.7)	70 (75.3)	
Peripheral Halo				
Absent or irregular, thick	111 (55.0)	76 (68.0)	35 (32.0)	**<0.0001**
Present, thin and regular	89 (45.0)	24 (27.0)	65 (73.0)	

5. Echogenicity - understood as hypoechogenicity, defined as a reduced ("darker") echogenicity (similar to the echogenicity of muscles, surrounding the thyroid); in contrast to normal thyroid echogenicity (isoechogenicity) in benign lesions.

6. Margin - blurred and poorly defined; in contrast to well-differentiated regular margin.

7. Halo - the absence of halo, or the presence of outer shell (rim) of uneven thickness that surrounds the lesion; in contrast to the presence of thin, regular halo which speaks for a benign nature of lesion.

Statistical analysis

The statistical analysis was performed with use of the Prism 5.0 software (GraphPad, La Jolla, USA). Fisher exact test was used to analyze distribution of the obtained results between the examined benign and malignant lesions. For each tested variable – the sensitivity, specificity, positive predictive values (PPV), negative predictive values (NPV) and odds ratios were estimated. Additionally, the 95% confidence intervals of these parameters were determined. The results were regarded as significant for $p < 0.05$.

Table 2 Values of sensitivity, specificity, PPV and NPV of the analyzed US characteristics (parameters)

Parameter	Sensitivity (%)	Specificity (%)	PPV (%)	NPV (%)
Vascularity	96 (90–99)	46 (36–56)	64 (56–72)	92 (80–98)
Microcalcifications	93 (86–97)	65 (54–74)	73 (64–80)	90 (80–96)
Orientation	86 (77–92)	98 (93–99)	97 (92–99)	87 (80–93)
Composition	94 (87–97)	21 (13–30)	54 (46–61)	77 (57–91)
Echogenicity	84 (75–90)	78 (68–85)	79 (70–86)	82 (73–89)
Margins	77 (67–84)	70 (60–78)	72 (62–80)	75 (65–83)
Peripheral Halo	76 (66–84)	65 (56–74)	68 (59–77)	73 (62–82)

The 95% confidence intervals are given in the brackets.

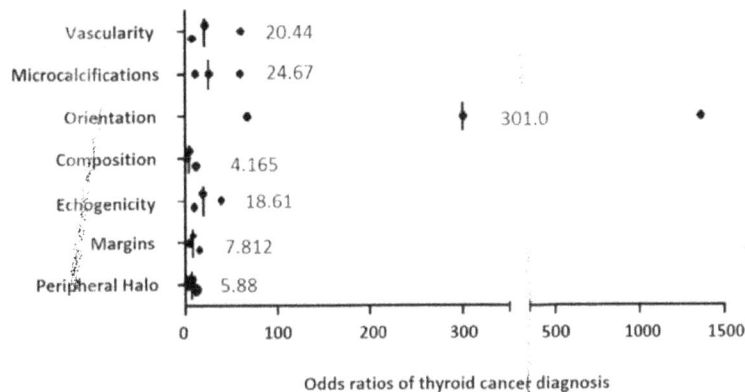

Figure 1 Odds ratios of analyzed US characteristics in diagnostics of malignant thyroid lesions. The values on the figure indicate the median odds ratio, with neighboring dots indicating the boundaries of 95% confidence intervals.

Results

The comparison of distribution of US characteristics, assessed in two (2) analyzed groups, showed the presence of significant statistical differences in the frequency of their occurrence, depending on the histopathological diagnosis (benign vs malignant lesions) (Table 1).

Table 2 presents the obtained values of sensitivity and specificity, also positive predictive values (PPV) and negative predictive values (NPV) of the analyzed parameters. Our results are comparable with data from reports of other authors [8,9,12-16].

Simultaneously, the assessment of the odds ratios of thyroid cancer diagnosis, in the presence of the particular characteristics evaluated in each case, showed the increased risk of malignancy. The highest values of odds ratios were recorded in case of lesions "taller-than-wide" in shape in transverse and/or longitudinal planes, also the presence of microcalcifications, the incorrect pattern of vascularisation (intranodular and increased or completely absent) and/or hypoechogenicity were related to the increased cancer risk. This also applied - but to a lesser extent - to the lesions such as solid composition, the absence of halo, and blurred margins (Figure 1).

In addition, data from numerous reports of other authors indicate an increased risk of malignancy, especially in the case of:

- the rapid growth of thyroid nodules/focal lesions [17] which is defined as a 20% increase in minimum two dimensions (at least - 2 mm) in the follow-up period shorter than 18 months [18];
- thyroid lesions coexisting with lymphadenopathy that may suggest nodal metastases [19,20].

It is to be recalled that cervical US is the optimal method for searching lymph node metastases [18]. This examination allows to reveal more than 90% of the current metastases [21], the presence of which is diagnosed in approximately 25% microcarcinomas and even more frequently, up to 50% in larger tumours, with significant extrathyroidal extension, *viz*. T_4 tumour stage in TNM scale [9,22]. However, it should be stressed that the simultaneous presence of the thyroid tumour and enlarged cervical lymph nodes does not necessarily constitute evidence of a direct causal relation;

Table 3 Summary of points awarded depending on the US characteristics

Most important characteristic (each feature – 3 points)	
G	Growth of nodules (resulting in rapid enlargement)
L	Pathologically altered lymph nodes
Major prognostic characteristic (each feature – 1 point)	
O	Orientation (shape)
C1	Calcifications (especially microcalcifications)
V	Vascularity (intranodular increased or absent)
E	Echogenicity (in particular hypoechogenicity)
Minor prognostic characteristic (each feature – 0.5 point)	
M	Margin (blurred and poorly defined)
H	Halo (absent or irregular and thick)
C2	Composition (solid)
D	Diameter (longer than 3.0 cm)

Table 4 The scoring system of US patterns, applied for thyroid nodules/focal lesions

Risk of malignancy, as assessed on the basis of US pattern	A total score
Low risk	0 < 4 points
Intermediate risk	≥ 4 < 7 points
High risk	≥ 7 points

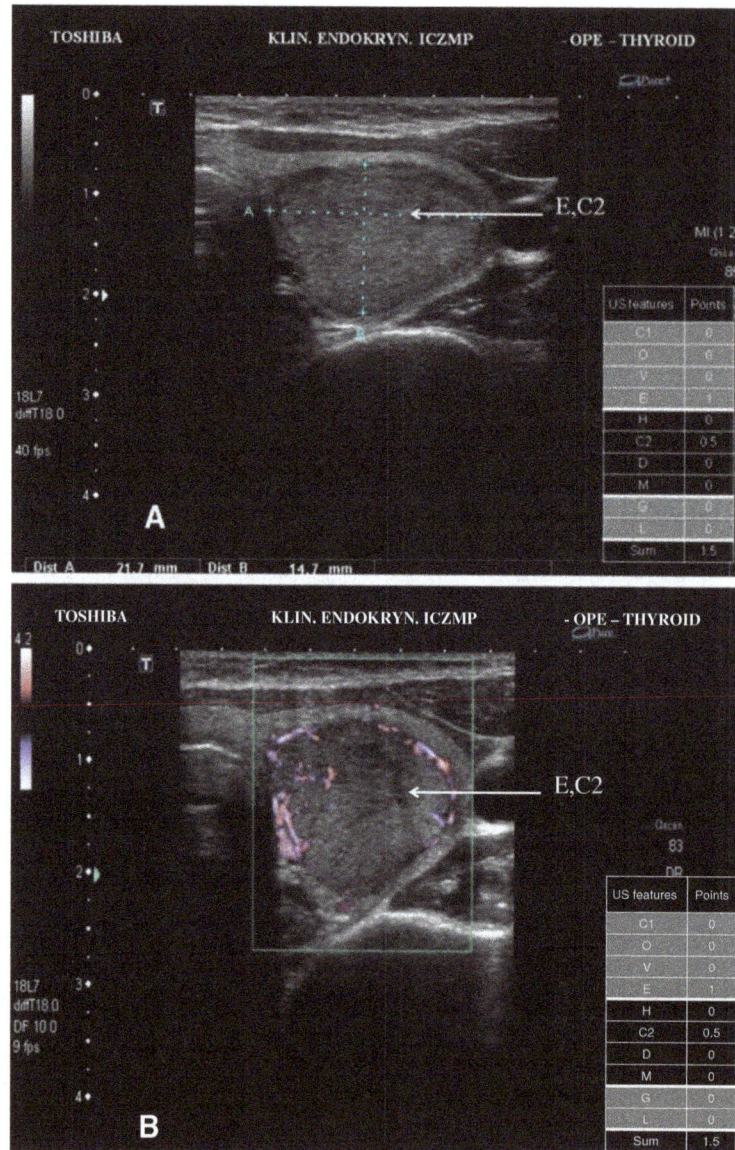

Figure 2 Low risk thyroid nodule/focal lesion US pattern. A. Ultrasound picture of the thyroid lesion (B-mode). The scoring system – 1.5 points (low risk US pattern 0 < 4 points); E – hypoechogenicity; C2 – solid composition; FNAB cytology in this case - category II TBSRTC; management - observation and repeat FNAB examination after 18 months. **B.** Ultrasound picture of the thyroid lesion (Power Doppler), peripheral blood flows.

– the presence of thyroid tumours with a diameter exceeding 3–4 cm [23]; in tumours of larger size - follicular carcinomas are diagnosed more frequently [23,24]. In these cases - FNAB, used as the sole diagnostic test, does not allow formulation of the final diagnosis and confirmation of malignant nature of tumours and its result always must be evaluated with reference to clinical and US examinations.

Three characteristics listed above (rapid growth, enlarged lymph nodes, tumour size) have not been evaluated or subjected to statistical calculations in our present study for

the reasons which we would like to explain. Follow-up of changes in the size of the analyzed lesions was not possible because the majority of US examinations were performed directly prior to surgery, and the patients submitted to surgical treatment were not previously hospitalised and diagnosed in our Department.

Due to the fact that the coexistence of thyroid lesions and of abnormal lymph nodes was found exclusively in case of malignant foci, we decided to exclude that feature from the statistical evaluation.

The diameter of all lesions examined by us did not exceed 3.0 cm, thus it was not possible to use the size of

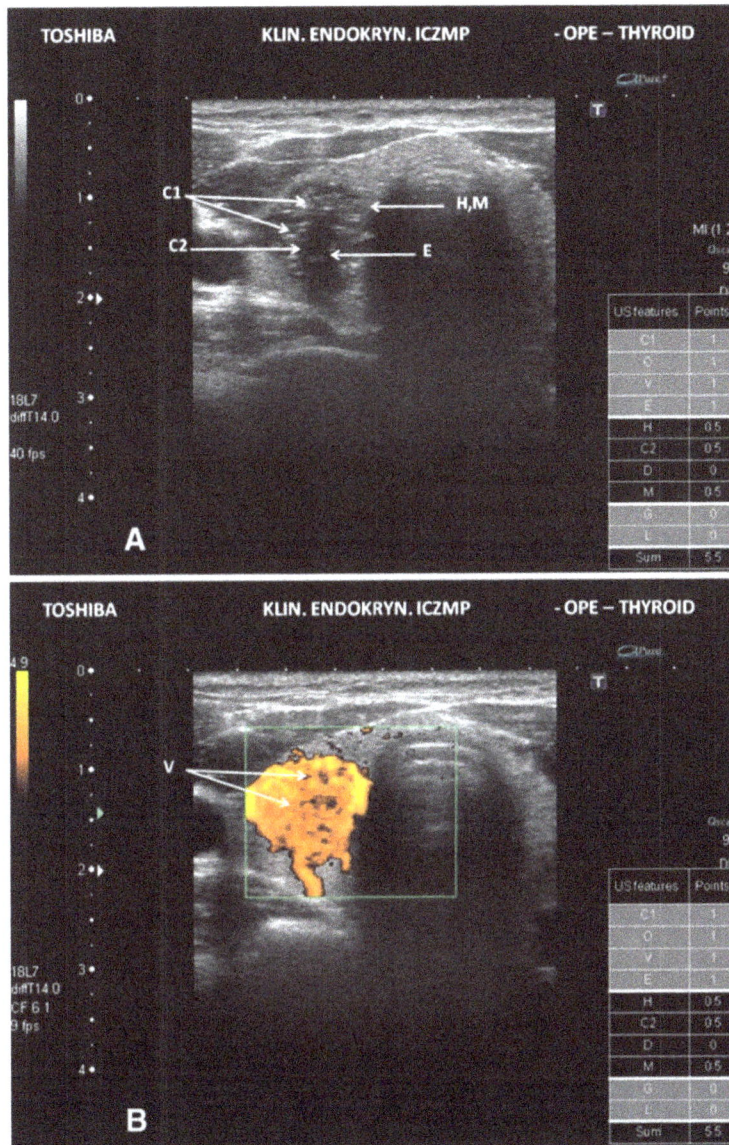

Figure 3 Intermediate risk thyroid nodule/focal lesion US pattern. A. Ultrasound picture of the thyroid lesion (B-mode). The scoring system - 5.5 points (intermediate risk US pattern ≥ 4 < 7 points); C1 – microcalcifications; O – orientation - "taller-than-wide" shape – not shown in the figure; E – hypoechogenicity; H – the absence of "halo"; C2 – solid composition; D – diameter - below 3 cm (not shown); M – irregular margin; FNAB cytology in this case - category IV TBSRTC; management - recommend surgery. **B.** Ultrasound picture of the thyroid lesion (Power Doppler). The scoring system - 5.5 points (intermediate risk US pattern ≥ 4 < 7 points); V – the increased intranodular blood flows.

lesions for differentiation of the studied groups (malignant vs benign).

Taking into account our own observations, in juxtaposition with the opinions of other authors [4,5,19,20,25-27], we propose a division of US features into 3 groups of different prognostic importance. Accordingly, microcalcifications, "taller-than-wide" orientation, the incorrect pattern of vascularisation, and hypoechogenicity constitute one group - each of the features in this group is awarded 1 point. In turn, the characteristics of minor prognostic importance, such as irregular margin, absence of halo, solid

composition, and large size (a diameter longer than 3.0 cm) - are associated with the granting 0.5 points each. The most important prognostic features – a rapid growth resulting in the enlargement of nodules/focal lesions, as well as a presence of pathologically altered lymph nodes are associated with the granting 3 points for each (Table 3).

Having assigned the points for each characteristics, we created the scoring system that is applied for better assessment of thyroid US patterns in whole.

A total score constitutes the basis to assign the patients to groups of varying degree of the risk of malignancy. Accordingly, patients with a total score ranging from 0 to less than 4 points belong to the group of low risk US pattern, patients with a score from 4 to less than 7 points represent US pattern of intermediate risk of malignancy, and in patients with a score 7 points and more – US pattern of a high risk of malignancy occurs (Table 4).

We have illustrated the practical application of our scoring system of the thyroid US patterns in Figures 2A, 2B, 3A, 3B, 4A and 4B.

Discussion

It is well known that none of the individual US features allows to differentiate malignant from benign thyroid lesions. However, finding in US image of nodule/focal lesion one (1) or more than one suspicious features, correlates well with the risk of malignancy. This fact is commonly used for the qualification of patients with nodules/focal lesions for FNAB cytology.

The current system of cytological diagnoses (TBSRTC) greatly facilitates therapeutic decisions (Table 5) [6]. This

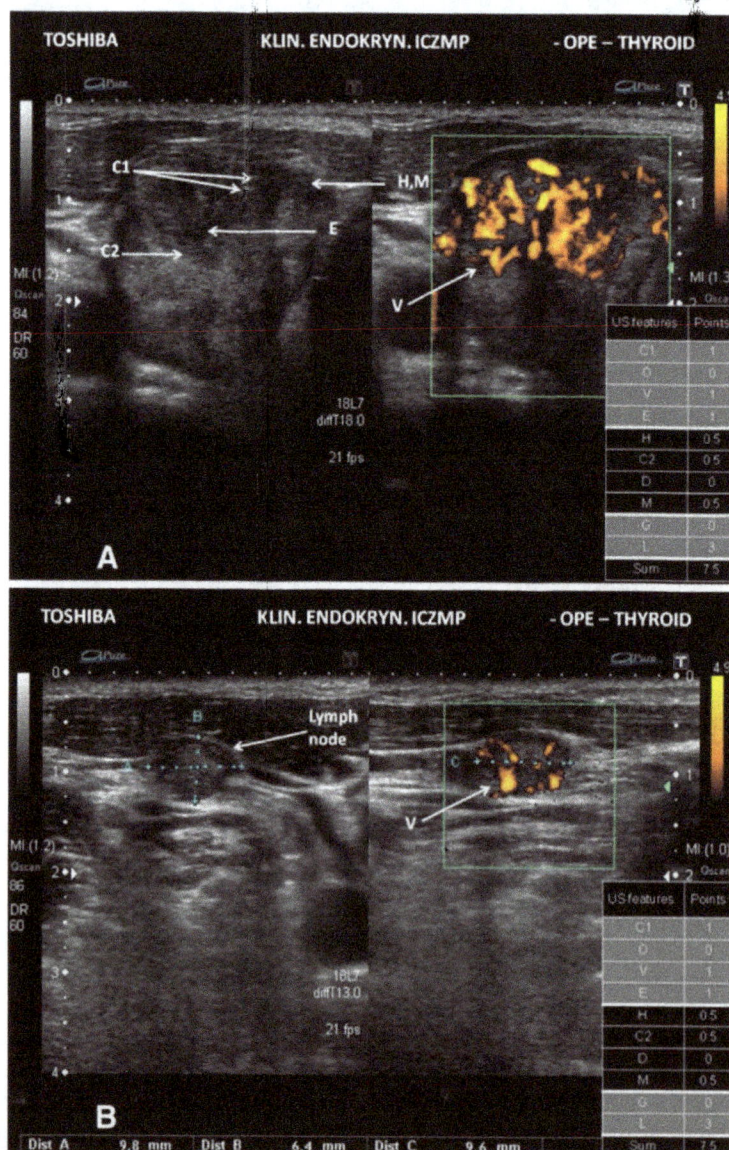

Figure 4 High risk thyroid nodule/focal lesion US pattern. A. Ultrasound picture of the thyroid lesion (B-mode, Power Doppler). The scoring system - 7.5 points (high risk US pattern ≥ 7 points); C1 – microcalcifications; O – orientation – shape other than "taller-than-wide" – not shown in the figure; V - the increased intranodular blood flows; E – hypoechogenicity; H – the absence of "halo"; C2 – solid composition; D – diameter - below 3 cm (not shown); M – irregular margin; FNAB cytology in this case - category V TBSRTC; management - recommend surgery.
B. Ultrasound picture of the metastatic lymph node in the same case (B-mode, Power Doppler). The scoring system - 7.5 points (high risk US pattern ≥ 7 points); the increased blood flows, mainly peripheral, in the metastatic lymph node.

Table 5 The Bethesda System for Reporting Thyroid Cytopathology (TBSRTC) – according to Cibas and Ali [6]

Diagnostic category	Risk of malignancy (%)
I Nondiagnostic or unsatisfactory	1-4
II Benign	0-3
III Atypia of undetermined significance or follicular lesion of undetermined significance	5-15
IV Follicular neoplasm or suspicious for a follicular neoplasm	15-30
V Suspicious for malignancy	60-75
VI Malignant	97-99

applies mainly to diagnoses of malignant lesions (category VI TBSRTC) or a suspicion of malignancy (category V TBSRTC) which both create the need for urgent referral for surgery, in order to perform a total thyroidectomy, except cases inoperable at the time of diagnosis.

Significantly more difficulties with making a therapeutic decision appear when FNAB belongs to the category IV TBSRTC - "follicular neoplasm or suspicious for a follicular neoplasm " or to category III TBSRTC - "follicular lesion of undetermined significance/atypia of undetermined significance". These diagnoses require a completely different clinical approach. Category IV TBSRTC is believed to be a final result, confirmed by the opinion of two independent pathologists. Repeating FNAB in such cases is not expected to provide additional benefits, thus, a repeated FNAB should be performed only in case of changes in the US pattern of lesions. The diagnosis of category III TBSRTC is "a category of exclusion" and should be treated as an optional diagnosis, thus, it can only ultimately be used. The main difference - when compared to category IV - is that category III requires a repeat

biopsy, like in case nondiagnostic or unsatisfactory FNAB results (category I TBSRTC). One cannot forget that even in the case of benign lesions (category II TBSRTC) false-negative results are still possible and a risk of malignancy in such cases reaches up to 3% [6].

However, it should be emphasized that the thyroid US and FNAB cytology are diagnostic tests that should not always decide about the fate of our patient and about recommending him/her the surgical treatment. Many clinical parameters have long been recognized as predictors of malignancy in patients with thyroid nodules/lesions. Such factors include family medical history (genetic background), age younger than 20 and older than 60 years, irradiation of the neck and head area (particularly in the childhood) and male sex [4,18,28]. Moreover, certain clinical circumstances, e.g., if the patient complains of hoarseness (which is not a result of *stricte* laryngeal disease), or of ache in the tumour and dysphagia - usually caused by a firm thyroid tumour, may indicate a malignant character of lesion and may require an inquisitive intense diagnostics of any type, and appropriate treatment, in most cases of the radical type.

Based on the results of our observations, in combination with data of other authors, we decided to stratify the risk of malignancy, depending on the ascertained signs and symptoms, US features, FNAB results according to TBSRTC categories, and – in consequence - we created the algorithm of diagnostic and therapeutic management, the use of which seems to be most favourable for patients with thyroid problems (nodules/focal lesions) (Figure 5).

We are aware of the fact that the assumption underlying of this study, namely comparison of distribution of US characteristics in the two groups of the same number of examined lesions, does not apply in the real epidemiological

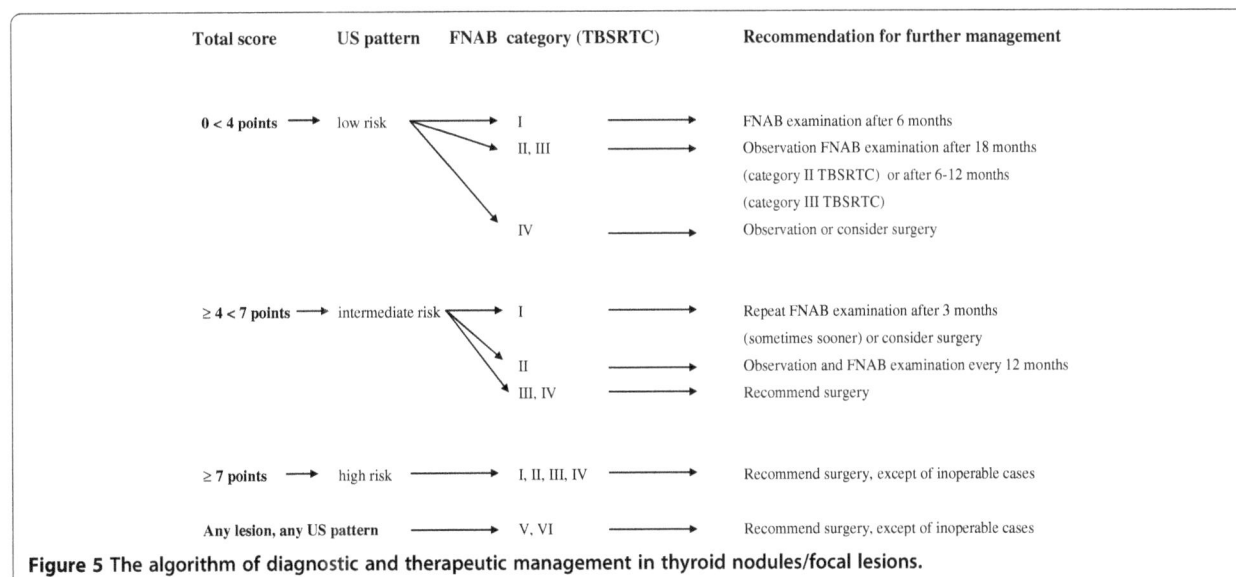

Figure 5 The algorithm of diagnostic and therapeutic management in thyroid nodules/focal lesions.

situation. However, we believe that such a design of the study highlights the most important US characteristics, the presence of which correlates - to the greatest extent - with the risk of malignancy. The presented algorithm of management in patients with thyroid problems is designed to highlight the complementarity of diagnostic procedures, such as US and FNAB. Simultaneously, we would like to stress that US is not only a tool used for selection of nodules which should be examined by FNAB but is also a diagnostic method, the outcomes of which can constitute a basis for the final therapeutic decision.

Conclusions

The presented algorithm, as many other previously developed to assess the nature of thyroid lesions, does not solve all the possible encountered clinical problems. However, by taking into consideration the important US characteristics, related to an increased risk of malignancy, in combination with cytological assessment of lesions, at the same time - by paying attention on the significance of clinical data from medical history and physical examination, it fulfils expectations in daily clinical practice and is helpful in making the proper diagnostic and therapeutic decisions.

Competing interests

The authors declare that they have no competing interests.

Authors' contributions

ZA designed the study, performed US examinations and participated in writing a manuscript. AL was involved in coordination of the study and supervised preparation of the final version of manuscript. Both authors read and approved the final manuscript.

Acknowledgments

This study was supported by statutory funds from the Medical University of Lodz, Poland (No. 503/1-107-03/503-01).

References

1. Frates MC, Benson CB, Charboneau JW, Cibas ES, Clark OH, Coleman BG, Cronan JJ, Doubilet PM, Evans DB, Goellner JR, Hay ID, Hertzberg BS, Intenzo CM, Jeffrey RB, Langer JE, Larsen PR, Mandel SJ, Middleton WD, Reading CC, Sherman SI, Tessler FN: Management of thyroid nodules detected at US: Society of Radiologists in Ultrasound consensus conference statement. *Ultrasound Q* 2006, **22:**231–238. discussion 239–240.
2. McCartney CR, Stukenborg GJ: Decision analysis of discordant thyroid nodule biopsy guideline criteria. *J Clin Endocrinol Metab* 2008, **93:**3037–3044.
3. Peli M, Capalbo E, Lovisatti M, Cosentino M, Berti E, Mattai Dal Moro R, Cariati M: Ultrasound guided fine-needle aspiration biopsy of thyroid nodules: Guidelines and recommendations vs clinical practice; a 12-month study of 89 patients. *J Ultrasound* 2012, **15:**102–107.
4. Horvath E, Majlis S, Rossi R, Franco C, Niedmann JP, Castro A, Dominguez M: An ultrasonogram reporting system for thyroid nodules stratifying cancer risk for clinical management. *J Clin Endocrinol Metab* 2009, **94:**1748–1751.
5. Kang HW, No JH, Chung JH, Min YK, Lee MS, Lee MK, Yang JH, Kim KW: Prevalence, clinical and ultrasonographic characteristics of thyroid incidentalomas. *Thyroid* 2004, **14:**29–33.
6. Cibas ES, Ali SZ: The Bethesda System for Reporting Thyroid Cytopathology. *Thyroid* 2009, **19:**1159–1165.
7. Moon WJ, Jung SL, Lee JH, Na DG, Baek JH, Lee YH, Kim J, Kim HS, Byun JS, Lee DH: Benign and malignant thyroid nodules: US differentiation–multicenter retrospective study. *Radiology* 2008, **247:**762–770.
8. Frates MC, Benson CB, Doubilet PM, Kunreuther E, Contreras M, Cibas ES, Orcutt J, Moore FD Jr, Larsen PR, Marqusee E, Alexander EK: Prevalence and distribution of carcinoma in patients with solitary and multiple thyroid nodules on sonography. *J Clin Endocrinol Metab* 2006, **91:**3411–3417.
9. Papini E, Guglielmi R, Bianchini A, Crescenzi A, Taccogna S, Nardi F, Panunzi C, Rinaldi R, Toscano V, Pacella CM: Risk of malignancy in nonpalpable thyroid nodules: predictive value of ultrasound and color-Doppler features. *J Clin Endocrinol Metab* 2002, **87:**1941–1946.
10. Alexander EK, Marqusee E, Orcutt J, Benson CB, Frates MC, Doubilet PM, Cibas ES, Atri A: Thyroid nodule shape and prediction of malignancy. *Thyroid* 2004, **14:**953–958.
11. Moon HJ, Kwak JY, Kim MJ, Son EJ, Kim EK: Can vascularity at power Doppler US help predict thyroid malignancy? *Radiology* 2010, **255:**260–269.
12. Bakhshaee M, Davoudi Y, Mehrabi M, Layegh P, Mirsadaee S, Rad MP, Leyegh P: Vascular pattern and spectral parameters of power Doppler ultrasound as predictors of malignancy risk in thyroid nodules. *Laryngoscope* 2008, **118:**2182–2186.
13. Fish SA, Langer JE, Mandel SJ: Sonographic imaging of thyroid nodules and cervical lymph nodes. *Endocrinol Metab Clin North Am* 2008, **37:**401–417.
14. Cappelli C, Pirola I, Cumetti D, Micheletti L, Tironi A, Gandossi E, Martino E, Cherubini L, Agosti B, Castellano M, Mattanza C, Rosei EA: Is the anteroposterior and transverse diameter ratio of nonpalpable thyroid nodules a sonographic criteria for recommending fine-needle aspiration cytology? *Clin Endocrinol (Oxf)* 2005, **63:**689–693.
15. Kim DL, Song KH, Kim SK: High prevalence of carcinoma in ultrasonography-guided fine needle aspiration cytology of thyroid nodules. *Endocr J* 2008, **55:**135–142.
16. Kim EK, Park CS, Chung WY, Oh KK, Kim DI, Lee JT, Yoo HS: New sonographic criteria for recommending fine-needle aspiration biopsy of nonpalpable solid nodules of the thyroid. *AJR Am J Roentgenol* 2002, **178:**687–691.
17. Hoang JK, Lee WK, Lee M, Johnson D, Farrell S: US Features of thyroid malignancy: pearls and pitfalls. *Radiographics* 2007, **27:**847–860. discussion 861–865.
18. Cooper DS, Doherty GM, Haugen BR, Kloos RT, Lee SL, Mandel SJ, Mazzaferri EL, McIver B, Pacini F, Schlumberger M, Sherman SI, Steward DL, Tuttle RM: Revised American Thyroid Association management guidelines for patients with thyroid nodules and differentiated thyroid cancer. *Thyroid* 2009, **19:**1167–1214.
19. Leboulleux S, Girard E, Rose M, Travagli JP, Sabbah N, Caillou B, Hartl DM, Lassau N, Baudin E, Schlumberger M: Ultrasound criteria of malignancy for cervical lymph nodes in patients followed up for differentiated thyroid cancer. *J Clin Endocrinol Metab* 2007, **92:**3590–3594.
20. Sohn YM, Kwak JY, Kim EK, Moon HJ, Kim SJ, Kim MJ: Diagnostic approach for evaluation of lymph node metastasis from thyroid cancer using ultrasound and fine-needle aspiration biopsy. *AJR Am J Roentgenol* 2010, **194:**38–43.
21. Krajewska J, Czarniecka A, Jarzab M, Kukulska A, Handkiewicz-Junak D, Hasse-Lazar K, Gubala E, Puch Z, Paliczka E, Roskosz J: Relapse of differentiated thyroid carcinoma in low-risk patients. *Pol J Endocrinol* 2006, **57:**386–391.
22. Czarniecka A, Jarzab M, Krajewska J, Chmielik E, Szcześniak-Klusek B, Stobiecka E, Kokot R, Sacher A, Poltorak S, Wloch J: Prognostic value of lymph node metastases of differentiated thyroid cancer (DTC) according to the local advancement and range of surgical excision. *Thyroid Res* 2010, **3:**8.
23. Mihai R, Parker AJ, Roskell D, Sadler GP: One in four patients with follicular thyroid cytology (THY3) has a thyroid carcinoma. *Thyroid* 2009, **19:**33–37.
24. Sillery JC, Reading CC, Charboneau JW, Henrichsen TL, Hay ID, Mandrekar JN: Thyroid follicular carcinoma: sonographic features of 50 cases. *AJR Am J Roentgenol* 2010, **194:**44–54.
25. Moon WJ, Baek JH, Jung SL, Kim DW, Kim EK, Kim JY, Kwak JY, Lee JH, Lee JH, Lee YH, Na DG, Park JS, Park SW: Ultrasonography and the ultrasound-based management of thyroid nodules: consensus statement and recommendations. *Korean J Radiol* 2011, **12:**1–14.

26. Park JY, Lee HJ, Jang HW, Kim HK, Yi JH, Lee W, Kim SH: **A proposal for a thyroid imaging reporting and data system for ultrasound features of thyroid carcinoma.** *Thyroid* 2009, **19**:1257–1264.

27. Hong YJ, Son EJ, Kim EK, Kwak JY, Hong SW, Chang HS: **Positive predictive values of sonographic features of solid thyroid nodule.** *Clin Imaging* 2010, **34**:127–133.

28. Bahn RS, Castro MR: **Approach to the patient with nontoxic multinodular goiter.** *J Clin Endocrinol Metab* 2011, **96**:1202–1212.

17

The impact of Lithium on thyroid function in Chinese psychiatric population

Kwan Yee Queenie Tsui

Abstract

Background: Lithium was known to cause thyroid dysfunction and most commonly subclinical hypothyroidism (SCH). The aim of this study is to determine the prevalence of Lithium associated thyroid dysfunction and to identify risk factors associated with development of SCH in patients receiving Lithium.

Methods: A retrospective cross-sectional study was conducted. Subjects who developed elated thyroid stimulating hormone (TSH) were compared with those who remained euthyroid with Lithium treatment. Logistic regression and survival analysis were applied to identify the significant factors associated with SCH.

Results: The prevalence of Lithium associated with SCH was 31.7 %. The significant risk factors associated with increased risk of SCH included being female, higher serum Lithium level, concomitant use of Valproate Sodium and use of antidepressant. Use of depot injection was associated with decreased risk of SCH.

Conclusions: Use of depot and avoidance of Valproate or antidepressant should be taken into account before starting patient on Lithium treatment. Thyroxine replacement should be considered when Lithium associated SCH was identified.

Keywords: Lithium, Thyroid, Subclinical, Hypothyroidism, Psychiatric

Background

Lithium, discovered in 1817, was initially used for treating gout. Throughout years of research since its introduction, Lithium has now been well established as an effective agent for treatment in acute mania, prophylaxis of bipolar disorder and augmentation in refractory depression. Possible long term side effects included renal insufficiency, thyroid dysfunction, persistent tremor, and dermatologic effects of acne and alopecia [1]. Among the possible side effects of Lithium, thyroid dysfunction especially subclinical hypothyroidism (SCH) was a common yet often neglected one. Lithium was reported to concentrate in thyroid gland and inhibit thyroidal iodine uptake. It also inhibits iodotyrosine coupling, alters thyroglobulin structure and inhibits thyroid hormone secretion. Lithium inhibits synthesis and release of thyroid hormones by stabilizing effect on thyroid microtubules, decreasing adenylate cyclase responsiveness to TSH and suppressing cyclic adenosine mono phosphate (c-AMP)

Correspondence: luna-1005@hotmail.com
Department of Psychiatry, Pamela Youde Nethersole Eastern Hospital, 3 Lok Man Road, Chai Wan, Hong Kong SAR, China

production. Lithium lowers de-iodination in the liver and decreases the clearance of free T4 [2].

According to ETA Guideline, SCH was characterized by TSH above the upper reference limit in combination with a normal free thyroxine (T4). Clinical hypothyroidism was characterized by TSH above the upper reference limit in combination with low free T4. Both situations were indicated by elated TSH.

The prevalence of clinical and subclinical hypothyroidism in the general population were 0.3 and 4.3 % respectively (NHANES III, 1988–1994). 36 % bipolar patients developed abnormal TSH with or without T4 abnormality while on Lithium [3]. The prevalence of clinical hypothyroidism while on Lithium was 10.4 % [4]. The prevalence of SCH while on Lithium was reported to be up to 20.3 % [5]. Bocchetta et al. noted only 1 case of hyperthyroidism among 150 patients on long term Lithium therapy during a 15 year follow up, suggesting Lithium induced hyperthyroidism was extremely rare [6]. Thus in this study, we would focus on mainly risk factors associated with development of elated TSH on Lithium.

Methods

This study was a retrospective cross-sectional analysis of case notes of all Chinese psychiatric patients, who were receiving Lithium treatment and had serum thyroid function test (TFT) and Lithium level taken in the past one year on 1st March 2014. It was conducted in the Department of Psychiatry of Pamela Youde Nethersole Eastern Hospital (PYNEH) in Hong Kong. The medical records of potential study sample were retrieved and screened from the Medical Record Office (MRO) and electronic Clinical Management System (e-CMS) of Hospital Authority in Hong Kong. The reference range of TSH and free T4 were 0.35–3.80mIU/L and 9.5–18.1pmol/L respectively in PYNEH. Patients who were not from Chinese origin and had thyroid dysfunction before starting Lithium treatment as indicated by TFT or documented in medical notes were excluded. Among 262 patients eligible for the study, 109 (41.6 %) patients were male and 153 (58.4 %) were female. The study population comprised of relatively balanced gender ratio of 1 male to 1.4 female. The mean age of the study population was 48.57 years old with standard deviation of 12.267 years.

A collection of important factors were indentified as independent variables that might predispose to the development of SCH in the participants, including demographic factors, clinical characteristics and characteristics of medications prescribed. The number of months between the date of starting Lithium and development of elated TSH would be calculated as "duration of Lithium use". If TSH remained normal throughout the study period, the number of months between the dates of starting Lithium till 1st March 2014 would then be calculated as "duration of Lithium use".

Data analysis

Comparison of demographic and clinical data between patients with normal and elated TSH while on Lithium treatment were done in univariate analysis. Variables showing statistically significant difference ($p < 0.05$) or marginally significant difference ($0.05 \leq p < 0.10$) would be indentified and multivariate logistic regression analysis would then applied. Variables having $p < 0.05$ after multivariate logistic regression were considered as significant. Survival analysis was further conducted to indentify factors associated with development of elated TSH while on Lithium treatment. Kaplan-Meier survival curve would be plotted to give graphical representation of the survival function. Data was analyzed through IBM Statistical Product and Service Solution (SPSS) software version 22.

Ethics approval

This study was approved by the Ethics Committee of Hong Kong East Cluster of Hospital Authority (HA) and the Chief of Service of the Department of Psychiatry of PYNEH.

Results

Total 304 cases that were on Lithium treatment at PYNEH on 1st March 2014 were indentified through CDARS. Ethnicity, availability of thyroid and Lithium monitoring in the past one year and presence of thyroid illness before starting Lithium treatment were screened. Total 42 cases were excluded. The overall number of patients eligible for study was 262. Among the recruited patients, 93 (35.5 %) cases developed elated TSH, of whom 10 (3.8 %) cases had clinical hypothyroidism and 83 (31.6 %) cases had SCH. TSH of the remaining 169 (64.5 %) patients remained non-elated while on Lithium treatment. 10 (3.8 %) patients developed decreased TSH, of whom 1 (0.4 %) case developed clinical hyperthyroidism and 9 (3.4 %) cases developed subclinical hyperthyroidism. 159 (60.7 %) patients remained euthyroid throughout the study. Figure 1 showed the forming of the study population.

Univariate analysis was preformed between patients with elated and non-elated TSH for demographic factors, clinical characteristics and characteristics of medications prescribed. Gender showed significant value of $p = 0.005$. Use of Valproate Sodium ($p < 0.001$) and use of depot injection ($p = 0.008$) were statistically significant and types of Lithium taking ($p = 0.073$) was marginally significant. Serum Lithium level ($p = 0.001$) was also statistically significant. The univariate test results were summarized in Table 1.

Multivariate logistic regression was then applied. Gender ($p = 0.001$) was significantly associated with development of elated TSH. Male gender was associated with lower odds of development of elated TSH, in which the odds of developing elated TSH would be 37 % of that in female. Serum Lithium level ($p = 0.007$) was also found to be associated with higher odds of development of elated TSH. One unit (1 µmol /L = 0.001 mEq/L) increase was associated with 0.2 % increase in the odds of developing elated TSH (OR = 1.002). Moreover, co-administration of depot injection with Lithium ($p = 0.013$) was shown to significantly lower risk of developing elated TSH. The odds of developing elated TSH for those on depot injection was 18.9 % of those not on depot injection (OR = 0.189). When Valproate Sodium was prescribed with Lithium ($p < 0.001$), there would be an increased risk of developing elated TSH. Patients on Valproate would have 4.522 times greater risk in having elated TSH than those not on Valproate (OR = 4.522). The multivariate logistic regression results were shown in Table 2.

After logistic regression analysis, survival analysis was further conducted to explore factors which correlated to the time to development of elated TSH. Univariate cox

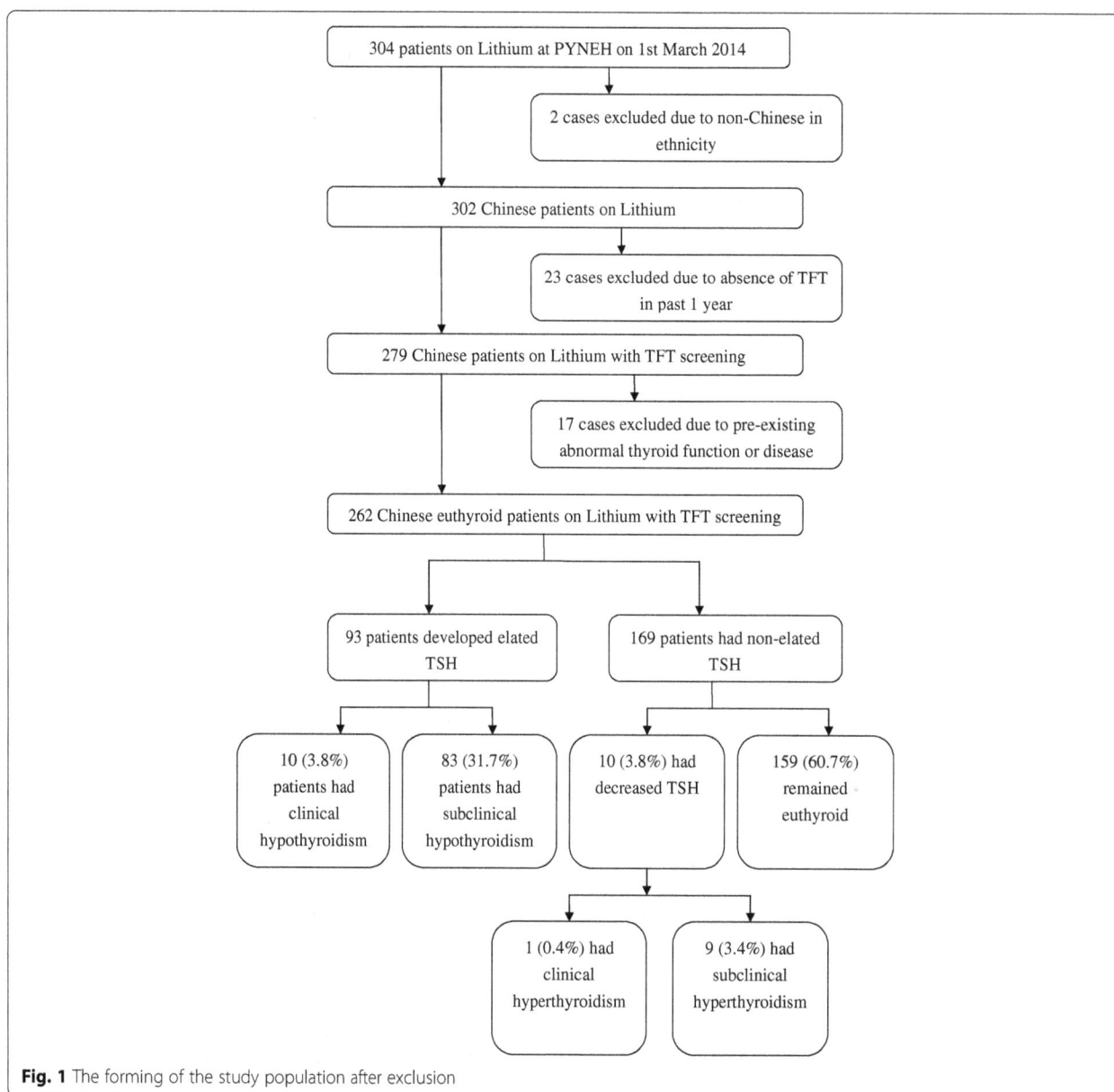

Fig. 1 The forming of the study population after exclusion

regression was applied to all the variables with results shown in Table 3. Multivariate cox regression was then applied to the factors having $p < 0.10$ in univariate cox regression. The multivariate cox regression identified the same four significant factors as the previous multivariate logistic regression analysis except one extra factor 'concomitant use of antidepressant' was identified as significant in survival analysis. The results of multivariate cox regression were presented as follows. Firstly, gender ($p = 0.008$) was statistically significant, and the hazard of male patients in developing elated TSH was 54.1 % of that in female patients (HR = 0.541). Secondly, serum Lithium level ($p = 0.015$) was associated with higher hazard in developing elated TSH, and one unit (1 μmol/L = 0.001 mEq/L) increase was

associated with 0.1 % raise in hazard of developing elated TSH (HR = 1.001). Thirdly, depot injection ($p = 0.046$) was shown to significantly lower the risk in developing elated TSH while on Lithium, and the hazard of patients using depot was 30.8 % of those not on depot injection (HR = 0.308). Fourthly, use of Valproate Sodium was significant ($p = 0.002$), and the hazard of patients on Valproate Sodium was 2.056 times greater in developing elated TSH than those not taking (HR = 2.056). Lastly, as described above, concomitant use of antidepressant with Lithium ($p = 0.04$) was noted to be a significant factor, and the hazard of patients using antidepressant in developing elated TSH was 1.576 times greater than those not on antidepressant treatment (HR = 1.576). The multivariate

Table 1 Univariate tests for factors between patient with non-elated and elated TSH

Factors	Non-elated TSH (N = 169)	Elated TSH (N = 93)	p
Male	81 (47.9 %)	28 (30.1 %)	0.005*[a]
Female	88 (52.1 %)	65 (69.9 %)	
Primary Psychiatric Diagnosis			0.573[b]
Schizophrenia/Schizoaffective Disorder/Psychosis	51 (30.1 %)	33 (35.5 %)	
Bipolar Affective Disorder/Mania	86 (50.9 %)	46 (49.5 %)	
Depression/Anxiety	26 (15.4 %)	11 (11.8 %)	
Mental Retardation	3 (1.8 %)	3 (3.2 %)	
Others	3 (1.8 %)	0 (0.0 %)	
Secondary Psychiatric Diagnosis			0.309[b]
Personality Disorder	1 (0.6 %)	1 (1.1 %)	
Mental Retardation	6 (3.5 %)	1 (1.1 %)	
Substance Abuse	5 (3.0 %)	1 (1.1 %)	
Autistic Spectrum Disorder	2 (1.2 %)	1 (1.1 %)	
Others	0 (0.0 %)	2 (2.1 %)	
Nil	155 (91.7 %)	87 (93.5 %)	
Physical Comorbidities			
Hypertension			0.505[a]
Yes	25 (14.8 %)	11 (11.8 %)	
No	144 (85.2 %)	82 (88.2 %)	
Diabetes			0.911[a]
Yes	21 (12.4 %)	12 (13 %)	
No	148 (87.6 %)	81 (87 %)	
Hyperlipidaemia			0.410[a]
Yes	18 (10.7 %)	7 (7.5 %)	
No	151 (89.3 %)	86 (92.5 %)	
Cardiovascular disorders			0.617[b]
Yes	2 (1.2 %)	2 (2.2 %)	
No	167 (98.8 %)	91 (97.8 %)	
Types of Lithium taking			0.073**[a]
Lithium CR	141 (83.4 %)	69 (74.2 %)	
Lithium IR	28 (16.6 %)	24 (25.8 %)	
Frequency of Lithium per day			0.311[b]
Once	147 (87.0 %)	75 (80.6 %)	
Twice	20 (11.8 %)	17 (18.3 %)	
Three times	2 (1.2 %)	1 (1.1 %)	
Use of depot injection			0.008*[b]
Yes	22 (13.0 %)	3 (3.2 %)	

Table 1 Univariate tests for factors between patient with non-elated and elated TSH *(Continued)*

No	147 (87.0 %)	90 (96.8 %)	
Use of oral antipsychotics			0.421[a]
Yes	129 (76.3 %)	75 (80.6 %)	
No	40 (23.7 %)	18 (19.4 %)	
Use of antidepressant			0.746[a]
Yes	62 (36.7 %)	36 (38.7 %)	
No	107 (63.3 %)	57 (61.3 %)	
Use of Benzodiazepine			0.742[a]
Yes	80 (47.3 %)	46 (49.5 %)	
No	89 (52.7 %)	47 (50.5 %)	
Use of Carbamazepine			0.669[b]
Yes	3 (1.8 %)	3 (3.2 %)	
No	166 (98.2 %)	90 (96.8 %)	
Use of Valproate Sodium			< 0.001*[a]
Yes	18 (10.7 %)	31 (33.3 %)	
No	151 (89.3 %)	62 (66.7 %)	
Use of other mood stabilizers			1.000[a]
Yes	5 (3.0 %)	2 (2.2 %)	
No	164 (97.0 %)	91 (97.8 %)	
Use of non-psychiatric medications			0.786[a]
Yes	77 (45.6 %)	44 (47.3 %)	
No	92 (54.4 %)	49 (52.7 %)	
Age, mean (SD)	48.47 (12.188)	48.76 (12.473)	0.852[c]
Serum Lithium Level (µmol /L), mean (SD)	541.30 (217.701)	639.14 (212.984)	0.001*[c]
Dosage of Lithium (mg), median (IQR)	800 (675–1000)	800 (600–800)	0.364[d]

*Note: *significant p < 0.05, **marginally significant 0.05 ≤ p < 0.10, [a]Chi-squared test, [b]Fisher's exact test, [c]Independent-sample-t-test, [d]Mann-Whitney U Test, SD Standard Deviation, IQR Interquartile Range*

cox regression results were also shown in Table 2. In addition, Kaplan-Meier survival curves were plotted for the significant results identified in survival analysis as shown in Fig. 2.

Discussion

In this study, 35.5 % patients developed elated TSH while on Lithium treatment and it was close to the rate (36 %) done in Pittsburgh study comprising of 143 patients [3]. Lithium induced clinical hyperthyroidism was shown to be a rare event as only 1 out of 262 patients developed clinical hyperthyroidism in this study.

It was found that the risk of developing SCH when on Lithium was significantly higher in women, which was also reported in other studies [4, 7]. Such difference was likely due to the exacerbating effect of estradiol in

Table 2 Significant factors identified in multivariate analysis

Multivariate Logistic Regression

Factors	OR (95 % CI)	p
Gender (Male)	0.370 (0.202–0.679)	0.001
Serum Lithium Level	1.002 (1.001–1.003)	0.007
Use of depot injection	0.189 (0.051–0.704)	0.013
Use of Valproate Sodium	4.522 (2.179–9.381)	< 0.001

Survival Analysis

Multivariate Cox Regression

Factors	HR (95 % CI)	p
Gender	0.541 (0.344–0.851)	0.008
Serum Lithium Level	1.001 (1.0–1.002)	0.015
Use of depot injection	0.308 (0.097–0.978)	0.046
Use of antidepressant	1.576 (1.021–2.435)	0.040
Use of Valproate Sodium	2.056 (1.311–3.224)	0.002

Note: Significant p < 0.05, OR Odds Ratio, HR Hazard Ratio, CI Confidence Interval

Table 3 Univariate cox regression for survival analysis

Demographic factors	p
Gender	0.011*
Age	0.726
Clinical Characteristics	
Primary Psychiatric Diagnosis	0.992
Secondary Psychiatric Diagnosis	0.296
Hypertension	0.136
Diabetes	0.405
Hyperlipidaemia	0.243
Cardiovascular disorders	0.833
Characteristics of medications prescribed	
Types of Lithium taking	0.109
Frequency of Lithium per day	0.298
Serum Lithium Level	0.028*
Dosage of Lithium	0.762
Use of depot injection	0.035*
Use of oral antipsychotics	0.908
Use of antidepressant	0.067**
Use of Benzodiazepine	0.588
Use of Carbamazepine	0.221
Use of Valproate Sodium	0.001*
Use of other mood stabilizers	0.577
Use of non-psychiatric medications	0.449

Note: *Significant p < 0.05, **Marginally Significant 0.05 ≤ p < 0.10

women and protective effect of testosterone in men. It has been demonstrated that estradiol would decrease iodide uptake in thyroid follicular cells [8]. Testosterone had also been shown to decrease thyroid enlargement and prevent the fall in free T4 levels in rats [9].

It was demonstrated in this study that there was a positive correlation between serum Lithium level and risk of developing elated TSH. A few studies had also reported on such finding [10, 11].

Antipsychotics were well known for their central activity on tuberoinfundibular dopaminergic pathway. The antagonism of dopamine 2 receptor could increase Thyroid Releasing Hormone stimulated TSH levels [12]. Use of depot injection had been shown to decrease risk of developing SCH. This was probably related to more stable plasma antipsychotics concentration with less fluctuation when using depot rather than oral administration [13].

When Valproate Sodium was taken concomitantly with Lithium, the risk of developing SCH would become greater. This showed that Lithium and Valproate Sodium had synergistic effect in inducing SCH. Valproate alone had been proven to induce SCH by several studies [14]. Valproate had been reported to increase serum Gamma-aminobutyric Acid (GABA) level [15]. GABA was also shown to inhibit TSH-stimulated thyroid hormone release from the thyroid gland [16]. Another mechanism proposed was Valproate induced SCH through blockage of N-methyl-D-aspartate (NMDA) synaptic transmission [17], while NMDA had been shown to increase serum thyroid hormone level [18]. Hence, both mechanisms would stimulate TSH release from the pituitary gland.

At last, use of antidepressant with Lithium was shown to increase risk of developing SCH. Such increased in risk was consistent with previous study results in which patients developed increased TSH while on Sertraline and Desipramine [19, 20]. Though the mechanism behind remained unclear. The possible explanation would be serotonin increased by antidepressant when administered in a chronic fashion induced lower plasma levels of thyroid hormones [21]. Thus, Lithium and antidepressant had synergistic effect in inducing SCH and such effect was only revealed by survival analysis when survival time was taken into account.

For patients who were at increased risk of developing thyroid dysfunction including being female, with personal or family history of thyroid disorders and with positive autoimmune markers or abnormal TFT in the initial blood taking prior to initiating Lithium, special caution in prescription regimen to avoid further exacerbation or development of thyroid dysfunction should be taken. According to this study, depot injection could be put at a higher priority than oral administration when antipsychotics were indicated. Simplification of regimen should be adopted, since co-administration of Valproate

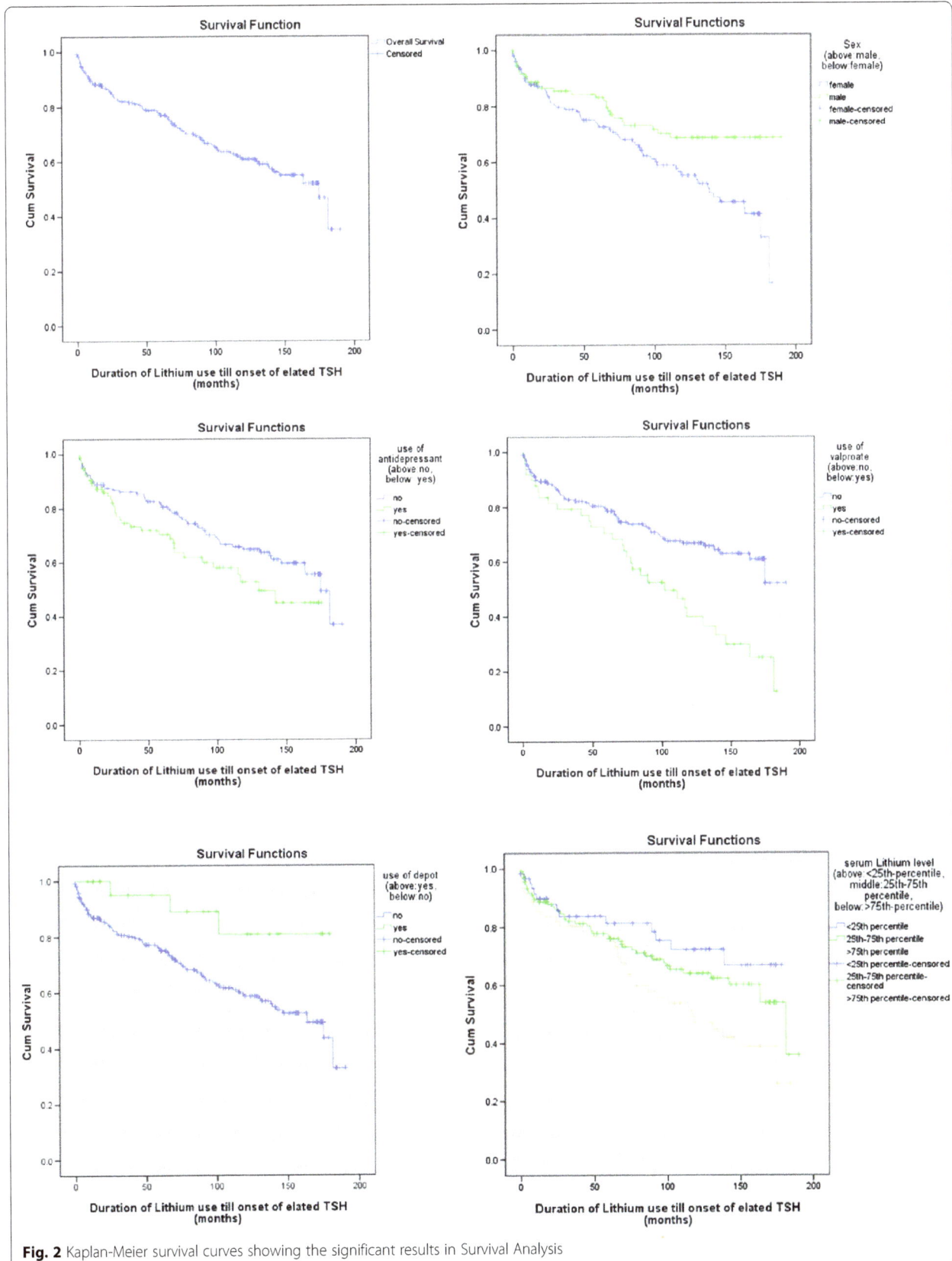

Fig. 2 Kaplan-Meier survival curves showing the significant results in Survival Analysis

Sodium or antidepressant had been shown to increase risk of developing SCH. When antidepressant was indicated, it should be prescribed for short term use if possible since chronic administration would have synergistic effect with Lithium in inducing SCH. Over-treatment should be avoided and lowering Lithium dosage after acute episode should be considered, since there was an increased in risk of developing SCH for every unit increase in serum Lithium level.

Discrepancy existed between different guidelines in reference to ongoing TFT monitoring in patients taking Lithium. National Institute for Health and Care Excellence (NICE), British National Formulary (BNF) and South London & Maudsley (SLAM) recommended TFT to be taken every 6 months while Best Practice review series and Drugs & Therapeutic Bulletin (DTB) recommended TFT to be taken every 12 months. Lithium had been shown to increase antibody titers, especially, when these antibodies had been present at the start of treatment [22]. However, among all the above guidelines, antiperoxidase and antithyroglobulin measurements had not been included in the initial blood tests recommended prior to start of Lithium. Also compliance to recommended guidelines were still difficult when requirements were too stringent, such as only 35 % of patients were compliant to the recommended guideline of three-monthly plasma Lithium level taking in 2013 NICE audit. Thus balance between theoretical recommendations and practical clinical scenarios remained for further discussion.

Patient's mental state should be closely monitored when put on Levothyroxine treatment since it had been reported that some patients would experience mania while on replacement therapy [23]. Levothyroxine treatment should be started prior to antidepressant trial for bipolar patients with depressive symptoms associated with SCH since thyroxine replacement might lead to improvement in mood.

To our knowledge, this is the first study to have extensively investigated on risk factors and predictors on Lithium associated SCH in Chinese patients. Apart from gender and age which had been widely investigated in previous studies, other risk factors including concomitant use of various psychiatric medications, comorbidities and serum Lithium level had been comprehensively investigated in this study by both logistic regression and survival analysis.

For the study results, consistent risk factors were found using both logistic regression and survival analysis meaning that these risk factors remained stable and significant despite employment of different statistical analyses. These risk factors not only showed statistical significance, but also gave clinical significance in further revision of current clinical guidelines and recommended treatment in terms of Lithium associated SCH.

There were several limitations in this study. The retrospective study design confined the collection of data to be only obtained from the case records. Other factors including infection, stress and smoking could also induce thyroid dysfunction but such information had not been recorded properly and consistently in case notes. Another limitation was this study was unable to develop causality between exposure of the risk factors in development of Lithium associated SCH. Besides, the severity of psychiatric diseases, which might had an effect on the results apart from the pharmacological action of drugs, had not been investigated in this study. The number of individuals having various severity levels of different psychiatric diagnoses would be too small and therefore they had been grouped together according to their mental disorders for statistical analysis.

Further research is required to establish and investigate on the effectiveness of depot in reducing development of SCH on Lithium when compared with use of oral antipsychotics. The effect of chronic administration of antidepressant and Lithium should also be further explored in development of SCH. Few studies had investigated on relationship with serum Lithium level and risk of SCH and further research might be required. With research in more comprehensive and deeper perspective, it was hoped that further improvement in current Lithium guidelines could be reached.

Conclusions

Despite various psychiatric medications had been discovered and manufactured throughout the century, Lithium remained the only drug with an established anti-suicidal efficacy for affective disorders. It was still widely advocated in patients with bipolar affective disorder and refractory depression. Thyroid dysfunction complicated by Lithium treatment had been investigated, but SCH with related risk factors was often neglected. Use of depot and avoidance of Valproate or antidepressant should be taken into account for patients receiving Lithium treatment. Serum Lithium level and thyroid function should be monitored regularly, and thyroxine replacement should be considered when Lithium associated SCH was identified. With increasing evidence in harm and risk of untreated SCH, further research and revision of current Lithium guidelines would be required.

Competing interests
The author declares that she has no competing interests.

Authors' contributions
Dr KYQT was solely responsible for designing of the study, data collection, statistical analysis and writing up of this paper. The work was part of the dissertation for completing the HKC Psych Part III Examination.

Acknowledgement
I would like to thank my parents, brother and especially my husband, Dr. Terry Wong, for their forever care, kindness and love whenever I was in need and throughout my years of learning.

References
1. Melvin GM. Lithium for bipolar disorder: a re-emerging treatment for mood instability. Curr Psychiatry. 2014;13(6):38–44.
2. Lazarus JH. The effects of lithium therapy on thyroid and thyrotropin-releasing hormone. Thyroid. 1998;8(10):909–13.
3. Fagiolini A, Kupfer DJ, Scott J, Swartz HA, Cook D, Novick DM, et al. Hypothyroidism in patients with bipolar I disorder treated primarily with lithium. Epidemiol Psychiatr Soc. 2006;15(2):123–7.
4. Johnston AM, Eagles JM. Lithium associated clinical hypothyroidism: prevalence and risk factors. Br J Psychiatry. 1999;175:336–9.
5. Choi HM, Chang JS, Kim J, Kim JH, Choi JE, Ha TH, et al. Subclinical hypothyroidism in patients with bipolar disorders managed by lithium or valproic acid. Korean J Biol Psychiatry. 2013;20(4):151–8. Korean.
6. Bocchetta A, Cocco F, Velluzzi F, Del-Zompo M, Mariotti S, Loviselli A. Fifteen-year follow-up of thyroid function in lithium patients. J Endocrinol Invest. 2007;30(5):363–6.
7. Kirov G, Tredget J, John R, Owen MJ, Lazarus JH. A cross-sectional and a prospective study of thyroid disorders in lithium-treated patients. J Affect Disord. 2005;87(2–3):313–7. doi:10.1016/j.jad.2005.03.010.
8. Furlanetto TW, Nunes Jr RB, Sopelsa AM, Maciel RM. Estradiol decreases iodide uptake by rat thyroid follicular FRTL-5 cells. Braz J Med Biol Res. 2001;34(2):259–63.
9. Bahrami Z, Hedayati M, Taghikhani M, Azizi F. Effect of testosterone on thyroid weight and function in iodine deficient castrated rats. Horm Metab Res. 2009;41(10):762–6. doi:10.1055/s-0029-1225629. Epub 2009 Jul.
10. Tellian FF, Rueda-Vasquez E. Effect of serum lithium levels on thyrotropin levels. South Med J. 1993;86(10):1182–3.
11. Gracious BL, Findling RL, Seman C, Youngstrom EA, Demeter CA, Calabrese JR. Elevated thyrotropin in bipolar youths prescribed both lithium and divalproex sodium. J Am Acad Child Adolesc Psychiatry. 2004;43(2):215–20. doi:10.1097/00004583-200402000-00018.
12. Bunevicius R, Steibliene V, Prange Jr AJ. Thyroid axis function after in-patient treatment of acute psychosis with antipsychotics: a naturalistic study. BMC Psychiatry. 2014;14:279. doi:10.1186/s12888-014-0279-7.
13. Barnes TR, Curson DA. Long-term depot antipsychotics. A risk-benefit assessment. Drug Saf. 1994;10(6):464–79.
14. Jerome MH, Kim SH, Chung HR, Kim SH, Kim H, Lim BC, et al. Valproic acid therapy causes subclinical hypothyroidism in children with epilepsy. Clin Thyroidol. 2012;24:15–6.
15. Loscher W, Schmidt D. Increase of human plasma GABA by sodium valproate. Epilepsia. 1980;21(6):611–5.
16. Wiens SC, Trudeau VL. Thyroid hormone and gamma-aminobutyric acid (GABA) interactions in neuroendocrine systems. Comp Biochem Physiol A Mol Integr Physiol. 2006;144(3):332–44. doi:10.1016/j.cbpa.2006.01.033.
17. Gean PW, Huang CC, Hung CR, Tsai JJ. Valproic acid suppresses the synaptic response mediated by the NMDA receptors in rat amygdalar slices. Brain Res Bull. 1994;33(3):333–6.
18. Alfonso M, Duran R, Arufe MC. Effect of excitatory amino acids on serum TSH and thyroid hormone levels in freely moving rats. Horm Res. 2000;54(2):78–83.
19. Eker SS, Akkaya C, Sarandol A. Effects of various antidepressants on serum thyroid hormone levels in patients with major depressive disorder. Neuropsychopharmacol Biol Psychiatry. 2008;32(4):955Y961.
20. Brady KT, Anton RF. The thyroid axis and desipramine treatment in depression. Biol Psychiatry. 1989;25(6):703–9.
21. Alessio S, Guglielmo B, Nicola M. Chronic peripheral administration of serotonin inhibits thyroid function in the rat. Muscles Ligaments Tendons J. 2011;1(2):48–50.
22. Calabrese JR, Gulledge AD, Hahn K, Skwerer R, Kotz M, Schumacher OP, et al. Autoimmune thyroiditis in manic-depressive patients treated with lithium. Am J Psychiatry. 1985;142(11):1318–21.
23. Josephson AM, Mackenzie TB. Thyroid-induced mania in hypothyroid patients. Br J Psychiatry. 1980;137:222–8.

18

Effect of perchlorate and thiocyanate exposure on thyroid function of pregnant women from South-West England: a cohort study

Bridget A. Knight[1,2]* iD, Beverley M. Shields[1], Xuemei He[3], Elizabeth N. Pearce[3], Lewis E. Braverman[3], Rachel Sturley[4] and Bijay Vaidya[5,6]

Abstract

Background: Iodine is important for thyroid hormone synthesis, and iodine deficiency in pregnancy may impair fetal neurological development. As perchlorate and thiocyanate inhibit sodium-iodide symporter reducing the transport of iodine from circulation into the thyroid follicular cells, environmental exposure to these substances in pregnancy may impair maternal thyroid hormone synthesis. We aimed to explore the impact of perchlorate and thiocyanate exposure on thyroid status in a cohort of pregnant mothers from South West England.

Methods: Urine samples were obtained from 308 women participating in a study of breech presentation in late pregnancy. They had no known thyroid disease and a singleton pregnancy at 36–38 weeks gestation. Samples were analysed for urinary concentrations of iodine (UIC), perchlorate (UPC) and thiocyanate (UTC). Blood samples were taken for free T4 (FT4), thyrotropin (TSH) and thyroid peroxidase antibodies (TPO-Ab). Baseline data included age, parity, smoking status, ethnicity and BMI at booking. Following delivery, data on offspring's sex, gestational age at birth and birthweight were collected.

Results: Participants had a mean (SD) age 31 (5) years, median (IQR) BMI 24.4 (22.0, 28.3) kg/m^2, 42% were primiparous, 10% were smokers, and 96% were Caucasian. Median UIC was 88 μg/l, and 174/308 (57%) women had UIC < 100 μg/l. Log transformed UPC negatively correlated with FT4, but not with TSH, in the whole cohort ($r = -0.12$, $p = 0.03$) and in the subgroup of women with UIC < 100 μg/l ($r = -0.15$, $p = 0.04$). Regression analysis with the potential confounders (TPO-Ab status, UIC and UTC) identified UPC to be negatively associated with FT4 ($p = 0.01$). There was no correlation between UTC and FT4 or TSH. Maternal UPC or UTC was not associated with offspring birthweight.

Conclusion: Environmental perchlorate exposure is negatively associated with circulating FT4 levels in third trimester pregnant women. This may have an adverse impact on neurocognitive development of the fetus.

Keywords: Perchlorate, Thiocyanate, Iodine, Thyroid, Pregnancy, Birth weight

* Correspondence: B.A.Knight@ex.ac.uk
[1]NIHR Exeter Clinical Research Facility, Royal Devon & Exeter Hospital,
University of Exeter Medical School, University of Exeter, Exeter EX2 5DW, UK
[2]Research & Development Department, Royal Devon and Exeter Hospital
NHS Foundation Trust, Exeter, UK
Full list of author information is available at the end of the article

Background

Optimal level of maternal thyroid hormone in pregnancy is important for fetal neurological development, and as iodine is an essential component of thyroid hormone, iodine deficiency in pregnancy may impair fetal neurological development [1]. In recent years, there has been increasing concern that exposure to environmental pollutants during pregnancy may result in reduced maternal thyroid hormone synthesis affecting fetal neurodevelopment [2, 3].

Perchlorate and thiocyanate are common environmental pollutants that can disrupt normal thyroid function by reducing the uptake of iodine from the circulation into the thyroid follicular cells through competitive inhibition at the sodium-iodide symporter [2]. Perchlorate can be found in water, milk and some food crops, including green leafy vegetables and fruits. It was found to be present in 77 out of 342 food items tested in the UK between 2014 and 15 [4]. It is also present in fertilisers, rocket fuels, explosives, fireworks, road flares and air bags. Cigarette smoke is the main source of thiocyanate, but it can also be found in some vegetables of the Cruciferae family, such as cabbage, broccoli and cauliflower. Perchlorate is about 15 times stronger than thiocyanate as an inhibitor of the sodium-iodide symporter [5], and in pharmacological doses is known to suppress thyroid hormone synthesis [2]. However, there is a concern that even a low-level exposure of perchlorate or thiocyanate could disrupt thyroid hormone synthesis, particularly in the presence of iodine deficiency. This could lead to health hazards that may be more pronounced in vulnerable populations, such as pregnant women. Several studies have examined the effect of perchlorate and thiocyanate exposure during pregnancy on maternal thyroid function, however these showed conflicting results, and the potential adverse impact of exposure remains controversial [6–12].

Therefore, we aimed to study the impact of perchlorate and thiocyanate exposure on thyroid function of pregnant mothers from South West England where iodine deficiency has been shown to be common [13].

Methods

Participants

We studied 308 women participating in a study of breech presentation in late pregnancy [14]. They were recruited during routine antenatal care at the Royal Devon and Exeter Hospital (RD&E), a secondary care hospital in South-West England serving a population of about 450,000. They had a singleton pregnancy at 36–38 weeks gestation. They had no known thyroid disease, and were not on any drugs which may affect thyroid function. We collected baseline clinical data (including age, parity, smoking status, ethnicity and body mass index (BMI) at booking), and blood and spot urine samples from the participants. Following delivery, we collected data on sex, gestational age at birth and birth-weight of the babies; these data were unavailable for one baby as their mother moved away out of area before delivery.

Sample analysis

Blood samples were analysed at the RD&E Blood Sciences department for serum thyroid stimulating hormone (TSH), free thyroxine (FT4) and thyroid peroxidase antibodies (TPO-Ab) using the electrochemiluminescent immunoassay, run on the Modular E170 Analyser (Roche, Burgess Hill, UK). Intra-assay coefficients of variations were < 5.3% for both TSH and FT4. The manufacturer's population reference ranges were: TSH 0.35–4.5 mIU/l and FT4 11–24 pmol/l. Serum TPO-Ab titre above 34 IU/l was considered positive.

Urine samples were analysed for iodine, perchlorate, and thiocyanate concentration using ion chromatography-mass spectrometry at the Iodine Research Laboratory (Boston University, Boston, Massachusetts) [15]. The inter-assay coefficient of variation ranges from 3.1–8.2% for the three analytes.

Statistical analysis

We assessed variables for normal distribution and log transformed (log) where appropriate. Where this did not result in a normal distribution, these data are presented as median (IQR). Correlations between two variables were assessed and results presented as Pearson correlation coefficients. Regression analysis was undertaken to identify independent predictors of thyroid status. As iodine deficiency may aggravate the effect of perchlorate and thiocyanate exposure, we also carried out subgroup analyses in women with urinary iodine concentration (UIC) less than 100 µg/l.

Table 1 Baseline Characteristics for total cohort (n = 308)

Characteristics	Figures
Age (years)[a]	31 (5)
Booking BMI (kg/m^2)[b]	24.4 (22.0, 28.3)
Gestation (weeks)[b]	37.0 (36.1, 37.6)
Primiparous	128 (42%)
Smoking	31 (10%)
Caucasian	295 (96%)
TSH (mIU/l)[b]	1.9 (1.4, 2.6)
Free T4 (pmol/l)[a]	12.0 (1.6)
TPO-Ab positive	16/305 (5%)
Urinary Iodine (µg/l)[b]	88 (55, 157)
Urinary Perchlorate (µg/l)[b]	2.1 (1.4,3.8)
Urinary Thiocyanate (µg/l)[b]	436 (302,683)

Data presented as [a]mean (SD), [b] median (IQR) or (n) %

We analysed correlations between offspring birthweight (corrected for sex and gestational age at birth) and maternal urinary perchlorate concentration (UPC) and urinary thiocyanate concentration (UTC). We also carried out subgroup analyses considering birthweight (corrected for gestational age) of male and female infants separately.

With a sample size of 300, we can detect correlation coefficients $r \geq 0.12$ as statistically significant at $p < 0.05$.

Statistical analysis was undertaken using SPSS (version 22).

Results
Baseline characteristics

Baseline clinical characteristics and thyroid function of the 308 participants are shown in Table 1. Ninety-six percent were Caucasian. The median UIC was 88 µg/l [13]. Fifty-seven percent (174 out of 308) women had UIC below 100 µg/l. The median UPC was 2.1 µg/l (IQR 1.4–3.8, range 0.3–143), and the median UTC was 436 µg/l (IQR 302–683, range 29–3290).

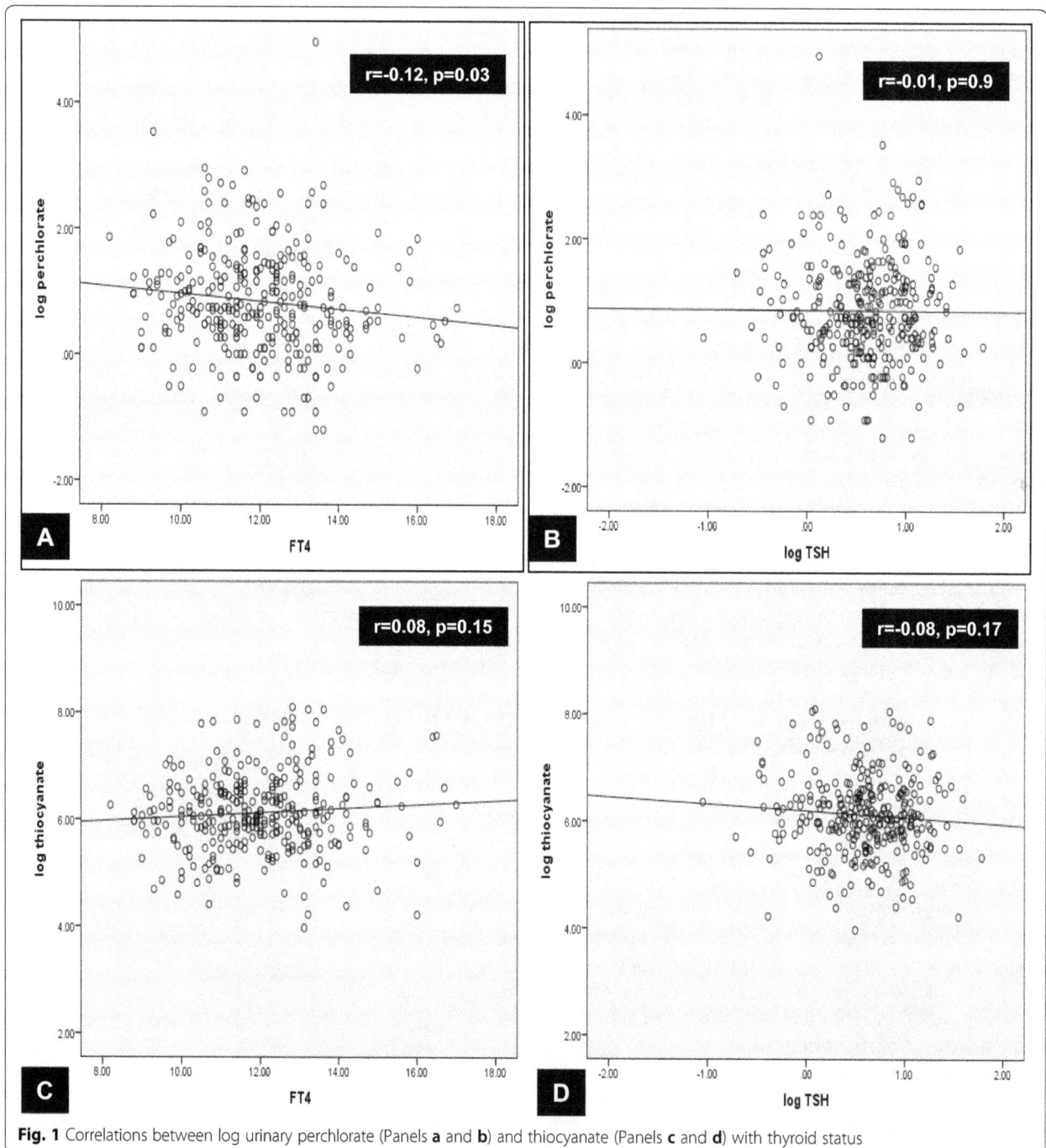

Fig. 1 Correlations between log urinary perchlorate (Panels **a** and **b**) and thiocyanate (Panels **c** and **d**) with thyroid status

Table 2 Regression analyses demonstrating the relationships between urinary perchlorate concentration and other potential confounding variables on serum FT4 and TSH (n = 308)

	β	SE	95% CI for β	t	p
Factors associated with serum FT4					
Urinary perchlorate[a]	−0.291	0.114	(− 0.515, − 0.066)	−2.55	**0.01**
Urinary iodine[a]	0.156	0.124	(−0.088, 0.401)	1.27	0.21
Urinary thiocyanate[a]	0.196	0.127	(−0.053, 0.446)	1.55	0.12
TPO antibody positive	−0.345	0.413	(−1.156, 0.467)	−0.84	0.4
Factors associated with serum TSH[a]					
Urinary perchlorate[a]	0.008	0.032	(−0.056, 0.071)	0.24	0.8
Urinary iodine[a]	−0.03	0.035	(−0.10, 0.039)	−0.85	0.4
Urinary thiocyanate[a]	−0.047	0.036	(−0.117, 0.24)	−1.31	0.2
TPO antibody positive	0.248	0.117	(0.02, 0.48)	2.126	**0.03**

[a]Denotes variable transformed using natural logs (allowing β coefficients to be interpreted in terms of percentage change)
Bold values are significant result in the table

Correlation between urinary perchlorate and maternal thyroid status

Log UPC was negatively correlated with FT4 ($r = − 0.12$, $p = 0.03$) but not with log TSH ($r = − 0.01$, $p = 0.9$) (Fig. 1, Panels a and b). In the subgroup of women with UIC less than 100 µg/l, log UPC remained negatively correlated with FT4 ($r = − 0.15$, $p = 0.04$) but not with log TSH.

Correlation between urinary thiocyanate and maternal thyroid status

There was no correlation between log UTC and FT4 ($r = 0.08$, $p = 0.15$) or log TSH ($r = − 0.08$, $p = 0.17$) (Fig. 1, Panels c and d). Likewise, in the subgroup of women with UIC less than 100 µg/l, there was no correlation between log UTC and FT4 ($r = 0.08$, $p = 0.17$) or log TSH ($r = − 0.08$, $p = 0.17$).

Multivariate analysis to assess the impact of potential confounders

We carried out multiple regression analysis to assess the impact of potential confounders (TPO-Ab, UIC, UPC and UTC). Maternal smoking was not included in the regression analysis because of its collinearity with thiocyanate levels (significant correlation between maternal smoking and log UTC, $r = 0.4$, $p < 0.001$). The regression analysis showed that only log UPC was significantly independently associated with FT4, with higher UPC associated with lower serum FT4 ($β = − 0.29$, 95% CI -0.52 to − 0.07, $p = 0.01$) (Table 2). The addition of smoking to the multivariable regression analysis did not change the association. The regression coefficient (β) of − 0.29 suggests that for every 10% increase in UPC, there will be a 0.03 pmol/l decrease in serum FT4.

Table 3 Regression analyses demonstrating the relationships between urinary perchlorate concentration and other potential confounding variables on serum FT4 and TSH in a subgroup of women with UIC < 100 µg/l ($n = 174$)

	β	SE	95% CI for β	t	p
Factors associated with serum FT4					
Urinary perchlorate[a]	−0.33	0.166	(−0.655, 0.001)	−1.97	**0.05**
Urinary iodine[a]	0.153	0.308	(−0.455, 0.762)	0.50	0.6
Urinary thiocyanate[a]	0.184	0.170	(−0.151, 0.520)	1.09	0.3
TPO-Ab positive	−0.316	0.512	(−1.328, 0.70)	−0.616	0.54
Factors associated with serum TSH[a]					
Urinary perchlorate[a]	0.04	0.043	(−0.046, 0.125)	0.91	0.4
Urinary iodine[a]	−0.06	0.081	(−0.214, 0.104)	−0.68	0.5
Urinary thiocyanate[a]	−0.044	0.044	(−0.131, 0.044)	−0.98	0.3
TPO-Ab positive	0.257	0.134	(−0.01, 0.52)	1.92	0.06

[a]Denotes variable transformed using natural logs (allowing â coefficients to be interpreted in terms of percentage change)
Bold value is significant result in the table

Table 4 Studies assessing the association between urinary perchlorate concentration and maternal thyroid status in pregnancy

Author (year)	Country	N	Gestation	Median UIC (µg/l)	Median UPC (range) (µg/l)	Association of UPC with	
						Maternal TSH	Maternal FT4
Pearce, 2010 [6]	Italy	787[a]	1st trimester	50–55	5 (0.04–168)	No	No
	Wales	854[b]	1st trimester	98–117	2 (0.02–368)	No	No
Pearce, 2011 [7]	USA	134	1st trimester	144	7.8 (0.4–284)	No	No
	Argentina	107	1st trimester	130	13.5 (1.1–676)	No	No
Pearce, 2012 [8]	Greece	134	1st trimester	120	4.1 (0.2–118.5)	No	Yes (negative)[c]
Charatcharoenwitthaya, 2014 [9]	Thailand	200	1st trimester	153.5	1.9 (0.1–35.5)	Yes (positive)	Yes (negative)
Horton, 2015 [10]	USA	284	1st trimester	235 (mean)[d]	3.54 (mean)[d]	Yes (positive)	No
Steinmaus, 2016 [11]	USA	1880	Median 7 weeks	155	6.5 (0.23–177)	Yes (positive)	TT4, FT4 (negative)
Mortensen, 2016 [12]	USA	359	3rd trimester	167	4.04 (geometric mean)	No	No
This study	England	308	3rd trimester	88	2.1 (0.3–143)	No	Yes (negative)

FT4 free T4, *TSH* thyroid stimulating hormone, *NK* not known, *UIC* urinary iodine concentration, *UPC* urinary perchlorate concentration
[a]Includes 261 women with hypothyroidism/hypothyroxinaemia (median UIC 55 µg/l) and 526 euthyroid women (median UIC 50 µg/l)
[b]Includes 374 women with hypothyroidism/hypothyroxinaemia (median UIC 98 µg/l) and 480 euthyroid women (median UIC 117 µg/l)
[c]Negative association on univariate analysis but no longer associated after adjustments in multivariate analysis
[d]Creatinine – adjusted (µg/g creatine)

Only TPO Ab positive was an independent predictor of serum TSH (Table 2). UPC or UTC was not an independent predictor of serum TSH.

The multiple regression analysis in the subgroup of women with UIC less than 100 µg/l also showed that log UPC was borderline significantly independently associated with serum FT4, with higher UPC associated with lower serum FT4 ($\beta = -0.33$, 95% CI -0.66 to 0.001, $p = 0.05$) (Table 3). UPC or UTC was not an independent predictor of serum TSH.

Effect of maternal perchlorate and thiocyanate exposure on offspring birthweight

There was no correlation between maternal UPC and offspring birthweight ($r = -0.07$, $p = 0.2$ for the whole cohort; $r = -0.04$, $p = 0.6$ for the subgroup of women with UIC less than 100 µg/l) or between maternal UTC and infant birthweight ($r = 0$, $p = 1.0$ for the whole cohort; $r = 0.03$, $p = 0.7$

for the subgroup of women with UIC less than 100 µg/l). Subgroup analyses using birthweight (corrected for gestational age) of male and female infants separately also failed to show association between offspring birthweight and maternal UPC ($r = -0.09$, $p = 0.3$) or maternal UTC ($r = 0.09$, $p = 0.3$).

Discussion

Our study has shown that environmental exposure to perchlorate and thiocyanate is ubiquitous and the exposure to perchlorate is associated with lower circulating FT4 levels in third trimester pregnant women. We did not identify an association between exposure to thiocyanate in pregnancy and maternal thyroid hormone. Maternal exposure of perchlorate or thiocyanate was not associated with offspring's birthweight.

Previous studies examining association between perchlorate exposure and maternal thyroid function in

Table 5 Studies assessing the association between urinary thiocyanate concentration and maternal thyroid status in pregnancy

Author (year)	Country	N	Gestation	Median UIC (µg/l)	Median UTC (range) (µg/l)	Association of UTC with	
						Maternal TSH	Maternal FT4
Pearce, 2010 [6]	Italy	787[a]	1st trimester	55–60	373 (132–6650)	No	Yes (negative)[c]
	Wales	854[b]		98–117	471 (34–3100)	No	No
Pearce, 2012 [8]	Greece	134	1st trimester	120	413 (0.6–1635)	Yes (positive)[d]	No
Charatcharoenwitthaya, 2014 [9]	Thailand	200	1 s trimester	153.5	510.5 (68–3525)	Yes (positive)	Yes (negative)
Horton, 2015 [10]	USA	284	1st trimester	235 (mean)[e]	1006 (mean)[e]	No	No
This study	England	308	3rd trimester	88	436 (29–3290)	No	No

FT4 free T4, *TSH* thyroid stimulating hormone, *NK* not known, *UIC* urinary iodine concentration, *UTC* urinary thiocyanate concentration
[a]Includes 261 women with hypothyroidism/hypothyroxinaemia (median UIC 55 µg/l) and 526 euthyroid women (median UIC 50 µg/l)
[b]Includes 374 women with hypothyroidism/hypothyroxinaemia (median UIC 98 µg/l) and 480 euthyroid women (median UIC 117 µg/l)
[c]Negative correlation in the euthyroid cohort on univariate analysis
[d]Positive association on univariate analysis but no longer associated after adjustments in multivariate analysis
[e]Creatinine – adjusted (µg/g creatine)

pregnancy have shown inconsistent results (Table 4). Although some studies [6–8, 12] found no association between UPC and maternal thyroid function, others have shown that UPC is associated with low maternal FT4 and/or high TSH [9–11]. Possible reasons for the discrepant results include diverse study populations, different iodine status, and variable gestational age at the time of perchlorate and thyroid function assessment. In our study, there was a 0.03 pmol/L decrease in maternal serum FT4 level with every 10% increase in UPC, providing additional evidence to support the association between perchlorate exposure and reduced maternal thyroid hormone levels. This is in keeping with observations outside pregnancy, where perchlorate exposure has been shown to be associated with decreased FT4 in the general population, including non-pregnant women and adolescent girls [16, 17].

The association between perchlorate exposure during pregnancy and reduced maternal serum FT4 could potentially have important clinical implications as maternal thyroid hormone insufficiency has been shown to be associated with impaired neurocognitive development of offspring and other adverse obstetric outcomes [18, 19]. In a recent study, pregnant women with subclinical hypothyroidism or hypothyroxinaemia and UPC in the upper 10% were found to have a 3-fold increased odds of having offspring with an intelligence quotient (IQ) in the lowest 10% at age of 3 years [20]. However, UPC was not associated with maternal thyroid hormone status in this cohort. Therefore, the mechanism for the association between maternal perchlorate exposure and reduced offspring IQ in this study remains uncertain although it may be due to the effect of perchlorate exposure on fetal thyroid function [20]. Another recent study has suggested that maternal perchlorate exposure in pregnancy could also affect obstetric outcomes, with maternal perchlorate exposure associated with increased birthweight in male infants, particularly in infants born prematurely [21]. However there was no assessment of maternal thyroid function in the cohort; therefore it is uncertain whether the association seen was mediated through changes in maternal thyroid hormone levels. Our study was unable to confirm the association between maternal perchlorate exposure and offspring birthweight in the whole cohort as well as in the subgroup of male infants. This is in keeping with a previous study which also found no association between perchlorate exposure in pregnancy and offspring's birthweight, birth length or gestational age at birth [22]. However, taken together, these observations highlight the need for further investigations to examine whether environmental exposure to perchlorate during pregnancy has adverse health outcomes beyond minor changes on maternal thyroid hormone levels.

In contrast to our findings on perchlorate exposure, we were unable to show an association between thiocyanate exposure and maternal thyroid hormone levels. This may

be because thiocyanate is a much weaker inhibitor of sodium-iodine symporter as compared to perchlorate [5]. However, a small number of previous studies have suggested potential effects of thiocyanate exposure on maternal thyroid status [6, 8, 9] (Table 5). Furthermore, it is also possible that co-exposure of thiocyanate with other environmental pollutants have more deleterious impact on maternal thyroid function than exposure to an individual pollutant [10].

We acknowledge several limitations of the study: urinary iodine, perchlorate and thiocyanate concentrations were measured on a single spot urine sample, and thyroid hormone assessments were carried out only once. Our cohort was predominantly Caucasian, from South West England, thereby limiting generalisability.

Conclusions

This study provides further evidence that environmental perchlorate exposure is associated lower circulating serum FT4 levels in pregnant women. This may have an adverse impact on neurocognitive development of the fetus and other pregnancy outcomes.

Abbreviations
BMI: Body mass index; CI: Confidence interval; FT4: Free thyroxine; IQ: Intelligence quotient; IQR: Inter-quartile range; RD&E: Royal Devon & Exeter hospital; SD: Standard deviation; TPO-Ab: Thyroid peroxidase antibodies; TSH: Thyroid stimulating hormone; UIC: Urinary iodine concentration; UPC: Urinary perchlorate concentration; UTC: Urinary thiocyanate concentration

Acknowledgements
Authors wish to thank the participants, and the midwives of Royal Devon & Exeter Hospital for their help in the recruitment of these study participants.

Funding
This study was funded by the Small Grants Scheme of the Research & Development Department, Royal Devon and Exeter Hospital NHS Foundation Trust. BAK and BMS are funded by the National Institute for Health Research (NIHR) as core members of the NIHR Exeter Clinical Research Facility. This article presents independent research supported by the NIHR Exeter Clinical Research Facility. The views expressed are those of the authors and not necessarily those of the NHS, the NIHR or the Department of Health.

Authors' contributions
BAK, BMS, RS and BV designed the study; XH, ENP and LEB were involved in the analysis of urinary iodine, perchlorate and thiocyanate; BAK and BMS carried out statistical analyses; BAK and BV wrote first draft; all authors reviewed, commented and approved the final version of the manuscript.

Competing interests
LEB and ENP have received research funding from Sociedad Química y Minera de Chile.

Author details

[1]NIHR Exeter Clinical Research Facility, Royal Devon & Exeter Hospital, University of Exeter Medical School, University of Exeter, Exeter EX2 5DW, UK. [2]Research & Development Department, Royal Devon and Exeter Hospital NHS Foundation Trust, Exeter, UK. [3]Section of Endocrinology, Diabetes & Nutrition, Boston University School of Medicine, Boston, USA. [4]Centre for Women's Health, Royal Devon and Exeter Hospital NHS Foundation Trust, Exeter, UK. [5]Department of Endocrinology, Royal Devon and Exeter Hospital NHS Foundation Trust, Exeter, UK. [6]University of Exeter Medical School, Exeter, UK.

References

1. Pearce EN, Lazarus JH, Moreno-Reyes R, Zimmermann MB. Consequences of iodine deficiency and excess in pregnant women: an overview of current knowns and unknowns. Am J Clin Nutr. 2016;104(Suppl 3):918S–23S.

2. Pearce EN, Braverman LE. Environmental pollutants and the thyroid. Best Pract Res Clin Endocrinol Metab. 2009;23(6):801–13.

3. Boas M, Feldt-Rasmussen U, Main KM. Thyroid effects of endocrine disrupting chemicals. Mol Cell Endocrinol. 2012;355(2):240–8.

4. The UK Food Standards Agency. An investigation of perchlorate levels in fruit and vegetables consumed in the UK (2016). [https://www.food.gov.uk/sites/default/files/fera-perchlorate-levels-report.pdf] (Accessed 23 Apr 2018).

5. Tonacchera M, Pinchera A, Dimida A, Ferrarini E, Agretti P, Vitti P, Santini F, Crump K, Gibbs J. Relative potencies and additivity of perchlorate, thiocyanate, nitrate, and iodide on the inhibition of radioactive iodide uptake by the human sodium iodide symporter. Thyroid. 2004;14(12):1012–9.

6. Pearce EN, Lazarus JH, Smyth PP, He X, Dall'amico D, Parkes AB, Burns R, Smith DF, Maina A, Bestwick JP, et al. Perchlorate and thiocyanate exposure and thyroid function in first-trimester pregnant women. J Clin Endocrinol Metab. 2010;95(7):3207–15.

7. Pearce EN, Spencer CA, Mestman JH, Lee RH, Bergoglio LM, Mereshian P, He X, Leung AM, Braverman LE. Effect of environmental perchlorate on thyroid function in pregnant women from Cordoba, Argentina, and Los Angeles, California. Endocr Pract. 2011;17(3):412–7.

8. Pearce EN, Alexiou M, Koukkou E, Braverman LE, He X, Ilias I, Alevizaki M, Markou KB. Perchlorate and thiocyanate exposure and thyroid function in first-trimester pregnant women from Greece. Clin Endocrinol. 2012;77(3):471–4.

9. Charatcharoenwitthaya N, Ongphiphadhanakul B, Pearce EN, Somprasit C, Chanthasenanont A, He X, Chailurkit L, Braverman LE. The association between perchlorate and thiocyanate exposure and thyroid function in first-trimester pregnant Thai women. J Clin Endocrinol Metab. 2014;99(7):2365–71.

10. Horton MK, Blount BC, Valentin-Blasini L, Wapner R, Whyatt R, Gennings C, Factor-Litvak P. CO-occurring exposure to perchlorate, nitrate and thiocyanate alters thyroid function in healthy pregnant women. Environ Res. 2015;143(Pt A):1–9.

11. Steinmaus C, Pearl M, Kharrazi M, Blount BC, Miller MD, Pearce EN, Valentin-Blasini L, DeLorenze G, Hoofnagle AN, Liaw J. Thyroid hormones and moderate exposure to perchlorate during pregnancy in women in Southern California. Environ Health Perspect. 2016;124(6):861–7.

12. Mortensen ME, Birch R, Wong LY, Valentin-Blasini L, Boyle EB, Caldwell KL, Merrill LS, Moye J Jr, Blount BC. Thyroid antagonists and thyroid indicators in U.S. pregnant women in the vanguard study of the National Children' study. Environ Res. 2016;149:179–88.

13. Knight BA, Shields BM, He X, Pearce EN, Braverman LE, Sturley R, Vaidya B. Iodine deficiency amongst pregnant women in south-West England. Clin Endocrinol. 2017;86(3):451–5.

14. Knight BA, Shields BM, Sturley R, Vaidya B. Maternal thyroid function in pregnant women with a breech presentation in late gestation. Clin Endocrinol. 2016;85(2):320–2.

15. Valentin-Blasini L, Mauldin JP, Maple D, Blount BC. Analysis of perchlorate in human urine using ion chromatography and electrospray tandem mass spectrometry. Anal Chem. 2005;77(8):2475–81.

16. McMullen J, Ghassabian A, Kohn B, Trasande L. Identifying subpopulations vulnerable to the thyroid-blocking effects of perchlorate and thiocyanate. J Clin Endocrinol Metab. 2017;102(7):2637–45.

17. Suh M, Abraham L, Hixon JG, Proctor DM. The effects of perchlorate, nitrate, and thiocyanate on free thyroxine for potentially sensitive subpopulations of the 2001-2002 and 2007-2008 National Health and nutrition examination surveys. J Exposure Sci Environ Epidemiol. 2014;24(6):579–87.

18. Thompson W, Russell G, Baragwanath G, Matthews J, Vaidya B, Thompson-Coon J. Maternal thyroid hormone insufficiency during pregnancy and risk of neurodevelopmental disorders in offspring: a systematic review and meta-analysis. Clin Endocrinol. 2018;88(4):575–84.

19. Korevaar TIM, Medici M, Visser TJ, Peeters RP. Thyroid disease in pregnancy: new insights in diagnosis and clinical management. Nat Rev Endocrinol. 2017;13(10):610–22.

20. Taylor PN, Okosieme OE, Murphy R, Hales C, Chiusano E, Maina A, Joomun M, Bestwick JP, Smyth P, Paradice R, et al. Maternal perchlorate levels in women with borderline thyroid function during pregnancy and the cognitive development of their offspring: data from the controlled antenatal thyroid study. J Clin Endocrinol Metab. 2014;99(11):4291–8.

21. Rubin R, Pearl M, Kharrazi M, Blount BC, Miller MD, Pearce EN, Valentin-Blasini L, DeLorenze G, Liaw J, Hoofnagle AN, et al. Maternal perchlorate exposure in pregnancy and altered birth outcomes. Environ Res. 2017;158:72–81.

22. Evans KA, Rich DQ, Weinberger B, Vetrano AM, Valentin-Blasini L, Strickland PO, Blount BC. Association of prenatal perchlorate, thiocyanate, and nitrate exposure with neonatal size and gestational age. Reprod Toxicol. 2015;57:183–9.

19

Concordance between the TIRADS ultrasound criteria and the BETHESDA cytology criteria on the nontoxic thyroid nodule

Hernando Vargas-Uricoechea[1], Ivonne Meza-Cabrera[2] and Jorge Herrera-Chaparro[3*]

Abstract

Background: Thyroid nodule is a common disorder of the thyroid. Despite their benign nature, they can be associated with multiple pathologic conditions, including thyroid cancer.

Methods: This cross-sectional study determined the concordance of Ultrasound (TIRADS criteria) and Fine Needle Aspiration Biopsy (FNA-BETHESDA system) in the assessment of the nontoxic thyroid nodule. A total of 180 subjects 18 years old or older underwent the two diagnostic tests and their results were compared using kappa index.

Results: Participants were mostly women, with average age of 57 years. The frequency of BETHESDA II was 65/180 versus 45/180 in TIRADS 2. In contrast, the highest frequency in category 4-IV was 62/180 for TIRADS 4 versus 41/180 for BETHESDA IV. The highest concordance was found among the category 2-II classification. The observed agreement was 87.2% with a linear weighted kappa of 0.69 (95% CI: 0.59-0.79). The heterogeneity analysis showed a trend towards a higher weighted kappa value in nodules ≥4 cm in males and individuals aged ≥50 years, with accelerated nodular growth, binding to adjacent structures, vocal folds paralysis, urban origin, and a history of head and neck radiation therapy.

Conclusions: The TIRADS criteria has a good concordance with the Bethesda system. The ultrasound findings of benign pathology are aligned with the cytology results. The correct interpretation of the two findings helps the clinician to reduce the risk of unnecessary invasive procedures in patients with a low probability of presenting thyroid cancer, while facilitating the identification of patients at higher risk of cancer.

Keywords: Thyroid, Nodule, TIRADS, Bethesda, Concordance

Background

A steady increase in the incidence rate of thyroid cancer has been noted in recent decades all over the world, and the causes of this increase are still controversial. Thyroid cancer is the most common endocrine malignancy (1.0–1.5% of all newly diagnosed cancers in the United States of America every year are originally thyroid). The increased frequency in thyroid cancer is almost exclusively due to the rise in the number of papillary cancers, with no significant changes in other histologic subtypes [1, 2].

The typical presentation is as small tumors, though there is a growing incidence of large tumors; it has been hypothesized that the rise in the incidence of thyroid cancer is mostly due to improved detection rather than to a real increase in frequency [3]. Thyroid nodule can be defined as a discrete lesion within the thyroid gland that is radiologically distinct from the surrounding thyroid parenchyma. It may be solitary, multiple, solid, or cystic, and may or not be functional. Thyroid nodules are frequent among the general population and thyroid Ultrasound (US) has considerably increased the number of cases identified. Thyroid nodules may be palpated in about 4–8% of the general population (however, neck palpation is

* Correspondence: hernandovargasuricoechea@gmail.com
[3]Department of surgery, Universidad del Cauca, Carrera 6 No 41 N-135 apto 202B terrazas del campestre, Popayán, Cauca, Colombia
Full list of author information is available at the end of the article

very imprecise in terms of determining the size and morphology). US identifies the presence of nodules in 19-67% of the cases, and is an accurate method for the detection of thyroid nodules; however, US has a low accuracy in differentiating between benign from malignant thyroid nodules [4]. The sonographic characteristics of a thyroid nodule associated with a higher likelihood of malignancy include hypoechogenicity, increased intranodular vascularity, irregular margins, microcalcifications, absent halo, and a taller-than-wide shape measured in the transverse dimension. Thus, several benign and malignant ultrasound gray scale and Doppler features have emerged over the last ten years that may be used in different ways to assign probabilities, together with a method based on the Breast Imaging Reporting and Data System (BIRADS). Likewise, several US Thyroid Imaging Reporting and Data Systems (TIRADS) have been proposed for risk stratification of thyroid nodules [5].

The nodules are usually divided into different categories based on TIRADS and are then referred for Fine-Needle Aspiration (FNA) Biopsy or follow-up, according to the variable risk of malignancy. The terminology of TIRADS was first used by Horvath et al. [6]. They described 10 US patterns of thyroid nodules and related the rate of malignancy based on the pattern. The initial purpose of TIRADS was to improve patient management and cost-effectiveness by avoiding unnecessary FNA Biopsies in patients with thyroid nodules (Table 1), with a sensitivity, specificity, positive predictive value, negative predictive value, and accuracy of 88, 49, 49, 88, and 94%, respectively. However, its clinical use is still very limited and its practical application in clinical practice is questioned. Moreover, FNA Biopsy is the most accurate method for determining malignancy, and is a fundamental part of current thyroid nodule evaluation. The Bethesda System for Reporting Thyroid Cytopathology is a standardized reporting system for classifying thyroid FNA Biopsy results that comprises six diagnostic categories with unique risks of malignancy and recommendations for clinical management. Since its inception, the Bethesda System has been widely adopted, each category conveys a risk of malignancy and recommended next steps, though it is unclear if each category also predicts the type and extent of malignancy (Table 1). Nevertheless, the implementation of this reporting system has shown significant diagnostic variability, both inter and intra pathologists, particularly when read as "atypical cells of undetermined significance, follicular lesion of undetermined significance, or follicular neoplasm" (also termed as Bethesda Category III, comprising a heterogeneous population of low-risk lesions that contain follicular cells exhibiting either architectural abnormalities or nuclear atypia that do not fit into other definitive

cytological categories). A recent meta-analysis evaluated the validity of the Bethesda reporting system and found 97% sensitivity, 50.7% specificity and 68.8% diagnostic accuracy; the negative and positive predictive values were 96.3 and 55.9%, respectively [7, 8]. Notwithstanding the fact that both US and FNA biopsy are widely recommended procedures to study patients with thyroid nodules, the value of the existing concordance between the two methods has not been established. Consequently, the purpose of this study was to assess the existing concordance between the two diagnostic methods used in the initial evaluation of individuals with non-toxic thyroid nodule (TIRADS and Bethesda systems).

Methods

The overall objective of the study was to determine the level of concordance between the ultrasound criteria established under TIRADS (The Thyroid Imaging Reporting and Data System for US of the thyroid); and the cytology criteria according to The Bethesda System for Reporting Thyroid Cytopathology [9, 10]. Additionally, the study population was characterized from the socio-demographic point of view, the concordance of the classification systems was estimated, and the heterogeneity of the factors influencing the consistency of the various classification systems was analyzed.

Ethics approval and consent to participate

All personal data were confidential and managed exclusively by the principal investigator, according to the legal standards on the confidentiality of the medical record and adhering to the rules of the Institutional Review Committee of Human Ethics (reference number: 221–011). Universidad del Valle, Valle del Cauca-Colombia.

Design of the study

This was a cross-sectional study to evaluate the concordance between two diagnostic systems (TIRADS and Bethesda), administered simultaneously to the same individual. The population consisted of consecutive patients consulting the outpatient endocrinology, internal medicine, or general surgery departments at a high complexity referral center, with a diagnosis of nodular or non-nodular "thyroid dysfunction". The inclusion criteria were as follows: male and females aged 18 years and older, with a non-toxic thyroid nodule (ranges for normal thyroid tests were Thyrotrophin (TSH): 0.4 to 4 mIU/L; Free thyroxine: 0.8 to 1.8 ng/dL, according to the National Academy of Clinical Biochemistry) identified either clinically or through imaging [11]. The exclusion criteria were: TIRADS 1 and Bethesda I (Table 1); Graves-Basedow–associated hyperthyroidism, patients with toxic thyroid nodular disease, chronic hypothyroidism (with

Table 1 Thyroid imaging reporting and data system (TIRADS) and the Bethesda System for Reporting Cytopathology (ref. 6, 8, 9)

TIRADS		BETHESDA	
Categories	Features	Diagnostic Categories	Risk of malignancy
TIRADS 1	Normal thyroid gland.	I. Nondiagnostic or unsatisfactory.	-
TIRADS 2	Benign conditions (0% malignancy).	Cyst fluid only.	
TIRADS 3	Probably benign nodules (5% malignancy).	Virtually acellular specimen.	
TIRADS 4	Suspicious nodules (5–80% malignancy rate). A subdivision into 4a (malignancy between 5 and 10%) and 4b (malignancy between 10 and 80%) was optional.	Other (obscuring blood, clotting artifact, etc.).	
TIRADS 5	Probably malignant nodules (malignancy >80%).	II. Benign.	0-3
TIRADS 6	Category included biopsy proven malignant nodules.	Consistent with a benign follicular nodule (includes adenomatoid nodule, colloid nodule, etc.).	
		Consistent with lymphocytic (Hashimoto) thyroiditis in the proper clinical context.	
		Consistent with granulomatous (subacute) thyroiditis.	
		III. Atypia of undetermined significance/follicular lesion of undetermined significance.	5-15
		IV. Follicular neoplasm/"suspicious" for follicular neoplasm. Specify if Hürthle cell type.	15-30
		V. Suspicious for malignancy.	60-75
		Suspicious for papillary carcinoma.	
		Suspicious for medullary carcinoma.	
		Suspicious for metastatic carcinoma.	
		Suspicious for lymphoma.	
		VI. Malignant.	97-99
		Papillary thyroid carcinoma.	
		Poorly differentiated carcinoma.	
		Medullary thyroid carcinoma.	
		Undifferentiated (anaplastic) carcinoma.	
		Squamous cell carcinoma.	
		Carcinoma with mixed features.	
		Metastatic.	

a minimum of six-months on treatment with levothyroxine sodium), iatrogenic hyperthyroidism resulting from high-dose sodium levothyroxine therapy regardless of the indication; a history of surgically resected thyroid cancer, and patients with a history of partial thyroidectomy (lobectomy) or subtotal/near total thyroidectomy under levothyroxine sodium therapy (the latter criterion is based on the fact that a constant high stimulus of thyroid hormones and the concomitant TSH suppression in patients with endogenous hyperthyroidism and levothyroxine management may impact the size of the thyroid nodules) [12, 13].

This study was supported by the Internal Medicine Department from The Faculty of medicina of the Universidad del Cauca (Popayán-Colombia), who provided funding to conduct the analysis and prepare the manuscript.

Sample size estimate and sampling

To estimate the sample size, matched categories in both reporting systems were considered. Based on the data from a pilot study with 32 subjects that met the above selection criteria, and using the formula below, the N value was established at 128 subjects:

$$n = \frac{P_e}{ee^2(1-P_e)}$$

Where:

P_e: Expected percentage of random concordance

Ee: Kappa index standard error [14–16].

A consecutive non-probabilistic sampling was used based on an initial review of 217 medical records; however the final analysis was limited to 180 patients and 37 patients were excluded due to:

1. Incomplete family history and missing socio-demographic information in 26 records.
2. The echography was not reported according to TIRADS criteria in 4 records.
3. The cytology results were not reported according to the Bethesda criteria in 5 cases.
4. The ultrasound examination had been done at a different institution or by a different radiologist in 2 cases.

The source of the information in this study is a registry of consecutive data from an outpatient center for patients with a diagnosis of thyroid dysfunction. A standard form collected socio-demographic information, family and personal history of diseases, in addition to the data available from the medical record. Patients undergoing thyroid ultrasound imaging and FNA Biopsy due to non-toxic nodular thyroid disease were analyzed in accordance with the medical opinion of the institution's study group on thyroid disease (endocrinology, pathology, radiology and surgery). All patients were informed about the procedure and after signing the informed consent, the thyroid ultrasound was performed, and the node(s) were sampled according to Crockett's FNA Biopsy protocol [17].

The same radiologist read all the tests. One out of every 20 patients was randomly selected to repeat the ultrasound examination. The principal researcher interpreted the results in accordance with the TIRADS criteria and if the second reading was inconsistent with the first, a second radiologist was asked for an opinion to arrive at a consensus between the two radiologists and establish a TIRADS-based ultrasonographic diagnosis. 9 of the 180 participants were randomly selected to assess the radiologists' agreement. One of the nine US results showed disagreement because the first radiologist reported TIRADS 3, while the second one reported TIRADS 2, based on the original classification. Upon further analysis the conclusion was TIRADS 3. The material obtained via the FNA Biopsy was placed on a glass slide previously impregnated with 96% alcohol and then a second glass slide was placed on top. The smear was again immersed in 96% alcohol and then stained using the Papanicolaou technique. To ensure the quality of the cytology specimens, the same experienced pathologist read the slides and reported a diagnosis based on the Bethesda criteria. One out every ten specimens was randomly selected to be analyzed by a second pathologist. In case of disagreement between the two pathologists, a pathologist meeting was convened (five pathologist). The second pathologist disagreed with two of the 18 specimens subject to a second evaluation; in both cases, the first pathologist classified the cytology specimen as Bethesda V, while the second pathologist classified the

specimens as Bethesda VI. Both specimens were further evaluated at a pathologist meeting, and the final classification was Bethesda VI. The radiologists and the pathologists were blinded to the patients' medical record data for both the ultrasound examination and the FNA biopsy.

Statistical analysis

The weighted Kappa statistical method with a 95% confidence interval and the statistical Z-test were used to estimate the level of concordance between the two systems. In order to pursue the Kappa analysis, categories 5 and 6 of both the TIRADS and the Bethesda classification were combined since the highest risk for malignancy is usually described in these two categories. Category 1 in both classifications was excluded from the selection process because a TIRADS 1 ultrasound examination is considered normal, and Bethesda I is considered an unsatisfactory specimen. The purpose of excluding category 1 was to avoid invalidating further comparisons since category 1 is inconclusive, particularly Bethesda I. Consequently, the analysis categories are as follows:

- TIRADS 2: "BENIGN"
- TIRADS 3: "PROBABLY BENIGN"
- TIRADS 4: "SUSPICIOUS"
- TIRADS 5: "PROBABLY MALIGNANT"
- Bethesda II: "BENIGN".
- Bethesda III: "PROBABLY BENIGN".
- Bethesda IV: "SUSPICIOUS".
- Bethesda V: "PROBABLY MALIGNANT"

Weighted Kappa statistic with linear weight was used to estimate the level of agreement between the two systems; Kappa with quadratic weighting was used for comparative purposes. A descriptive analysis was used to indicate the distribution of the quantitative variables. Based on that distribution, the average represented the central trend and the scatter represented the standard deviation. The qualitative variables were defined in terms of percentages by category. A stratified analysis was performed to explore heterogeneity factors, resulting in a linear weighted Kappa for the following categories: Gender, age, nodule size, urban/non-urban origin, accelerated nodule growth, vocal folds paralysis, hard nodule, attached to underlying structures, history of head and neck radiation therapy, and family history of thyroid cancer. All the analyses used STATA 10.1

Results

The average age was 57 years old. Over 75% of the participants were females and 68.9% came from the urban area; however, there was a remarkable high frequency of risk factors for thyroid cancer. (Table 2) The frequency

Table 2 Socio-demographic characteristics and risk factors for thyroid cancer

Characteristic	Frequency
Mean age	57 y (SD:±14y)
Sex	Fem: 141 (78.3%)
	Male: 39 (21.7%)
Origin	Urban: 124 (68.9%).
	Non-Urban: 56 (31.1%).
Thyroid cancer family backgrounds	N (%)
No	119 (66.1%)
Yes	61 (33.9%)
Accelerated Growth of the Thyroid Nodules	
No	121 (67.2%)
Yes	59 (32.8%)
Head Radiation	
No	163 (90.6%)
Yes	17 (9.4%)
Firm Nodule	
No	94 (51.7%)
Yes	86 (47.8%)
Adjacent structure Attachment	
No	130 (72.2%)
Yes	50 (27.8%)
Vocal Chord Paralysis	
No	130 (72.2%)
Yes	50 (27.8%)
≥4 cm nodule	
No	109 (60.6%)
Yes	71 (39.4%)

Table 3 Joint distribution of BETHESDA & TIRADS categories

Diagnostic categories		TIRADS				Total
		2	3	4	5	
BETHESDA	II	42	19	2	2	65
		23.33%	10.56%	1.11%	1.11%	
	III	3	21	14	1	39
		1.67%	11.67%	7.78%	0.56%	
	IV	0	1	33	7	41
		0%	0.56%	18.33%	3.89%	
	V	0	0	13	22	35
		0%	0%	7,22%	12,22%	
	Total	45	41	62	32	180

distribution according to the scales was strikingly different for categories 2-II and 4-IV. The frequency of category II in Bethesda was 65/180 versus 45/180 in TIRADS 2. In contrast, the highest frequency in category 4-IV was 62/180 for TIRADS 4 versus 41/180 for Bethesda IV. (Table 3) The highest concordance was found for categories TIRADS 2-Bethesda II (23.33%). None of the patients classified as TIRADS 2 were rated as Bethesda IV or V. In contrast, 4 subjects classified as Bethesda II were classified as TIRADS 4 ($n = 2$) or V ($n = 2$). Of the 35 patients classified as Bethesda V none were classified as TIRADS 2 or 3, but 3 of the 32 subjects with TIRADS 5 were classified as Bethesda II ($n = 2$) or III ($n = 1$). The weighted Kappa value according to the linear weights was 0.69 (95% CI: 0.59–0.79). The overall Kappa and the Kappa with quadratic weighting were also estimated for comparative purposes. (Table 4) The heterogeneity analysis showed a trend towards a higher weighted kappa

value in nodules ≥4 cm in males and individuals aged ≥50 years, with accelerated nodular growth, binding to adjacent structures, vocal folds paralysis, urban origin, and a history of head and neck radiation therapy (Tables 5 and 6).

Discussion

This study evaluated the concordance between the TIRADS and the Bethesda reporting systems on the non-toxic thyroid nodule. The result showed a "good or substantial" concordance and the most frequent consistency was found for categories II and IV. The kappa index measures the level of inter-observer concordance, or as in this particular case, the concordance between two diagnostic methods rather than the "quality" of the observation, so it is not possible to establish the validity of the resulting classifications. This study addresses the level of discrepancy, the report categories, and which categories tend to exhibit a higher frequency of discrepancies between the two methods. When particular types of disagreements are more frequent, this information shall be kept in mind when developing the kappa index [18, 19]. For this reason, the weighted kappa analysis was used, without neglecting the fact that although using weights is logical and attractive, it introduces a component of subjectivity since assigning weights is subjective and may impact the interpretation of the data when used for a different population –the weights assigned may vary based on the frequency of the disease-. This is evidenced through the variation in the kappa estimates when weighing is used, and depends on the weighing method used. The weighted kappa estimate with linear weights assigned to the categories shows a value of 0.69. The weighted kappa value based on quadratic weights was higher than the overall kappa or the linear weighted kappa (the quadratic weighted kappa value was 0.80). The difference is based on the fact that the linear and quadratic methods are based on the relative separation among the classification categories but

Table 4 Kappa comparison according to the estimation method

Kappa	Observed Agreement	Expected agreement	Kappa	Standard error	IC 95%	Z	Value p
Global	65.56%	25.27%	0.5391	0.0425	0.46–0.62	12.68	<0.001
Weighted (linear weights)	87.22%	58.76%	0.6901	0.0528	0.59–0.79	13.07	<0.001
Estimated (quadratic weights	94.63%	72.86%	0.8021	0.0731	0.66–0.94	10.97	<0.001

the quadratic approach uses square differences, while the linear approach uses absolute values [20, 21]. Consequently, quadratic weights tend to assign a higher weight to disagreements that were relatively few in this study; when the kappa interpretation is based on quadratic weights, the level of concordance remains unchanged versus the interpretation of the linear weighted kappa; but if analyzed as an absolute value, it is evidently overestimated. Since the kappa value is affected by the prevalence of the characteristic studied, caution is of the essence when generalizing the results of inter-observer comparisons in the presence of varying prevalence. The prevalence of malignancy based on cytology findings (Bethesda V in the matched scale) was reported at 19.4% (35/180); however, using the TIRADS scale (maximum value of 5 in the matched scale), the prevalence of malignancy was 17% (32/180), showing a non-significant difference between the two methods. This is extremely relevant when considering that a prevalence of close to 50% results in a higher kappa value for the same proportion of agreements observed [22, 23]. Thus, the interpretation of the kappa index requires identifying the value of the marginal frequencies on the table (prevalence observed per observer). Since the difference between the prevalence estimated by both methods is not significant, the conclusion is than that the prevalence of the event did not affect the kappa value reported. When evaluating heterogeneity based on characteristics such as gender, age, size of the nodule, place of origin, accelerated nodular growth, vocal folds paralysis, hard nodule, binding to adjacent structures, a history of head and

neck radiation therapy, a family history of thyroid cancer, the trend indicates a stronger concordance (expressed as a weighted kappa value). This is also the case for variables such as nodule size ≥4 cm, male gender, and age ≥50 years. Despite this trend, the study failed to show statistically significant differences. The TIRADS classification attempts to improve the interpretation of the findings of a thyroid nodule by defining categories that in the end are exclusive, although the original classification indicates a risk of malignancy between 5-80% for TIRADS 4, and this fact makes it difficult to clinically define a follow-up and management strategy. Notwithstanding this consideration, from the clinical perspective, in a subject with low probability of having thyroid cancer (and a TIRADS 2 or 3) the US negative predictive value will be greatly enhanced. The best US diagnostic performance is probably with extreme results of the classification (TIRADS 2–3 and TIRADS 5–6 of the original classification). Depending on the clinical probability of malignancy, the US findings may be more or less useful and applicable [24].

Previous studies have evaluated the diagnostic performance of both US and FNA Biopsy in the initial study of thyroid nodules. A recent study was aimed at developing a diagnostic algorithm using the data reported in the US (in accordance with a scoring system evaluating the risk of malignancy based on several US patterns) and the results of the FNA Biopsy (according to Bethesda). This study showed that classifying an individual in accordance with the presence of different US patterns as low, intermediate or high risk, together with the results of the FNA Biopsy, enables optimal clinical decision-making with regards to treatment strategies [25]. Along the same lines, other studies classify the risk of malignancy in accordance with the US characteristics and based on such risk, establish the need to perform a FNA Biopsy. The higher the risk of malignancy (according to the US) the greater the need to do the FNA Biopsy, and vice-versa –the lower the risk of malignancy based on the US, the lower the indication for a FNA Biopsy– [26–28].

Our study showed that the highest concordance was found among both the lowest risk (TIRADS 2 and Bethesda II) and the higher risk categories (TIRADS 4 and Bethesda IV), which is consistent with the previously described trials. This indicates that the US characteristics suggesting a higher or lower risk of malignancy, will be associated with higher

Table 5 Stratification according to nodule size, sex, and age in order to assess heterogeneity

Strata	Observed Agreement	Expected Agreement	Kappa	Standard Error	IC 95%
Nodule Size					
<4 cm	85.63%	65.15%	0.5876	0.067	0.46-0.72
≥4 cm	89.67%	66.26%	0.6938	0.083	0.53-0.86
Sex					
Men	89.74%	58.32%	0.7539	0.117	0.53-0.98
Women	86.52%	59.30%	0.6689	0.059	0.55-0.78
Age					
<50 years old	82.49%	59.91%	0.5632	0.092	0.38-0.74
≥50 years old	89.53%	59.18%	0.7435	0.064	0.62-0.87

Table 6 Heterogeneity assessment by stratifying the variables according to: thyroid cancer family history, accelerated growth of the nodules, firm nodule, underlying structure, vocal chords paralysis, origins, and history of radiation

Strata	Observed Agreement	Expected Agreement	Kappa	Standard Error	95% CI
Thyroid Cancer Family history					
Yes	87.98%	60.71%	0.694	0.086	0.53–0.86
No	86.83%	58.81%	0.680	0.066	0.55–0.81
Accelerated Growth of the nodule					
Yes	90.40%	60.12%	0.759	0.090	0.58–0.94
No	85.67%	59.89%	0.643	0.065	0.52–0.77
Firm Nodule					
Yes	86.82%	58.55%	0.682	0.076	0.53–0.83
No	87.59%	60.10%	0.689	0.073	0.55–0.83
Adjacent Structure Attachment					
Yes	94.00%	65.52%	0.826	0.096	0.64–1.01
No	84.62%	59.42%	0.621	0.062	0.50–0.74
Vocal Chords Paralysis					
Yes	94.67%	66.11%	0.843	0.096	0.65–1.03
No	84.36%	58.52%	0.623	0.062	0.50–0.74
Origin					
Urban (exclusive)	88.70%	58.99%	0.7245	0.065	0.60–0.85
Urban or Rural	84.41%	58.26%	0.6265	0.0881	0.45–0.8
Head and neck radiation therapy					
Yes	96.08%	61.48%	0.8982	0.1689	0.57–1.23
No	86.30%	58.55%	0.6695	0.0557	0.56–0.78

or lower probability of malignancy according to the FNA Biopsy report (Bethesda), respectively.

Finally, the interpretation of the results in this study requires acknowledging that over two thirds of the subjects were women. Probably this trend is due to the fact that autoimmune thyroid disease is significantly more frequent in females than in males, so these patients with autoimmune thyroid disease visit the physician more often increasing the probability of detecting the nodules either through palpation or ultrasound; clinically this situation may be defined as a "medical surveillance bias" [29, 30]. The geographical distribution indicates that most of the patients were from urban areas and those from the rural areas were mostly from municipalities with accessible specialized care. The participants in the study had information about exposure/disease since they had been referred for a study of the thyroid nodule with a probable diagnosis of malignancy. In cross-section studies the participants may be more prone to participate based on their knowledge about exposure and disease and the convenience of their geographical location leading to a higher "selection bias" that in turn could overestimate the frequency of malignancies [31, 32]. This study highlights the high frequency of factors that have been historically associated with thyroid cancer. Those factors were evaluated with the survey administered to the

study subjects that had been previously referred for tests to rule out malignancies, so these participants were more likely to recall past exposures (accurate or vague) potentially leading to a "recall bias" [30, 33]. Furthermore, since the data collection from the participants was not masked (they had been previously identified as nodular thyroid disease patients screened for malignancies), the interviewer's interest in evaluating the exposure factors could have resulted in an "interviewer bias" [34, 35].

Conclusions

The thyroid ultrasound report using the TIRADS criteria has a good concordance with the Bethesda cytology findings using FNA Biopsy. The ultrasound findings of benign pathology are aligned with the cytology results and viceversa; ultrasound findings of malignancy shall be consistent with cytology-identified malignant disease. The correct interpretation of the two findings helps the clinician to reduce the risk of unnecessary invasive procedures in patients with a low probability of presenting thyroid cancer, while facilitating the identification of patients at higher risk of cancer. There is a need to develop study and monitoring protocols for cases classified as "discordant", particularly when extreme categories are identified (TIRADS 5-Bethesda II, TIRADS 2-Bethesda V).

Abbreviations

BIRADS: Breast Imaging Reporting and Data System; FNA: Fine-Needle Aspiration; TIRADS: The Thyroid Imaging Reporting and Data System for US of the thyroid; TSH: Thyrotrophin; US: Ultrasound

Acknowledgements

None.

Funding

This study was supported by the Internal Medicine Department from The Faculty of medicina of the Universidad del Cauca (Popayán-Colombia), who provided funding to conduct the analysis and prepare the manuscript.

Authors' contributions

H V-U, I M-C and J H-Ch were involved in study design, acquisition of data, analysis and interpretation of data and drafting and revising the manuscript. H V-U, and I M-C were involved in data collection and analysis and manuscript drafting. All authors read and approved the final manuscript.

Competing interests

All authors declare no financial competing interests, nor any other type of conflicts of interest.

Author details

[1]Department of Internal Medicine, Division of Endocrinology and Metabolism, Universidad del Cauca, Popayán, Colombia. [2]Laboratory of Pathology, Hospital Universitario San José, Popayán, Cauca, Colombia. [3]Department of surgery, Universidad del Cauca, Carrera 6 No 41 N-135 apto 202B terrazas del campestre, Popayán, Cauca, Colombia.

References

1. Ferlay J, Soerjomataram I, Dikshit R, Eser S, Mathers C, Rebelo M, Parkin DM, Forman D, Bray F. Cancer incidence and mortality worldwide: sources, methods and major patterns in GLOBOCAN 2012. Int J Cancer. 2015;136(5): 359–86.
2. Torre LA, Bray F, Siegel RL, Ferlay J, Lortet-Tieulent J, Jemal A. Global cancer statistics, 2012. CA Cancer J Clin. 2015;65(2):87–108.
3. Wiltshire JJ, Drake TM, Uttley L, Balasubramanian SP. Systematic review of trends in the incidence rates of thyroid cancer. Thyroid. 2016;26(11):1541–52.
4. Gharib H, Papini E, Garber JR, Duick DS, Harrell RM, Hegedüs L, Paschke R, Valcavi R, Vitti P, AACE/ACE/AME Task Force on Thyroid Nodules. American Association Of Clinical Endocrinologists, American College Of Endocrinology, And Associazione Medici Endocrinologi Medical Guidelines For Clinical Practice For The Diagnosis And Management Of Thyroid Nodules–2016 Update. Endocr Pract. 2016;22(5):622–39.
5. Yoon JH, Lee HS, Kim EK, Moon HJ, Kwak JY. Malignancy risk stratification of thyroid nodules: comparison between the thyroid imaging reporting and data system and the 2014 American thyroid association management guidelines. Radiology. 2016;278(3):917–24.
6. Horvath E, Majlis S, Rossi R, Franco C, Niedmann JP, Castro A, Dominguez M. An ultrasonogram reporting system for thyroid nodules stratifying cancer risk for clinical management. J Clin Endocrinol Metab. 2009;94(5):1748–51.
7. Pusztaszeri M, Rossi ED, Auger M, Baloch Z, Bishop J, Bongiovanni M, Chandra A, Cochand-Priollet B, Fadda G, Hirokawa M, Hong S, Kakudo K, Krane JF, Nayar R, Parangi S, Schmitt F, Faquin WC. The Bethesda system for reporting thyroid cytopathology: proposed modifications and updates for the second edition from an international panel. Acta Cytol. 2016;60(5):399–405.
8. Garg S, Desai NJ, Mehta D, Vaishnav M. To establish bethesda system for diagnosis of thyroid nodules on the basis of fnac with histopathological correlation. J Clin Diagn Res. 2015;9(12):EC17–21.
9. Russ G, Bigorgne C, Royer B, Rouxel A, Bienvenu-Perrard M. The Thyroid Imaging Reporting and Data System (TIRADS) for ultrasound of the thyroid. J Radiol. 2011;92(7–8):701–13.
10. Cibas ES, Ali SZ. NCI Thyroid FNA State of the Science Conference. The Bethesda System for reporting thyroid cytopathology. Am J Clin Pathol. 2009;132:658–65.
11. Baloch Z, Carayon P, Conte-Devolx B, Demers LM, Feldt-Rasmussen U, Henry JF, LiVosli VA, Niccoli-Sire P, John R, Ruf J, Smyth PP, Spencer CA, Stockigt JR, Guidelines Committee, National Academy of Clinical Biochemistry. Laboratory medicine practice guidelines. Laboratory support for the diagnosis and monitoring of thyroid disease. Thyroid. 2003;13(1):3–126.
12. Zelmanovitz F, Genro S, Gross JL. Suppressive therapy with levothyroxine for solitary thyroid nodules: a double-blind controlled clinical study and cumulative meta-analyses. J Clin Endocrinol Metab. 1998;83:3881–5.
13. Grussendorf M, Reiners C, Paschke R, Wegscheider K. Reduction of thyroid nodule volume by levothyroxine and iodine alone and in combination: a randomized, placebo-controlled trial. J Clin Endocrinol Metab. 2012;96:2786–95.
14. Kramer M, Feinstein AR. Clinical Biostatistics. The biostatistics of concordance. Clin Pharmacol Ther. 1981;29:111–23.
15. Cantor AB. Sample-size calculation for Cohen's kappa. Psychol Methods. 1996;1:150–3.
16. Sim J, Wrigth CC. The Kappa statistic in reliability studies: Use, interpretation, and sample size requirements. Phys Ther. 2005;85:257–68.
17. Crockett JC. The thyroid nodule fine-needle aspiration biopsy technique. J Ultrasound Med. 2011;30:685–94.
18. Landis JR, Koch GG. The measurement of observer agreement for categorical data. Biometrics. 1977;33:159–74.
19. Barnhart HX, Williamson JM. Weighted least-squares approach for comparing correlated kappa. Biometrics. 2002;58(4):1012–109.
20. McHugh ML. Interrater reliability: the kappa statistic. Biochem Med (Zagreb). 2012;22(3):276–82.
21. Cyr L, Francis K. Measures of clinical agreement for nominal and categorical data: the kappa coefficient. Comput Biol Med. 1992;22(4):239–46.
22. Brenner H, Kliebsch U. Dependence of weighted kappa coefficients on the number of categories. Epidemiology. 1996;7(2):199–202.
23. Guggenmoos-Holzmann I, Vonk R. Kappa-like indices of observer agreement viewed from a latent class perspective. Stat Med. 1998;17(8):797–812.
24. Rosario PW. Thyroid Nodules with Atypia or Follicular Lesions of Undetermined Significance (Bethesda Category III): Importance of Ultrasonography and Cytological Subcategory. Thyroid. 2014;24:1115–20.
25. Adamczewski Z, Lewiński A. Proposed algorithm for management of patients with thyroid nodules/focal lesions, based on ultrasound (US) and fine-needle aspiration biopsy (FNAB); our own experience. Thyroid Res. 2013;6:6. doi:10.1186/1756-6614-6-6.
26. Cavaliere A, Colella R, Puxeddu E, Gambelunghe G, Falorni A, Stracci F, d'Ajello M, Avenia N, De Feo P. A useful ultrasound score to select thyroid nodules requiring fine needle aspiration in an iodine-deficient area. J Endocrinol Invest. 2009;32(5):440–4.
27. Petrone A, Mannucci E, De Feo ML, Parenti G, Biagini C, Panconesi R, Vezzosi V, Bianchi S, Boddi V, Di Medio L, Pupilli C, Forti G. A simple ultrasound score for the identification of candidates for fine needle aspiration of thyroid nodules. J Endocrinol Invest. 2012;35(8):720–4.
28. Remonti LR, Kramer CK, Leitão CB, Pinto LC, Gross JL. Thyroid ultrasound features and risk of carcinoma: a systematic review and meta-analysis of observational studies. Thyroid. 2015;25(5):538–50.
29. Haut ER, Pronovost PJ. Surveillance bias in outcomes reporting. JAMA. 2011;305(23):2462–3.
30. Hoppin JA, Tolbert PE, Taylor JA, Schroeder JC, Holly EA. Potential for selection bias with tumor tissue retrieval in molecular epidemiology studies. Ann Epidemiol. 2002;12(1):1–6.
31. Holford TR, Stack C. (1995) Study design for epidemiologic studies with measurement error. Stat Methods in Med Res. 1995;4(4):339–58.
32. Flanders WD, Eldridge RC. Summary of relationships between exchangeability, biasing paths and bias. Eur J Epidemiol. 2015;30(10):1089–99.
33. Sanderson S, Tatt ID, Higgins JP. Tools for assessing quality and susceptibility to bias in observational studies in epidemiology: a systematic review and annotated bibliography. Int J Epidemiol. 2007;36(3):666–76.
34. Wynder EL. Investigator bias and interviewer bias: the problem of reporting systematic error in epidemiology. J Clin Epidemiol. 1994;47(8):825–7.
35. Davis RE, Couper MP, Janz NK, Caldwell CH, Resnicow K. Interviewer effects in public health surveys. Health Educ Res. 2010;25(1):14–26.

20

Ultrasound criteria for risk stratification of thyroid nodules in the previously iodine deficient area of Austria - a single centre, retrospective analysis

Christina Tugendsam[1], Veronika Petz[2], Wolfgang Buchinger[3], Brigitta Schmoll-Hauer[1,4], Iris Pia Schenk[1,5], Karin Rudolph[1], Michael Krebs[1,6] and Georg Zettinig[1*]

Abstract

Background: We aimed to study the validity of six published ultrasound criteria for risk stratification of thyroid nodules in the former severely iodine deficient population of Austria.

Methods: Retrospective, single centre, observer blinded study design. All patients with a history of thyroidectomy due to nodules seen in the centre between 2004 and 2014 with preoperative in-house sonography and documented postoperative histology were analyzed ($n = 195$). A board of five experienced thyroidologists evaluated the images of 45 papillary carcinomas, 8 follicular carcinomas, and 142 benign nodules regarding the following criteria: mild hypoechogenicity, marked hypoechogenicity, microlobulated or irregular margins, microcalcifications, taller than wide shape, missing thin halo.

Results: All criteria but mild hypoechogenicity were significantly more frequent in thyroid cancer than in benign nodules. The number of positive criteria was significantly higher in cancer (2.79 ± 1.35) than in benign nodules (1.73 ± 1.18; $p < 0.001$). Thus, with a cut-off of two or more positive criteria, a sensitivity of 85% and a specificity of 45% were reached to predict malignancy in this sample of thyroid nodules. As expected, the findings were even more pronounced in papillary cancer only (2.98 ± 1.32 vs. 1.73 ± 1.18, $p < 0.001$). The six ultrasound criteria could not identify follicular cancer.

Conclusion: Our findings support the recently published EU-TIRADS score. Apart from mild hypoechogenicity, the analyzed ultrasound criteria can be applied for risk stratification of thyroid nodules in the previously severely iodine deficient population of Austria.

Keywords: TIRADS, Sonography, Ultrasound, Nodule, Hypoechogenicity, Microcalcifications, Halo

Background

Thyroid nodules are a common finding in any given population, with an estimated prevalence of 20-76% on ultrasound examination [1]. The vast majority of these nodules – regardless of whether they were initially palpable or incidental findings (e.g. upon carotid artery sonography) – are benign [2].

Therefore it is of high importance to discern truly benign thyroid nodules from those at higher risk [3].

Thyroid cancer is a tumor entity with steep increase in incidence, albeit with the majority of new cases belonging to the group of low risk tumor stages [4]. How to select the thyroid nodules for further assessment by fine needle aspiration is currently still a matter of debate [5]. Especially with the widespread use of high resolution neck ultrasound, many thyroid nodules are detected as incidentalomas [1, 2].

There is no typical sonographic pattern of thyroid cancer. Various sonographic criteria have been proposed to estimate the risk of malignancy in thyroid nodules. In 2009, two different proposals for a so-called TIRADS

---

* Correspondence: georg.zettinig@meduniwien.ac.at
[1]Schilddruesenpraxis Josefstadt, Laudongasse 12/8, Vienna AT-1080, Austria
Full list of author information is available at the end of the article

scoring system based on ultrasound nodule patterns were published [6, 7]. The concept was inspired by the widely used BIRADS system for assessing breast lesions, but partly been criticized for its complexity. It is still under debate whether this system can easily be applied to routine clinical use [5], and several modifications have been proposed during the last years [8–10].

In August 2017, the European Thyroid Association Guidelines for Ultrasound Malignancy Risk Stratification of Thyroid Nodules in Adults have been published [11]. Prior to this, the British Thyroid Association has published ultrasound features indicative of malignant nodule in its Guidelines for the management of thyroid cancer in 2014 [12], and the American Thyroid Association presented sonographic patterns suspicious for thyroid cancer in their 2015 guidelines [13], leading to some modifications of the Korean Thyroid Association guidelines in 2016 [14].

A number of studies evaluated the sensitivity and specificity of various criteria in patient samples from e.g. Korea [8, 15, 16], France [9, 10], or Poland [17]. We selected the following six criteria: mild hypoechogenicity [7–9, 11, 12], marked hypoechogenicity [7–9, 11, 12], microlobulated or irregular margins [7, 8, 9, 11, 12,], microcalcifications [7–9, 11, 12], taller than wide shape [7–9, 11, 12], and the absence of a thin halo [7, 12].

The presence of two or more of the six ultrasound criteria mild hypoechogenicity, marked hypoechogenicity, microlobulated or irregular margins, microcalcifications, taller than wide shape, and a solid component have been proposed to identify nodules at risk in a large Korean study evaluating more than 1600 patients including follow-up data which was the basis for the TIRADS Kwak score [8]. In the TIRADS French score system the four criteria irregular shape, irregular margins, microcalcifications, and marked hypoechogenicity are classified as highly suspect whereas mild hypoechogenicity in the absence of any of the four high suspicious features is the criterion for intermediate risk [11].

Comparable to France and several other European countries, Austria has been a moderately to even severely iodine depleted area with a high prevalence of endemic goiter, functional autonomies and cretinism, especially in the alp regions, for a long time [18]. In Austria, table salt has been iodized by federal law since 1963. The initial concentration of 10 mg KI per kg salt was increased to 20 mg/kg in 1990 when urine iodine secretion was still found to be in the mildly deficient range, currently it is 15-20 mg/kg. This strategy proved to be successful in greatly reducing the incidence of the above mentioned consequences of iodine deficiency [19].

Yet recent data indicate that iodine intake is still insufficient in at least part of the Austrian population, especially in pregnant women [20]. Due to decreased intake of table salt (as advocated for preventing hypertension) and the widespread use of not iodinated industrial salt, iodine intake might be insufficient even in the general population [20, 21].

The aim of our study was to assess six ultrasound criteria indicating thyroid cancer mainly published in the TIRADS Kwak score [8] and the TIRADS French score [9, 10] in the former iodine deficient Greater Vienna area. The study was conducted as a single centre, retrospective analysis of all nodules with postoperative histologic data available over the time course of 10 years (2004-2014). Five blinded experts rated the sonographic images according to the presence of published criteria. Diagnostic values of these criteria were then determined and compared to the published literature.

Methods
Setting and Study sample
The thyroid centre "Schilddruesenpraxis Josefstadt" is the largest private thyroid centre in Vienna and has been founded in 2004. We analysed all patients who were seen in this secondary care centre between October 2004 and December 2014 and identified all patients with the diagnosis of "history of thyroidectomy". Among these 491 patients, 47 were operated due to Graves' disease and excluded from analysis. There were 91 patients with thyroid cancer and 353 with benign thyroid nodules. Of the 444 patients seen postoperatively, 223 had preoperative thyroid sonography at the centre. From this sample another 28 patients were excluded due to the following reasons: poor image quality (12), very small microcarcinoma (14), original histological data not available (2).

Thus the initial study sample consisted of 195 patients: 45 papillary thyroid carcinomas (PTC), 8 follicular thyroid carcinomas (FTC), and 142 benign nodules (BN). Considering the medical history of each patient, the two unblinded investigators (GZ and VP) assigned all preoperative ultrasound images either to the thyroid cancer group or to the benign nodules group and anonymized all ultrasound images using the individual patient numbers given to all patients at the initial visit at the centre. GZ also selected the nodule that led to surgery in all patients with multinodular goitre. Images were available as electronic files since 2009, and before 2009 as prints.

Retrospective expert review of the ultrasound images
Five experienced Austrian thyroidologists (CT, WB, BSH, KR, MK) met in April 2016 to review all preoperative sonographic patterns in a single session. They all have their focus on treating thyroid patients for many years, and their experience in thyroid sonography is up to 27 years.

Table 1 Detailed characteristics of the subgroups

	BN	PTC	FTC
Females	127/142 (89%)	36/45 (80%)	6/8 (75%)
Age (mean ± SD)	49 ± 11 years	42 ± 12 years	36 ± 11 years
Date of birth after 1 January 1963	63/142 (44%)	36/45 (80%)	6/8 (75%)
Maximum diameter of the nodule (mean ± SD)	28 ± 11 mm	20 ± 12 mm	31 ± 7 mm

The experts reviewed each nodule regarding the presence or absence of six ultrasound criteria given below. In a second step, they ranked the nodule as benign or malignant. Each expert wrote his or her assessment in an evaluation form (criterion 1-6 present or absent, nodule benign or malignant). Thereafter, the experts decided on the presence or absence of all six criteria and categorized the nodule as benign or malignant together. In case of disagreement between the experts, consensus was reached by discussion.

Definition of ultrasound criteria of suspicion

The study was designed to evaluate the presence or absence of the following six criteria:

Mild hypoechogenicity

The nodule was classified as mildly hypoechogenic if the echogenicity was less than the thyroid parenchyma but more than the surrounding strap muscle.

Marked hypoechogenicity

The nodule was classified as marked hypoechogenic if the echogenicity was less than that of the surrounding strap muscle.

Microlobulated or irregular margins

The margin had many small lobules on the surface of a nodule or was infiltrative.

Microcalcifications

Defined as calcifications that were equal to or less than 1 mm in diameter and visualized as tiny punctate hyperechoic foci, either with or without acoustic shadows.

Taller than wide shape

The nodule was greater in its anteroposterior dimension than in its transverse dimension.

No thin halo

Absence of a thin hypoechoic rim around the nodule.

In partly cystic lesions, always the solid component was evaluated. Mild hypoechogenicity excluded marked hypoechogenicity and vice versa. Therefore, a maximum number of five criteria were possible in a single nodule.

Statistics

Demographic data and nodule size are presented as mean ± standard deviation (SD). We compared them by chi-square statistics for categorical data and unpaired students t-test for continuous variables. The number of positive criteria was added for all nodules resulting in a minimum score of 0 and a maximum of 5 positive criteria (with mild hypoechogenicity and marked hypoechogenicity being mutually exclusive). Mean number of positive criteria in benign versus malignant lesions were compared by unpaired student's t-test. A $p < 0.05$ was considered statistically significant. One-way ANOVA, followed by multiple t-tests with Bonferroni correction as post-hoc test (if appropriate), was used to compare mean numbers of positive criteria in the three subgroups of BN, PTC, and FTC.

The ability of the six ultrasound criteria to significantly discriminate between benign and malignant lesions was assessed by chi-square tests with Bonferroni correction for multiple testing. Thus, a p-value of < 0.0083 (0.05/6) was considered statistically significant.

Additionally the diagnostic values sensitivity, specificity, positive and negative predictive values (together with their respective 95% intervals) for each parameter and the expert opinion were calculated to predict the

Table 2 Chi-square statistics: Number (%) of positive criteria - BN versus cancer

BN vs. cancer:	BN	Cancer	x^2	p-value
Mild hypoechogenicity	55/142 (39%)	19/53 (36%)	0.136	0.712
Marked hypoechogenicity	26/142 (18%)	22/53 (42%)	11.194	0.001
Microlobulated/ irregular margins	39/142 (27%)	29/53 (55%)	12.621	0.0004
Microcalcifications	10/142 (7%)	16/53 (30%)	17.894	0.00002
Taller than wide	17/142 (12%)	15/53 (28%)	7.503	0.006
No thin halo	99/142 (70%)	47/53 (89%)	7.375	0.007

Table 3 Chi-square statistics: Number (%) of positive criteria - BN versus PTC

BN vs.PTC:	BN	PTC	x^2	p-value
Mild hypoechogenicity	55/142 (39%)	17/45 (38%)	0.013	0.909
Marked hypoechogenicity	26/142 (18%)	20/45 (44%)	12.583	0.0004
Microlobulated/ irregular margins	39/142 (27%)	27/45 (60%)	15.839	0.00007
Microcalcifications	10/142 (7%)	15/45 (33%)	20.394	0.00001
Taller than wide	17/142 (12%)	15/45 (33%)	10.993	0.001
No thin halo	99/142 (70%)	40/45 (89%)	6.582	0.010

risk of cancer and PTC. The same diagnostic values were also calculated to compare the risk of malignancy in nodules with less than 2 vs. 2 or more criteria and less than 3 vs. 3 or more criteria, respectively. Statistical analysis was performed using SPSS Version 24 statistic software package.

Results

Demographic characteristics
Patients with cancer were significantly younger compared to the BN group (41 ± 11.9 vs. 49 ± 11.4 years; $p < 0.001$), and there was a lower rate of females among the cancer patients (79% vs. 89%, $p = 0.063$). An overview of the demographic characteristics of the subgroups (BN, PTC, FTC) is given in Table 1. PTC were significantly smaller than the nodules from the other groups.

The study sample included 103 patients (53%) born after 1963 (the year when iodization of table salt became mandatory in Austria). All but one patient were born before 1990 (when iodine content of table salt was increased from 10 to 20 mg/kg salt).

Ultrasound criteria
Of the investigated malignancy suspicious criteria, all but mild hypoechogenicity were statistically different between benign and malignant lesions when compared by chi-square statistics. When comparing subgroups, the criterion no thin halo reached only borderline significance to predict PTC after Bonferroni correction for multiple comparisons ($p = 0.01$). Table 2 and 3 provide a detailed overview. Noteworthy, 23% of the carcinomas were isoechogenic.

The sensitivity, specificity, positive predictive value, and negative predictive value of each of the six criteria is given in Table 4 and 5 for both analyses (BN vs. cancer and the subgroup analysis). Sensitivity for the criterion no thin halo was 89%, all other criteria showed sensitivities of 60% and less. Several criteria showed a specificity of > 80%, whereas the most sensitive criterion no thin halo showed a specificity of only 30%.

Mean number of positive criteria
Mean number of positive criteria were statistically different between BN and cancer ($1,73 \pm 1,18$ versus $2,79 \pm 1,35$, respectively; $p < 0.001$, unpaired student's t-test). There was also a significant difference between the three subgroups BN, PTC, and FTC ($p < 0.001$, one-way ANOVA). In the post-hoc tests (multiple t-tests with Bonferroni correction), PTC were statistically significantly different from BN ($p < 0.001$) as well as from FTC ($p = 0.026$), while mean number of criteria were comparable in BN and FTC. See Table 6 for details.

Calculated sums of positive criteria
Three out of 45 PTC (6.6%) did not show any of the criteria published in the literature. Of those, two were T1b and one was T1a. All three were labelled benign by the expert panel.

With a cut-off value of two or more positive criteria, 45 out of 53 malignant lesions (89%) were labelled correctly and 78 out of 142 benign lesions (55%) incorrectly as cancer. Thus, this cut-off resulted in a sensitivity of 89%[76-96], specificity of 45%[37-55], PPV of

Table 4 Diagnostic parameters for cancer

Cancer	Sensitivity	Specificity	PPV	NPV
Mild hypoechogenicity	36%	61%	26%	72%
Marked hypoechogenicity	42%	82%	46%	79%
Microlobulated/ irregular margins	55%	73%	43%	81%
Microcalcifications	30%	93%	62%	78%
Taller than wide	28%	88%	47%	77%
No thin halo	89%	30%	32%	88%

Table 5 Diagnostic parameters for PTC

PTC	Sensitivity	Specificity	PPV	NPV
Mild Hypoechogenicity	38%	61%	24%	76%
Marked hypoechogenicity	44%	82%	44%	82%
Microlobulated/ irregular margins	60%	73%	41%	85%
Microcalcifications	33%	93%	60%	82%
Taller than wide	33%	88%	47%	81%
No thin halo	89%	30%	29%	90%

Table 6 Mean number of positive ultrasound criteria in BN and in all cancer patients as well as in the subgroups of PTC and FTC

	BN (n = 142)	Cancer (n = 53)	PTC (n = 45)	FTC (n = 8)
Mean number of criteria	1.73 ± 1.18	2.79 ± 1.35*	2.98 ± 1.32*	1.75 ± 1.04 **

* BN vs. Cancer: p < 0.001
* PTC vs. BN: p < 0.001, PTC vs. FTC: p = 0.026
** FTC vs. BN: p > 0.99, FTC vs. PTC: p = 0.026

34%[30-38], and NPV of 93%[85-97] to detect cancer based on ultrasound criteria when compared to benign lesions.

When increasing the threshold to three or more criteria, correct assignment of cancer to benign decreased while incorrect labelling of benign lesions as cancer dropped. See Tables 7, 8, 9, and 10 for details for both the PTC as well as the cancer group.

With this criterion, 16 nodules with a postoperative diagnosis of PTC were rated as benign. Those nodules were staged pT1a (7 nodules), pT1a(m) (2 nodules), pT1b (5 nodules), pT2 (1 nodule), pT3 (1 nodule).

Pooled expert opinion
The experts diagnosed cancer with a specificity of 84%[76-90] and a sensitivity of 52%[38-65]. PPV was 58%[47-69] and NPV 80%[75-84]. The diagnostic values of the pooled expert opinion for PTC were: sensitivity 64%[49-78], specificity 78%[70-85], PPV 48%[39-58], NPV 87%[82-91]. Of the 16 PTC falsely labelled as benign by the experts staging was pT1a in 7, pT1b in 5, pT1b(m) in 1, and pT3 in 1 lesion. 6 fulfilled 3 or more positive ultrasound criteria. On the other hand experts rated 7 lesions fulfilling only 2 ultrasound criteria correctly as carcinomas. 8 lesions were missed by both methods (5 fulfilling 1 and 3 fulfilling 2 ultrasound criteria).

Discussion
In light of the widespread use of ultrasonography and frequent findings of thyroid incidentalomas, strategies that systematically and reliably identify those thyroid nodules with a higher risk of malignancy are highly warranted.

In iodine deficient areas like Austria the spectrum of thyroid malignancies differs from iodine sufficient areas with a relatively higher proportion of follicular carcinomas and the occurrence of anaplastic carcinomas in multinodular goiters (which almost disappeared after the introduction of iodization of table salt) [22].

We therefore conducted a retrospective analysis of sonographic images from thyroid nodules with available postoperative histological data from Austrian patients (mainly from Vienna and surroundings). Since the published sonographic criteria relate to papillary carcinomas only, we also calculated a statistical analysis restricted to PTC vs. benign lesions.

At the time the study was designed, several criteria were repeatedly studied and published [7–9, 12]. According to previously published reports, we analyzed mild hypoechogenicity, marked hypoechogenicity, microlobulated or irregular margins, microcalcifications, and a taller than wide shape. As retrospective assessment of the composition of a nodule (solid, mainly solid, mainly cystic) in two dimensional images seemed problematic to us, we decided not to include this criterion in our analysis. These five criteria are also among the proposals for the TIRADS French [9] and the recently published EU-TIRADS scoring system [11] and are included in the system proposed in the recently published ATA 2015 guidelines [13]. Due to the rather small sample size, however, we decided to restrict our analysis to applying the most widely used criteria without applying a formal scoring system. In addition, we evaluated the absence of a thin perinodular halo. There is no hard evidence from studies, but the halo sign traditionally has been regarded as an important ultrasound sign for the risk stratification of thyroid nodules in central Europe [23, 24] and is still discussed as a suggested feature for thyroid cancer in several diagnostic algorithms [12, 25, 26]. Noteworthy, the halo sign has also recently been discussed also in the European Thyroid Association Guidelines for Ultrasound Malignancy Risk Stratification of Thyroid Nodules in Adults [11] and is one of the nine sonographic features initially identified in the white paper

Table 7 Chi-square statistics of calculated sums of positive criteria – BN vs. cancer

BN vs. cancer	BN	Cancer	X^2	p-value
≥1 criterion	120/142 (85%)	49/53 (93%)	2.10869	0.14646
≥2 criteria	78/142 (55%)	45/53 (85%)	14.89056	0.00011
≥3 criteria	36/142 (25%)	31/53 (59%)	18.79224	0.00001
≥4 criteria	10/142 (7%)	19/53 (36%)	25.29781	0.0000005
5 criteria	2/142 (1%)	4/53 (8%)	4.87687	0.02722

Table 8 Chi-square statistics of calculated sums of positive criteria – BN vs. PTC

BN vs. PTC	BN	PTC	X^2	p-value
≥1 criterion	120/142 (85%)	42/45 (93%)	2.29850	0.12950
≥2 criteria	78/142 (55%)	40/45 (89%)	16.92502	0.00004
≥3 criteria	36/142 (25%)	29/45 (64%)	23.02780	0.000002
≥4 criteria	10/142 (7%)	19/45 (42%)	32.27589	0.00000001
5 criteria	2/142 (1%)	4/45 (9%)	6.15697	0.01309

Table 9 Sensitivity, specificity, PPV, and NPV of the number of criteria for cancer

Cancer	≥1 criterion	≥2 criteria	≥3 criteria	≥4 criteria	5 criteria
Sensitivity	93%	85%	59%	36%	8%
Specificity	16%	45%	75%	93%	99%
PPV	29%	37%	46%	66%	67%
NPV	85%	89%	83%	80%	74%

of the ACR TIRADS Committee [26]. Our findings indicate that the absence of a thin halo is also helpful for the diagnosis of thyroid cancer, at least in the former severely iodine depleted population of Austria.

Overall we found a good accordance of the published risk markers with the lesions evaluated in this sample. Our findings support the validity of the TIRADS Kwak criteria [8], the ATA 2015 criteria [13] as well as the TIRADS French [10] and the EU-TIRADS [11] criteria for the former severely iodine deficient area of Austria. One notable exception is the criterion of mild hypoechogenicity. In contrast to marked hypoechogenicity, mild hypoechogenicity could not discriminate between benign and malignant lesions in our sample. This is different to TIRADS Kwak [8]. ATA 2015 does not discriminate between mild and marked hypoechogenicity. In EU-TIRADS, mild hypoechogenicity indicates intermediate risk but no high risk for thyroid cancer [11], indicating that also in the previously iodine deficient population of France, mild hypoechogenicity is not that strict criterion for malignancy as in iodine sufficient regions such as Korea.

There are several possible reasons for this finding. Firstly, all the nodules included in this sample were considered to be reason enough to operate on the patient. Reasons leading to the operation decision were not systematically recorded, but included suspicious results in fine needle aspiration, nodule size, local complaints, patient's wish, and also suspicion of malignancy in ultrasound. Thus, unambiguously benign lesions were underrepresented or (e.g. simple cysts) even absent from the study sample.Yet another possible reason for this finding is the effect of iodine deficiency that might results in changes in thyroid tissue that are only partially reversible upon iodine supplementation. In a large French sample (France being a formerly iodine deficient region), mild

Table 10 Sensitivity, specificity, PPV, and NPV of the number of criteria for PTC

PTC	≥1 criterion	≥2 criteria	≥3 criteria	≥4 criteria	5 criteria
Sensitivity	93%	89%	64%	42%	9%
Specificity	16%	45%	75%	93%	99%
PPV	26%	34%	45%	66%	67%
NPV	88%	93%	87%	84%	77%

hypoechogenicity conferred only intermediate risk for thyroid cancer [27], in contrast to the iodine sufficient region of Korea.

Of note, 48% of the patients included in the study were born before the year 1963, when iodization of table salt was introduced in Austria and therefore spent at least parts of their early lives in severe iodine deficiency. Only one of the patients was born after 1990 when iodization of table salt in Austria was doubled to 20 mg/kg, because iodine supplementation was still considered insufficient [27]. The different iodine status in Austria and France could also be the explanation mild hypoechogenicity being classified as an intermediate risk factor in the TIRADS French study, but not discriminating in our sample.

A third European country with former iodine deficiency is Poland [28]. Recently an evaluation of four TIRADS classification systems in Polish multinodular goiter patients was published suggesting TIRADS Kwak as a suitable and practicable tool for this patient group. [17].

There is no single ultrasound feature which could reliably distinguish benign from malignant lesions. Some markers (e.g. microcalcifications) have a high specificity but insufficient sensitivity and vice versa. Thus, the combination of several features enhances the diagnostic value of sonography. In a recent Korean study [15], performed on a very large sample of thyroid nodules 10-19 mm in size, a head to head comparison of six risk stratification systems proposed in the literature was performed and yielded, as would be expected, different diagnostic values. Application of TIRADS French (using the number of positive criteria with a cut-off of two or more criteria being present for proposing fine needle aspiration) resulted in a sensitivity of 95% and a specificity of 52%, respectively. In the sample presented here, the cut-off value of two or more positive criteria for PTC resulted in a roughly comparable diagnostic performance (with slightly lower sensitivity of 89% and specificity of 45%). Other stratification systems resulted in even higher sensitivity at the cost of lower specificity.

On the other hand, the pooled expert estimation of malignancy risk yielded sensitivity and specificity very similar to the 3 criteria cut-off condition. Thus, 35% of PTC were mislabelled as benign from the expert panel (although the PTC misjudged as benign were all but one postoperatively staged as pT1).

The experts diagnosed cancer with a specificity of 84%, but the sensitivity was only 52%. For the diagnosis of PTC, the expert's sensitivity of 64% was only slightly higher. These findings indicate that in real life setting, the accurate differential diagnosis of nodules still remains difficult. Our five thyroidologists, who have longtime experience in interpreting thyroid ultrasound, did not predict malignancy accurately. Using a number of at least two positive ultrasound criteria to define the risk of malignancy yields a higher sensitivity but a lower specificity than expert judgement.

Our findings suggest that mild hypoechogenicity should be clearly differentiated from marked hypoechogenicity. The role of mild hypoechogenicity as a malignancy marker has to be clarified in relation to iodine status: In the sample studied here, in opposition to marked hypoechogenicity - which was significantly more frequent in PTC - mild hypoechogenicity didn't even show a trend towards higher frequency in PTC. On the other hand, the absence of a thin halo added diagnostic value in the sample presented here and might be worthy of consideration when evaluating nodules for possible malignancy.

The 2015 American Thyroid Association Management Guidelines for Adult Patients with Thyroid Nodules and Differentiated Thyroid Cancer [13] have been published after a long debate including a revised concept for ultrasonographic risk stratification of thyroid nodules. These guidelines do not distinguish between mild and marked hypoechogenicity. Hypoechogenic solid nodules without other risk patterns are classified as intermediately suspicious with a malignancy risk of 10-20%. In our study sample, however, the criterion hypoechogenicity was not found more often in cancer than in benign lesions.

The six criteria were not helpful for diagnosing follicular cancer. As presented in Table 6, the mean number of ultrasound criteria of FTC did not differ from BN, but from PTC. In these patients, the "nodule in nodule sign" could be a criterion for future studies [29]. If, as sometimes is suggested, the scintigraphic pattern (with reduced versus isointense activity) would be helpful in risk stratification of those nodules, is currently unclear. The sample did not include any patient with medullary thyroid cancer. Most probably this is because in Vienna nearly all patients with medullary thyroid cancer are followed up in a single tertiary centre after surgery.

Strengths of the study include the assessment by five thyroid experts in a systematic way and the availability of histological data of all the included nodules. Limitations of the study include the retrospective study design, that only B-mode images were used, the lack of information on the actual iodine status of the patients, the rather small sample size and the single center study design.

Conclusions

In conclusion, we report validity of published ultrasound malignancy risk markers of thyroid nodules in the formerly severely iodine deficient area of Austria for the first time. Our findings support the EU-TIRADS scoring system. With the exception of hypoechogenicity, ultrasound criteria as described in the literature were applicable with good sensitivity for risk adjustment of thyroid nodules in this secondary care setting. Additionally, the missing halo sign was a sensitive malignancy marker in this sample, which might be useful in a screening setting.

Abbreviations

BN: Benign nodules; FTC: Follicular thyroid cancer; PTC: Papillyry thyroid cancer; SD: Standard deviation

Authors' contributions

CT was involved in the study design, analysis, and writing of the manuscript, and reviewed all preoperative sonographic patterns. VP collected the data and was involved in the study design and analysis. WB reviewed all preoperative sonographic patterns and was involved in the study design and writing of the manuscript. BSH and KR reviewed all preoperative sonographic patterns. IPS was involved in collecting the data. MK was involved in the study design, analysis, and writing of the manuscript, and reviewed all preoperative sonographic patterns. GZ was involved in the study design, analysis, and writing of the manuscript, and reviewed all preoperative sonographic patterns. All authors read and approved the final manuscript.

Competing interests

The authors declare that they have no competing interests.

Author details

[1]Schilddruesenpraxis Josefstadt, Laudongasse 12/8, Vienna AT-1080, Austria. [2]Division of Nuclear Medicine, Department of Biomedical Imaging and Image-guided Therapy, Medical University of Vienna, Vienna, Austria. [3]Schilddrueseninstitut Gleisdorf, Gleisdorf, Austria. [4]Department of Nuclear Medicine, Krankenanstalt Rudolfstiftung, Vienna, Austria. [5]Department of Nuclear Medicine, Sozialmedizinisches Zentrum Hietzing, Vienna, Austria. [6]Clinical Division of Endocrinology, Department of Medicine III, Medical University of Vienna, Vienna, Austria.

References

1. Russ G, Leboulleux S, Leenhardt L, Hegedues L. Thyroid incidentalomas: epidemiology, risk stratification with ultrasound and workup. Eur Thyroid J. 2014;3:154–63.
2. Buchinger W, Petnehazy E, Pap A, Kaserer K, Zettinig G. Der Schilddrüsenfall: Leitliniengerechte Knotenabklärung. J Klin Endokrinol Stoffw. 2016;9:16–17.
3. Zafon C, Díez JJ, Galofré JC, Cooper DS. Nodular Thyroid Disease and Thyroid Cancer in the Era of Precision Medicine. Eur Thyroid J. 2017;6:65–74.
4. Lim H, Devesa SS, Sosa JA, Check D, Kitahara CM. Trends in Thyroid Cancer Incidence and Mortality in the United States, 1974-2013. JAMA. 2017;317:1338–48.
5. Negro R, Attanasio R, Grimaldi F, Frasoldati A, Guglielmi R, Papini E. A 2016 Italian Survey about Guidelines and Clinical Management of Thyroid Nodules. Eur Thyroid J. 2017;6:75–81.
6. Horvath E, Majlis S, Rossi R, Franco C, Niedmann JP, Castro A, Dominguez M. An ultrasonogram reporting system for thyroid nodules stratifying cancer risk for clinical management. J Clin Endocrinol Metab. 2009;94:1748–51.
7. Park JY, Lee HJ, Jang HW, Kim HK, Yi JH, Lee W, Kim SH. A proposal for a thyroid imaging and data system for ultrasound features of thyroid carcinoma. Thyroid. 2009;19:1257–64.

8. Kwak JY, Han KH, Yoon JH, Moon HJ, Son EJ, Park SH, Jung HK, Choi JS, Kim BM, Kim EK. Thyroid imaging reporting and data system for US features of nodules: a step in establishing better stratification of cancer risk. Radiology. 2011;260:892–9.

9. Russ G, Royer B, Bigorgne C, Rouxel A, Bienvenu-Perrard M, Leenhardt L. Prospective evaluation of thyroid imaging reporting and data system on 4550 nodules with and without elastography. Eur J Endocrinol. 2013; 168:649–55.

10. Russ G, Bigorgne C, Royer B, Rouxel A, Bienvenu-Perrard M. Le système TIRADS en échographie thyroïdienne. J Radiol. 2011;92:701–13.

11. Russ G, Bonnema SJ, Erdogan MF, Durante C, Ngu R, Leenhardt L. European Thyroid Association Guidelines for Ultrasound Malignancy Risk Stratification of Thyroid Nodules in Adults: The EU-TIRADS. Eur Thyroid J. 2017;6:225–37.

12. Perros P, Colley S, Boelaert K, Evans C, Evans RM, Gerrard GE, Gilbert JA, Harrison B, Johnson SJ, Giles TE, Moss L, Lewington V, Newbold KL, Taylor J, Thakker RV, Watkinson J, Williams GR. British Thyroid Association Guidelines for the Management of Thyroid Cancer. Clin Endocrinol. 2014;81(1):1–122.

13. Haugen BR, Alexander EK, Bible KC, Doherty GM, Mandel SJ, Nikiforov YE, Pacini F, Randolph GW, Sawka AM, Schlumberger M, Schuff KG, Sherman SI, Sosa JA, Steward DL, Tuttle RM, Wartofsky L. 2015 American Thyroid Association Management Guidelines for Adult Patients with Thyroid Nodules and Differentiated Thyroid Cancer: The American Thyroid Association Guidelines Task Force on Thyroid Nodules and Differentiated Thyroid Cancer. Thyroid. 2016;26:1–133.

14. Yi HK. The Revised 2016 Korean Thyroid Association Guidelines for Thyroid Nodules and Cancers: Differences from the 2015 American Thyroid Association Guidelines. Endocrinol Metab (Seoul). 2016;31:373–8.

15. Yoon JH, Han K, Kim EK, Moon HJ, Kwak JY. Diagnosis and Management of Small Thyroid Nodules: A Comparative Study with Six Guidelines for Thyroid Nodules. Radiology. 2017;283:560–9.

16. Yoon JH, Lee HS, Kim EK, Moon HJ, Kwak JY. Malignancy Risk Stratification of Thyroid Nodules: Comparison between the Thyroid Imaging Reporting and Data System and the 2014 American Thyroid Association Management Guidelines. Radiology. 2016;278:917–24.

17. Migda B, Migda M, Migda AM, Bierca J, Slowniska-Srzednicka J, Jakubowski W, Slapa RZ. Evaluation of Four Variants of the Thyroid Imaging Reporting and Data System (TIRADS) Classification in Patients with Multinodular Goiter. Endokrynol Pol. 2018;69:142–9.

18. Weissel M. Legal augmentation of iodine content in table salt from 10 to 20 mg KI/kg: documented effects a decade later. Exp Clin Endocrinol Diabetes. 2003;111:187–90.

19. Heinisch M, Kumnig G, Asböck D, Mikosch P, Gallowitsch HJ, Kresnik E, Gomez I, Unterweger O, Lind P. Goiter prevalence and urinary iodide excretion in a formerly iodine-deficient region after introduction of statutory Iodization of common salt. Thyroid. 2002;12:809–14.

20. Lindorfer H, Krebs M, Kautzky-Willer A, Bancher-Todesca D, Sager M, Gessl A. Iodine deficiency in pregnant women in Austria. Eur J Clin Nutr. 2015; 69:349–54.

21. Buchinger W, Lorenz-Wawschinek O, Semlitsch G, Langsteger W, Binter G, Bonelli RM, Eber O. Thyrotropin and thyroglobulin as an index of optimal iodine intake: correlation with iodine excretion of 39,913 euthyroid patients. Thyroid. 1997;7:593–7.

22. Passler C, Scheuba C, Prager G, Kaczirek K, Kaserer K, Zettinig G, Niederle B. Prognostic factors of papillary and follicular thyroid cancer: differences in an iodine-replete endemic goiter region. Endocr Relat Cancer. 2004;11:131–9.

23. Zettinig G, Buchinger W, Gessl A. Schilddruesen Ultraschall Kursbuch. 1st ed. Vienna: facultas.wuv; 2013. p. 50–1.

24. Dietlein M, Kobe C, Schmidt M, Schicha H. The incidentaloma of the thyroid. Over- or underuse of diagnostic procedure for an epidemiologic finding? Nuklearmedizin. 2005;44:213–24.

25. Andrioli M, Carzaniga C, Persani L. Standardized Ultrasound Report for Thyroid Nodules: The Endocrinologist's Viewpoint. Eur Thyroid J. 2013;2:37–48.

26. Grant EG, Tessler FN, Hoang JK, Langer JE, Beland MD, Berland LL, Cronan JJ, Desser TS, Frates MC, Hamper UM, Middleton WD, Reading CC, Scoutt LM, Stavros AT, Teefey SA. Thyroid Ultrasound Reporting Lexicon: White Paper of the ACR Thyroid Imaging, Reporting and Data System (TIRADS) Committee. J Am Coll Radiol. 2015;12:1272–9.

27. Lind P, Kumnig G, Heinisch M, Igerc I, Mikosch P, Gallowitsch HJ, Kresnik E, Gomez I, Unterweger O, Aigner H. Iodine supplementation in Austria: methods and results. Thyroid. 2002;12:903–7.

28. Zygmunt A, Lewinski A. Iodine prophylaxis in pregnant women in Poland - where we are? (update 2015). Thyroid Res. 2015;8:17.

29. Kobayashi K, Ota H, Hirokawa M, Yabuta T, Fukushima M, Masuoka H, Higashiyama T, Kihara M, Ito Y, Miya A, Miyauchi A. "Nodule in Nodule" on Thyroid Ultrasonography. Possibility of Follicular Carcinoma Transformed from Benign Thyroid Tumor. Eur Thyroid J. 2017;6:101–7.

21

Characteristics and natural course of hypoechoic thyroid lesions diagnosed as possible thyroid lymphomas by fine needle aspiration cytology

Tomoe Nakao[1*], Mitsushige Nishikawa[1], Mako Hisakado[1], Toshihiko Kasahara[1], Takumi Kudo[1], Eijun Nishihara[1], Mitsuru Ito[1], Shuji Fukata[1], Hirotoshi Nakamura[1], Mitsuyoshi Hirokawa[2] and Akira Miyauchi[3]

Abstract

Background: There is little information regarding the natural course of hypoechoic thyroid lesions that are probable or possible thyroid lymphoma based on fine needle aspiration cytology (FNAC) results.

Methods: Sixty-five patients who were diagnosed as probable or possible thyroid lymphoma by ultrasonography (US) and FNAC were investigated. Forty-three patients with strong suspicion underwent thyroid surgery for the diagnosis at our hospital, and 22 patients were followed up with periodic US examination. Thyroid lymphoma was definitely diagnosed in 41 out of 43 patients who underwent thyroid surgery, and such patients were defined as Group A. The outcomes of 22 patients who were followed up without an immediate therapy were analyzed. Their hypoechoic lesions decreased in size ($n = 10$) or disappeared ($n = 2$) in 12 of 22 patients, and such patients were defined as Group B. Patients in Group A and B were compared using the Kuma Hospital-US classification (USC), the diagnostic categories of the Bethesda System for Reporting Thyroid Cytopathology, and the κ/λ deviation of the immunoglobulin light chain in the FNAC specimens. Mann-Whitney U-test and chi-squared test (with Yate's continuity correction) were used to compare the two groups.

Results: The USC of < 3.5 [9/12 (75.0%) in Group B; 10/41 patients (24.4%) in Group A] and the κ/λ deviation ratio of < 3.40 [11/12 (91.7%) in Group B; 17/41 patients (41.5%) in Group A] were significantly more frequent ($p < 0.01$), and the FNAC of 'benign' or 'atypia of undetermined significance or follicular lesion of undetermined significance (AUS)' with a comment of possible lymphoma [9/12 (75.0%) in Group B; 12/41 patients (29.3%) in Group A] was significantly more frequent ($p < 0.05$) in Group B than Group A.

Conclusions: Our study suggests that some hypoechoic thyroid lesions that are possible thyroid lymphoma based on US and FNAC might decrease in size or disappear during the careful observation.

Keywords: Thyroid lymphoma, Hypoechoic thyroid lesion, Regression, Fine needle aspiration cytology, κ/λ deviation

* Correspondence: tomoenakao@gmail.com
[1]Department of Internal Medicine, Kuma Hospital, Centre for Excellence in Thyroid Cares, 8-2-35 Shimoyamate-dori, Chuo-ku, Kobe 650-0011, Japan
Full list of author information is available at the end of the article

Background

Primary thyroid lymphoma is a rare cause of malignancy, accounting for 2–5% of all thyroid malignancies [1] and < 2% of extranodal lymphomas [2, 3]. A rapidly enlarging mass was the most common clinical manifestations in earlier series, but recently small lesions are found at the early stage [4]. It is a potentially lethal disease, but often responds well to appropriate treatments [5]. Thyroid lymphoma is not always diagnosed easily, especially in its early phase, because most of the cases are associated with Hashimoto's thyroiditis.

Ultrasonography (US) of the thyroid is initially used for the diagnosis of thyroid lymphoma. On US, lymphoma is shown as hypoechoic lesions, but subacute thyroiditis, focal chronic thyroiditis, some thyroid cancers, and metastatic thyroid cancer is also shown as hypoechoic lesions mimicking thyroid lymphoma. Based on US findings of internal echo levels, borders, and posterior echoes, thyroid lymphoma can be classified as the nodular, diffuse, or mixed type [6]. Although the nodular type often resembles follicular tumor or adenomatous nodule and the mixed type often resembles adenomatous goiter on US, these lesions can be often distinguished by an enhancement of posterior echoes. The diffuse type shows homogeneous and hypoechoic internal echoes, but these findings are also typical for severe chronic thyroiditis [6, 7].

Fine needle aspiration cytology (FNAC) is the next diagnostic strategy for thyroid lymphoma, but is challenging, particularly due to its histological similarities with mucosa-associated lymphoid tissue (MALT) lymphoma and chronic thyroiditis [8, 9]. The flow cytometry with CD45 gating on the FNAC specimen can be used to analyze the proportions of lymphocytic cells with κ and λ immunoglobulin light chains. The κ/λ deviation ratio of the light chain assessment is an important criterion for discriminating between polyclonal reactive processes such as chronic thyroiditis and monoclonal lymphomas. Strong deviation in the κ/λ ratio is regarded as suggestive monoclonal growth of lymphocytes, thus indicating thyroid lymphoma [10].

Even with these modalities, a definite diagnosis is not established easily. A surgical interventions is often needed for the histopathological diagnosis, but it might be unnecessary for the benign lesions. This is especially true for the small or moderate-size lesions. Needle biopsy is usually useful for the diagnosis of diffuse large B-cell type lymphoma, but is often insufficient in the case of MALT lymphoma.

We have observed some hypoechoic lesions that were diagnosed as possible thyroid lymphoma based on the FNAC decrease in size or disappear during their clinical courses without definitive treatment. However, there is little information regarding the natural course of such hypoechoic lesions that were possible thyroid lymphoma based on FNAC findings. We conducted the present study to (1) clarify the natural course of hypoechoic thyroid lesions that were possible thyroid lymphoma, and (2) identify clinical features that might be used to discriminate benign non-progressive lesions from those with progressive character.

Methods

Between April 2012 and July 2016, 136 patients were suspected of having thyroid lymphoma on US examination at Kuma Hospital, where approximately 15,000 new patients with thyroid diseases are evaluated annually. US examinations were routinely performed by our well-experienced operators. US was performed using an APLIO 500 TUS-A500 system (Toshiba Medical Systems Co., Ltd., Otawara, Japan) with a PLT-805AT (Toshiba) or PLT-1005BT probe (Toshiba). Patients with systemic lymphoma or previously diagnosed lymphoma were excluded. Of these 136 patients, 122 were diagnosed as having probable or possible thyroid lymphoma by FNAC (Fig. 1). The remaining 14 patients were excluded from the study, because they had other diagnoses based on FNAC findings (eight specimens were normal or benign, one anaplastic carcinoma of the thyroid, one subacute thyroiditis or thyroid papillary carcinoma, and one metastatic renal cell carcinoma; the remaining three specimens were inadequate for diagnosis). Among the 122 patients, 57 were excluded from the study, because 56 were referred to other hospitals for the definitive diagnosis and chemo radiotherapy, and one patient dropped out from the follow-up study. Thus, the remaining 65 patients were investigated in this study. Forty-three patients strongly suspected of having thyroid lymphoma underwent thyroid surgery at our hospital for the definite diagnosis and 22 patients with comments of possible lymphoma on cytology were followed up with periodic US examination for 1–41 (median 11.5) months. Whether surgery or follow-up examination was determined by each doctor in charge based on clinical and radiological findings, including the rapidity of the enlargement of the thyroid mass, and the US and FNAC findings. Of 43 patients who underwent thyroid surgery at our hospital, 41 (95.3%) were diagnosed as definite thyroid lymphoma, and the other two (4.7%) were diagnosed as chronic thyroiditis (Fig. 1). Among the 41 patients who were diagnosed as definite thyroid lymphoma, 34 were diagnosed as MALT lymphoma and seven were diagnosed as diffuse large B-cell lymphoma. Whether the lesions of all 41 patients were limited to the thyroid was not known because all were referred to other hospitals to undergo further diagnostic examinations, including the determination of the disease stage, and treatment.

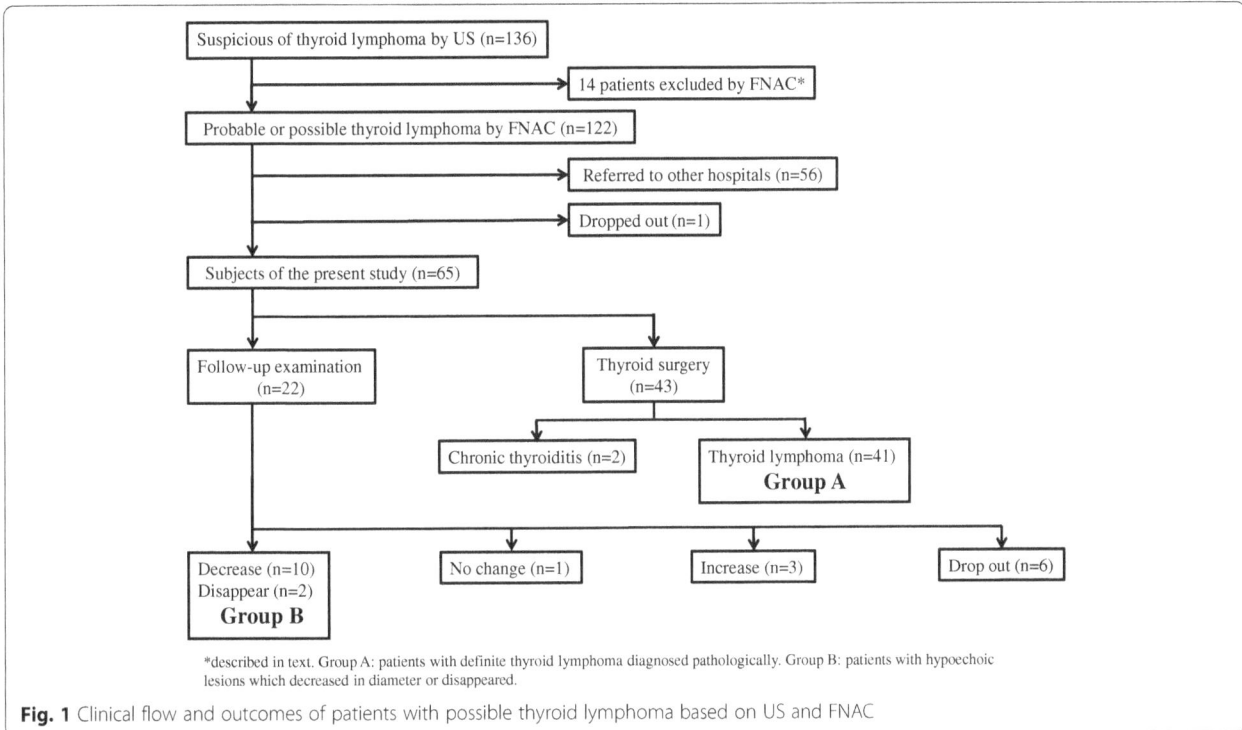

Fig. 1 Clinical flow and outcomes of patients with possible thyroid lymphoma based on US and FNAC

Hypoechoic lesions of the periodically followed-up 22 patients were analyzed. The US examination was repeated 1–3 month-interval at first and then 6 month-interval when no deterioration was observed. None of 22 patients were treated with steroids or immunosuppressive drugs during the follow-up examination. Other medications or supplementations, or dietary habit including iodine intake were not known in detail. When the maximum diameter of a hypoechoic lesion increased by ≥3 mm, we defined the case as an "increase" of the hypoechoic lesion. When

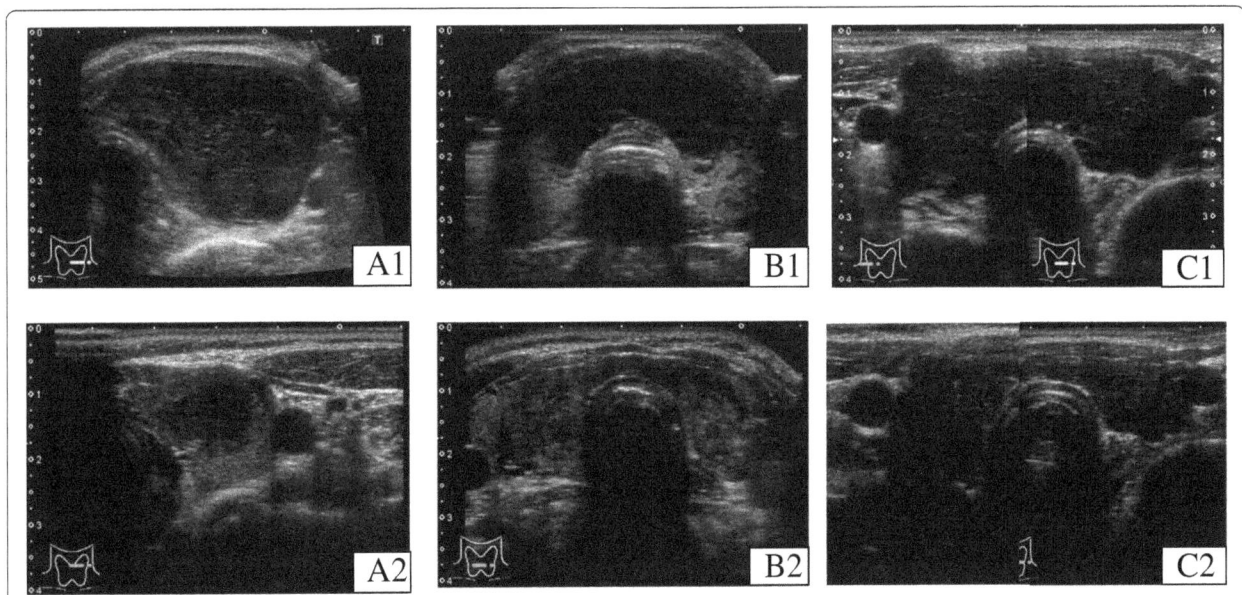

Fig. 2 Echograms of three representative patients whose hypoechoic lesions decreased or disappeared on careful follow-up examination. **a** A 74-year-old woman with a nodular hypoechoic lesion at presentation (A1) that had markedly decreased in size one month later (A2) (case No. 9 in Table 2). **b** A 69-year-old woman with a severely hypoechoic lesion involving the both thyroid lobes (B1) that had almost disappeared 10 months later (B2), although the irregularity remained possibly due to underlying chronic thyroiditis (case No. 4 in Table 2). **c** A 53-year-old woman with a diffuse severely hypoechoic lesion involving the whole thyroid (C1) that had markedly decreased in size 27 months later (C2) (case No. 1 in Table 2)

the maximum diameter of a hypoechoic lesion reduced by ≥3 mm, we defined the case as a "decrease." When the hypoechoic lesions were not detected clearly at follow-up examination, it was defined as "disappeared." We established this parameter because, in our previous study, plus or minus 2 mm was recognized as an observation variation [11]. In the present study, in some cases in which the entire thyroid volume was observed to have decreased, the maximum diameter of the hypoechoic lesions was measured and analyzed.

Representative US images showing "decrease" and "disappearance" are shown in Fig. 2. Our hospital uses its own ultrasound classification system for the diagnosis of thyroid nodules, which consists of five US classes (USC) based on the characteristics of thyroid nodules, such as a regular or irregular shape, solid or cystic content, the presence or absence of microcalcifications, extraglandal invasion, and other factors. The classification consists of five classes from 1 to 5. Intermediate classes from class 2 to class 4 (designated as classes 2.5 and 3.5) are also used (Table 1) [12]. Some cases of lymphoma with diffuse or mixed lesion are hardly classified according to USC, because this classification is mainly scored to thyroid nodules. However, in the present study, the US classification was applied to the hypoechoic lesions. The present study was approved by the Institutional Review Board of Kuma Hospital and the Ethics Committee in Kuma Hospital.

The hypoechoic lesions in 22 patients who were followed up with periodic US examination decreased in size ($n = 10$), disappeared ($n = 2$), showed no change ($n = 1$) or increased in size ($n = 3$). The remaining six patients dropped out from the follow-up examination. Of the three patients whose hypoechoic lesions increased in size, one patient was referred to another hospital and diagnosed as diffuse large B-cell lymphoma; the other two patients were carefully followed up without further progression (Fig. 1).

Forty-one patients with histopathologically diagnosed thyroid lymphoma were defined as Group A, and 12 patients whose hypoechoic lesions decreased in diameter or disappeared as defined Group B (Fig. 1). Their clinical features, the diameter of hypoechoic lesions, US features at the first presentation, and the diagnostic categories of the Bethesda System for Reporting Thyroid Cytopathology (BethSys categories) were compared between Group A and B. Mann-Whitney U-test and chi-squared test (with Yate's continuity correction) were used to compare the two groups.

Results

Table 2 summarizes the clinical features of 16 patients who underwent follow-up US examinations of hypoechoic lesions that were diagnosed as possible thyroid lymphoma. Thyroid function tests at presentation showed hypothyroid ($n = 1$), subclinical hypothyroid ($n = 4$) and euthyroid ($n = 11$). Some patients were taking levothyroxine (LT4) before and during the follow-up examination. However, whether LT4 supplementation was involved in the decrease or disappearance of the hypoechoic lesions is unclear, because of the small number of the cases. All Group B patients were thyroglobulin antibody (TgAb)- and/or thyroid peroxidase antibody (TPOAb)-positive. As a result of FNAC, 'atypia of undetermined significance or follicular lesion of undetermined significance (AUS)' was diagnosed in eight, 'suspicious for 'malignancy' in two, 'malignancy' in one, and 'benign' in one patient. The pathological report of case 2 in Table 2 said that it was probably benign; however, lymphoma could not be completely excluded. On flow cytometry of the fine needle aspirations, the κ/λ ratio varied from 0.31 to 4.61. When κ/λ ratio was lower than 1.00, we converted κ/λ ratio to λ/κ ratio (deviation ratio) to discriminate between the polyclonal reactive process and the monoclonal reactive process that is characteristic to lymphomas.

There were no significant differences in age, sex, thyroid function, TgAb, TPOAb, echo pattern of hypoechoic lesions, USC, BethSys, the diameter of hypoechoic lesions, κ/λ deviation ratio, LT4 supplementation or TSH between the patients whose hypoechoic lesions decreased in size or disappeared and patients whose lesions were unchanged or increased in size.

There were no significant differences in patient age, sex, or the diameter of the hypoechoic lesions between Groups A and B (Mann-Whitney U-test) (Table 3). The USC and the κ/λ deviation ratio were significantly lower in Group B than Group A ($p < 0.001$ and $p < 0.02$, respectively). The USC of < 3.5 [9/12 (75.0%) in Group B; 10/41 patients (24.4%) in Group A] was significantly more frequent ($p < 0.01$), and the FNAC finding of 'benign' or 'AUS' [9/12 (75.0%) in Group B; 12/41 patients

Table 1 Ultrasonographic classification for thyroid nodule at Kuma Hospital

Class	Description
1	Round or anechoic lesion.
2	Regular-shaped nodule with cystic change. The echo level of solid lesion is similar to that of normal thyroid.
3	Solid and regular-shaped nodule. Internal echo is homogeneous, or may have strong echoes internally or at the capsule.
4	Solid and irregular-shaped nodule. Internal echo is usually low and may have fine strong echogenic spots.
5	Solid and irregular-shaped nodule with extrathyroid extension.

Intermediate classes from class 2 to class 5 (designated as classes 2.5,3.5 and 4.5) are also used

Table 2 Clinical features of 16 patients who underwent follow-up US examinations of hypoechoic lesions that were diagnosed as possible thyroid lymphoma

Case	Age	Sex	Thyroid function[a]	TgAb (IU/mL)	TPOAb (IU/mL)	Echo pattern of hypoechoic lesions	US class	BethSys[b]	Duration of follow-up (months)	Before (mm)	After (mm)	κ/λ deviation ratio[c]	LT4 supplementation (μg/day)	TSH during follow-up	Outcome
1	53	F	subclinical hypothyroid (with LT4 50 μg/day)	4000≦	535	diffuse	3	AUS[d]	27	61	47	1.21	75	normal	decrease
2	62	F	hypothyroid	4000≦	600≦	diffuse	3.5	benign[e]	30	120	80	1.50	112.5	suppressed	decrease
3	66	F	euthyroid	28	89	nodular	3.5	AUS	12	25	11	4.61	50	normal	decrease
4	69	F	euthyroid	120.7	600≦	nodular	3	AUS	10	37	disappearance	3.14	–	normal	disappearance
5	70	M	euthyroid	54	118	nodular	3	AUS	37	15	12	1.84	–	normal	decrease
6	71	M	subclinical hypothyroid	1171	–	nodular	3	malignancy	6	37	23	3.20	50	normal	decrease
7	72	F	euthyroid	906	–	nodular	2.5	Suspicious for malignancy	3	27	14	2.90	50	normal	decrease
8	74	F	euthyroid	512.9	151	nodular	3	AUS	41	12	disappearance	2.75	–	normal	disappearance
9	74	F	euthyroid	688.8	16	nodular	3	Suspicious for malignancy	1	105	25	1.72	–	normal	decrease
10	74	F	euthyroid	121.8	–	nodular	3	AUS	7	16	9	2.06	75	suppressed	decrease
11	77	F	subclinical hypothyroid	1402	–	diffuse	3	AUS	25	46	40	1.53	50	normal	decrease
12	83	F	euthyroid	89.9	–	nodular	3.5	AUS	6	23	19	3.21	–	normal	decrease
13	66	F	euthyroid	235.5	–	nodular	4	AUS	22	22	22	0.86	75	suppressed	no change
14	46	F	euthyroid	609.6	–	nodular	3	Suspicious for malignancy	7	22	30	–	–	normal	increase
15	87	M	euthyroid	750.4	≦16	nodular	3	Suspicious for malignancy	6	19	23	4.09	–	normal	increase
16	94	F	subclinical hypothyroid	586.3	26.5	diffuse	3	Suspicious for malignancy	11	65	160	1.81	62.5	normal	increase

The normal range of TgAb is ≤39.9 U/mL; TPOAb: ≤27.9 U/mL. –: TPOAb not done or no levothyroxine (LT4) supplementation

Intermediate US classes from class 2 to class 4 (designated as classes 2.5 and 3.5) are also used

[a]Thyroid function at the first examination and diagnosis as possible thyroid lymphoma by FNAC

[b]The Bethesda System for Reporting Thyroid Cytopathology

[c]The κ/λ deviation ratio was calculated by λ/κ ratio when the κ/λ ratio was < 1.00

[d]Atypia of undetermined significance or follicular lesion of undetermined significance

[e]Lymphoma cannot be denied

Table 3 Comparison of clinical features of Group A and B

	Group A (n = 41)	Group B (n = 12)	p-value
Age (year)	67 (48–91)	72 (53–83)	0.35
Sex (Male, number)	11	2	0.48
Diameter of hypoechoic lesions (mm)	35 (16–75)	38 (12–120)	0.51

Group A is the patients with thyroid lymphoma diagnosed histopathologically following thyroid surgery. Group B is the patients whose hypoechoic lesions decreased or disappeared. Data are median and (ranges). The p-values were calculated by Mann-Whitney U-test

(29.3%) in Group A] was significantly more frequent ($p < 0.05$) in Group B than Group A (Tables 4 and 5). Lastly, the κ/λ deviation ratio of the immunoglobulin (Ig) light chain in the FNAC specimens of < 3.40 [11/12 (91.7%) in Group B; 17/41 patients (41.5%) in Group A] was significantly more frequent in Group B than Group A ($p < 0.01$) (Table 6).

Discussion

The characteristics and natural course of hypoechoic lesions that were diagnosed as possible thyroid lymphoma based on the FNAC findings were investigated. Careful US examinations were repeatedly performed in 22 of 65 patients, and hypoechoic lesions decreased in diameter in 10 patients (10 of the 22; 45.5% or 10 of 65 patients; 15.4%), and disappeared in two patients (two of 22; 9.1% or two of 65 patients; 3.1%).

The USC and the κ/λ deviation ratio were significantly lower in Group B than Group A, and the FNAC finding of 'benign' or 'AUS' was significantly more frequent in Group B than Group A. Although thyroid lymphoma typically presents with a rapidly enlarging neck mass leading to compressive symptoms [4], some hypoechoic lesions diagnosed as possible thyroid lymphoma might regress in their natural courses in the present study.

Several studies have demonstrated that *Helicobacter pylori* infection is associated with low-grade gastric MALT lymphoma, and that the eradication of *Helicobacter pylori* can cause histological regression of the lymphoma [13, 14]. Uohashi et al. reported that a hypoechoic lesion in the right lobe disappeared spontaneously after being diagnosed pathologically as non-Hodgkin's lymphoma following a contralateral lobe resection, and suggested spontaneous regression of acute inflammation [15]. Okamoto et al. reported a patient whose primary thyroid lymphoma of cytotoxic T-cell origin regressed spontaneously [16]. Although its cause remains unknown, it may be attributable to an association of acute inflammation [17, 18], and immune mechanisms such as those involving T-helper cells or natural killer cells of the peripheral blood [19].

However, to our best knowledge, there has been no report that the natural course of hypoechoic lesions suspected of being possible thyroid lymphoma was studied extensively. With the combination of US, FNAC, and CD gating analysis for κ/λ deviation, candidate for the surgery could be accurately selected in 41 out of 43 patients (95%) as demonstrated in Group A. However, the management of not strongly suggestive of lymphoma may be controversial. In the present study, the hypoechoic lesion decreased in size in 10, and disappeared in two out of 22 patients, suggesting the careful observation for such lesions.

The limitation of the present study concerns the retrospective analysis that may eliminate the ability to obtain the strong conclusions. Selection of open surgery or careful observation depends on various factors including the results of FNAC and patients' previous courses. Therefore, the proper diagnostic rate of Group A was higher than in that of Group B, and the selection bias might cause the difference of the course of the two groups. The nature of the hypoechoic lesions that regressed during the follow-up examination is unclear in the present study, because open biopsies were not performed in these patients. Some could be actually low-grade thyroid lymphoma, but others could be focal or regional lymphocytic thyroiditis, atypical subacute thyroiditis, or other etiology-unknown lesion(s). Further prospective studies including histopathology and factor(s) involved in the regression or progression of the

Table 4 Comparisons of US classification between the Group A (n = 41) and Group B (n = 12)

US class	Group A	Group B
2.5	1	1
3	9	8
3.5	9	3
4	21	0

P < 0.01

Classes 2.5 and 3.5 designate intermediate classes between 2 &3 and 3 & 4, respectively

Table 5 Comparisons of the diagnostic categories of the Bethesda System for Reporting Thyroid Cytopathology between the Group A (n = 41) and Group B (n = 12)

Diagnostic categories	Group A	Group B
Benign	1	1
AUS	11	8
Suspicious for malignancy	22	2
Malignant	7	1

P < 0.02

US: ultrasound. AUS: atypia of undetermined significance or follicular lesion of undetermined significance

Benign: benign, but with the comment that lymphoma cannot be denied

Characteristics and natural course of hypoechoic thyroid lesions diagnosed as possible thyroid lymphomas...

199

Table 6 Comparisons of Groups A and B regarding the κ/λ deviation ratio of Ig light chain

κ/λ deviation ratio	Group A	Group B	Total
≥3.40	24	1	25
< 3.40	17	11	28
Total	41	12	53

The κ/λ deviation ratio of < 3.40 was significantly more frequent in Group B compared to Group A ($p < 0.01$, chi-square test (with Yate's continuity correction)). When the κ/λ deviation ratio was lower than 1.00, we converted it to the λ/κ ratio (deviation ratio)

lesions are needed to investigate the true nature of such lesions, and to clarify the best method of managing such patients.

Hypoechoic lesions suspected of having possible lymphoma decreased in size or disappeared in 12 out of 22 patients (55%), and such a regression should be emphasized in the present study. Because most of these lesions cannot be diagnosed definitely by core needle biopsy, open surgery might be considered. But unnecessary surgeries for benign lesions might be avoided.

Conclusion

Our study suggests that some hypoechoic thyroid lesions that are possible thyroid lymphoma based on US and FNAC might decrease in size or disappear during the careful observation. A careful observation before surgery is suggested for those lesions such as USC < 3.5, a κ/λ deviation ratio < 3.4, and the FNAC classification of 'benign' or 'atypia of determined significance or follicular lesions of undetermined significance'. However, an open biopsy or thyroid surgery should be considered in case of the increasing lesion in diameter on follow-up US examination.

Abbreviations
AUS: Atypia of undetermined significance or follicular lesion of undetermined significance; BethSys categories: Bethesda System for Reporting Thyroid Cytopathology; FNAC: Fine needle aspiration cytology; Ig: Immunoglobulin; MALT: Mucosa-associated lymphoid tissue; TgAb: Thyroglobulin antibody; TPOAb: Thyroid peroxidase antibody; US: Ultrasonography; USC: US classification

Authors' contributions
TN and MN were involved in study design, acquisition of data, analysis and interpretation of data and drafting and revising the manuscript. TN, MN, MH, TK, TK, EN, MI, SF, HN, MH and AM were involved in data collection and manuscript drafting. All authors read and approved the final manuscript.

Competing interests
The authors declare that they have no competing interests.

Author details
[1]Department of Internal Medicine, Kuma Hospital, Centre for Excellence in Thyroid Cares, 8-2-35 Shimoyamate-dori, Chuo-ku, Kobe 650-0011, Japan. [2]Department of Diagnostic Pathology and Cytology, Kuma Hospital, Centre for Excellence in Thyroid Cares, 8-2-35 Shimoyamate-dori, Chuo-ku, Kobe 650-0011, Japan. [3]Department of Surgery, Kuma Hospital, Centre for Excellence in Thyroid Care, 8-2-35 Shimoyamate-dori, Chuo-ku, Kobe 650-0011, Japan.

References
1. Klopper JP, Kane MA, Haugen BR. Anaplastic thyroid cancer and miscellaneous tumors of the thyroid. In: Braverman LE, Cooper DS, editors. Werner & Ingbar's The Thyroid. 10th ed; 2013. p. 765–74.
2. Freeman C, Berg JW, Occurrence CSJ. Prognosis of extranodal lymphomas. Cancer. 1972;29:252–60.
3. Thieblemont C, Mayer A, Dumontet C, Barbier Y, Callet-Bauchu E, et al. Primary thyroid lymphoma is a heterogeneous disease. J Clin Endocrinol Metab. 2002;87:105–11.
4. Matsuzuka F, Miyauchi A, Katayama S, Narabayashi I, Ikeda H, et al. Clinical aspects of primary thyroid lymphoma: diagnosis and treatment based on our experience of 119 cases. Thyroid. 1993;3:93–9.
5. Watanabe N, Noh JY, Narimatsu H, Takeuchi K, Yamaguchi T, et al. Clinicopathological features of 171 cases of primary thyroid lymphoma: a long-term study involving 24553 patients with Hashimoto's disease. Brit J Hematol. 2011;153:236–43.
6. Ota H, Ito Y, Matsuzuka F, Kuma S, Fukata S, et al. Usefulness of ultrasonography for diagnosis of malignant lymphoma of the thyroid. Thyroid. 2006;16:983–7.
7. Mizokami T, Hamada K, Maruta T, Higashi K, Yamashita H, et al. Development of primary thyroid lymphoma during an ultrasonographic follow-up of Hashimoto's thyroiditis: a report of 9 cases. Intern Med. 2016;55:943–8.
8. Sangalli G, Serio G, Zampatti C, Lomuscio G, Colombo L. Fine needle aspiration cytology of primary lymphoma of the thyroid: a report of 17 cases. Cytopathology. 2001;12:257–63.
9. Aleskow S, Wartofsky L. Primary thyroid lymphoma: a clinical review. J Clin Endocrnol Metab. 2013;98:3131–8.
10. Zeppa P, Cozzolino I, Peluso AL, Troncone G, Lucariello A, et al. Cytologic, flow cytometry, and molecular assessment of lymphoid infiltrate in fine-needle cytology samples of Hashimoto thyroiditis. Cancer Cytopathology. 2009;117:174–84.
11. Ito Y, Miyauchi A, Inoue H, Fukushima M, Kihara M, et al. An observational trial for papillary thyroid microcarcinoma in Japanese patients. World J Surg. 2010;34:28–35.
12. Ito Y, Amino N, Yokozawa T, Ota H, Ohshita M, et al. Ultrasonographic evaluation of thyroid nodules in 900 patients: comparison among ultrasonographic, cytological, and histological findings. Thyroid. 2007;17:1269–76.
13. Montalban C, Manzanal A, Boixeda D, Redondo C, Alvarez I. Helicobacter pylori eradication for the treatment of low-grade gastric MALT lymphoma: follow-up together with sequential molecular studies. Ann Oncol. 1997;2:37–9.
14. Grgov S, Katić V, Krstić M, Nagorni A, Radovanović-Dinić B. Treatment of low-grade gastric MALT lymphoma using Helicobactert pylori eradicateon. Vojnosanit Pregl. 2015;72:431–6.
15. Uohashi A, Imoto S, Matsui T, Murayama T, Okimura Y, et al. Spontaneous regression of diffuse large-cell lymphoma associated with Hashimoto's thyroiditis. Am J Hematol. 1996;53:201–11.
16. Okamoto A, Namura K, Uchiyama H, Kajita Y, Inaba T, et al. Cytotoxic T-cell non-Hodgkin's lymphoma of the thyroid gland. Am J Hematol. 2005;80:77–8.
17. Drobyski WR, Qazi R. Spontaneous regression in non-Hodgkin's lymphoma. Clinical and pathologic considerations. Am J Hematol. 1989;31:138–41.
18. Seachrist L. Spontaneous cancer remissions spark questions. J Natl Cancer Inst. 1993;85:1892–5.
19. Papac RJ. Spontaneous regression of cancer: possible mechanisms. In Vivo. 1998;12:571–8.

22

Study of Optimal Replacement of Thyroxine in the Elderly (SORTED) – results from the feasibility randomised controlled trial

Salman Razvi[1,2]* [ID], Lorna Ingoe[2], Vicky Ryan[3], Simon H. S. Pearce[1] and Scott Wilkes[4]

Abstract

Background: Hypothyroidism is a common condition, particularly in the older population. Thyroid hormone requirements change with age and serum TSH levels also alter, especially in older patients. However, in practice laboratory reference ranges for thyroid function are not age-specific and treatment in older patients aims to achieve a similar target thyroid function level as younger age groups.

Methods: A dual centre, single blind, randomised controlled trial was conducted to determine the feasibility of a future definitive RCT in hypothyroid individuals aged 80 years or older who were treated with levothyroxine. Potential participants were identified from 17 research-active GP practices ($n = 377$), by opportunistic invitations ($n = 9$) or in response to publicity ($n = 4$). Participants were randomly allocated to either usual (0.4–4.0 mU/L) or a higher (4.1–8.0 mU/L) target serum TSH range. Information on participants' willingness to enter the trial, acceptability of study design, length of time to complete recruitment and dose titration strategy was collected.

Results: Fifteen percent (57/390) of potentially eligible hypothyroid individuals consented to participate in this trial and 48 were randomised to trial medication for 24 weeks, giving a recruitment rate of 12 %. Recruitment averaged 5.5 participants per month over approximately 9 months. Eight participants withdrew (3/24 and 5/24 in the usual and higher TSH arms, respectively) with the commonest reason cited (5 patients) being tiredness. Interestingly, 3/5 participants withdrew from the site that required a visit to a Research Facility whereas only 5/43 participants withdrew from the site that offered home visits. In the higher TSH arm, of those participants who completed the study, approximately half of participants (10/19) reached target TSH.

Conclusions: It is feasible to perform a randomised controlled trial of thyroid hormones in hypothyroid patients aged 80 or older. A definitive trial would require collaboration with a large number of General Practices and the provision of home visits to achieve recruitment to time and target. Power calculations should take into account that approximately 12 % of those approached will be randomised and 1 in 6 participants are likely to withdraw from the study. Finally, several dose adjustments may be required to achieve target serum TSH levels in this age group.

Keywords: Hypothyroidism, Older age, Feasibility

* Correspondence: salman.razvi@newcastle.ac.uk
[1]Institute of Genetic Medicine and Queen Elizabeth Hospital, International Centre for Life, Newcastle University, Central Parkway, Newcastle upon Tyne NE1 3BZ, UK
[2]Department of Endocrinology, Queen Elizabeth Hospital, Gateshead NE9 6SX, UK
Full list of author information is available at the end of the article

Background

Thyroid hormones regulate metabolism and impact on several organs in the body. Hypothyroidism (underactive thyroid) is a common endocrine condition in which the thyroid gland produces insufficient thyroid hormones. Hypothyroidism is more prevalent in women and in older individuals with rates of up to 16 % reported in those aged over 80 years [1, 2]. Hypothyroidism is diagnosed based on results of blood tests with low thyroid hormone levels in the presence of high serum Thyroid Stimulating Hormone (TSH) concentrations (usually > 4.0 mU/L). Treatment with the synthetic form of thyroxine (Levothyroxine or LT4) is the treatment of choice in these patients and patients are generally managed in primary care. LT4 is prescribed to 3–4 % of the general population and its use is increasing [3–5]. Thyroid function changes with age and several reports suggest that the upper limit of the TSH reference range increases with age [6–10]. In addition, observational studies have shown that older individuals with a slightly raised serum TSH level have no adverse consequences [11–16]. In fact, one report suggests that a slightly raised TSH may be beneficial for survival in 85-year old individuals followed up for four years [17]. Despite this, all patients are treated uniformly with the aim of achieving a serum TSH target level (usually 0.4–4.0 mU/L) and age-specific ranges are not used. Moreover, evidence obtained from General Practice records suggests LT4 is increasingly being prescribed for older individuals and for minimally raised serum TSH levels [18]. This issue is of increasing importance as the populations in most developed – and many developing – countries are ageing and diagnoses of hypothyroidism are therefore likely to rise. Before a definitive randomised controlled trial (RCT) in the older hypothyroid population can be conducted it would be highly desirable to assess its feasibility. We, therefore, designed a feasibility RCT to investigate lower dose LT4 (aiming for a higher than usual serum TSH) versus usual dose LT4 (aiming for the currently utilised serum TSH range) in hypothyroid individuals aged 80 years or more. We report the feasibility of this trial in this paper.

Methods

The detailed protocol has been published previously [19]. Briefly, a dual-centre single-blind RCT of elderly (≥80 years) individuals with primary hypothyroidism and good biochemical control (as demonstrated by serum TSH levels within the reference range in the preceding 3 months) was organised. After providing written informed consent, participants were randomised in a 1:1 ratio to either usual dose LT4 (aiming to continue to keep serum TSH between 0.4 and 4.0 mU/L) or lower dose LT4 (reduced by 25 mcg daily initially and a further 25 mcg daily, if required at 12 weeks) to aim for a

slightly higher serum TSH level of 4.1–8.0 mU/L. After randomisation participants were assessed at 12 and 24 weeks, with a final follow-up phone call at 25 weeks. The inclusion criteria required participants of either gender, aged 80 years or older, living independently in the community, who had been prescribed LT4 (at least 50 mcg daily) for at least 6 months and whose serum TSH was between 0.4 and 4.0 mU/L in the preceding 3 months. Patients were excluded if they were deemed to not have capacity to provide written informed consent, had severe chronic medical conditions that would prevent participation, thyroid cancer, on medications affecting thyroid function, non-English speakers, had participated in another RCT in the previous 3 months or had lactose intolerance.

The primary objectives were to demonstrate that recruitment to such a trial is possible; to gauge participants' acceptability of being part of the study; to assess the length of time required to complete recruitment; to assess the dose titration strategy and the length of time required to achieve desired TSH levels; and to gauge medication compliance.

The design and analysis followed published recommendations for feasibility studies [20, 21]. As such, no formal sample size calculation was performed; a target sample size of 50 randomised participants was deemed sufficient to assess the feasibility of the trial. The data analyses were descriptive, and statistical comparisons between randomised treatment groups were not undertaken.

Results

Screening and recruitment

Participants were screened for their eligibility to participate in the trial via one of three possible routes: from participating GP practices, hospital endocrine clinics or self-referral responding to posters in hospitals and participating GP practices. (See Fig. 1)

Twenty research-active practices agreed to identify potential patients for the trial. These GP practices were identified by the then National Institute for Health Research, Primary Care Research Network. Of these, two practices did not have the capacity to identify patients for the study and a third responded late in the recruitment process. The remaining 17 GP practices facilitated the identification of potential participants and posted letters of invitation (Table 1). The prevalence of treated hypothyroid patients aged ≥ 80 years ranged from 0.5 to 1.4 % of the total number of patients registered in those practices (Table 1). A total of 377 invitation letters (with a reply slip and stamped addressed envelope) were sent by practice staff and 233/377 (62 %) responded, of which 66 (18 % of total invitations) agreed to participate. The protocol allowed the participating GP practices to send reminder letters to patients that had not replied but this

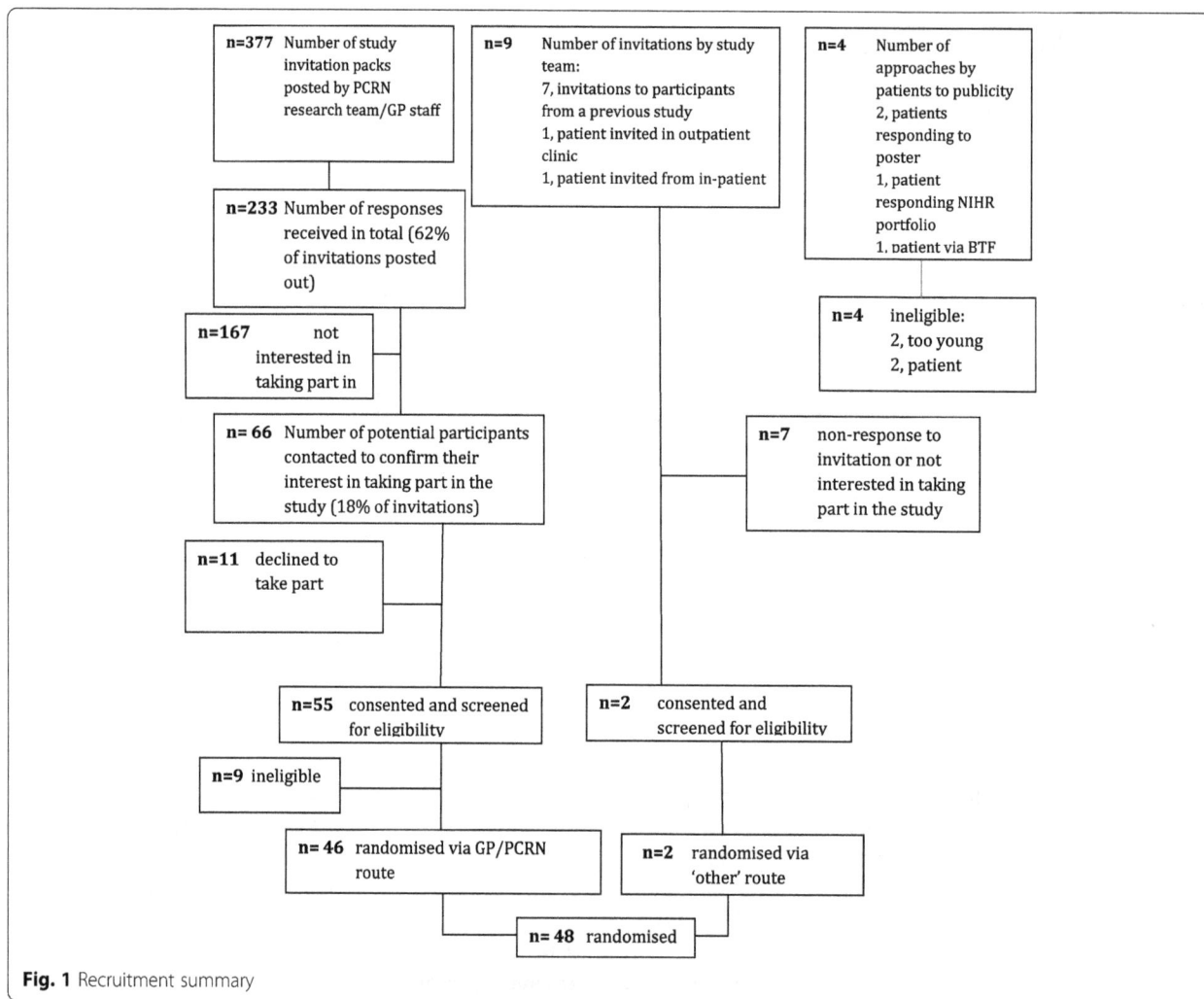

Fig. 1 Recruitment summary

was not followed. Subsequently, 11 individuals changed their mind and declined participation. The reasons given for changing their mind related to either not understanding the study requirements or due to change in circumstances (such as illness). A further 9 patients were deemed ineligible after study-specific screening as either their serum TSH was too low ($n = 6$) or too high ($n = 3$). Therefore, a total of 46 patients (12 % of the 377 potentially eligible participants) were randomised via this route.

Another 13 participants were invited by either the study team or self referred in response to publicity posters in hospitals, the NIHR portfolio or via the patient-led charity the British Thyroid Foundation newsletter. Of these, 2 (15 %) participants were screened and subsequently randomised.

Randomisation process
Participants were randomised in a ratio of 1:1, using random permuted blocks. Randomisation was stratified by usual (pre-study) LT4 dose (50, 75, 100 and 125 mcg daily) and administered by the Newcastle Clinical Trials Unit using a secure password-protected web-based system (Table 2).

Baseline characteristics
The median age of the participants was 83 years (range: 80 to 93 years) and majority (71 %) were women (Table 3).

Primary outcome measures
This feasibility trial had five primary outcome measures.

1. Participants' willingness to enter the trial (as gauged by the ratio of those who consented to participate to those who were potentially eligible and approached): 57 out of 390 (15 %) potentially eligible patients consented to participate but, as stated above, 9 individuals (16 % of the potentially eligible group) were not eligible due to abnormal thyroid function at screening.

Table 1 Number of participants approached and randomised by each GP practice

Practices [a]	Total registered patients (n) (A)	Potentially eligible hypothyroid patients aged ≥ 80 year (% of A)	Invites sent [c] (n) (B)	Replies received (% of B)	Consented to be screened (n) (% of B)	Randomised (n) (% of B)
A	16,340	112 (0.7 %)	112	63 (56 %)	20 (18 %)	13 (12 %)
B	5475	42 (0.8 %)	42	25 (60 %)	6 (14 %)	6 (14 %)
C	8830	75 (0.9 %)	14	14 (100 %)	7 (50 %)	5 (36 %)
D	9230	58 (0.6 %)	39	23 (59 %)	5 (13 %)	3 (8 %)
E	11,019	63 (0.6 %)	20	15 (75 %)	3 (15 %)	3 (15 %)
F	10,141	28 [b]	11	10 (91 %)	4 (36 %)	3 (30 %)
G	5960	82 (1.4 %)	20	14 (70 %)	4 (20 %)	3 (15 %)
H	6875	52 (0.8 %)	10	6 (50 %)	3 (30 %)	3 (30 %)
I	4478	57 (1.3 %)	4	4 (100 %)	2 (50 %)	2 (50 %)
J	7460	36 (0.5 %)	36	20 (50 %)	6 (17 %)	1 (3 %)
K	3728	7 [b]	7	4 (57 %)	1 (14 %)	1 (14 %)
L	11,788	31 [b]	20	14 (70 %)	1 (5 %)	1 (5 %)
M	6893	9 [b]	9	3 (33 %)	1 (11 %)	1 (11 %)
N	19,223	20 [b]	10	7 (70 %)	1 (10 %)	1 (10 %)
O	3274	3 [b]	3	1 (33 %)	1 (33 %)	0 (0 %)
P	3296	12 [b]	5	2 (40 %)	1 (20 %)	0 (0 %)
Q	5565	15 [b]	15	8 (53 %)	0 (0 %)	0 (0 %)
Total	139,575	703	377	233 (62 %)	66 (18 %)	46 (12 %)

[a]The names of the GP practices are not shown to protect identity
[b]For these practices the total number of potentially eligible patients was not provided
[c]Some practices were asked to only send invites to a random selection of patients to be able to obtain a wide spread of responses from GP practices as possible

2. Participants' acceptability of study design (as measured by the completion rate of participants in each randomised group): 21 out of 24 (87.5 %) and 19/24 (79.2 %) randomised participants completed the trial in the usual and higher TSH arms, respectively.

3. Participant recruitment rate (as measured by the number of patients randomised divided by the length of the recruitment period): Participants were recruited between 17th October 2012 and 10th July 2013 with the first participant randomised on 9th November 2012 and the last one on 10th July 2013. The projected recruitment was 5 or 6 participants/month. Over the 267 days that trial recruitment was open 48 participants were recruited (5.5 participants/month) (See Fig. 2).

4. Dose titration strategy and length of time required to achieve desired TSH levels (as calculated by number of participants in each group that reach target TSH range at both 12 and 24 weeks): For the 40 participants who remained in the study until their final study assessment, most participants in the usual dose arm stayed within their target TSH range of 0.4–4.0 mU/L whereas half of the higher target TSH arm achieved their target TSH range (Table 4).

5. Medication compliance (tablet count at each visit): At the end of visits 2 and 3, participants were asked to return any surplus study drug in the original packaging to the study team, who verified and documented compliance. Compliance was deemed to be generally good. In participants who completed the trial, $n = 40$, compliance was 100 and 95 % at

Table 2 Distribution of patients by randomisation strata (pre-study dose of Levothyroxine) and allocated treatment group

Pre-study dose of Levothyroxine	Treatment group		Total randomised
	Target TSH range 0.4–4.0 mU/L	Target TSH range 4.1–8.0 mU/L	
50 μg daily	5	5	10
75 μg daily	9	9	18
100 μg daily	8	7	15
125 or more μg daily	2	3	5
Total	24	24	48

Table 3 Baseline characteristics

	Total n =48
Sex	
Female (n,% of females)	34 (71 %)
Male (n, % of males)	14 (29 %)
Age (years) Median (range)	83.0 (80.0 – 93.0)
Blood pressure (mmHg) Median (IQR)	
Systolic	154.5 (141.0 – 168.5)
Diastolic	85.0 (77.0 – 92.5)
Physical examination Mean (sd)	
Height (cm)	158.8 (8.8)
Weight (kg)	68.5 (13.1)
BMI (kg/m^2)	27.1 (4.7)
Pulse (bpm)	67.9 (9.8)
Chronic conditions n (%)	
Type 2 diabetes mellitus	4 (8.3)
Hypertension	24 (50)
Ischaemic heart disease	13 (27.1)
Cerebrovascular disease	7 (14.6)
COPD	6 (12.5)
Blood results Median (IQR)	
TSH (mU/L)	1.43 (0.88 – 2.64)
FT4 (pmol/L)	18.8 (16.7 – 19.7)
FT3 (pmol/L)	3.8 (3.6 – 4.2)
Total Cholesterol (mmol/L)	4.9 (4.4 – 6.2)
HDLc (mmol/L)	1.6 (1.5 – 1.9)
Triglycerides (mmol/L)	1.3 (1.0 – 1.9)
Serum CTX (pg/mL)	0.27 (0.17 – 0.37)
TPO antibodies	
< 35 IU/ml (n, %)	28 (58 %)
≥ 35 IU/ml (n, %)	20 (42 %)

IQR interquartile range, *sd* standard deviation, *bpm* beats per minute, *COPD* chronic obstructive pulmonary disease, *TSH* thyroid stimulating hormone, *FT4* free thyroxine, *FT3* free triiodothyronine, *HDLc* high density lipoprotein cholesterol, *CTX* carboxy-terminal collagen crosslinks, *TPO* thyroid peroxidase

both visits in the usual TSH and higher target TSH arms, respectively (Table 4).

Adverse Events (AEs) and Serious Adverse Events (SAEs): There were 119 AEs reported by 37 patients; 16 patients in the usual TSH arm reporting 49 AEs (mean = 3.1 per patient, sd = 2.1) and 21 patients in the higher TSH arm reporting 70 AEs (mean = 3.3, sd = 2.2). Patients reported between 1 and 10 AEs over the course of the study. The frequency of AEs with regards to the various organ-systems appeared to be broadly similar. For example, the frequency of participants reporting new-onset or worsening tiredness/fatigue was 41.7 % vs 50 % in the usual and higher TSH arms, respectively. Muscle aches and pains (29.2 % vs 16.7 %), dizziness (20.8 % vs 25 %) and constipation (16.7 % vs 29.2 %) were comparable in the two groups.

There were three SAEs, two in the usual TSH arm and one in the higher TSH arm. (See Table 5 for details).

Site of follow-up: At baseline 71 % of patients (34/48) chose to have their first study visit at home and 29 % (14/48) chose to come into hospital out-patients. At visit 2, four patients switched from out-patient visits to home visits with one patient switching in the other direction (this patient had become a hospital inpatient). Of the 40 patients still in the study at visit 3, 80 % (32/40) had their visit at home and 20 % (8/40) had their visit as an out-patient.

Phone contacts: Over the course of the 24 week study period a total of 27 telephone contacts were made by 20 participants and discussed with the research staff. The majority (20/27) were made in the first 12 weeks; of which 15 were in the first 4 weeks. The queries were with regards to new or existing symptoms (20 contacts by 14 participants; n = 8 in usual TSH arm and n = 6 in higher TSH arm), query relating to study drug (4 phone calls by 3 participants, all in usual TSH arm), and one phone call each for taking study drug in addition to usual dose levothyroxine (usual TSH arm) and problems in swallowing study drug (usual TSH arm).

Withdrawals and reasons: Eight patients withdrew from the study; three from the usual TSH arm and five from the higher TSH arm (Table 6). Five patients withdrew before visit 2 (two usual TSH, three higher TSH), one patient withdrew at visit 2 (higher TSH arm), and two patients withdrew after visit 2 but before visit 3 (one usual TSH and 1 higher TSH arm, respectively). Three of the five participants withdrew (60 %) from the site that required a visit to a Research Facility whereas only 5/43 participants (12 %) withdrew from the site that offered home visits. In seven participants, the reasons cited for withdrawal were AEs (mainly tiredness or constipation in six and infected foot and wrist pain in a seventh). One participant was withdrawn from the study by the research team for safety reasons as she was found to be taking the study drug in addition to her usual levothyroxine medication.

Discussion

It is currently unclear what the best practice for managing hypothyroidism is in older people. There is good evidence that thyroid hormone requirements change with age and that the current practice of treating everyone in a uniform fashion may not be appropriate. This feasibility RCT has demonstrated that reducing the dose of the synthetic thyroid hormone levothyroxine is possible and that patients are willing to participate.

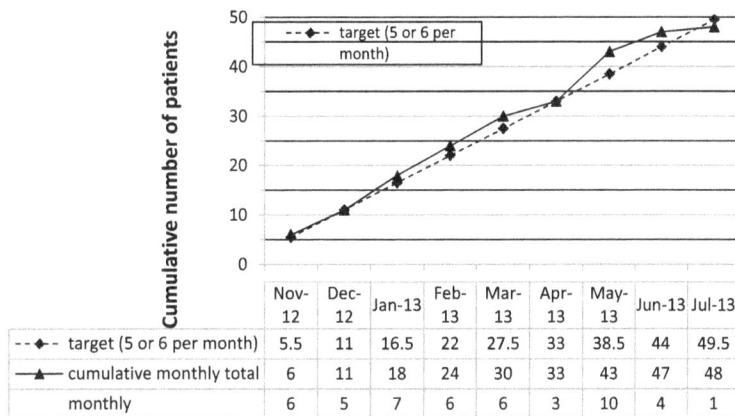

	Nov-12	Dec-12	Jan-13	Feb-13	Mar-13	Apr-13	May-13	Jun-13	Jul-13
target (5 or 6 per month)	5.5	11	16.5	22	27.5	33	38.5	44	49.5
cumulative monthly total	6	11	18	24	30	33	43	47	48
monthly	6	5	7	6	6	3	10	4	1

Fig. 2 Plot of cumulative number of patients randomised, target versus actual

The population of the western world - including the United Kingdom - is ageing. Ageing of the population refers to both the increase in the median age as well as the increase in the absolute number and proportion of older individuals. The number of people aged 75 and over has increased by 89 % over the period 1974 to 2014 and now makes up 8 % of the total population [22]. Between 2015 and 2020, when the general population is expected to increase by 3 %, it is estimated that people aged 65 years or more will rise by 12 % to 1.1 million; those over 85 years by 18 % to 300,000; and the number of centenarians by 40 % (7000) [22]. Similar demographic changes are occurring across much of the Western world. For instance, in the United States it is estimated that there are now about six million persons aged 85 years and older and this number may reach 19 million in 2050 [23]. Data from this feasibility study suggests that the prevalence of treated hypothyroidism in the over 80 age group is between 0.5 and 1.4 % of the entire population. It is also apparent that the majority of hypothyroid patients in this age group are on modest doses of LT4 – which is indicative that treatment was commenced for borderline raised TSH levels. This has significant implications for the management of hundreds of thousands of older hypothyroid individuals in the United Kingdom. Furthermore, as the number of older individuals increases then the absolute number of older people with treated hypothyroidism is also likely to grow.

The result of this feasibility trial has shown that it is possible to recruit participants into an interventional trial to aim for a higher than usual target serum TSH. The randomisation rate was approximately 5.5 participants per month from the 17 GP practices that identified patients and from the other sources of referral. Overall, 12 % of potentially eligible patients consented to participate and were randomised. This feasibility data suggests that a large-scale RCT would have to recruit from hundreds of GP practices. Furthermore, allowance would have to be made for 16 % (possibly even higher in a study of a longer duration) of participants to withdraw from the study. Any subsequent full RCT would have to be of longer duration (probably several years) and designed to be able to answer the important question of the optimum target serum TSH to aim for in older hypothyroid patients. Such a trial would require hard clinical end points including cardiovascular events and fractures as its main outcome measures.

One of the limitations of this trial is that we are unable to assess the characteristics of individuals who refused to participate. This is because study invitations were sent by individual GP practices and the responses were received in an anonymised form by the study team.

Table 4 Dose titration strategy and compliance with study medications

Dose titration strategy: Participants who remained in the study until their final study assessment (i.e. excluding withdrawals), n = 40	Usual TSH range (0.4–4.0 mU/L) n = 21	Higher TSH range (4. 1–8.0 mU/L) n = 19
Percent achieving target TSH range at week 12 (visit 2)	18/21 (85.7 %)	6/19 (31.6 %)
Percent achieving target TSH range at week 24 (visit 3)	18/21 (85.7 %)	10/19 (52.6 %)
Percent compliant at week 12 (visit 2)	21/21 (100 %)	18/19 (94.7 %)
Percent compliant at week 24 (visit 3)	21/21 (100 %)	18/19 (94.7 %)

Table 5 Chronological listing of serious adverse events

Treatment allocation	Randomisation date	Date of initial report	Description	Onset Date	Severity	SAE reason	Outcome
Usual TSH arm	01/03/2013	26/04/2013	Stroke	22/04/2013	mild	Involved patient hospitalisation	Recovered with sequelae
Usual TSH arm	20/03/2013	13/06/2013	Possible overdose on levothyroxine	12/06/2013	mild	Other significant medical event	Completely recovered
Higher TSH arm	21/01/2013	01/07/2013	Cardiac arrest due to acute myocardial infarction	25/06/2013	severe	Life threatening	Death (after study completion: 05/08/2013)

Therefore, it is not possible to assess differences between responders and non-responders.

Adverse events and serious adverse events did appear to be similar in both the usual TSH arm as well as the higher TSH arm in our study. However, this feasibility trial was not powered to detect a significant difference in any effect size. It is therefore possible that there may be a higher incidence of adverse events in a larger trial over a longer follow-up period. This would require support to be available for study participants. In this trial telephone support was made use of by a number of participants and may have contributed to their retention. The telephone contacts were made mostly in the first few weeks after randomisation and related to either symptoms or study drug. It is important to consider providing telephone support in a full large RCT particularly in the first 4 weeks after commencing study drug. In

addition, it is also evident that participants in this age group prefer to have home visits rather than to have to come to a hospital research facility. It is unclear how participants would view visits to their local GP practice.

It is important to consider strategies that would help retain participants in the trial and lead to high completion rates. Approximately 4 out of 5 randomised participants completed this trial. This was achieved by offering flexible study dates, times and venue, providing alternative appointments at short notice, being seen by the same member of staff at each visit and availability of telephonic support.

This feasibility trial revealed that of the patients randomised to a higher TSH range, who remained in the study until their final study assessment, only half reach their target. This is not surprising given that up to half the hypothyroid population, irrespective of age does not

Table 6 Chronological listing of withdrawals

Subject ID	Treatment allocation	Randomisation date	Withdrawal date	Days in the study	Reason (severity and relation to study drug)
709	Reduced dose	07/12/2012	09/01/2013	34	Withdrew due to AEs experienced whilst on the study: constipation, tiredness and generally unwell (mild, possibly related)
103	Usual dose	11/01/2013	23/01/2013	13	Withdrew due to "feeling unwell" (mild, possibly related)
104	Reduced dose	11/01/2013	27/03/2013	76	Withdrew due to infected right foot (moderate, not related), loose stools (moderate, unknown relationship to study drug) and sore wrist (mild, unknown relationship to study drug)
509	Reduced dose	26/11/2012	22/04/2013	148	6 weeks after Visit 2 withdrew from the study due to tiredness (moderate, possibly related)
205	Usual dose	01/03/2013	22/04/2013	53	Withdrew due to fatigue which started 2 weeks after commencing the study drug. The patient was hospitalised with a mild stroke on 22/04/13, reported to be linked to ongoing hypertension (severe, not related).
515	Reduced dose	18/02/2013	08/05/2013	80	Withdrew after experiencing several AEs: dry skin, dry hair, feeling cold, weight gain and tiredness (mild, possibly related), and swollen face with itching (mild, not related) - unscheduled home visit: thyroid function normal, weight gain of 0.3kgs.
521	Reduced dose	15/05/2013	12/06/2013	29	Withdrew after experiencing several AEs: nausea and loss of appetite (mild, not related), vertigo (mild, not related) and confusion (mild, not related)
614	Usual dose	20/03/2013	27/06/2013	100	At Visit 2 patient reported that she had been taking her prescribed dose of LT4 as well as the study medication. Patient reported no AEs. Serum thyroid function was normal (TSH 0.60, FT4 20.8). Subsequently the patient changed her mind and withdrew.

AEs adverse events, *LT4* levothyroxine

have good biochemical control as evidenced by their serum TSH level [24, 25]. The implications of this are that more frequent or smaller dose adjustments of levothyroxine may be required in the full trial to be able to achieve a higher proportion of participants in the desired relaxed TSH range.

Conclusion

In conclusion, this feasibility trial has shown that it is possible to recruit and retain patients with levothyroxine treated hypothyroidism aged 80 years or older into a RCT. Several important lessons have been learnt that would help to design a trial that should be able to successfully recruit and retain patients into a longer-term study.

Abbreviations

AEs: Adverse events; BMI: Body mass index; COPD: Chronic obstructive pulmonary disease; CTX: Carboxy-terminal collagen crosslinks; FT3: Free triiodothyronine; FT4: Free thyroxine; GP: General practitioner; IQR: Interquartile range; LT4: Levothyroxine; PCRN: Primary Care Research Network; RCT: Randomised control trial; SAEs: Serious adverse events; sd: Standard deviation; TPO: Thyroid peroxidase; TSH: Thyroid stimulating hormone

Acknowledgments

Primary Care Clinical Research Network Staff, especially Norah Phipps; TSC members: Dr Catherine Watson (trial manager), Mrs Janis Hickey (BTF member) as well as SR, SW, SP, VR and LI); independent DMEC members: Dr Ramzi Ajian (chair), Dr Petros Perros (expert), Dr Barbara Gregson (statistician). This report is independent research arising from a NIHR RfPB award PB-PG-0610 22139 supported by the National Institute for Health Research. The views expressed in this publication are those of the author(s) and not necessarily those of the NHS, the NIHR or the Department of Health.

Funding

This project is funded by the NIHR RfPB (http://www.nihr.ac.uk/funding/fundingdetails.htm?postid=1572, reference PB-PG-0610 22139).

Authors' contributions

The study was designed by SR, SP, VR and SW. LI performed study visits. SR wrote the first draft, and all authors reviewed, commented and approved the final version of the manuscript.

Authors' information

Dr Salman Razvi is Senior Lecturer and Consultant Endocrinologist, Newcastle University, UK.
Ms Lorna Ingoe is a research nurse, Gateshead Health NHS Foundation Trust.
Ms Vicky Ryan is a senior statistician, Institute of Health and Society, Newcastle University, UK.
Prof Simon Pearce is a Professor of Endocrinology, Newcastle University, UK.
Prof Scott Wilkes is a Professor of Primary Care, Sunderland University, UK.

Competing interests

The authors declare that they have no competing interests.

Author details

[1]Institute of Genetic Medicine and Queen Elizabeth Hospital, International Centre for Life, Newcastle University, Central Parkway, Newcastle upon Tyne NE1 3BZ, UK. [2]Department of Endocrinology, Queen Elizabeth Hospital, Gateshead NE9 6SX, UK. [3]Institute of Health & Society, Newcastle University, Baddiley Clark Building, Richardson Road, Newcastle upon Tyne NE2 4AX, UK. [4]Department of Pharmacy, Health and Wellbeing, Faculty of Applied Sciences, University of Sunderland, Sunderland SR1 3SD, UK.

References

1. Canaris GJ, Manowitz NR, Mayor G, Ridgway EC. The Colorado thyroid disease prevalence study. Arch Intern Med. 2000;160(4):526–34.
2. Hollowell JG, Staehling NW, Flanders WD, Hannon WH, Gunter EW, Spencer CA. Serum TSH, T(4), and thyroid antibodies in the United States population (1988 to 1994): National Health and Nutrition Examination Survey (NHANES III). J Clin Endocrinol Metab. 2002;87(2):489.
3. Leese GP, Flynn RV, Jung RT, Macdonald TM, Murphy MJ, Morris AD. Increasing prevalence and incidence of thyroid disease in Tayside, Scotland: the Thyroid Epidemiology Audit and Research Study (TEARS). Clin Endocrinol (Oxf). 2008;68(2):311–6.
4. Flynn RW, MacDonald TM, Morris AD, Jung RT, Leese GP. The thyroid epidemiology, audit, and research study: thyroid dysfunction in the general population. J Clin Endocrinol Metab. 2004;89(8):3879–84.
5. Mitchell AL, Hickey B, Hickey JL, Pearce SH. Trends in thyroid hormone prescribing and consumption in the UK. BMC Public Health. 2009;9:132.
6. Surks MI, Hollowell JG. Age-specific distribution of serum thyrotropin and antithyroid antibodies in the US population: implications for the prevalence of subclinical hypothyroidism. J Clin Endocrinol Metab. 2007;92(12):4575–82.
7. Vadiveloo T, Donnan PT, Murphy MJ, Leese GP. Age- and gender-specific TSH reference intervals in people with no obvious thyroid disease in Tayside, Scotland: the Thyroid Epidemiology, Audit, and Research Study (TEARS). J Clin Endocrinol Metab. 2013;98(3):1147–53.
8. Ehrenkranz J, Bach PR, Snow GL, Schneider A, Lee JL, Ilstrup S, Bennett ST, Benvenga S. Circadian and circannual rhythms in thyroid hormones: determining the TSH and free T4 reference intervals based upon time of day, age, and sex. Thyroid. 2015;25(8):954–61.
9. Bremner AP, Feddema P, Leedman PJ, Brown SJ, Beilby JP, Lim EM, Wilson SG, O'Leary PC, Walsh JP. Age-related changes in thyroid function: a longitudinal study of a community-based cohort. J Clin Endocrinol Metab. 2012;97(5):1554–62.
10. Atzmon G, Barzilai N, Hollowell JG, Surks MI, Gabriely I. Extreme longevity is associated with increased serum thyrotropin. J Clin Endocrinol Metab. 2009;94(4):1251–4.
11. Virgini VS, Wijsman LW, Rodondi N, Bauer DC, Kearney PM, Gussekloo J, den Elzen WP, Jukema JW, Westendorp RG, Ford I, Stott DJ, Mooijaart SP, PROSPER Study Group. Subclinical thyroid dysfunction and functional capacity among elderly. Thyroid. 2014;24(2):208–14.
12. Simonsick EM, Newman AB, Ferrucci L, Satterfield S, Harris TB, Rodondi N, Bauer DC, Health ABC Study. Subclinical hypothyroidism and functional mobility in older adults. Arch Intern Med. 2009;169(21):2011–7.
13. Blum MR, Wijsman LW, Virgini VS, Bauer DC, den Elzen WP, Jukema JW, Buckley BM, de Craen AJ, Kearney PM, Stott DJ, Gussekloo J, Westendorp RG, Mooijaart SP, Rodondi N, PROSPER study group. Subclinical thyroid dysfunction and depressive symptoms among the elderly: a prospective cohort study. Neuroendocrinology. 2016;103(3-4):291–9.
14. Hyland KA, Arnold AM, Lee JS, Cappola AR. Persistent subclinical hypothyroidism and cardiovascular risk in the elderly: the cardiovascular health study. J Clin Endocrinol Metab. 2013;98(2):533–40.
15. Waring AC, Arnold AM, Newman AB, Bůžková P, Hirsch C, Cappola AR. Longitudinal changes in thyroid function in the oldest old and survival: the cardiovascular health study all-stars study. J Clin Endocrinol Metab. 2012;97(11):3944–50.
16. Pearce SH, Razvi S, Yadegarfar ME, Martin-Ruiz C, Kingston A, Collerton J, Visser TJ, Kirkwood TB, Jagger C. Serum thyroid function, mortality and disability in advanced old age: The Newcastle 85+ study. J Clin Endocrinol Metab. 2016;23:jc20161935.
17. Gussekloo J, van Exel E, de Craen AJ, Meinders AE, Frolich M, Westendorp RG. Thyroid status, disability and cognitive function, and survival in old age. JAMA. 2004;292(21):2591–9.

18. Taylor PN, Iqbal A, Minassian C, Sayers A, Draman MS, Greenwood R, Hamilton W, Okosieme O, Panicker V, Thomas SL, Dayan C. Falling threshold for treatment of borderline elevated thyrotropin levels – balancing benefits and risks. Evidence from a large community-based study. JAMA Intern Med. 2014;174(1):32–9.

19. Wilkes S, Pearce S, Ryan V, Rapley T, Ingoe L, Razvi S. Study of Optimal Replacement of Thyroxine in the ElDerly (SORTED): protocol for a mixed methods feasibility study to assess the clinical utility of lower dose thyroxine in elderly hypothyroid patients: study protocol for a randomized controlled trial. Trials. 2013;14:83.

20. Lancaster GA, Dodd S, Williamson PR, et al. Design and analysis of pilot studies: recommendations for good practice. J Eval Clin Pract. 2004;10:307–12.

21. Thabane L, Ma J, Chu R, et al. A tutorial on pilot studies: the what, why and how. BMC Med Res Methodol. 2010;10:1.

22. UK National Statistics. http://www.ons.gov.uk/ons/rel/pop-estimate/population-estimates-for-uk–england-and-wales–scotland-and-northern-ireland/mid-2014/sty-ageing-of-the-uk-population.html. Accessed 17 June 2016.

23. 2014 National Population Projections. 2014; https://www.census.gov/population/projections/data/national/2014/summarytables.html. Accessed 17 June 2016.

24. Parle JV, Franklyn JA, Cross KW, Jones SR, Sheppard MC. Thyroxine prescription in the community: serum thyroid stimulating hormone level assays as an indicator of undertreatment or overtreatment. Br J Gen Pract. 1993;43(368):107–9.

25. Flynn RW, Bonellie SR, Jung RT, MacDonald TM, Morris AD, Leese GP. Serum thyroid-stimulating hormone concentration and morbidity from cardiovascular disease and fractures in patients on long-term thyroxine therapy. J Clin Endocrinol Metab. 2010;95(1):186–93.

23

The largest reported papillary thyroid carcinoma arising in struma ovarii and metastasis to opposite ovary

Mohamed S. Al Hassan[1], Tamer Saafan[1*] ⓘ, Walid El Ansari[2,3], Afaf A. Al Ansari[4], Mahmoud A. Zirie[5], Hanan Farghaly[6] and Abdelrahman Abdelaal[1]

Abstract

Background: Malignant struma ovarii (MSO) is a very rare, germ cell tumor of the ovary, histologically identical to differentiated thyroid cancers. Struma ovarii (SO) is difficult to diagnose on clinical basis or imaging and is mostly discovered incidentally, with few published cases in the literature.

Case presentation: A 42-year old primiparous woman presented with abdominal pain and midline pelvic palpable firm mass arising from the pelvis. Imaging showed pelvic solid cystic mass. Total abdominal hysterectomy, bilateral salpingo-oopherectomy (TAH BSO) and infracolic omentectomy were performed. Histopathology revealed left ovary papillary thyroid carcinoma (PTC) arising in SO (11 cm) and metastatic papillary thyroid carcinoma in the right ovary. Thyroid functions tests were all normal, ultrasound thyroid showed two complex nodules in the left thyroid lobe. Total thyroidectomy was decided, but the patient refused further surgical management and was lost to follow up as she left the country. We undertook a comprehensive literature search, and MSO and thyroid management data from 23 additional publications were analyzed and tabulated. This PTC MSO is probably the largest reported in the literature.

Conclusions: Among the different surgeries for MSO, TAH + BSO appears to have the best clinical outcome. However, unilateral salpingo-oopherectomy/ unilateral oophorectomy and bilateral salpingo-oopherectomy also seem effective. Ovarian cystectomy alone seems associated with higher recurrence. There remains no consensus on the associations between MSO tumor size and potential extent of metastasis, and about the management of thyroid gland. However, surveillance and thyroid gland work up to detect concurrent thyroid cancer are recommended.

Keywords: Total abdominal hysterectomy, Oopherectomy, Salipingo-oopherectomy, Thyroid cancer, Malignant struma ovarii, Papillary thyroid carcinoma, Follicular thyroid carcinoma

* Correspondence: tsaafan@gmail.com
[1]Department of General Surgery, Hamad General Hospital, Doha, Qatar
Full list of author information is available at the end of the article

Background

Struma ovarii (SO) is a specialized or monodermal teratoma predominantly composed of mature thyroid tissue (thyroid tissue must comprise > 50% of overall tissue) [1]. SO accounts for ≈5% of all ovarian teratomas [2–4]. Histologically, SO can be benign or malignant [5], although malignant struma ovarii (MSO) is rare (< 5% of cases), and metastasis is rare (0.3–0.5%) [6, 7]. SO is difficult to diagnose on basis of clinical manifestations or imaging, and most cases are incidental findings in patients aged 40–60 years, with a mean age of diagnosis of 43 years [4, 5, 8].

Common presenting symptoms include abdominal pain (20.6%), palpable lower abdominal mass (23.5%), vaginal bleeding (8.8%), or asymptomatic (41.2%, tumor discovered by routine ultrasound). Tachycardia and ascites are sometimes present (12%, 16% of patients respectively). Clinical and biochemical features of hyperthyroidism are uncommon in women with SO (< 5–8% of cases) [3, 5, 6], and whilst some reports observed no SO patients with overt hyperthyroidism symptoms (hence no thyroid function tests undertaken), others found 5–8% incidence of hyperthyroidism with SO [4, 9, 10]. SO women with hyperthyroidism can also have goiter and/or Grave's disease, but the incidence is very rare [11, 12]. Seldom, seeding of the peritoneum by a benign tumor can occur (strumosis), which may present with ascites with or without pleural effusion [13, 14].

As for imaging, ultrasound appearance of SO may be as heterogeneous uni/multilocular solid mass or multilocular cystic masses [15–17]. An ultrasound feature of SO is the presence of one or more well circumscribed roundish areas of solid tissue with smooth surface 'struma pearls', often vascularized at Doppler examination, but otherwise similar (but not identical) to the 'white ball' comprising hair and sebum usually seen at ultrasound of dermoid cysts [17].

In women presenting with a pelvic mass, SO is typically diagnosed postoperatively based upon histologic findings of thyroid follicles in the resected ovary, where the histological pattern may show micro/macrofollicular or oxyphil adenoma, with/without papillary hyperplasia [12, 18]. As in thyroid gland follicular tumors, the thyroid epithelium in the teratoma may be organized in a solid, embryonal or pseudotubular pattern, rather than thyroid follicles [19].

We present an extraordinary case of a primiparous woman with large SO containing papillary thyroid carcinoma, with metastasis to the contralateral ovary. To the best of our knowledge, this narrate is the first published case report of possibly the largest papillary thyroid carcinoma in SO with metastasis to the opposite ovary. Ethics approval and consent to publish were provided (Medical Research Centre review board, IRB, #16024/16, Hamad Medical Corporation, Doha, Qatar).

Case presentation

A 42-year-old Indonesian female, presented at Hamad General Hospital in Doha, Qatar complaining of an on and off lower abdominal pain mainly in the right iliac fossa. She had a normal delivery 15 years ago, had regular menstrual cycles, and no previous medical illnesses.

General examination

She was vitally stable, with no significant lymphadenopathy or pedal edema. Abdominal examination revealed midline palpable firm mass with mild tenderness. The mass arose from the pelvis, extending 2 cm below the umbilicus. There was no ascites. Complete blood picture, renal and liver function tests were normal except for hemoglobin of 11.7 g/dl, and CA 125 was elevated (251 KU/L).

Investigations

Abdominal ultrasound showed a large solid cystic mass in the right adnexa region, reaching the midline (≈6 × 13 cm) with mild vascularity in the solid component. Both ovaries were not separately visualized. There was mild left hydrosalpinx and mild ascites. Transvaginal ultrasound did not show the left ovary, but the right ovary was visualized separately (2.5 × 2.1 cm) and confirmed the presence of complex solid cystic mass in the middle of the pelvis. The mass (13.5 × 9.8 cm) extended to the left adnexa, with cystic area (9.2 × 5.9 cm) and a solid component (9.1 × 7 cm) that had increased vascularity. Further chest/abdomen/pelvis CT and MRI (Fig. 1) confirmed the size and solid/ cystic nature of the mass and showed no metastatic lesions, and also deviation of uterus to the left side.

Management

The patient's clinical picture was discussed at our gynecologic multidisciplinary meeting and total abdominal hysterectomy (TAH), bilateral salpingo-oopherectomy (BSO) and lymphadenectomy were decided. Patient underwent TAH + BSO plus infracolic omentectomy. During surgery, a freely mobile left ovarian mass was found with irregular surface and intact capsule. Right adnexa and uterus were normal. Patient had a smooth post-operative recovery and was discharged. Microscopic examination revealed an 11.0 cm left ovarian papillary thyroid carcinoma arising in SO (Figs. 2 and 3), with metastatic papillary thyroid carcinoma to the right ovary. No malignancy was found in right fallopian tube, uterus or cervix and there were negative lymph nodes. Following the histopathology results, patient had thyroid

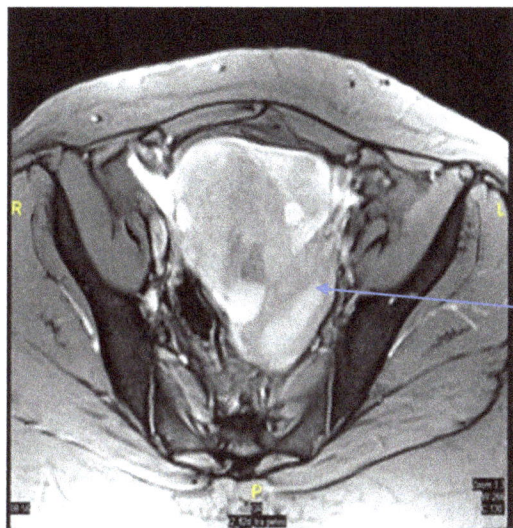

Fig. 1 Transverse T2 MRI section. The section shows well-defined complex lesion (arrow) with solid and cystic contents in the pelvis, extending on either side of the midline reaching to both sides of adnexa and measuring 13 × 9.4 × 8.1 cm. Ovaries are not seen separately from the lesion. Uterus shows mild deviation to the left side due to pressure effect from the mass. No obvious lymph nodes or signs of metastasis

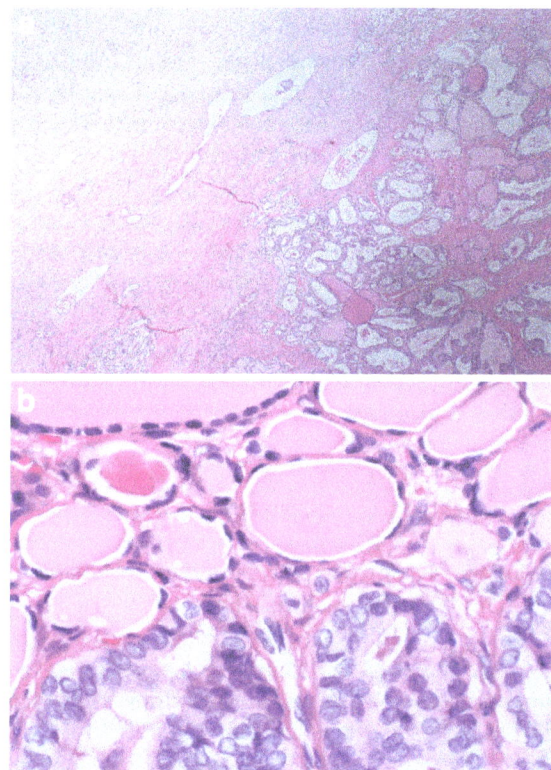

Fig. 2 Low and High power hematoxylin and eosin-stained section. **a** Low power hematoxylin and eosin-stained section (4×) demonstrates thyroid follicles of papillary carcinoma arising in benign thyroid follicles of SO. **b** High power hematoxylin and eosin-stained section (60×) demonstrates papillary thyroid carcinoma with follicular pattern. Nuclear features including nuclear groves, clearing, overlapping and enlargement, consistent with papillary thyroid carcinoma arising in a SO

function tests (TSH, free T4, thyroglobulin) that were all normal. Thyroid ultrasound revealed 7 × 11 mm complex nodule, a 6 × 6 mm complex nodule and a 3 × 4 mm cyst in the left thyroid lobe. No lesions were observed in the right thyroid lobe. The patient's clinical findings were discussed at our thyroid multidisciplinary meeting where total thyroidectomy and radioactive iodine therapy were decided; however the patient refused further surgical management, and was lost to follow up as she left the country.

Pathologic findings

Upon histopathologic examination, a papillary thyroid carcinoma was identified arising in SO tumor (11.0 cm in greatest dimension) of the left ovary (Figs. 1, 2a and b), and a small metastatic focus measuring 0.1 cm in the right ovary. There was no malignancy in right fallopian tube, uterus or cervix and negative lymph nodes. Thyroglobulin immunohistochemical stained section highlighted the thyroid tissue in a background of ovarian tissue with SO, and confirmed the origin from thyroid tissue (Fig. 3). AJCC Pathologic tumor staging was p T1b and FIGO stage was IB.

Discussion

SO is an uncommon ovarian tumor with < 5% malignancy, 5–23% metastasis, and 7.5–35% recurrence rates [3, 6, 15, 20]. Our comprehensive literature review of MSO, details

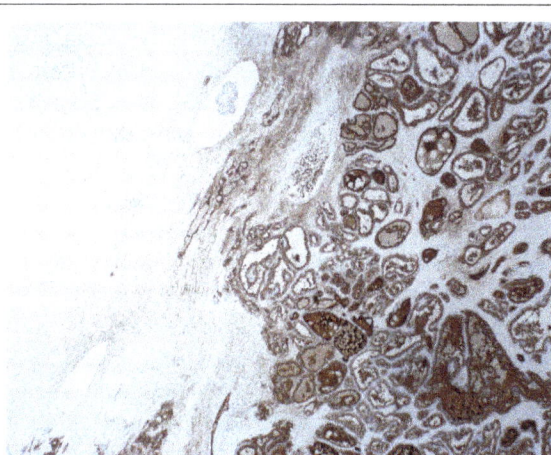

Fig. 3 Thyroglobulin immunohistochemical stain. Low power thyroglobulin immunohistochemical stained section (4×) highlights the thyroid tissue in a background of ovarian tissue with SO

a wide range of parameters in relation to MSO that include: size, histopathological categories, type of gynecological surgery, thyroid gland workup and management, and MSO follow up and recurrence (Table 1).

Regarding the tumor size of MSO, a range of dimensions (0.1–4.2 cm) has been reported (Table 1), and an analysis of large series of 68 MSO patients observed a mean tumor size of 5.28 cm [8]. To the best of our knowledge, our MSO is the possibly the largest (11 cm) reported MSO with PTC tumour confirmed by histopathology to date. Others found a MSO measuring 20 cm, but did not report the tumor histopathology; hence we are unable to judge their tumor subtype [8]. Our MSO is also first to be reported from the Middle East and North Africa region. Such a large sized tumor is likely to cause pressure effects (as observed in our patient who had deviation of uterus to the left side) (Fig. 1).

As for the relationship between tumour size and metastasis, research [21] reported that a larger sized tumor was associated with higher probability of metastasis. We are in agreement, as our tumour (11 cm) showed PTC metastasis to the contralateral ovary. Nonetheless, it remains to be established whether the relationship between primary tumour size and metastasis is consistent for all MSO. For instance, others [22] reported two patients with metastasis despite their small primary tumors (first was 8 mm MSO tumour with contralateral ovarian metastasis; second comprised multiple small tumour foci in left ovary with metastasis to the liver).

In terms of management of the primary (ovarian) tumour, no standard guidelines exist for treatment of papillary thyroid carcinoma arising in MSO due to its scarcity. TAH + BSO and omentectomy are considered optimal, however due to the permanent infertility associated with this procedure, unilateral salpingo-oopherectomy/unilateral oophorectomy in order to preserve the patients' fertility is suggested, as more aggressive approaches did not decrease the tumour's recurrence rate [8, 20, 23]. Our patient received TAH + BSO, in agreement with the published literature [18, 24].

As for recurrence, our primary tumour was in the left ovary with PTC metastasis to the right ovary, but we are unable to report on recurrence as our patient left Qatar (lost to follow up). Treatments for the primary ovarian tumor include: TAH + BSO (considered ideal), with no recurrence over 6 months - 4 years follow up [22, 24]; hysterectomy and unilateral oophorectomy/ unilateral salpingo-oopherectomy with no recurrence over 1– 7 years [22, 25–27]; bilateral salpingo-oophrerectomy with no recurrence over 2–5 years [28, 29]; and unilateral oophorectomy/ unilateral salpingo-oophorectomy with no recurrence over 1–25 years [22, 30–35]. Our

patient received TAH + BSO that has good reported outcomes [22, 24, 29].

Whilst the role of ovarian cystectomy alone in managing MSO is unclear due to lack of data, ovarian cystectomy alone may be suboptimal as the patient may subsequently present with recurrences/ metastasis. For instance, a patient received ovarian cystectomy for SO with PTCF, but follow up and recurrence were not known [36]; another patient had right salpigo-oopherectomy for SO with mature cystic teratoma and enucleation of left ovarian cyst for PTCF, where multiple metastasis were subsequently found [37]; and two patients who had ovarian cystectomy as initial operations, both subsequently presented with metastasis [22]. Nevertheless, for patients with unilateral adnexal mass (unilateral MSO), both unilateral salpingo-oophrecetomy /unilateral oophorectomy and TAH seem effective. However, careful pre/operative assessment of the contralateral side and consistent post-operative follow up are recommended, as it may also harbor (benign or malignant) SO. Others found contralateral benign SO associated with unilateral SO tumor (not described whether malignant or benign) (4 cases) [18]; contralateral MSO PTCF associated with unilateral benign SO [37]; while both the current study and other reports [22] observed contralateral malignant metastatic deposits from the unilateral primary MSO tumour.

As for management of the thyroid gland itself, debate remains about the role of thyroidectomy and radioactive iodine ablation (T + RIA) for MSO. Most authors support aggressive treatment by surgical removal of the tumour followed by radiotherapy, chemotherapy and radioactive iodine therapy regardless of metastasis at time of diagnosis [4, 6, 38–41] (see also Table 1), and our MDT decision in managing our patient was in agreement with such an approach. Conversely, others hold that surgical removal of the ovarian tumour only is sufficient, and thyroidectomy and radioactive iodine to be undertaken in case of metastases or recurrent disease [42]. Certain SO characteristics may necessitate thyroidectomy and radioactive iodine therapy (e.g. tumor size ≥1 cm, disease outside ovary, or histopathological features of aggressive tumor) [3, 43]. Moreover, MSO may actually increase the risk of additional thyroid cancer [23], where, among 68 MSO, 9% had primary thyroid cancer in the neck, and 67% had invasive thyroid cancer disease [8]. Early genomic instability and gene mutations may provide a common pathogenesis for all papillary thyroid cancers irrespective of their body locations [21, 40].

Conclusion

This report is a comprehensive literature review of MSO, detailing the sizes and histopathological

Table 1 Case studies of malignant Struma Ovarii

Study*	Country	Tumor Type	Size (mm)	Type of Gynecological Surgery	Thyroid Workup	Thyroid Nodule	Thyroid Management	Follow up	Recurrence
Middelbeek 2017 [29]	USA	PTCF	12	LBSO	a	a	HT then TT	a	a
Pineyro 2017 [30]	Uruguay	PTCF	4	Right ovarian cystectomy, left adnexectomy	TFT Normal U/S	4x2x4 mm FNA NC	Conservative	Lost follow up	Lost follow up
Fernández 2016 [35]	Spain	PTC	25	UO	U/S HN	1.5 cm FNA BFN	TT, HP PTC, RAI, LT	6 y	Nil
Wei 2015 [44]	USA	PTCF (8 cases)	1–42	—	—	—	TC	1 m-11 y	—
		PTC (2 cases)	4–30	—	—	—		8-15 y	—
		HDFCO	—	—	—	—		17 y	Nil
		PTCT and OM (2 cases)	—	—	—	—		NC	—
Monti 2015 [45], Goffredo 2015 [8]	Italy USA	PTC 68 (HP NC)	— mean 52.8 (1–200)	UO UO, BO,oophorectomy and omentectomy, debulking surgery	U/S, TFT, TgAb NC	Nil NR	Prophylactic TC, RAI TT	NC 2 m- 34 y (mean 8 y)	— —
Kumar 2014 [27]	India	PTCF	—	UO,TAH, omentectomy, appendectomy	TFT, U/S	Nil	TT, HP lymphocytic thyroiditis	1 y	Nil
Mardi 2013 [46]	India	PTCT	—	Cystectomy	—	—	—	6 m	Nil
Leite 2013 [31]	Portugal	PTC	—	USO	—	—	Complete thyroidectomy, HP PTCF	2 y	Nil
Meringolo 2012 [47]	Italy	PTC	3	Monolateral annessectomy	TFT, TgAb, TPO ab	Yes, FNA benign	LT	—	—
Barrera 2012 [24]	Philippines	PTC	—	TAH BSO	TFT, U/S, HNs	No FNA done	RIA, LT	6 m	Nil
Stanojevic 2012 [32]	Japan	PTCF	10	USO, contralateral cystectomy(HP benign)	TFT, Tg, TgAb U/S	6×4 mm	Patient planned for FNA and TT	—	—
O'Neill 2012 [33]	Ireland	PTC	—	USO	NC	—	TT, HP normal, RAI	—	—
Jean 2012 [28]	USA	PTC	25	BSO, peritoneal biopsy, lymph node sampling	TFT, U/S	2.7 cm nodule	TT (HP benign), RAI	2y	Nil

Table 1 Case studies of malignant Struma Ovarii (Continued)

Study*	Country	Tumor Type	Size (mm)	Type of Gynecological Surgery	Thyroid Workup	Thyroid Nodule	Thyroid Management	Follow up	Recurrence
Tanaka 2011 [26]	Japan	PTCF	30	Total hysterectomy + USO	–	–	–	14 m	Nil
Shaco-Levy 2010 [48]	USA	FTC	–	–	–	–	–	–	Yes in 15 patients[b]
		PTC (24 cases, 4 re classified as AC)	All NR except one (2)	–	–	–	RAI	–	
		FA (60)		–	–	–	RAI	–	
Sibio 2010 [25]	Italy	PTC	1	Hysterectomy, UA, peritoneal implants removal, LL	Patient had previous Total Thyroidectomy	–		7 y	Nil
Coyne 2010 [36]	USA	PTCF	–	Unilateral ovarian cystectomy	TFT, U/S, CT	Patient planned for final pregnancy followed by TT + RAI		–	–
Robboy 2009 [18]	USA	FTC (3 cases)	–	UO /TAH BSO/tumor debulking	–	–	Thyroidectomy/ biopsy in 14 patients	25 y; 10 y survival 89, 84% at 25 y	Yes in 10 patients[c]
		PTC (20 cases)	–	"	"	"	"		
		PTCF (1 case)	–	"	"	"	"		
		PTC + MA (4 cases)	–	"	"	"	"		
		Adenomatous patterns (58)	–	"	"	"	"		
Garg 2009 [22]	USA	PTC (2 cases) PTCF(4 cases) PTCF and PTC Bilateral PTCF Poorly differentiated carcinoma (2 cases)	1.1–80	Cystectomy, USO, TAH BSO, hysterectomy with USO	Radioactive iodine scan, thyroglobulin	–	TT(HP benign) and RAI in two patients,	1 to 14 y	2 cases[d]
Roth 2008 [34]	USA	PTC (3 case)	–	e	e	e	e	e	e

Table 1 Case studies of malignant Struma Ovarii (*Continued*)

Study*	Country	Tumor Type	Size (mm)	Type of Gynecological Surgery	Thyroid Workup	Thyroid Nodule	Thyroid Management	Follow up	Recurrence
		FTC poorly differentiated (1 case)	–	e	e	e	e	e	e
Salvatori 2008 [37]	Italy	PTCF	–	f	f	f	f	f	f
Yassa 2008 [3]	USA	PTC	9	–	TSH, TG, TG ab, U/S	1 cm FNA benign	Thyroxine therapy	1 y	none

AC Anaplastic carcinoma, *BFN* Benign follicular nodule, *CT* Computerized tomography, *FA* Follicular adenoma, *FTC* Follicular thyroid carcinoma, *HDFCO* (Highly differentiated follicular carcinoma of ovarian origin): tumor involved extra ovarian tissues without nuclear features of PTC, *HN* Hypoechoic nodule, *HP* Histopathology, *HT* Hemithyroidectomy, *LBSO* Laparoscopic bilateral salpingo-oophorectomy, *LL* Locoregional lymphadenectomy, *LT* Levothyroxine, *m* months, *MNS* Microcarcinoma focus size not specific, *MA* Mucinous adenocarcinoma, *PTC + OM* Primary papillary thyroid carcinoma + ovarian metastasis, *PTC* Papillary thyroid cancer, *PTCF* PTC follicular variant, *PTCT* Tall cell variant, *RAI* Radioactive iodine, *SO* struma ovarii, *TAH BSO* Total abdominal hysterectomy and bilateral salpingo-oophorectomy, *TAH* Total abdominal hysterectomy, *TFT* Thyroid function tests, *TgAb* Anti-thyroglobulin antibody, *TPO ab:* thyroperoxidase antibody, *TT* Total thyroidectomy, *U/S* Ultrasound, *UA* Unilateral adnexectomy, *UO* Unilateral oophorectomy, *USO* Unilateral salpingo-oophorectomy, *y* years

*Due to space considerations, only first author is cited; ": same as above; –: not reported, cannot be inferred

^aPatient diagnosed initially as thyroid PTCF, had HT followed by TT, thyroid scan and SPECT (right adnexal mass uptake), histopathology: PTCF within SO suggestive of primary disease not metastatic, radio iodine treatment given postoperative, no recurrence features over 5 years

^b15 patients with recurrences (11 FA, 4 PTC)

^c10 patients with recurrences, initial gynecological operation for each is not clear

^dFirst patient had left ovarian cystectomy, HP later found to be SO + PTCF. On 3 years follow up right ovarian tumor 2.4 cm detected, during surgery cul de sac and omentum implants found, HP was PTC. Patient then had RAI scan (diffuse uptake in abdomen), TT done, then RAI therapy given. Second patient had left ovarian cyst, ovarian cystectomy done. Caesarian section four years later (uterus, pelvis, cul-de-sac lesions found, TAH BSO done, PTCF lesions), RAI scan done (diffuse uptake in chest/ abdomen), patient had TT + RAI. Also had metastatic liver mass 8 cm (PTCF) that was resected. It is noted that recurrences in both patients occurred with well-differentiated and small foci of their primary tumors

^eOne PTC case had unilateral adnexal excision, paraortic LNs dissection + radiation therapy postoperative. Thyroid workup/ management NC. Follow up/ recurrence NC. One PTC case had right oophorectomy, left ovarian cystectomy and uterine curettage. Thyroid workup/ management NC. Follow up 25 years and patient is well. One PTC case had TAH BSO and pelvic node dissection, died soon after surgery. One poorly differentiated FTC had TAH BSO and peritoneal biopsies, then total TT, RAI and chemotherapy. Died 3years after primary operation

^fInitial operation was right salpingo-oopherectomy for right ovarian cyst, HP was SO with mature cystic teratoma, patient then had enucleation of left ovarian cyst (HP: PTCF) and multiple biopsies from pink nodules in abdomen and pelvis (HP: endometriosis). Then patient had TT and RAI scan (multiple liver, abdominal, pelvic uptakes), CT and MRI (multiple abdominal/ pelvic nodules). Patient underwent debulking of nodular mass, partial omentectomy and partial excision of ovarian cortex (due to patient's wish), followed by RAI therapy

categories, types of gynecological surgery, thyroid gland workup and management, and follow up and recurrence. Our case report is possibly the largest MSO PTC in the literature. TAH + BSO seems to be best in terms of curative outcome, however, hysterectomy with unilateral salpinogo-oophrectomy/unilateral oophorectomy, bilateral salpingo-oopherectomy and unilateral salpingo-oopherectomy/unilateral oophorectomy seem also effective treatment options. Fertility may be preserved with unilateral salpingo-oopherectomy/ unilateral oophorectomy, as this has great impact on the patient's psychology and social life. When unilateral removal of adnexal mass in undertaken, the contralateral side should be carefully assessed with surveillance for metastatic MSO. Ovarian cystectomy alone is associated with recurrences/ metastasis. Debate remains as to the association between MSO tumor size and potential extent of metastasis, and about the management of thyroid gland, however, surveillance and thyroid gland work up to detect concurrent thyroid cancer are recommended.

Abbreviations

AJCC: American Joint Committee on Cancer; CT: Computerized tomography; MDT: Multi disciplinary team; MRI: Magnetic resonance imaging; MSO: Malignant struma ovarii; PTC: papillary thyroid carcinoma; PTCF: papillary thyroid carcinoma follicular variant; SO: Struma ovarii; T + RIA: thyroidectomy and radioactive iodine ablation; T4: Thyroxine; TAH BSO: Bilateral salpingo-oopherectomy; TAH + BSO: Total abdominal hysterectomy and bilateral salpingo-oopherectomy; TAH: Total abdominal hysterectomy; TSH: Thyroid-stimulating hormone

Acknowledgements

Not applicable.

Authors' contribution

MSA, TS and WEA wrote the first draft of the manuscript. AA contributed to the writing of the manuscript. MSA, TS, AA, HF, AAA and MZ contributed to the acquisition of the clinical data. WEA, AA, and TS jointly developed the structure and arguments of the paper. WEA, TS, AA, HF and MSA made critical revisions and approved the final version of the manuscript. All authors agreed with the manuscript results and conclusions and reviewed and approved the final manuscript.

Funding

Not applicable.

Competing interests

The authors declare that they have no competing interests.

Author details

[1]Department of General Surgery, Hamad General Hospital, Doha, Qatar. [2]Department of Surgery, Hamad General Hospital, Doha, Qatar. [3]College of Medicine, Qatar University, Doha, Qatar. [4]Department of Gynecologic Oncology, Hamad General Hospital, Doha, Qatar. [5]Department of Endocrinology, Hamad General Hospital, Doha, Qatar. [6]Department of Pathology, Hamad General Hospital, Doha, Qatar.

References

1. Dunzendorfer T, deLas Morenas A, Kalir T, Levin RM. Struma ovarii and hyperthyroidism. Thyroid. 1999;9:499.
2. Kondi-Pafiti A, Mavrigiannaki P, Grigoriadis C, et al. Monodermal teratomas (struma ovarii). Clinicopathological characteristics of 11 cases and literature review. Eur J Gynaecol Oncol. 2011;32:657.
3. Yassa L, Sadow P, Marqusee E. Malignant struma ovarii. Nat Clin Pract Endocrinol Metab. 2008;4:469.
4. Yoo SC, Chang KH, Lyu MO, Chang SJ, Ryu HS, Kim HS. Clinical characteristics of struma ovarii. J Gynecol Oncol. 2008;19:135–8.
5. Kraemer B, Grischke EM, Staebler A, et al. Laparoscopic excision of malignant struma ovarii and 1 year follow-up without further treatment. Fertil Steril. 2011;95(6):2124.e9–12.
6. DeSimone CP, Lele SM, Modesitt SC. Malignant struma ovarii: a case report and analysis of cases reported in the literature with focus on survival and I131 therapy. Gynecol Oncol. 2003;89:543–8.
7. McGill JF, Sturgeon C, Angelos P. Metastatic Struma ovarii treated with total thyroidectomy and radioiodine ablation. Endocr Pract. 2009;15(2):167–73.
8. Goffredo P, Sawka AM, Pura J, Adam MA, Roman SA, Sosa JA. Malignant struma ovarii: a population-level analysis of a large series of 68 patients. Thyroid. 2015;25(2):211–5.
9. Salman W, Singh M, Twaij Z. A case of papillary thyroid carcinoma in struma ovarii and review of the literature. Patholog Res Int. 2010;2010: 352476.
10. Tomee JF, van der Heijden PF, van den Hout JH, Brinkhuis M, Veneman TF. Papillary carcinoma in struma ovarii: an unusual presentation. Neth J Med. 2008;66(6):248–51.
11. Sussman SK, Kho SA, Cersosimo E, Heimann A. Coexistence of malignant struma ovarii and Graves' disease. Endocr Pract. 2002;8(5):378–80.
12. Teale E, Gouldesbrough DR, Peacey SR. Graves' disease and coexisting struma ovarii: struma expression of thyrotropin receptors and the presence of thyrotropin receptor stimulating antibodies. Thyroid. 2006;16(8):791–3.
13. Talerman A. Germ cell tumors of the ovary. In: Kurman RJ, editor. Blaustein's pathology of the female genital tract. 3rd ed. New York: Springer Verlag; 2001. p. 967–1033.
14. Roth LM, Talerman A. The enigma of struma ovarii. Pathology. 2007;39(1):139–46.
15. Makani S, Kim W, Gaba AR. Struma Ovarii with a focus of papillary thyroid cancer: a case report and review of the literature. Gynecol Oncol. 2004;94:835.
16. Zalel Y, Seidman DS, Oren M, et al. Sonographic and clinical characteristics of struma ovarii. J Ultrasound Med. 2000;19:857.
17. Savelli L, Testa AC, Timmerman D, Paladini D, Ljungberg O, Valentin L. Imaging of gynecological disease (4): clinical and ultrasound characteristics of struma ovarii. Ultrasound Obstet Gynecol. 2008;32:210–9.
18. Robboy SJ, Shaco-Levy R, Peng RY, Snyder MJ, Donahue J, Bentley RC, Bean S, Krigman HR, Roth LM, Young RH. Malignant struma ovarii: an analysis of 88 cases, including 27 with extraovarian spread. Int J Gynecol Pathol. 2009; 28(5):405–22.
19. Nalbanski A, Pŭnevska M, Nalbanski B. Stromal ovary in 14 years old girl. Akush Ginekol (Sofiia). 2007;46(6):44–6. Bulgarian
20. Marti JL, Clark VE, Harper H, Chhieng DC, Sosa JA, Roman SA. Optimal surgical management of well-differentiated thyroid cancer arising in Struma ovarii: a series of 4 patients and a review of 53 reported cases. Thyroid. 2012;22:400–6.
21. Schmidt J, Derr V, Heinrich MC, Crum CP, Fletcher JA, Corless CL, Nose´ V. BRAF in papillary thyroid carcinoma of ovary (struma ovarii). Am J Surg Pathol. 2007;31:1337–43.
22. Garg K, Soslow RA, Rivera M, Tuttle MR, Ghossein RA. Histologically bland "extremely well differentiated" thyroid carcinomas arising in struma ovarii can recur and metastasize. Int J Gynecol Pathol. 2009;28(3):222–30.
23. Boyd JC, Williams BA, Rigby MH, Kieser K, Offman S, Shirsat H, Trites JRB, Taylor SM, Hart RD. Malignant Struma ovarii in a 30-year old nulliparous patient. Thyroid Res. 2017;30(10):3.
24. Barrera JR, Manalo LA, Ang FL. Papillary thyroid-type carcinoma arising from struma ovarii. BMJ Case Rep. 2012 11; 2012.
25. Sibio S, Borrini F, Sammartino P, Accarpio F, Biacchi D, Caprio G, Iafrate F, Baccheschi AM, Cornali T, Di Giorgio A. Predominant Brenner tumor combined with struma ovarii containing a papillary microcarcinoma associated with benign peritoneal strumosis: report of a case and histologic features. Endocr Pathol. 2010;21(3):199–203.
26. Tanaka H, Sakakura Y, Kobayashi T, Yoshida K, Asakura T, Taniguchi H. A case of thyroid-type papillary carcinoma derived from ovarian mature cystic teratoma, resected by laparoscopic surgery. Asian J Endosc Surg. 2011;4(2):86–9.

27. Kumar SS, Rema P, R AK, Varghese BT. Thyroid type papillary carcinoma arising in a mature teratoma. Indian J Surg Oncol. 2014;5(3):168–70.

28. Jean S, Tanyi JL, Montone K, et al. Papillary thyroid cancer arising in struma ovarii. J Obstet Gynaecol. 2012;32:222.

29. Middelbeek RJW, O'Neill BT, Nishino M, Pallotta JA. Concurrent thyroid Cancer in Struma Ovarii: a case report and literature review. J Endocr Soc 2017 23;1(5):396–400.

30. Pineyro MM, Pereda J, Schou P, de Los Santos K, de la Peña S, Caserta B, Pisabarro R. Papillary thyroid microcarcinoma arising within a mature OvarianTeratoma: case report and review of the literature. Clin Med Insights Endocrinol Diabetes. 2017;10 https://doi.org/10.1177/1179551417712521.

31. Leite I, Cunha TM, Figueiredo JP, Félix A. Papillary carcinoma arising in struma ovarii versus ovarian metastasis from primary thyroid carcinoma: a case report and review of the literature. J Radiol Case Rep. 2013 Oct; 7(10):24–33.

32. Stanojevic B, Dzodic R, Saenko V, Milovanovic Z, Krstevski V, Radlovic P, Buta M, Rulic B, Todorovic L, Dimitrijevic B, Yamashita S. Unilateral follicular variant of papillary thyroid carcinoma with unique KRAS mutation in struma ovarii in bilateral ovarian teratoma: a rare case report. BMC Cancer. 2012;8(12):224.

33. O'Neill JP, Burns P, Kinsella J. Papillary type thyroid carcinoma in an ovarian struma. Ir J Med Sci. 2012;181(1):115–7.

34. Roth LM, Karseladze AI. Highly differentiated follicular carcinoma arising from struma ovarii: a report of 3 cases, a review of the literature, and a reassessment of so-called peritoneal strumosis. Int J Gynecol Pathol. 2008; 27(2):213–22.

35. Fernández Catalina P, Rego Iraeta A, Lorenzo Solar M, Sánchez Sobrino P. Sincronous malignant struma ovarii and papillary thyroid carcinoma. Endocrinol Nutr. 2016;63(7):366–7.

36. Coyne C, Nikiforov YE. RAS mutation-positive follicular variant of papillary thyroid carcinoma arising in a struma ovarii. Endocr Pathol. 2010;21(2):144–7.

37. Salvatori M, Dambra DP, D'Angelo G, Conte LL, Locantore P, Zannoni G, Campo V, Campo S. A case of metastatic struma ovarii treated with 131I therapy: focus on preservation of fertility and selected review of the literature. Gynecol Endocrinol. 2008;24(6):312–9.

38. Zhu Y, Wang C, Zhang GN, Shi Y, Xu SQ, Jia SJ, He R. Papillary thyroid cancer located in malignant struma ovarii with omentum metastasis: a case report and review of the literature. World J Surg Oncol. 2016;20(14):1–17.

39. Shrimali RK, Shaikh G, Reed NS. Malignant struma ovarii: the west of Scotland experience and review of literature with focus on postoperative management. J Med Imaging Radiat Oncol. 2012;56:478–82.

40. Leong A, Roche PJ, Paliouras M, Rochon L, Trifiro M, Tamilia M. Coexistence of malignant struma ovarii and cervical papillary thyroid carcinoma. J Clin Endocrinol Metab. 2013;98:4599–605.

41. Matysiak-Grzes M, Fischbach J, Gut P, Klimowicz A, Gryczynska M, Wasko R, Ruchala M. Struma ovarii maligna. Neuro Endocrinol. 2013;34:97–101.

42. Zhang X, Axiotis C. Thyroid-type carcinoma of Struma ovarii. Arch Pathol Lab Med. 2010;34:786–91.

43. Janszen EW, van Doorn HC, Ewing PC, de Krijger RR, de Wilt JH, Kam BL, et al. Malignant Struma ovarii: good response after thyroidectomy and I ablation therapy. Clin Med Oncol. 2008;2:147–52.

44. Wei S, Baloch ZW, LiVolsi VA. Pathology of Struma Ovarii: a report of 96 cases. Endocr Pathol. 2015;26(4):342–8.

45. Monti E, Mortara L, Zupo S, Dono M, Minuto F, Truini M, Naseri M, Giusti M. Papillary thyroid cancer in a struma ovarii: a report of a rare case. Hormones (Athens). 2015;14(1):154–9.

46. Mardi K, Gupta N. Tall cell variant of papillary carcinoma arising from strumaovarii: a rare case report. J Cancer Res Ther. 2013;9(1):119–21.

47. Meringolo D, Bianchi D, Capula C, Costante G. Papillary thyroid microcarcinoma in struma ovarii. Endocrine. 2012;41(1):164–5.

48. Shaco-Levy R, Bean SM, Bentley RC, Robboy SJ. Natural history of biologically malignant struma ovarii: analysis of 27 cases with extraovarian spread. Int J Gynecol Pathol. 2010;29(3):212–27.

24

Thyroid hormones increase stomach goblet cell numbers and mucin expression during indomethacin induced ulcer healing in Wistar rats

Jackline Namulema[1]* (iD), Miriam Nansunga[1,4], Charles Drago Kato[2,5], Muhammudu Kalange[1] and Samuel Babafemi Olaleye[3]

Abstract

Background: Gastric ulcers are mucosal discontinuities that may extend into the mucosa, submucosa or even deeper. They result from an imbalance between mucosal aggressors and protective mechanisms that include the mucus bicarbonate layer. Thyroid hormones have been shown to accelerate gastric ulcer healing in part by increasing the adherent mucus levels. However, the effects of thyroid hormones on goblet cell numbers and expression of neutral and acidic mucins during ulcer healing have not been investigated.

Methods: Thirty six adult male Wistar rats were randomly divided into six groups each with six animals. Group 1 (normal control) and group 2 (negative control) were given normal saline for eight weeks. Groups 3 and 4 were given 100 μg/kg per day per os of thyroxine so as to induce hyperthyroidism. Groups 5 and 6 received 0.01% (w/v) Propylthiouracil (PTU) for 8 weeks so as to induce hypothyroidism. After thyroid hormonal levels were confirmed using radioimmunoassay and immunoradiometric assays, ulcer induction was done using 40 mg/kg intragastric single dose of Indomethacin in groups 2, 3 and 5. Stomachs were extracted after day 3 and 7 of ulcer induction for histological examination. Histochemistry was carried out using Periodic Acid Shiff and Alcian Blue. The number of acidic and neutral goblet cells were determined by counting numbers per field. Mucin expression (%) was determined using Quick Photo Industrial software version 3.1.

Results: The numbers of neutral goblet cells (cells/field) increased significantly ($P < 0.05$) in the ulcer+thyroxine (14.67 ± 0.33), thyroxine (17.04 ± 1.71) and ulcer+PTU (12.89 ± 1.06) groups compared to the normal control (10.78 ± 1.07) at day 3. For the acidic goblet cells, differences between treatment groups were more pronounced at day 7 between the ulcer+thyroxine (22.56 ± 1.26) and thyroxine (22.89 ± 0.80). We further showed that percentage expression of both neutral and acidic mucins was significantly higher in the ulcer+thyroxine (9.23 ± 0.17 and 6.57 ± 0.35 respectively) and thyroxine groups (9.66 ± 0.21 and 6.33 ± 0.38 respectively) as compared to the normal control group (4.08 ± 0.20 and 4.38 ± 0.11 respectively) at day 3 after ulcer induction.

Conclusion: This study confirms the role played by thyroid hormones in healing of indomethacin induced gastric ulcers. The study further demonstrates increased numbers of both neutral and acidic goblet cells and the increase in expression of both neutral and acidic mucins during healing of indomethacin induced ulcers.

Keywords: Thyroid hormones, Goblet cells, Mucins, Indomethacin, Ulcer healing

---

* Correspondence: jacklineemily@gmail.com
[1]Department of Physiology, Faculty of Biomedical Sciences, Kampala International University, P.O BOX 71, Ishaka, Bushenyi, Uganda
Full list of author information is available at the end of the article

Background

Stomach or peptic ulcers are the most common gastrointestinal tract ailments that affect half of the world's population [1]. The highest burden of this disease both in morbidity and mortality occurs in developing countries [2]. In Uganda, the rate of death from these ulcers is 2.81 per 100,000 individuals [3]. An ulcer of the gastrointestinal tract is defined as a discontinuity in the muscularis mucosae into the submucosa or deeper [4]. Along the length of the gastrointestinal tract, ulcers commonly occur in the stomach and the duodenum [5]. They are due to an imbalance between the protective and aggressive mechanisms including pepsin, *Helicobacter pylori* infection and gastric acid [6].

Normally, the epithelial cells of the stomach are protected from various aggressive factors by a mucus-bicarbonate-phospholipid barrier which conserves the continuity of the surface epithelium [7, 8] thus preventing the ulcers from occurring. The adherent mucus layer, a very important component of the barrier is secreted by surface epithelial cells (goblet cells) [9–11]. The mucous covers the stomach epithelial cells and serves as the first line of defense against mucosal aggressors [10, 12].The mucus is formed by gel-forming mucin glycoproteins (MUCs) and water [13]. In order for the levels of mucus to increase after any stress, the cell surface mucins first detect the changes in the external environment and signal these changes to the goblet cell [14]. This is followed by increase in the adherent mucus levels that promote ulcer healing.

Four mucins are found in the stomach MUC1, MUC4, MUC5AC and MUC6 [15]. These mucins are histochemically classified into acidic and neutral mucins [16, 17]. The expression of the different mucin types depends on the type of mucosal aggressor [13, 18].

Ulcer healing depends on the removal of the aggressive mechanisms and increase in the protective mechanisms [19, 20]. Since the adherent mucus layer is the first line of defenses against ulcers [10], it follows that mucus secretion increases as ulcer healing progresses. In secretory organs and tissues, thyroid hormones have been associated with increased body fluid secretion [21]. In the stomach, these hormones have been shown to accelerate ulcer healing when given before or at the beginning of the stress [21]. Ulcer healing has been associated with an increase in adherent mucus content [22], accelerated reepithelization [23] and angiogenesis [24]. The increase in the mucus levels could be attributed to the increase in the number of goblet cells or in their individual secretion rate. Therefore, the present study aimed at determining the effect of thyroid hormones on goblet cell numbers and expression of both neutral and acidic mucins in the stomach of wistar rats during healing of indomethacin induced ulcers.

Methods

Experimental design

Thirty six adult male Wistar albino rats with an average weight 180 ± 21.4 g were procured from the Department of Pharmacology, Kampala International University-Western Campus. The rats were housed in standard rat cages in the animal house at the Department of Pharmacology with access to food and water for two weeks before the beginning of the experiment. Animals were grouped into six groups each having six rats that were careful matched for weight (Additional file 1: Table S1). Group one (normal control) and group two (negative control) were given normal saline for eight weeks. Hyperthyroidism was induced in group three and group four by administering thyroxine (Leehpl ventures, India) at a dose of 100 µg/kg per day per os for eight weeks [25]. Hypothyroidism was induced in group five and group six through the administration of Propylthiouracil, PTU (Macleod, India) as described previously [26]. Thyroid hormone levels were confirmed using radioimmunoassay for thyroxine and triiodothyronine and immunoradiometric assay for thyroid stimulating hormone as described previously [23] (results shown in Additional file 2: Table S2). After an overnight fast but with access to water, ulcers were induced in groups 2, 3 and 5 using 40 mg/kg intragastric single dose of Indomethacin (Sun Pharma, India) as previously described [27]. After ulcer induction, treatment with respective drugs were stopped.

Histochemistry studies

From each group, three rats were sacrificed on day three and the remaining three rats sacrificed at day 7 after ulcer induction under diethyl ether anaesthesia. The abdomens were opened along the greater curvature and the stomach excised. The stomachs were rinsed with saline water and later fixed in 10% formalin. Prior to any staining procedures, sections were cut at 5 µm using a microtome and placed on glass slides. The sections were deparaffinised in xylene and rehydrated in a graded alcohol series. Six slides were prepared for each rat; three for acidic goblet cells and expression of acidic mucins and the other three for neutral goblet cells and expression of neutral mucins.

Determination of neutral goblet cells and mucins was by a method described by Forder et al. [28]. Briefly, following the deparaffinization and rehydration, the sections were subjected to mild acid hydrolysis to eliminate the contribution of acid residues. They were incubated in 0.5% Periodic Acid (PA) for 20 min and washed and incubated with Schiff's reagent for 20 min. After rinsed in tap water for 10 min, were dehydrated and then mounted on a light microscope.

Determination of acidic goblet cells and mucins was by a method described by Uni et al. [29]. Briefly, following the deparaffinization and rehydration, sections were incubated in 3% acetic acid for 3 min and then Alcian Blue solution (1% in 3% acetic acid, pH 2.5). Slides were rinsed in water, dehydrated and mounted on a light microscope.

Image analysis

After examination, selected slides were photographed using a digital camera (Canon, China) mounted on a light microscope (Carl Zeiss, Germany). Images were acquired from the slides using Zoom browser Ex, version 2 Imaging software. Goblet cells were counted according to the method described by [30] with slight modification. Briefly, goblet cells that stained with Periodic Acid Schiff (PAS) and Alcian Blue (AB) were counted using a calibrated microscope in five randomly selected areas of the gastric mucosal tissue and presented as numbers per field. Counts were done in triplicate for each slide. The mean value was calculated for each group and represented as Mean ± SEM.

Determination of the levels of mucin expression was carried out using a method described by Nonose et al. [31]. The expression of neutral and acid mucins was quantified by means of computer-assisted image processing. The images selected were captured on a video camera that was coupled to an optical microscope. These images were processed and analyzed using the Quick PHOTO INDUSTRIAL software version 3.1. The software determined the color intensity in number of pixels in each field selected, and transformed the final data into percentage expressions by analyzed fields. The final value taken for each field measured in the segments was the mean of the values found from evaluating three different fields. Data was presented as Mean ± SEM in percentage.

Statistical analysis

Statistical analysis was done using Graph pad Prisms Version 6. Mean values for the number of the goblet cells and mucin intensity (%) were obtained for each group of rats. Data was presented as Mean ± SEM (Standard Error of Mean). Within treatment groups comparisons were made for each group of rats at day 3 and 7 after ulcer induction using a Student's t-test. Comparisons of the means across treatment groups were done using one way ANOVA followed by Tukey's multiple comparison tests. Significant differences in the means for both statistical tests were considered at $P < 0.05$ level.

Results

Effect of thyroid hormones on ulcer healing

In order to demonstrate ulcer induction and the effect of thyroid hormones on ulcer healing, the histopathology of the stomach was analyzed among experimental animals. At day 3 after ulcer induction, the results showed that the ulcer+normal saline and ulcer+PTU (hypothyroid) groups

had regions of mucosal injury characterized by discontinuity of the mucosal epithelium, lymphocyte infiltration, erosions in the lamina propria, tissue hemorrhages and necrosis (Fig. 1). By day 7, there was marked improvement in the ulcer+normal saline group to levels comparable to the normal control. The ulcer+PTU group still had lymphocyte infiltration and erosions by day 7. In the ulcer+thyroxine group, there was minimal mucosa injury by day 3 and by day 7, the mucosal integrity was restored and comparable to that of the normal control group (Fig. 1).

Effect of thyroid hormones on the number of goblet cells

In order to measure the effect of thyroid hormones on goblet cell numbers during ulcer healing, we enumerated the number of acidic and neutral goblet cells. The results showed that both neutral and acidic goblet cell numbers significantly differed across treatment groups at both day 3 (F $_{[5, 12]}$ = 4.09, $P = 0.02$ and F $_{[5, 12]}$ = 16.74 $P < 0.0001$ respectively) and day 7 (F $_{[5, 12]}$ = 24.63, $P < 0.0001$ and F $_{[5, 12]}$ = 20.19, $P < 0.0001$ respectively).

The numbers of neutral goblet cells (cells/field) increased significantly ($P < 0.05$) in the ulcer+thyroxine (14.67 ± 0.33), thyroxine (17.04 ± 1.71) and ulcer+PTU (12.89 ± 1.06) groups compared to the normal control (10.78 ± 1.07) at day 3 (Fig. 2a). However, by day 7, only the ulcer+thyroxine (20.07 ± 1.56) and thyroxine (19.44 ± 2.70) groups showed significant differences ($P < 0.05$) compared to the normal control (11.56 ± 0.40) (Fig. 2b). For the acidic goblet cells, differences between treatment groups were more pronounced at day 7 (Fig. 2d) between the ulcer+thyroxine (22.56 ± 1.26) and thyroxine (22.89 ± 0.80) as compared to the normal control (15.23 ± 0.69). On comparison of goblet cells at day 3 and 7 within the treatment groups, the number of neutral goblet cells was significantly increased in the ulcer+thyroxine ($P < 0.02$) group with no significant differences in the other groups. There were no significant differences in numbers of acidic goblet cells within treatment groups at both days (Table 1).

Effect of thyroid hormones on the expression of neutral and acidic mucins during ulcer healing

In order to determine the effect of thyroid hormones on the expression of neutral and acidic mucins during ulcer healing, the intensity of the stains as an indicator of mucin intensity was measured. The results showed that thyroid hormones significantly increased the expression of both neutral and acidic mucins at both day 3 (F $_{(5, 12)}$ = 308, $P < 0.0001$ and F $_{(5, 12)}$ = 32, P value < 0.0001 respectively) and day 7 (F $_{(5, 12)}$ = 308.5, $P < 0.0001$ and F $_{(5, 12)}$ = 32.65, $P < 0.0001$ respectively) after ulcer induction with indomethacin. Comparisons between the different groups showed that the percentage expression of both neutral (Fig. 3a) and acidic (Fig. 3c) mucins was significantly higher in the ulcer+thyroxine (9.23 ± 0.17 and 6.57 ± 0.35

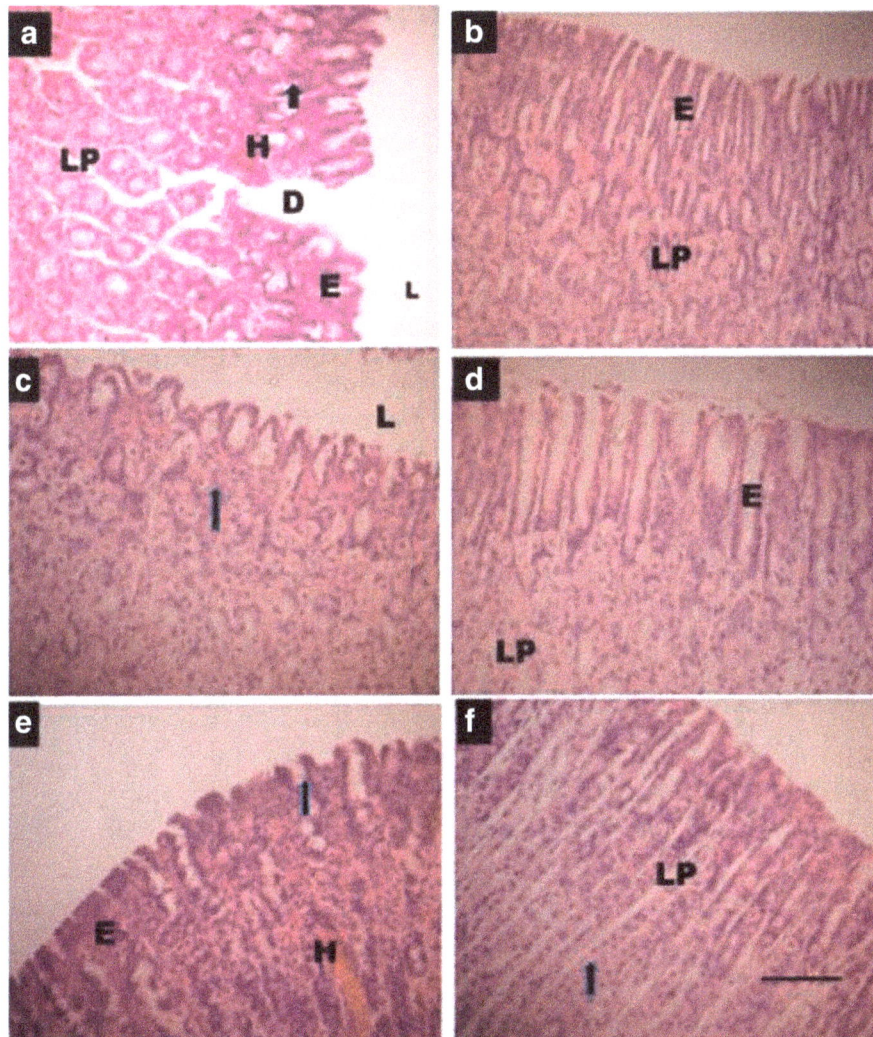

Fig. 1 Effect of thyroid hormones on the healing of indomethacin induced gastric ulcers at days 3 (**a**, **c** and **e**) and 7 (**b**, **d** and **f**) after ulcer induction. Mucosal injury characterized by, discontinuity in the mucosa (**d**), lymphocyte infiltration (arrows) and erosions (R) in the epithelium (**e**) and lamina propria (LP), hemorrhage (H) can be seen in Plate **a** and **e**. **a** and **b**, ulcer+normal saline, **c** and **d**, ulcer+thyroxine and **e** and **f**, ulcer+PTU. L-lumen

respectively) and thyroxine groups (9.66 ± 0.21 and 6.33 ± 0.38 respectively) as compared to the normal control group (4.08 ± 0.20 and 4.38 ± 0.11 respectively) at day 3 after ulcer induction. By day 7 after ulcer induction, the expression of both neutral (Fig. 3b) and acidic (Fig. 3d) mucins in the ulcer+thyroxine (12.9 ± 0.18 and 16 ± 1.26 respectively) and thyroxine (9.73 ± 0.21 and 14.89 ± 0.80 respectively) treated groups remained significantly elevated as compared to the normal control (4.58 ± 0.28 and 7.23 ± 0.69 respectively). Comparison of the number of goblet cells within treatment groups at days 3 and 7 after ulcer induction showed a significant increase in the expression of neutral goblet cells in the ulcer+saline (3.00 ± 0.35 at day 3 to 3.80 ± 0.27 at day 7, $P < 0.0004$). In addition, to the ulcer+thyroxine group (9.23 ± 0.21 at day 3 to 9.73 ± 0.21 at day 7, $P < 0.00001$). Only the ulcer

+thyroxine (4.70 ± 0.28 at day 3 to 16.97 ± 0.18 at day 7, $P < 0.00001$) group showed a significant increase in the expression of acidic mucins (Table 2).

Discussion

The results of the study showed that increased thyroid hormone levels accelerated healing of Indomethacin induced ulcers by day 7 after ulcer induction. This gastro-protective effect was indicated by the clearance of inflammatory cells and restoration of mucosal integrity by day 7 after ulcer induction in the ulcer+thyroxine (hyperthyroid) group yet these persisted in the ulcer +PTU (hypothyroid) group compared to the normal (euthyroid) control. This is in agreement with other studies that showed that high levels of thyroid hormones accelerated the healing of acetic acid [23, 25] and indomethacin

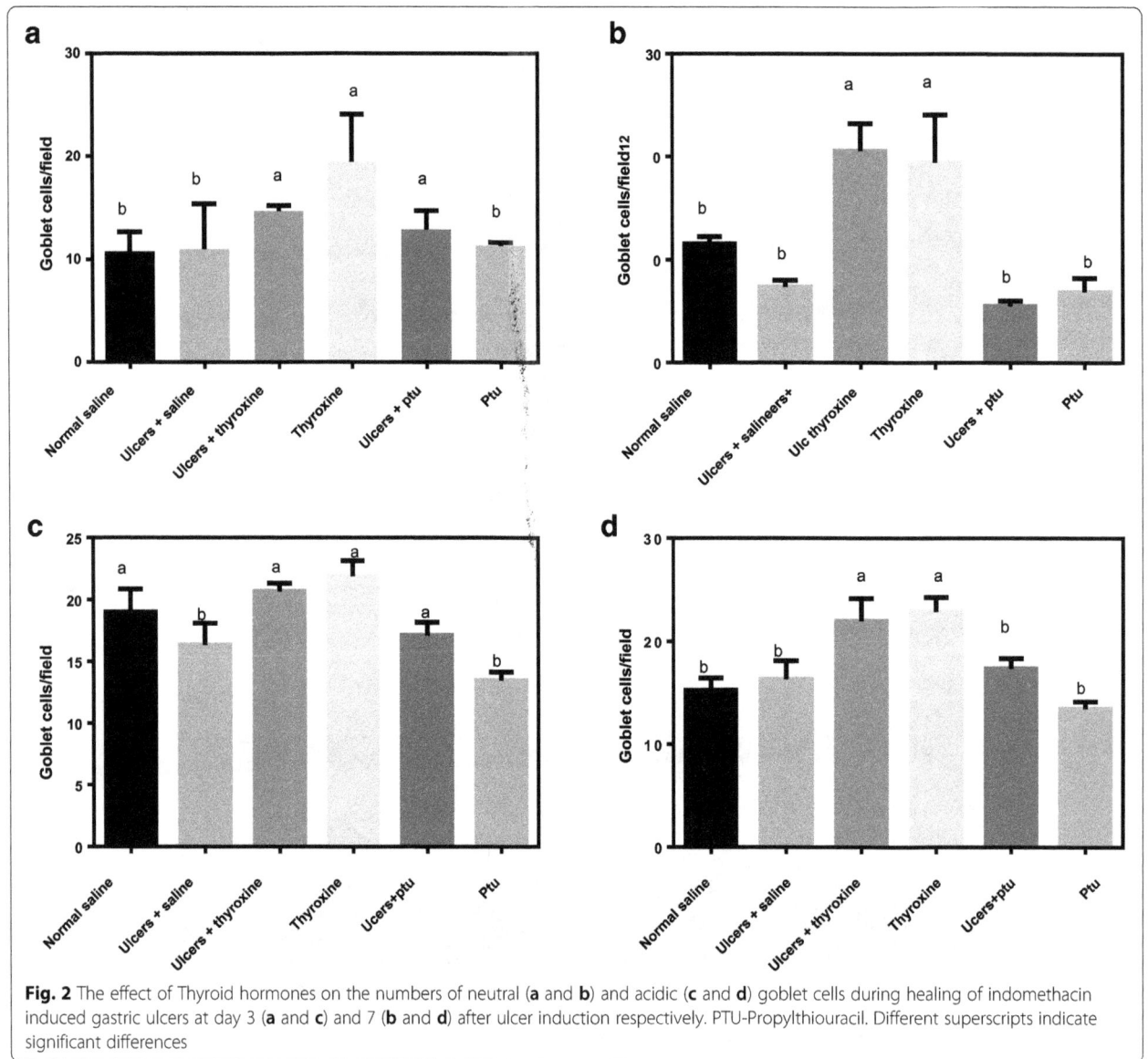

Fig. 2 The effect of Thyroid hormones on the numbers of neutral (**a** and **b**) and acidic (**c** and **d**) goblet cells during healing of indomethacin induced gastric ulcers at day 3 (**a** and **c**) and 7 (**b** and **d**) after ulcer induction respectively. PTU-Propylthiouracil. Different superscripts indicate significant differences

induced ulcers when given before or after induction of the stress [21]. The faster clearance of inflammatory cells by thyroid hormones indicates that thyroid hormones speed up the inflammatory phase of gastric ulcer healing. The early clearance of these cells by thyroid hormones provides room for their replacement by fibroblasts and angiogenesis, processes that are also promoted by thyroid hormones [32]. Thyroid hormones also increase blood flow [33] to supply essential nutrients that promote ulcer healing. The ulcer+thyroxine and thyroxine groups showed significant

Table 1 Comparison of goblet numbers at day 3 and 7 during ulcer healing

Treatment	N	Neutral			Acidic		
		Day		P-value	Day		P-value
		3	7		3	7	
Normal control	6	10.78 ± 1.09	10.62 ± 0.9	0.32	19 1.07	15.23 0.69	0.41
Ulcer + Normal saline	6	11.00 ± 2.55	7.33 ± 0.38	0.23	16.33 1.02	17.33 0.39	0.37
Ulcer + Thyroxine	6	14.67 ± 0.33	20.56 ± 1.56	0.02*	20.67 0.38	22.56 1.26	0.07
Ulcer + PTU	6	8.00 ± 1.06	11.78 ± 0.40	0.39	17.11 0.62	17.33 0.58	0.16

Asterisks indicate significant differences at $P<0.05$

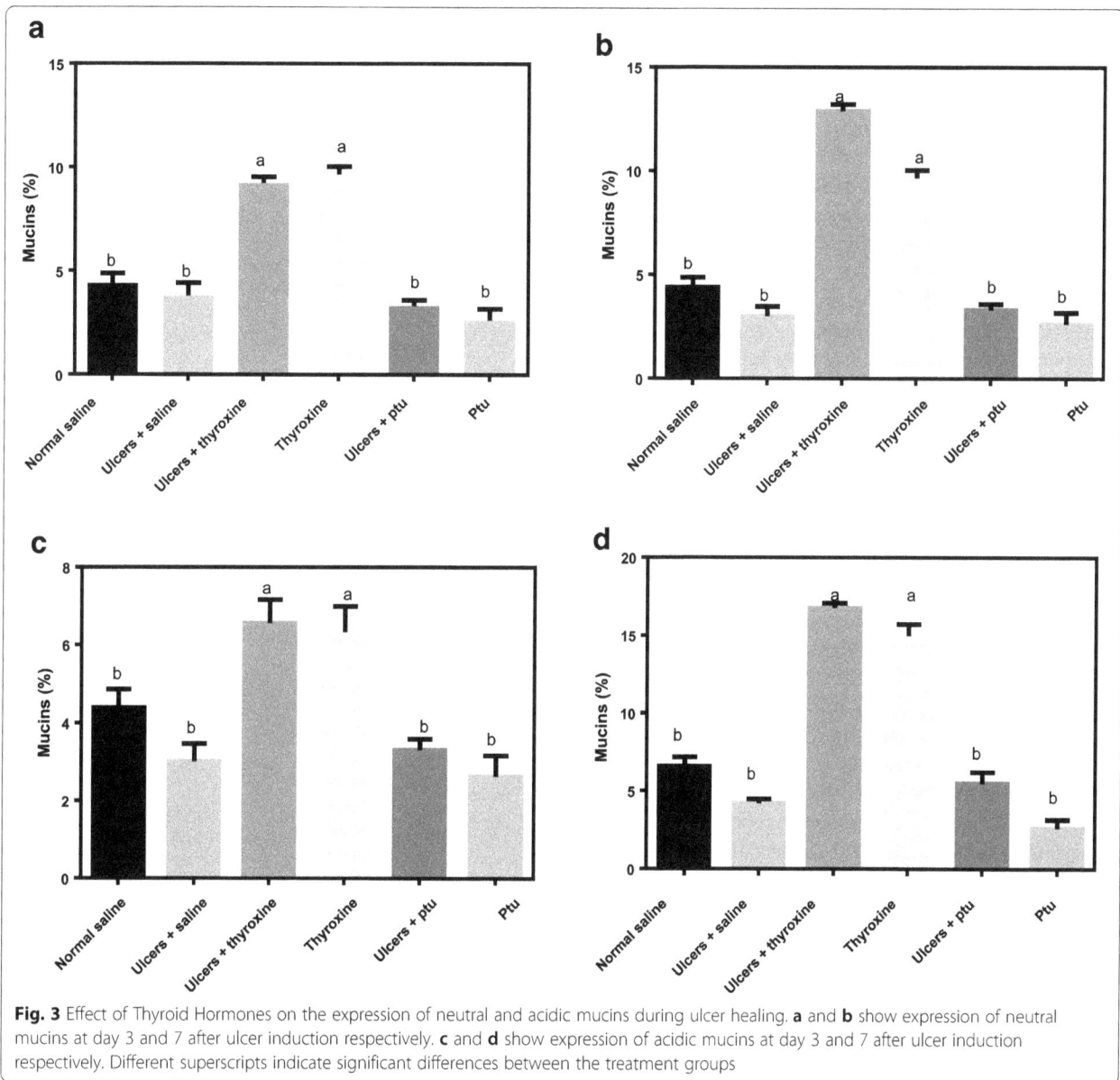

Fig. 3 Effect of Thyroid Hormones on the expression of neutral and acidic mucins during ulcer healing. **a** and **b** show expression of neutral mucins at day 3 and 7 after ulcer induction respectively. **c** and **d** show expression of acidic mucins at day 3 and 7 after ulcer induction respectively. Different superscripts indicate significant differences between the treatment groups

Table 2 Comparison of the expression of neutral and acidic mucins at day 3 and 7

Treatment	N	Neutral mucins			Acidic mucins		
		Day		P-value	Day		P-value
		3	7		3	7	
Normal control	6	4.08 ± 0.20	4.58 ± 0.28	0.04	12.81 ± 0.19	7.23 ± 0.69	0.07
Ulcer + Normal saline	6	3.00 ± 0.35	3.80 ± 0.27	0.0004*	9.66 ± 0.22	4.73 ± 0.43	0.08
Ulcer + Thyroxine	6	9.23 ± 0.21	9.73 ± 0.21	0.00001*	4.70 ± 0.28	16.97 ± 0.18	0.01*
Ulcer + PTU	6	3.31 ± 0.16	2.31 ± 0.11	0.06	3.26 ± 0.16	5.87 ± 0.42	0.12

Asterisks indicate significant differences at $P < 0.05$

increase in the number of goblet cells compared to the normal control by both days after ulcer induction. This is in agreement with other studies that have showed thyroid hormones to increase the rate of differentiation [34] and mitotic activity in different parts of the body [35] and that the hormones promote re-epithelization of the gastric mucosa during ulcer healing [25]. Since goblets cells are part of the cells that make up the gastric mucosa, it follows that thyroid hormones also increase their numbers.

The results of the study also showed that there was an increase in the expression of neutral mucins in the ulcer +thyroxine and thyroxine groups as compared to the normal control group at day 3 after ulcer induction. However, the increase in neutral mucins was more pronounced. This study confirms the findings that thyroid hormones increase the rate of activity of almost all cells [36], including the goblet cells. This is also in line with other studies that have showed that thyroid hormones increase the levels of adherent mucus during ulcer healing [23]. Thyroid hormones have been associated with a decrease in the pH of luminal contents that prevents exacerbation of the ulcers [22]. This could be attributed to their ability to increase the secretion of neutral mucins since they neutralize the acid thus reducing the pH [10]. On the other hand, the increase in the secretion of acidic mucins is important for the healing of the ulcers to progress since they contain chelating groups [29] and therefore act as antibacterial and antiviral agents [28]. Acidic mucins are also thick and viscous and thus form the major part of the protective mucus layer for both protection and lubrication [37], factors that are associated with healing of gastric ulcers. Studies have shown the stomach contains only two secreted mucins; MUC5AC (acidic) and MUC6 (neutral) [38]. It follows that thyroid hormones probably increase the expression of both gastric secreted mucins during ulcer healing.

Conclusion

We show in here that thyroid hormones accelerate healing of Indomethacin induced gastric ulcers by increasing the numbers of both neutral and acidic goblets cells and the expression of both neutral and acidic mucins during healing of indomethacin induced ulcers in wistar rats. Therefore, in order to accelerate healing of indomethacin induced gastric ulcers, thyroid hormones increase the number of neutral and acidic goblet cells which is followed by an increase in the expression of both neutral and acidic mucins. Since in study histochemistry was used to show the expression of the mucins, other studies should be done using advanced molecular biology techniques to ascertain the effect of thyroid hormones on the exact mucin levels of the different types of stomach mucins during healing of indomethacin induced ulcers.

Abbreviations

IRMA: Immunoradiometric assay; LMICs: Low and Middle Income countries; MUC: Mucin; NSAIDs: Non-steroid anti-inflammatory drugs; PTU: Propylthiouracil; PUD: Peptic Ulcer Disease; RIA: Radioimmunoassay; SEM: Standard Error of Mean; T3: Triiodothyronine; T4: Thyroxine; THs: Thyroid Hormones; TSH: Thyroid Stimulating Hormone

Acknowledgements

The authors are grateful to Kisekka Majid of College of Veterinary Medicine, Animal Resources and Bio-security, Makerere University for technical assistance during histochemistry.

Author's contributions

SBO conceptualized and made the initial design, MN, CDK and JN were involved in acquisition, analysis and interpretation of the data and MK was involved in data analysis and interpretation. All the authors were involved in drafting and writing the final manuscript.

Competing interests

The authors declare that they have no competing interests.

Author details

[1]Department of Physiology, Faculty of Biomedical Sciences, Kampala International University, P.O BOX 71, Ishaka, Bushenyi, Uganda. [2]Department of Immunology and Microbiology, Faculty of Biomedical Sciences, Kampala International University, P.O BOX 71, Ishaka, Bushenyi, Uganda. [3]Laboratory for Gastrointestinal Secretion and Inflammation Research, Department of Physiology, College of Medicine, University of Ibadan, Ibadan, Nigeria. [4]Department of Physiology, Faculty of Biomedical Sciences, St Augustine International University, P.O BOX 88, Kampala, Uganda. [5]School of Biosecurity, Biotechnical & Laboratory Sciences, College of Veterinary Medicine, Animal Resources and Biosecurity, Makerere University, P.O Box 7062, Kampala, Uganda.

References

1. Mustafa M, et al. Risk factors, diagnosis, and Management of Peptic ulcer disease. J Dent Med Sci. 2015;14:40–6.
2. Stewart, B. et al. Global disease burden of conditions requiring emergency surgery. 9–22 (2014). https://doi.org/10.1002/bjs.9329
3. WHO. Peptic Ulcer Disease. World Health Rankings (2014).
4. Tootian Z, et al. Histological and mucin histochemical study of the small intestine of the Persian squirrel (Sciurus anomalus). Anat Sci Int. 2013;88:38–45.
5. Sung JJY, Kuipers EJ, El-serag HB. Systematic review : the global incidence and prevalence of peptic ulcer disease. Aliment Pharmacol Ther. 2009;29: 938–46.
6. Akpamu U, Owoyele V, Ozor M, Osifo U. Indomethacin-induced gsatric ulcers: Model in female wistar rats. Int. J. Basic, Appl. Innov. Res. 2013;2:78–84.
7. Allen A, Flemström G. Gastroduodenal mucus bicarbonate barrier: protection against acid and pepsin. Am J Physiol Cell Physiol. 2005;288:C1–C19.
8. Holm L, Phillipson M. Methods in Molecular Biology; 2012. p. 217–27. https://doi.org/10.1007/978-1-61779-513-8.
9. Birchenough GMH, Johansson ME, Gustafsson JK, Bergström JH, Hansson GGC. New developments in goblet cell mucus secretion and function. Mucosal Immunol. 2015;8:1–8.

10. Pelaseyed T, et al. The mucus and mucins of the goblet cells and enterocytes provide the first defense line of the gastrointestinal tract and interact with the immune system. Immunol Rev. 2014;260:8–20.

11. Johansson MEV, Sjövall H, Hansson GC. The gastrointestinal mucus system in health and disease. Nat Rev Gastroenterol Hepatol. 2013;10:352–61.

12. Latif II. Cytoprotective effects of Bauhinia purpurea leaf extract against ethanol-induced gastric mucosal ulcer in rats. Sci Res Essays. 2011;6:5396–402.

13. Gustafsson JK, Birchenough GMH, Johansson MEV, Hansson GC. New developments in goblet cell mucus secretion and function. Mucosal Immunol. 2015;32:1–8.

14. Linden SK, Sutton P, Karlsson NG, Korolik V, McGuckin MA. Mucins in the mucosal barrier to infection. Mucosal Immunol. 2008;1:183–97.

15. Sternberg LR, Bresalier RS. Inhibition of gastric mucin synthesis by helicobacter pylori. Gastroenterology. 2000;118:1072–9.

16. Boonzaier J, Van der Merwe EL, Bennett NC, Kotzé SH. A comparative histochemical study of the distribution of mucins in the gastrointestinal tracts of three insectivorous mammals. Acta Histochem. 2013;115:549–56.

17. Prathima S, Kumar HML. Mucin profile of upper gastrointestinal tract lesions. J Clin Biomed Sci. 2012;2:185–91.

18. Schenk M, Mueller C. The mucosal immune system at the gastrointestinal barrier. Best Pract Res Clin Gastroenterol. 2008;22:391–409.

19. Sarkar S, Guha D. Effect of ripe fruit pulp extract of Cucurbita pepo Linn in aspirin induced gastric and duodenal ulcer in rats. Indian J Exp Biol. 2008;46:639–45.

20. Gege-Adebayo G, Igbokwe VU, Shafe M, Akintayo C, Mbaka D. Anti-ulcer effect of ocimum gratissimum on indomethacin induced ulcer and percentage of superoxide dismutase on wistar rats. J Med Med Sci. 2013;4:8–12.

21. Koyuncu A, et al. Effect of thyroid hormones on stress ulcer formation. ANZ J Surg. 2002;72:672–5.

22. Oluwale FS, Saka MT. Effects of thyroid hormone on gastric mucus secretion around indomethacin induced gastric ulcers in rats. J MedSci. 2007;7:678–81.

23. Olaleye SB, Adeniyi OS, Emikpe BO. Thyroxine accelerates healing of acetic acid- induced gastric ulcer in rats. Arch Bas App Med. 2013;1:77–85.

24. Davis PJ, Davis FB, Moussa SA. Thyroid Hormones-induced angiogenesis. Curr. Cardiol. Rev. 2009;5:12–6.

25. Adeniyi OS, Emikpe BO, Olaleye SB. Gastric mucosa re-epithelisation, Oxidative Stress and Apoptosis During Healing of Acetic Acid-Induced Ulceration in Thyroxine Treatment and Thyroidectomy on Rats. J Afr Ass Physiol Sci. 2007;2:57–66.

26. Bruck R, et al. Induced hypothyroidism accelerates the regression of liver fibrosis in rats. J Gastroenterol Hepatol. 2006;22:2189–94.

27. Bhattacharya S, Chaudhuri SR, Chattopadhyay S, Bandyopadhyay SK. Healing properties of some Indian medicinal plants against indomethacin-induced gastric ulceration of rats. J Clin Biochem Nutr. 2007;41:106–14.

28. Forder REA, Howarth GS, Tivey DR, Hughes RJ. Bacterial modulation of small intestinal goblet cells and mucin composition during early posthatch development of poultry. Poult. Sci. 2007;86:2396–403.

29. Uni Z, Smirnov A, Sklan D. Pre- and posthatch development of goblet cells in the broiler small intestine: effect of delayed access to feed. Poult Sci. 2003;82:320–7.

30. Chinedu O, Buhari A. Evaluation of the anti-gastric ulcer effect of Methanolic extract of Pennisetum purpureum (Schumach) in male Wistar rats. Int J Curr Microbiol App Sci. 2015;4:466–74.

31. Nonose R, et al. Tissue quantification of neutral and acid mucins in the mucosa of the colon with and without fecal stream in rats. Acta Cir Bras. 2009;24:267–75.

32. Davis FB, Moussa SA, O'Connor L, Mohamed S. Proangiogenesis action of thyroid Hormoes is fibroblast growth factor dependent and is initiated at the cell surface. Circ Res. 2004;94:1500–6.

33. Tarnawski A, Szabo I, Husain S, Soreghan B. Regeneration of gastric mucosa during ulcer healing is triggered by growth factors and signal transduction pathways. J Physiol. 2001;95:337–44.

34. Zhang J, Lazar M. a. The mechanism of action of thyroid hormones. Annu Rev Physiol. 2000;62:439–66.

35. Tarım Ö. Thyroid hormones and growth in health and disease. J Clin Res Pediatr Endocrinol. 2011;3:51–5.

36. Hulbert AJ. Thyroid hormones and their effects: a new perspective. Biol. Rev. Camb. Philos. Soc. 2000;75:519–631.

37. Padra JT, et al. Aeromonas salmonicida binds differentially to mucins isolated from skin and intestinal regions of Atlantic salmon in an N-acetylneuraminic acid-dependent manner. Infect Immun. 2014;82:5235–45.

38. Marques T, David L, Reis C, Nogueira A. Topographic expression of MUC5AC and MUC6 in the gastric mucosa infected by helicobacter pylori and in associated diseases. Pathology. 2005;201:665–72.

25

A rare malignant thyroid carcinosarcoma with aggressive behavior and DICER1 gene mutation

Jing Yang, Carmen Sarita-Reyes, David Kindelberger and Qing Zhao*⬤

Abstract

Background: Malignant biphasic tumor also known as carcinosarcoma is an uncommon neoplasm that is composed of both malignant epithelial and mesenchymal components. Most reported cases of carcinosarcoma affect the female genital tract; however, other sites including head and neck, lung, and breast have been described. Carcinosarcoma of the thyroid is an extremely rare and aggressive malignancy with an ominous clinical course similar to anaplastic carcinoma.

Case presentation: We report a case of a 45-year-old female who was found to have a biphasic thyroid carcinosarcoma. Her clinical course declined significantly shortly after she underwent a total thyroidectomy and she developed distant metastases to the lungs. Histopathological features of the primary and metastatic tumor were identical. The tumor is composed of an intimately intermixed epithelial component of poorly differentiated follicular thyroid carcinoma and a spindle cell sarcoma with rhabdomyosarcoma differentiation. Molecular analysis using a next-generation sequencing based assay revealed a *DICER1* (E1705K) point mutation in neoplastic cells.

Conclusion: To our knowledge, the E1705K point mutation within the *DICER1* gene is the first reported mutation in carcinosarcoma of the thyroid. A comprehensive review of the relevant literature is also included for discussion.

Keywords: Thyroid, Carcinosarcoma, Biphasic tumor, Lung metastasis, DICER1 mutation

Background

Thyroid carcinosarcoma is a rare and aggressive malignant thyroid tumor [1]. These tumors are usually found to infiltrate the surrounding soft tissue at the time of diagnosis. The overall survival rate for these patients is only a few months and most of the cases occur in women who are older than 50 years of age. To date, less than 30 cases of thyroid carcinosarcoma have been reported in the literature (Table 1) [1–8]. According to the latest World Health Organization (WHO 2017) classification for thyroid tumors, carcinosarcoma is considered to be a variant of anaplastic carcinoma [9]. Recently, Agrawal et al. proposed that, with the presence of both malignant epithelial and mesenchymal cells, 'thyroid

carcinosarcoma' should be considered a distinct entity from anaplastic carcinoma [6].

The pathogenesis of thyroid carcinosarcoma is not fully understood. Carcinosarcoma of the thyroid has been suggested to originate from both malignant epithelial (carcinoma) and mesenchymal (sarcoma) elements of the thyroid [1, 6]. Positive immunohistochemical (IHC) staining for thyroglobulin in carcinomatous cells, and positive staining for vimentin in mesenchymal cells supports a diagnosis of carcinosarcoma [1]. In contrast, studies from anaplastic thyroid carcinoma suggested a monoclonal origin of the tumor [2]. The sarcoma-like morphology of the tumor is thought to be de-differentiated from the epithelial component during the process of carcinogenesis.

In 2013, Agrawal et al. reviewed 25 cases reported in the literature as carcinosarcoma of the thyroid. Since

* Correspondence: Grace.Zhao@bmc.org
Department of Pathology and Laboratory Medicine, Boston University
Medical Center, 670 Albany St. Biosquare III, Boston, MA 02118, USA

Table 1 Summary of all reported cases of thyroid carcinosarcoma in English literature

Author; year; Ref [#]	Morphology	Metastasis	Treatment	Survival (months)
Rasheed; 2017; [8]	Follicular carcinoma with sarcoma	none	total thyroidectomy, chemotherapy	3
Ekici; 2015; [7]	Papillary carcinoma with sarcoma	none	total thyroidectomy	2
Agrawal; 2013; [6]	Papillary carcinoma with sarcoma	lymph nodes	total thyroidectomy, right neck dissection	12
Naqiyah; 2010; [5]	Follicular carcinoma with sarcoma	none	total thyroidectomy, radiation	8
Guiffrida; 2000; [1]	Follicular carcinoma with sarcoma	bilateral lung, lymph nodes	total thyroidectomy lymph node dissection and chemoradiation therapy	6
Al-Sobhi; 1997; [4]	Follicular carcinoma with sarcoma	lung	total thyroidectomy, radiation	8
Cooper; 1989; [3]	Follicular carcinoma with chondrosarcoma	N/A	subtotal thyroidectomy	5
Donnell; 1987; [2]	Follicular carcinoma with osteosarcoma and chondrosarcoma	lung	subtotal thyroidectomy	26

then, there have been two additional cases reported. Among the reported cases, most were described as fibrosarcoma or osteosarcoma with co-existing differentiated thyroid carcinoma, such as follicular or papillary carcinoma [1–8]. In most of the cases, the tumors behaved aggressively, with death from disease occurring within 2 months to 26 months following diagnosis [1–8]. No specific molecular signatures or genetic alteration have been reported. The current report presents a case of a young female patient with a biphasic thyroid carcinosarcoma. Next generation sequencing (NGS) analysis revealed a novel point mutation in the *DICER1* gene (E1705K) in neoplastic cells.

Case presentation

A 45-year-old woman presented to our hospital with multiple lung nodules. She had a history of poorly differentiated thyroid carcinoma, diagnosed 7 months prior to admission, at an outside hospital. The patient was healthy otherwise and reported no radiation exposure or any family history of thyroid cancer. The initial work-up at the time of discovery of the right thyroid nodule included fine needle aspiration and core biopsy, with findings consistent with poorly differentiated thyroid carcinoma. The patient then underwent a total thyroidectomy and central neck lymph node dissection. The pathologic diagnosis from the outside hospital reported a 2.8 × 2.4 × 1.1 cm tumor in the right thyroid without extrathyroidal extension or lymph node metastasis. However, both capsular invasion and extensive vascular space invasion were noted. Based on the tumor size, tumor extension and lymph node status, the tumor was designated as Stage II (pT2 pN0 pMx). IHC staining showed that the tumor cells were positive for thyroglobulin and thyroid transcription factor 1 (TTF1). An immunostain for p53 was also performed at the outside hospital and showed a small focus (< 1 cm) with p53 positivity, suggesting a diagnosis of anaplastic thyroid carcinoma.

At our institution, the diagnosis was revised, based on review of both the primary thyroid tumor and the current lung metastases. Both tumors were remarkable for biphasic malignant components: the carcinoma and the sarcoma. The carcinoma component showed a poorly differentiated microfollicular type thyroid carcinoma, composed of sheets and islands of tightly packed thyroid follicles with dense colloid. The tumor nuclei were small and round with vesicular chromatin, resembling those of typical poorly differentiated follicular thyroid carcinoma. Admixed with the epithelial component were malignant spindle cells with small round blue cell type morphology. Focally, rhabdomyosarcoma-like cells with eosinophilic cytoplasm were appreciated. No heterologous cartilage or bone components were identified. The IHC staining performed at the outside hospital showed that the thyroid carcinoma (epithelial) component was positive for thyroglobulin, PAX8 and TTF1 (Fig. 1). The sarcoma (spindled) component was negative for all thyroid carcinoma markers (TTF-1, thyroglobulin and PAX8), but was positive for vimentin and focally positive for myogenin (supporting skeletal muscle differentiation) consistent with mesenchymal differentiation. Interestingly, the foci of vascular space invasion contained both epithelial and mesenchymal components as well.

The patient received Taxol with Carboplatin for 7 weeks followed by radiation therapy. Her thyroglobulin level rose from 1.2 ng/mL to 25.40 ng/mL 5 months after completion of the chemo-radiation therapy, suggesting progression of the disease. A follow-up CT scan of the chest showed multiple newly developed nodules (ranging from 1 to 2 cm) in the right lung, highly suspicious for metastases. The patient underwent a right thoracotomy, right lung resection/metastasectomy. The surgery was uneventful with negative resection margins. However, the patient's general condition deteriorated and she succumbed to the disease 4 months later.

Histological examination of the lung nodules revealed similar tumor morphology and tumor differentiation

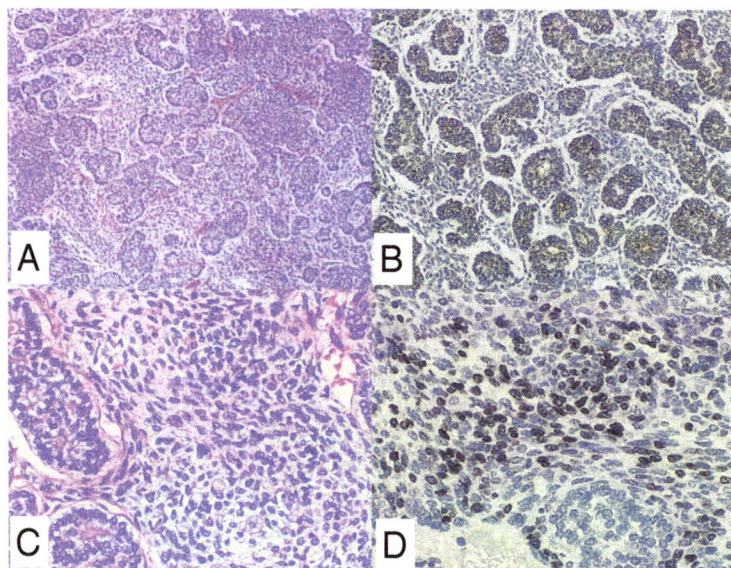

Fig. 1 Immunohistochemical stains demonstrated biphasic components. The carcinoma component (**a**) showed positivity for thyroglobulin (**b**). The sarcoma component (**c**) showed positivity for myogenin (**d**). All pictures are at 200×

when compared to the original thyroid tumor, which is somewhat unusual for a biphasic carcinosarcoma (Fig. 2). Tumor necrosis was also present. Mutational analysis using a next-generation sequencing based assay showed that the neoplastic cells from the lung metastasis were devoid of genomic alterations for known thyroid cancers, including *BRAF, RAS* family (*KRAS, NRAS* and *HRAS*), *EGFR, PTEN, TERT, PI3Kinase* or *RET. BRAF* or *RAS* family are known as the most commonly altered genes in papillary thyroid cancers. Other molecular mutations reported in the development of anaplastic thyroid carcinoma include p53, *PAX8/PPAR* gamma rearrangement [10]. None of the mentioned gene mutations were identified in our patient.

However, an interesting finding in this case is the presence of a point mutation in *DICER1* (E1705K*)* that has

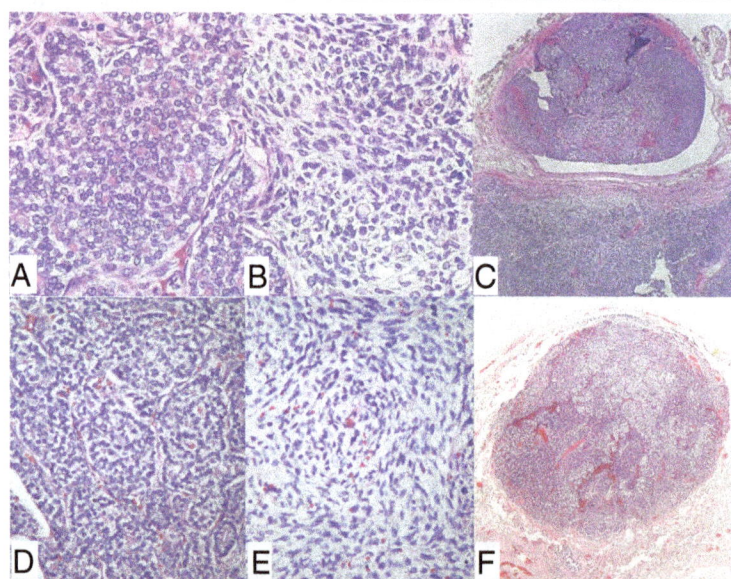

Fig. 2 Histological features of primary thyroid cancer and metastatic lung nodules. The epithelial component in the thyroid cancer (**a**) is morphologically similar to the epithelial component in the lung nodule (**d**). The sarcomatous component is composed of spindle cells both in the thyroid cancer (**b**) and in the lung nodule (**e**). There is vascular invasion in the thyroid cancer (**c**). Low power review of a small lung nodule (40×) in (**f**)

previously been associated with differentiated thyroid carcinoma [11, 12]. Whether the *DICER1* (E1705K) mutation is the underlying genetic event leading to the initiation of tumorigenesis or is downstream to other gene alterations in tumor development is largely unknown. Additional mutations of unknown significance were also detected in this tumor including *FLCN* (R239H), *POLD1* (Q684H) and *SYK* (R217L). These variants have not been adequately characterized in the scientific literature and their prognostic and therapeutic significance is unclear.

Discussion and conclusions

Thyroid carcinosarcoma is a very aggressive malignant tumor with a clinical course similar to that of anaplastic thyroid carcinoma [4]. All reported thyroid carcinosarcoma cases have resulted in patients only surviving a few months after initial diagnosis [1–8]. To our knowledge, there is no previously published molecular analysis of thyroid carcinosarcoma. This is the first report to describe potential gene alterations identified using next generation sequencing. The DICER1 protein is a member of the ribonuclease III (RNase III) family that plays an important role in the post-transcriptional regulation of gene expression. Heterozygous germline *DICER* mutations are described in the so-called DICER1 syndrome, which leads to a predisposition to develop a variety of tumors in children, including pleuropulmonary blastoma, cystic nephroma, rhabdomyosarcoma, ovarian Sertoli-Leydig tumors and multinodular goiter. A recent case study reported that a germline *DICER1* mutation (S1814 L) is associated with an increased risk of thyroid follicular carcinoma [11]. A somatic *DICER1* hotspot mutation at E1705K was reported in a case of anaplastic sarcoma of the kidney and in approximately 60% of Sertoli-Leydig cell tumors [12, 13]. The presence of this point mutation of *DICER1* at E1705K in thyroid carcinosarcoma has never been reported. The presence of a *DICER1* mutation in this case provides further evidence that development of the carcinosarcoma may not be a random occurrence, but is a likely due to a specific genetic alteration. Due to the highly aggressive nature of thyroid carcinosarcomas, the identification of specific genetic signatures for these tumors becomes critical in identifying effective treatments. However, there are still many questions regarding the pathogenesis and tumorigenesis of thyroid carcinosarcoma. Further studies will be of great benefit for the diagnosis and treatment.

Other mutations that were identified in this tumor include *POLD1* (Q684H), *FLCN* (R239H) and *SYK* (R217L). *POLD1* (Q684H) is a recently described mutation that had been reported in a patient with colorectal cancer [14]. Germline mutations in the folliculin (FLCN) gene, encoding the folliculin tumor-suppressor protein, are reported to be associated with Birt Hogg Dubé

syndrome [15]. Spleen tyrosine kinase (SYK) is an essential enzyme required for signaling involving multiple classes of immune receptors [16]. SYK functions as a modulator of tumorigenesis and has been reported in association with leukemia and breast cancers [16]. The clinical significance of *FLCN* (R239H) and *SYK* (R217L) mutations in thyroid carcinosarcoma is unknown.

The differential diagnosis of thyroid carcinosarcoma includes anaplastic carcinoma. P53 point mutations are present in 60–80% of anaplastic thyroid carcinomas. Patients develop anaplastic carcinoma from a pre or co-existent differentiated carcinoma after a multistep process of dedifferentiation associated with loss of the p53 oncogene suppressor. Due to the similarities between anaplastic carcinoma and carcinosarcoma of the thyroid gland, it has been proposed that p53 mutation may contribute to the pathogenesis of carcinosarcoma. In our patient, a less than 1 cm focus within the anaplastic area showed p53 IHC positivity. No P53 mutation was detected by next generation sequencing. Molecular pathogenetic mechanisms of p53 involvement in the transformation of carcinosarcoma are not well understood. Other mutations reported in anaplastic thyroid carcinoma include *RAS, BRAF, PTEN, TERT,* and PIK3-kinase which were not identified in this patient. Thus, the diagnosis of anaplastic carcinoma is not supported by our studies.

The clinical course of thyroid carcinosarcoma is similar to anaplastic carcinoma. Some case reports have recommended following the standard treatment approach for anaplastic carcinoma. Multimodality treatment for anaplastic carcinoma, consisting of radical surgery followed by radiotherapy and chemotherapy is reported to be associated with better clinical outcomes. However, there is no uniform consensus about the treatment approach for thyroid carcinosarcoma due to its very low incidence, its aggressive nature with poor prognosis, and the consequent lack of large clinical series. Most reported cases were treated with total or subtotal thyroidectomy. Adjuvant chemotherapy, radiation therapy and immunotherapy have not proven to be beneficial. However, NGS performed on collected thyroid carcinosarcoma cases could be of great benefit for the identification of targeted treatments.

In conclusion, the present study reports a rare case of primary thyroid carcinosarcoma with metastasis to the lung in a 45-year-old female patient who ultimately succumbed to the disease after receiving surgeries for primary and metastatic tumors and adjuvant chemoradiation therapy. Her total survival time was 11 months from the time of diagnosis and her total disease free survival was 7 months. A *DICER1* (E1705K) gene mutation was identified in this patient. Primary thyroid carcinosarcoma is extremely rare and can be diagnostically challenging.

Immunohistochemical staining may be useful for establishing a diagnosis and for distinguishing the disease from anaplastic carcinoma. Although the overall survival is dismal despite aggressive treatment, careful evaluation and the use of NGS to detect specific gene alterations may lead to the development of effective targeted therapies.

Abbreviations

BRAF: B-Raf Proto-Oncogene; DICER1: Ribonuclease III; EGFR: Epidermal growth factor receptor; IHC: Immunohistochemical; NGS: Next generation sequencing; PAX8: Paired box gene 8; PIK3kinase: Phosphatidylinositol-4, 5-bisphosphate 3-kinase; RET: Proto-oncogene encodes a receptor tyrosine kinase; TTF1: Thyroid transcription factor 1; WHO: World health organization

Acknowledgements

Not applicable.

Funding

Not applicable.

Author's contributions

All authors were directly involved in the care of this patient. JY and QZ contributed to the acquisition of data, writing and revision of the manuscript; all authors have read and approved the final version of the manuscript for publication.

Competing interests

The authors declare that they have no competing interests.

References

1. Giuffrida D, Attard M, Marasa L, Ferrau F, Marletta F, et al. Thyroid carcinosarcoma, a rare and aggressive histotype: a case report. Ann Oncol. 2000;11:1497–9.
2. Donnell C, Pollock W, Sybers W. Thyroid carcinosarcoma. Arch Pathol Lab Med. 1987;111:1169–72.
3. Cooper K, Barker E. Thyroid carcinosarcoma. A case report. S. Afr J Surg. 1989;27:192–3.
4. Al-Sobhi S, Novosolov F, Sabançi U, et al. Management of thyroid carcinosarcoma. Surgery. 1997;122:548–52.
5. Naqiyah I, Zulkarnaen AN, Rohaizak M, Das S. Carcinosarcoma of the thyroid: a case report. Hippokratia. 2010;14:141–2.
6. Agrawal M, Uppin SG, Challa S, Prayaga AK. Carcinosarcoma thyroid: an unusual morphology with a review of the literature. South Asian J Cancer. 2013;2:226.
7. Ekici M, Kocak C, Bayhan Z, et al. Carcinosarcoma of the thyroid gland. Case Rep Surg; 2015. https://doi.org/10.1155/2015/494383.
8. Rasheed R, Saeed N, Naqvi A, Rasheed S, et al. Sporadic carcinosarcoma of thyroid gland resistant to chemotherapy: a case report. J Endocrinol. Thyroid Res. 2017;1:1–3.
9. El-Naggar A, Baloch Z, Eng C, et al. Anaplastic thyroid carcinoma. In: Lloyd RV, Osamura RY, Kloppel G, Rosai J, editors. World Health Organization classification of tumors, pathology and genetics of tumors of endocrine organs. Lyon, France: IARC Press; 2017. p. 104–6.
10. Xing M. Molecular pathogenesis and mechanisms of thyroid cancer. Nat Rev Cancer. 2013;13:184–99.
11. Rutter M, Jha P, Schultz K, et al. DICER1 mutations and differentiated thyroid carcinoma: evidence of a direct association. J Clin Endocrinol Metab. 2016; 101:1–5.
12. Yoshida M, Hamanoue S, Seki M, et al. Metachronous anaplastic sarcoma of the kidney and thyroid follicular carcinoma as manifestations of DICER1 abnormalities. Hum Pathol. 2017;61:205–9.
13. Conlon N, Schultheis A, Piscuoglio S, et al. A survey of DICER1 hotspot mutations in ovarian and testicular sex cord-stromal tumors. Mod Pathol. 2015;28:1603–12.
14. Raskin L, Guo Y, Du L, et al. Targeted sequencing of established and candidate colorectal cancer genes in the colon cancer family registry cohort. Oncotarget. 2017;8:93450–63.
15. Schmidt L, Linehan W. FLCN: the causative gene for Birt-Hogg-Dubé syndrome. Gene. 2018;640:28–42.
16. Krisenko M, Geahlen R. Calling in SYK: SYK's dual role as a tumor promoter and tumor suppressor in cancer. Biochim Biophys Acta. 1853;2015:254–63.

26

Management of hypothyroidism with combination thyroxine (T4) and triiodothyronine (T3) hormone replacement in clinical practice: a review of suggested guidance

Colin Dayan[1] and Vijay Panicker[2*] (iD)

Abstract

Background: Whilst trials of combination levothyroxine/liothyronine therapy versus levothyroxine monotherapy for thyroid hormone replacement have not shown any superiority, there remains a small subset of patients who do not feel well on monotherapy. Whilst current guidelines do not suggest routine use of combination therapy they do acknowledge a trial in such patients may be appropriate. It appears that use of combination therapy and dessicated thyroid extract is not uncommon but often being used by non-specialists and not adequately monitored. This review aims to provide practical advice on selecting patients, determining dose and monitoring of such a trial.

Main body: It is important to select the correct patient for a trial so as to not delay diagnosis or potentially worsen an undiagnosed condition. An appropriate starting dose may be calculated but accuracy is limited by available formulations and cost. Monitoring of thyroid function, benefits and adverse effects are vital in the trial setting given lack of evidence of safe long term use. Also important is that patients understand set up of the trial, potential risks involved and give consent.

Conclusion: Whilst evidence is lacking on whether a small group of patients may benefit from combination therapy a trial may be indicated in those who remain symptomatic despite adequate levothyroxine monotherapy. This should be undertaken by clinicians experienced in the field with appropriate monitoring for adverse outcomes in both short and long term.

Keywords: Levothyroxine, Liothyronine, T4, T3, Thyroid hormone replacement

Background

Since the 1970s levothyroxine (LT4) has become the standard of care for thyroid hormone replacement in subjects unable to produce their own thyroid hormones due to congenital, autoimmune or iatrogenic causes. Levothyroxine has become one of the most widely used drugs worldwide, it is the most commonly prescribed drug in the United States (US), the third most in the United Kingdom (UK), and there is evidence that its use

is steadily increasing [1, 2]. Despite this, there remains controversy as to the best way to therapeutically replace thyroid hormones, with a small group of people on LT4 monotherapy not feeling as though they have achieved their premorbid well-being [3, 4] and hence a significant push for other therapies including combination LT4/ liothyronine (LT3) therapy, LT3 alone or extracts from animal thyroids.

Possible reasons for some patients not responding to levothyroxine monotherapy and evidence for efficacy of mono- and combination therapy have been well covered in recent systematic reviews by both the American Thyroid Association (ATA) [5] and European Thyroid Association

* Correspondence: Vijay.Panicker@health.wa.gov.au
[2]Department of Endocrinology, Sir Charles Gairdner Hospital, Nedlands, WA 6009, Australia
Full list of author information is available at the end of the article

(ETA) [6]. Both guidelines suggest that in select cases, a trial of therapy including LT3 can be considered, carefully supervised by an expert in the field. The purpose of this review, therefore, is not to repeat the analysis in these recent reports, but to provide a more practical approach to the use of combination therapy in clinical practice including safety aspects and cost, where a trial is considered appropriate.

The target audience for this review is clinicians who incorporate or would consider incorporating trials of combination LT4/LT3 therapy in their practice, or who have patients who have questions about this therapy. The review was performed by literature search in each area, review of published articles and studies and practical experience.

Thyroid hormone replacement

Although the thyroid gland produces T4 and T3, LT4 monotherapy has been the mainstay of thyroid hormone replacement since the 1970s replacing desiccated thyroid extract (DTE) which had been used for many years prior. This is because it is easily administered, well absorbed by the oral route and its long half-life allows for once daily dosing with very stable serum levels. It was also shown to be converted to T3 within the body [7] alleviating the need to add LT3 which does not have the same stable pharmacological profile. Furthermore, it has also been shown that the majority of circulating T3 comes from peripheral conversion of T4 to T3 and not secretion of T3 from the thyroid [8], hence a T4:T3 secretion ratio of approximately 14:1 appears average in humans, suggesting only a small role for secreted T3. However, there is a small group of patients who do not feel back to their euthyroid wellbeing despite having thyroid function tests suggestive of adequate replacement on LT4 [3, 9, 10]. There are also several studies showing that on LT4 monotherapy serum T3 levels are significantly lower for the same TSH in euthyroid patients [11–16], although the clinical significance of this is unknown. Another study showed it was not possible to normalise serum TSH, T3 and T4 levels or tissue T3 levels in laboratory animals giving them LT4 monotherapy [17].

Because of this there have now been at least 13 randomized controlled trials (RCT) comparing efficacy of combination LT4/LT3 therapy versus LT4 monotherapy for thyroid hormone replacement [18–30]. There has also been one trial comparing DTE to LT4 monotherapy [31]. The trials differ significantly in study population size, method of substituting LT3 for LT4, dose, length of study and outcomes measured. There have now been 4 systematic reviews/meta-analyses of these studies attempting to clarify the findings [32–35]. Overall these

meta-analyses have suggested there is no significant benefit of combination LT4/LT3 therapy compared to LT4 monotherapy in terms of mood, health-related quality of life or cognitive function. This provides reasonable evidence that at a population level there is no benefit of using combination therapy over monotherapy. However, the different methods of replacing LT4 with LT3 (some resulting in raised TSH suggestive of under replacement) and small size and hence power of some studies should be considered. There was no increase in adverse events in the combination groups in this admittedly short period of follow up. There is one randomized cross-over trial comparing DTE with levothyroxine monotherapy in 70 patients for 16 weeks each arm [31]. This did not show any significant benefit of DTE over LT4 in symptoms and neurocognitive markers. There was an increase in preference for DTE over LT4 however it is unclear what this signifies given an overall lack of improvement in symptoms. The study was too small to pick up subgroups responding to T3 and future studies in this area may consider having a synthetic T4/T3 arm also to determine if any benefit is due to the addition of T3 or DTE itself.

Whilst this evidence is convincing there remains a possibility that a small subset of hypothyroid patients will do better on combination therapy; this group may get lost in the larger group of patients with no benefit. Practicing clinicians will be able to identify a group of patients not satisfied on LT4 monotherapy which makes up a small subset of all their patients on LT4. There is also one study suggesting that a polymorphism in the DIO2 gene which codes for the deiodinase 2 enzyme (Thr92Ala), important for conversion of T4 to T3 in many tissues including the brain may suggest the group which will respond to therapy (rare homozygotes approximately 12% of the Caucasian population) [36]. These findings remain controversial however, particularly with inconsistent findings of the functional effect of this polymorphism [37–39].

After extensive review of available literature on this topic guidelines were produced by both the ATA and ETA related to thyroid hormone replacement with LT4 and alternatives. Both guidelines suggest there is insufficient or no strong evidence of superiority of combination LT4/LT3 therapy over LT4 monotherapy in patients with hypothyroidism. However, both acknowledge that there are patients who have persistent symptoms or sub-optimal health despite LT4 therapy guided by normal thyroid biochemistry and suggest possible reasons for this include inadequacy of LT4 monotherapy to normalise serum and tissue T4 and T3 levels. Thus, both suggest that in an appropriate clinical setting (see below) combination therapy may be trialled to determine if it is beneficial for the individual patient [5, 6]. The remainder of this review will consider practical issues related to such a trial/long term therapy.

As in all clinical practice, clinicians should only offer treatments that they are comfortable using. The experience is, however, that patients wishing for a trial are often frustrated at the lack of specialists willing to provide such, and therefore often obtain combination therapy from health practitioners with little training in the area, who do not monitor for complications, can give incorrect doses/dose ratios and offer ongoing treatment without assessing the benefits. In some instances, patients self-treat with medications obtained online. Until more is known of benefits and risks, LT3 should not be offered routinely. LT3 should only be trialled in pts. who specifically request it, who have marked persisting symptoms, and who fully understand and accept (with written/documented information if possible) the unknown potential for long-term harm. Endocrinologists are clearly best suited to provide this.

Current practice

One of the reasons for this review was that despite recommendations and guidelines from various specialist bodies, use of combination T4/T3 therapy appears significant in most developed countries. In a survey of specialist members of The Endocrine Society, The American Thyroid Association and The American Association of Clinical Endocrinologists spread internationally, but mostly in North America; showed that 3.6% of the 880 respondents would trial adding LT3 to LT4 in the setting of a hypothyroid patient with persistent symptoms despite a TSH within the target range [40]. De Jong and colleagues from the Netherlands using data from a sample of Dutch pharmacies showed that use of combination T4/T3 was 0.82% of thyroid hormone users in 2005 and this slowly rose to 0.90% by 2011 [41]. In the TEARS study population sampled from an area in Scotland 0.95% of those on thyroid hormone replacement were taking combination T4/T3 therapy and 0.21% T3 only [42]. A study by Michaelsson and colleagues from Denmark which elicited survey responses from patients known to be on T4/T3 combinations did not estimate the frequency of combination use, but did show that in the responding population of 293 on combination therapy slightly more patients had received their treatment from their GP (42%) than had from their endocrinologist (39%), 50% were on DTE with 43% on T4/T3 and 28% were adjusting their own dose [43]. This study suffers from selection bias associated with internet surveys particularly on a topic which has been strongly debated publicly recently in Denmark, however, it does highlight that methods other than LT4 monotherapy for thyroid hormone replacement may frequently not be monitored by specialists.

Practice point: Alternatives to LT4 monotherapy for thyroid hormone replacement are being used in a small percentage of hypothyroid patients and it appears frequently without specialist oversight and appropriate monitoring. If specialists are willing to discuss the available evidence, possible benefits and adverse effects of such therapy with patients, it is likely to make this practice safer.

Patient selection

Patient selection is important to determine pre-trial whether the patient is likely to gain benefit from the treatment and prevent harm to the patient. There are circumstances in which a trial may delay another treatable diagnosis or put the patient at significant risk without possibility of benefit in which it may be inappropriate.

Collect evidence that there is thyroid dysfunction

The first important step in this age of accessibility to thyroid function testing is to clarify the diagnosis of hypothyroidism requiring thyroid hormone replacement. There is good evidence from the UK that the median TSH level at which LT4 therapy was commenced is relatively low (Taylor et al. 7.8 mU/L in 2009 [2], Leese et al. 6.2 mU/L in 2001 [44]). It is therefore important to clarify the initial diagnosis, if possible with access to diagnosis thyroid function/antibody levels and presenting symptoms. It is also worthwhile considering if there was an initial response to LT4 therapy which was subsequently lost or if there was never a response.

Ensure adequate dose of LT4 has been used

It is important to ensure that the patient is on adequate T4 dosage prior to a trial of combination therapy. Most guidelines would suggest returning the serum TSH level to the population reference range as an indication of adequate replacement [45, 46], as clinical symptoms have not been shown to be accurately predict serum levels [47]. However, even with these guidelines studies have shown that a high percentage of patients on T4 have serum TSH above the reference range, even those on for many years [2, 3, 47, 48]. Furthermore, many would suggest a serum TSH in the lower part of the reference range is appropriate, given the skewed distribution of TSH values in the reference population [49], and the concept that individual TSH levels within the reference range vary little in health and therefore each person may have a genetically derived set point [50]. There are however no trials suggesting this improves any measurable clinical markers compared with TSH within the entire reference range and this practice is not accepted by all [51]. Furthemore a trial looking at slight alterations in LT4 dose in hypothyroid patients did not show any difference between clinical symptoms or measurable parameters despite clear differences in TSH on the different treatment regimens [52].

Exclude co-morbidities

Given the generalised nature of hypothyroid symptoms it is possible another condition may be causing them, or that the two conditions may co-exist, given the high prevalence of hypothyroidism in the population. Typical conditions which may lead to a mis-diagnosis are Depression, Chronic Fatigue Syndrome and Fibromyalgia. As the majority of hypothyroidism has an autoimmune origin and these conditions frequently occur with other autoimmune conditions [53–55] it is worthwhile considering whether there may be another diagnosis present with careful history taking, examination and targeted investigations if appropriate. The question of whether thyroid autoimmunity itself can cause symptoms is a more complicated one. A large population study from Norway suggests not [56], however, two smaller studies suggest an association unrelated to thyroid hormone levels [57, 58] giving it some plausibility. The answer is therefore not clear. Again, if persisting symptoms are related to thyroid autoimmunity then these would not be expected to resolve with combination therapy but should improve as antibody levels subside. However, due to the tenuous link it would appear inadvisable to be measuring thyroid antibody levels and using this as a deciding factor to initiate a trial of combination therapy.

Be aware of psychological comorbidities

This is important because psychological comorbidities may confuse the diagnosis (depressive symptoms versus hypothyroid symptoms), affect the response to treatment and in some cases be worsened by the addition of LT3 (for example anxiety).

Exclusions

Although there is little clear evidence most practitioners would exclude patients with significant cardiovascular disease or arrhythmia for a trial, given the potential to cause life-threatening side effects. Furthermore, given the importance of tight control of thyroid hormone levels, particularly T4, for the normal development of the foetus and progression of pregnancy, and lack of data showing LT3 can be safely used in pregnancy, it is not recommended in pregnant women or woman actively trying to conceive. Patients with poorly controlled anxiety and thyroid cancer requiring suppression of serum TSH may also fall into a worrying area. It is unclear whether combination therapy in disseminated thyroid cancer can adequately suppress TSH across a 24 h period, and therefore the individual patients' prognosis and need for TSH suppression needs to be considered and discussed in this setting.

Not currently useful

Is *genetic testing* a useful aid to patient selection? On current evidence there is no clear genetic test which will determine patients who will respond to therapy. Use of an unvalidated test may preclude some patients receiving a trial who may benefit and therefore it is not recommended. Further studies are required to delineate the actual genetic markers which may be useful for patient selection. In a similar way trials have not suggested a biochemical marker (including thyroid hormone levels) which will predict who will respond (Table 1).

Pharmacology and formulations

Studies using both older [59–61] and newer [62] thyroid hormone assays have suggested a diurnal rhythm of free T3 and TSH in healthy subjects with no thyroid disease. These studies suggest a peak of T3 at around 4 am with a nadir between 3 to 5 pm; this appears to lag behind TSH levels by about 90 mins [62]. Given its long half-life it is not surprising that in most studies free T4 levels remain very stable throughout the day. Despite a statistically measurable diurnal variation in T3 the actual difference in T3 levels is low (11.2%) and the levels are effectively stable over a 24 h period. It would appear reasonable to mimic these levels if trying to appropriately replace thyroid hormones, particularly as there are few biomarkers which reliably suggest complete thyroid hormone replacement. However, currently this is limited by formulations of T3 which are available (Table 2 for a non-exhaustive list). In many countries, the 20μg table of liothyronine is the only available making accurate dosing very difficult. This is reflected in the combination T4/T3 trials which were not uniform in their method of replacing LT4 with T3, either using a 10:1 or 5:1 LT4:LT3 ratio, or replacing an amount of LT4 with from a fifth to a whole dose of LT3.

Studies looking at the pharmacology of LT3 replacement all show a significant peak of serum T3 2–4 h after dose and wearing off after 12 h in those on a single daily dose, these include hypothyroid patients on combination therapy [63] (Fig. 1), LT3 monotherapy [64, 65], and

Table 1 Pre-trial assessment of potential patients

1. Collect evidence of thyroid dysfunction
2. Ensure adequate dosage of levothyroxine has been trialled
3. Exclude co-morbidiies
4. Be aware of psychological co-morbidities
5. Exclusions

Not currently useful	
	Genetics
	Biochemistry
	Symptom profile

Table 2 Available formulations of LT3 and combination LT3/LT4

Name	T3 dose	T4 dose	Available
Cytomel	5, 25, 50mcg		US, Canada, Netherlands
Thybon	20, 100mcg		UK
Tertroxin	20 mcg		Australia, South Africa
Liotyr	5 mcg (soft gel)		Italy
Prothyroid	10 mcg	100 mcg	Germany
Novothyral	5/15/20 mcg	25/75/100 mcg	Several Europe
Thyreotom forte	10/30 mcg	40/120 mcg	Czech republic

even euthyroid subjects taking LT3 only [66]. The profiles are very different to those in patient with normal endogenous thyroid function, and depending on the dose of LT3 the peak level is often above the reference range, and/or the serum TSH is raised/suppressed compared to T4 treatment [67]. Figure 1 suggests that to sample the peak serum T3 level a test taken 2–4 h after ingestion of the T3 would be appropriate. There is a study showing equivalent TSH responsiveness to TRH in patients on either T3 or T4 monotherapy [68], suggesting the rise in TSH seen in some of these studies is an indication of under replacement. Almost all the combination trials used once daily LT3 dosing with one using twice daily.

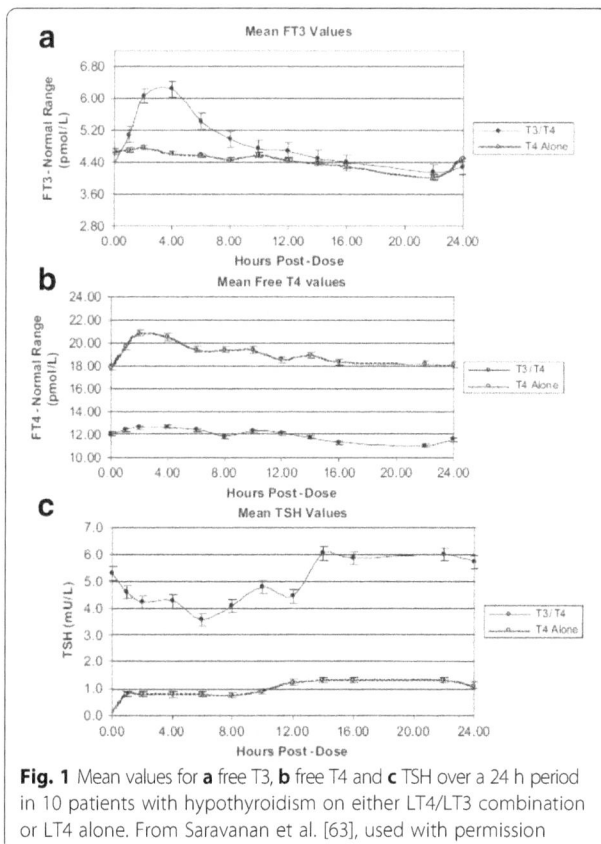

Fig. 1 Mean values for **a** free T3, **b** free T4 and **c** TSH over a 24 h period in 10 patients with hypothyroidism on either LT4/LT3 combination or LT4 alone. From Saravanan et al. [63], used with permission

To truly mimic the normal production of T3 patients would have to split the dose of T3 and take it two or three times a day, however, the large dose size of the available products may preclude this in patients with a lower requirement for thyroid hormone. Comparison of the figures from Saravanan et al. [63] and Russell et al. [62] would suggest that to mimic serum T3 levels in euthyroid individuals the LT3 dose should be split with the second dose given approximately 8 h after the first. This may prevent the insomnia reported by some patients when they take LT3 prior to bed which is presumably secondary to a serum T3 peak whilst trying to sleep. What effect this will have on the steady state of the drug is unclear as there are no studies looking at serum levels in multiple daily dosing, and even the half-life of T3 is debated with a wide range of opinions. Saravanan et al. did not find any difference in cardiovascular parameters (pulse rate and blood pressure) between their groups on T4/T3 and T4 only despite the clear peak in T3 levels at approximately 4 h. This interesting finding reminds us that serum hormone levels do not necessarily reflect action in tissues due to the presence of thyroid hormone transporters and deiodinases in different tissues which may influence the effect of these hormones in individual tissues [69]. Furthermore, most actions of thyroid hormone take several hours to have effect as they require the synthesis of new mRNA and protein.

There are no commercially available slow release T3 formulations currently. Hennemann and colleagues tested their own slow release T3 preparation in combination with T4 and found that compared to once daily T3 there was a lower peak of T3 and smoother profile [70]. They suggested all future trials use slow release T3 but a commercially available product has not been forthcoming. Doubts have been raised as to whether this study showed a product that could be used as a once a day dosage and what actual effect it had given no change in TSH levels for either formulation [71]. Compounding pharmacies will provide compounded formulations of slow release T3, however the ATA do not recommend the use of compounded preparations except in cases of clear allergic reactions to commercial preparations [5]. This is because there are few studies on these products that meet scientific criteria for rigorous peer review showing that they can be used to provide adequate thyroid hormone replacement, are equivalent to approved preparations or have a long-term safety profile. Furthermore, the preparations need to be used relatively quickly after synthesis to prevent loss of efficacy due to degradation [72], requiring regular compounding of new products. In addition, compounded preparations are generally higher in cost and not standardised between different pharmacies. There have also been reports of thyrotoxicosis [73, 74] and hypothyroidism [75] caused by errors in compounding.

Practice point: be aware of formulations of LT3 and LT4/LT3 available locally and if possible their pharmacokinetics. Errors in the preparations of compounded preparations have been reported.

Dosage

Wiersinga et al. in their review suggest 3 different methods for calculating appropriate dosages for combination T4/T3 therapy [6]. These are based on the assumptions that persisting symptoms are due to LT4 monotherapy being unable to deliver normal serum and tissue T4 and T3 levels in humans as shown in rats [17] and that mimicking the normal thyroid secretion of T4 and T3 will correct this [76]. The methods are based on using the dose of LT4 which gives the target TSH in the patient, then replacing a small amount of T4 with T3 using a 3:1 equivalence ratio derived from a study in thyroidectomized patients [77] to give the appropriate ratio. The three methods give a final dose T4:T3 ratio between 13:1 and 20:1, much closer to normal human thyroid secretion [8] but in generally lower than those used in the T4/T3 studies, in some cases significantly lower. Furthermore, many of the studies had variable ratios due to a fixed substitution (eg. 10μg T3 for 50μg T4). This dose ratio is also significantly lower than that of animal thyroid extracts in which the T4:T3 ratio is generally around 4:1 (see later). Note also however that for a patient previously on 100μg of T4 a day the T3 dose from these methods is between 4 and 6μg a day which with most current formulations would be difficult to deliver in a split dose.

Practice point: starting dose in a patient on adequate LT4 monotherapy will always require removal of part of the LT4 dose and replacement with LT3. In practice the dose of LT3 will usually be a dose of 5 – 20 mcg a day in a split dose, by necessity often determined by the availability of low dose formulations of LT3.

Length of trial

Again, there is very little evidence to determine how long a trial of combination therapy should be, the RCTs ranged from 5 weeks to 52 weeks. Most of those who showed a benefit had shown this by 3 months, and it is generally advised that 6 weeks to 3 months are waited until LT4 dose is adjusted to allow a steady state to develop in all tissues. It would therefore be reasonable to give a 3–6 month trial before deciding if it has been beneficial to the patient symptoms. If there is clear benefit it would be reasonable to continue the trial further, however, given the significant placebo effect seen in trials of thyroid hormone replacement [26] and the fact that LT3 may initially give a feeling of euphoria, clinicians should be encouraged to continue to assess the treatment as the benefit may disappear. The fixed term nature of the trial should be agreed with the patient prior to beginning and there should be agreement that there will be a return to LT4 monotherapy if no significant benefit is seen, given its easier dosing and better evidence of its safety. Figure 2 displays a proposed timeline for a trial.

Practice point: initial trial 6 months, and then confirm benefit is still present at least 1 year before planning long-term therapy

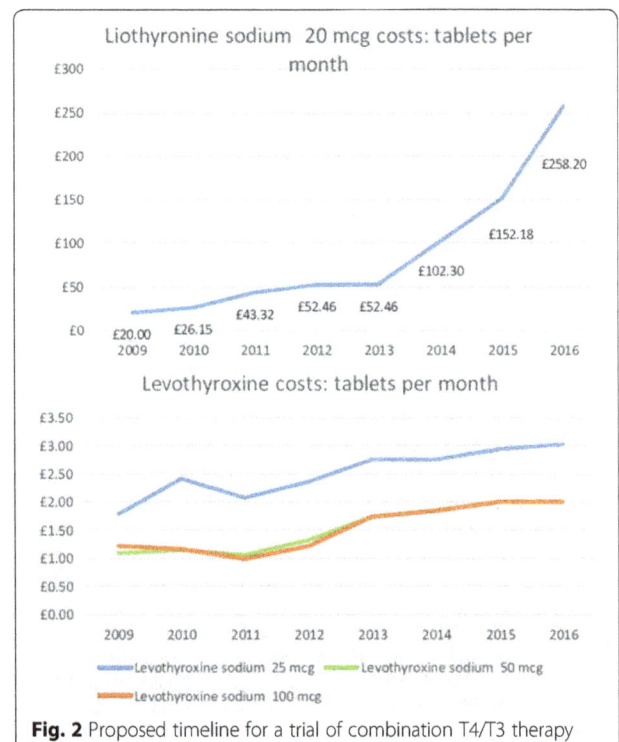

Fig. 2 Proposed timeline for a trial of combination T4/T3 therapy

Monitoring

There are no long term studies which link serum levels of T3 to adverse outcomes and therefore are able to direct monitoring of combination T4/T3 therapy. Given evidence for poorer outcomes with raised thyroid hormone levels/suppressed TSH levels in both subjects not on thyroid hormone replacement and on LT4 monotherapy it is reasonable to measure TSH, free T4 and free T3 2–4 h post dose as this is the expected peak of serum T3 post dose. Keeping both the serum T3 and TSH within the reference range at this point would suggest that the patient is at the least risk of developing both short and long term complications. Monitoring of these would include clinical assessment of pulse rate and rhythm, blood pressure, mood (particularly anxiety) and as clinically appropriate (depending on individual patient characteristics): ECG, echocardiogram and Bone Densitometry. Whilst studies in patients on LT4 would suggest that dose changes can be seen in end organ markers such as serum cholesterol and sex hormone binding globulin (SHBG), these changes are so small that they are often contained in the normal variance in the population.

Practice point: Patients should be monitored indefinitely for cardiovascular, psychological and bone adverse effects.

Safety

Given the relatively small number of patients using combination T4/T3 therapy safety data has until recently been lacking. None of the 13 RCTs comparing combination therapy to T4 monotherapy showed any increase in adverse events in the combination group, however the follow up was generally short ranging from 5 to 52 weeks. Leese et al. have recently reported safety data in their observational cohort in the TEARS study [42]. In this study a subgroup of patients on thyroid hormone placement were considered with outcomes for those who had ever been taking LT3 ($n = 400$) compared to those who had only ever taken LT4 ($n = 33,955$). The study showed no increase in cardiovascular disease, atrial fibrillation or fractures (outcomes previously shown to be associated with levothyroxine overtreatment [78]) with a median follow-up of 9 years. There was an increased risk for new prescriptions of anti-psychotic medications of unclear significance. There was also a possible association with an increased risk of breast cancer in subjects who had taken LT3. Although there is some data on T3 augmentation of breast cancer cell line proliferation and higher endogenous T3 being associated with more aggressive breast cancers, the authors point out that this association was of borderline statistical significance and not related to number of prescriptions of LT3,

arguing against a causal relationship. This potential association should be assessed in other large cohorts. The data from Leese et al. are from an observational study and so carry a risk of bias and self-selection; in addition the duration of LT3 use was not quantified. However, this may be the largest and longest duration study of its type for some time and offers some reassurance that the risks of taking T3 are not greater than expected.

Cost

Lack of regulation of the cost of unbranded Liothyronine in the UK has seen the price rise markedly in recent years, currently 28 tablets of 20mcg costs around £258.20, therefore 10mcg bd for a year would cost around £3365 per patient. This represents a greater than 4000% increase from the branded 'Tertroxin' (just over £13 for 100 tablets) which precipitated a 'black listing' of the use of LT3 in several health trusts (Fig. 3) and has now attracted the attention of the UK regulatory and competition and markets authority. Synthetic T4 as Levothyroxine 100mcg once daily costs approximately £25 per patient per year. Whilst the government looks to close the loophole allowing companies to do this, many patients who had been maintained on LT3/LT4 for many years have been forced to come off LT3 or source it from overseas.

In Australia a similar dose of Liothyronine would cost $142 Australian dollars for a year on a private prescription, it is available on a government subsidized prescription for half that cost, available for patients who 'have a documented intolerance or resistance to thyroxine', which is open to the interpretation of the treating physician. A 100mcg tablet of thyroxine would cost around $58 Australia dollars a year on the government scheme.

In the US for patients not covered by health insurance, hypothyroid treatment typically costs $15–$100 per month – or $180–$1200 per year – for the synthetic thyroid hormone typically prescribed. For example, Drugstore.com charges about $15–$20, depending on the dose, for a one-month supply of the brand-name drug Levothroid, or $25–$45 for a one-month supply of the brand-name drug Synthroid. Drugstore.com charges

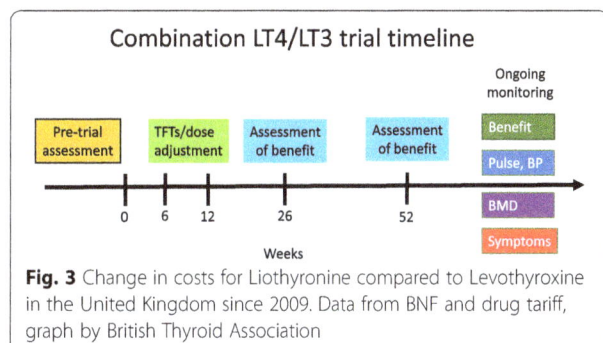

Fig. 3 Change in costs for Liothyronine compared to Levothyroxine in the United Kingdom since 2009. Data from BNF and drug tariff, graph by British Thyroid Association

up to $100 or more for a one-month supply, depending on dosage, of the brand-name drug Cytomel (LT3). Therefore in most countries combination therapy is comes at increased cost to the patient (or government) and this needs to be taken into consideration when planning a trial.

Practice point: be aware and make patients aware of costs and availability of formulations prior to prescribing.

Dessicated thyroid extract

Many patients and alternative physicians prefer to use forms of dessicated thyroid extract (DTE) for thyroid hormone replacement. DTE is described as "the cleaned, dried, and powdered thyroid gland previously deprived of connective tissue and fat. It is obtained from domesticated animals that are used for food by humans" by the United States Pharmacopeia. Extracts of animal thyroids have been used for hypothyroid symptoms for many centuries in different cultures, and as a form similar to what is used today for over 110 years [79]. Most formulations are from porcine thyroid; however some from bovine thyroid or a combination of the two exist. Initially it was titrated to improvement in clinical symptoms and avoidance of hyperthyroid symptoms. The development of Levothyroxine and ability to assay serum TSH, T4 and T3 levels in the 1980's led to calls for removal of DTE for treatment of hypothyroidism because of supraphysiological levels of T3 post dose, hyperthyroid symptoms and complications, and fluctuating levels of T3 as compared to very stable TSH, T3 and T4 levels with levothyroxine dosing [80–83]. Despite continuing concerns about these issues and also the consistency of the various preparations it continues to be used. Whilst the dramatic cases of thyroxtoxicosis on these preparations are mainly historical, there remain concerns about frequency of adverse events and calls for greater standardization of these preparations [84].

DTE is often prescribed in grains: 1 grain is typically around 60-65 mg of DTE and most commonly contains 38μg of T4 and 9μg of T3. Bioavailability has been shown to be different to synthetic LT4 and LT3 preparations [81]. Table 3 displays commonly available brands and doses contained. The doses above give a T4:T3 ratio

Table 3 Dessicated thyroid extract formulations

Name	T3 dose	T4 dose	Available
Nature thyroid per 65 mg grain	9mcg	38mcg	US
Westhroid pure per 65 mg grain	9mcg	38mcg	US
NP thyroid per 60 mg grain	9mcg	38mcg	US
Thyroid (erfa) per 60 mg grain	8mcg	35mcg	Europe/Canada
Armour thyroid per 60 mg grain	9mcg	38mcg	US

of 4.2:1 significantly more T3 than the 14:1 secreted by the normal thyroid and the doses recommended above. This makes dosing difficult as displayed by several studies which have shown supraphysiological T3 doses post dose, fluctuating T3 levels during the day and more hyperthyroid symptoms in subjects taking DTE compared to LT4 monotherapy [80, 82, 85, 86]. As with combination T4/T3 therapy, there are no longer term trials or safety data available on long term use of DTE. This is important as there are concerns that regular supraphysiological levels of T3 may induce hyperthyroidism-like complications over the longer term. Given lack of safety data, difference and variability in the various preparations and no studies showing clear benefit over T4 monotherapy, all major endocrine and thyroid societies currently advise against the routine use of DTE for thyroid hormone replacement [5, 6].

Amour thyroid is the most commonly used formulation, also the most expensive, and in the US costs around $1 per 60 mg grain.. Price varies across the UK mostly around £1 per grain. These formulations are not available in Australia and therefore most users import them from the US at similar cost plus postage.

DTE formulations contain unmeasured quantities of diiodothyronine and monoiiodothyronine which many of its supporters believe make it a more suitable replacement for thyroid hormone, although there are no studies suggesting these are required for normal functioning, or that they are secreted in significant quantities from a normal human thyroid. These products also contain other thyroid-related proteins and antigens which could potentially invoke immune responses; these have not been studied to date.

Practice point: whilst all major endocrine and thyroid societies advise against the use of DTE for hypothyroidism, it is clear that its use remains significant. Better regulated formulations and trials are required to determine its role, if any. Until these are available patients who continue to use DTE should be advised on appropriate safety monitoring as for using T4/T3.

Conclusion

Although there is convincing evidence that there is no benefit of combination T4/T3 therapy over T4 monotherapy for management of hypothyroidism at a population level, there remains a population of patients who do not feel well on T4 monotherapy. There are several possible reasons for this, one of which is an inability to use T4 effectively in a group of patients who may respond better to combination T4/T3 therapy. This will remain a possibility until large RCTs in an appropriately targeted population can confirm or refute it, and whilst it does a trial of combination therapy in such patients may be indicated. It is important that this be performed by a clinician with adequate knowledge and experience in the area, with appropriate patient selection, clear explanation of risks and benefits to the patient for consent and careful monitoring and follow-up. Possible ways to do this are covered in this review although it is clear that further research into this area and possible methods of delivering T3 are required.

Abbreviations

ATA: American Thyroid Association; DTE: Dessicated Thyroid Extract; ECG: Electrocardiogram; ETA: European Thyroid Association; LT3: Liothyronine; LT4: Levothyroxine; mg: Milligram; RCT: Randomised Controlled Trial; SHBG: Sex Hormone Binding Globulin; T3: Tri-iodothyronine; T4: Thyroxine; TRH: Thyrotropin Releasing Hormone; TSH: Thyroid Stimulating Hormone; µg: Micrograms; UK: United Kingdom; US: United States (of America)

Acknowledgements

Not applicable.

Funding

Not applicable.

Authors' contributions

VP performed literature search and drafted manuscript. CD help draft manuscript, added additional references. Both authors read and approved the final manuscript.

Competing interests

The authors declare that they have no competing interests.

Author details

[1]Thyroid Research Group, School of Medicine, Cardiff University, Cardiff, UK. [2]Department of Endocrinology, Sir Charles Gairdner Hospital, Nedlands, WA 6009, Australia.

References

1. Rodriguez-Gutierrez R, Maraka S, Ospina NS, Montori VM, Brito JP. Levothyroxine overuse: time for an about face? Lancet Diabetes Endocrinol. 2016;5(4):246–8.
2. Taylor PN, Iqbal A, Minassian C, Sayers A, Draman MS, Greenwood R, Hamilton W, Okosieme O, Panicker V, Thomas SL, et al. Falling threshold for treatment of borderline elevated thyrotropin levels-balancing benefits and risks: evidence from a large community-based study. JAMA Intern Med. 2014;174(1):32–9.
3. Saravanan P, Chau WF, Roberts N, Vedhara K, Greenwood R, Dayan CM. Psychological well-being in patients on 'adequate' doses of l-thyroxine: results of a large, controlled community-based questionnaire study. Clin Endocrinol. 2002;57(5):577–85.
4. Engum A, Bjøro T, Mykletun A, Dahl AA. An association between depression, anxiety and thyroid function–a clinical fact or an artefact? Acta Psychiatr Scand. 2002;106(1):27–34.
5. Jonklaas J, Bianco AC, Bauer AJ, Burman KD, Cappola AR, Celi FS, Cooper DS, Kim BW, Peeters RP, Rosenthal MS, et al. Guidelines for the treatment of hypothyroidism: prepared by the american thyroid association task force on thyroid hormone replacement. Thyroid. 2014;24(12):1670–751.
6. Wiersinga WM, Duntas L, Fadeyev V, Nygaard B, Vanderpump MP. 2012 ETA guidelines: the use of L-T4 + L-T3 in the treatment of hypothyroidism. Eur Thyroid J. 2012;1(2):55–71.
7. Braverman LE, Vagenakis A, Downs P, Foster AE, Sterling K, Ingbar SH. Effects of replacement doses of sodium L-thyroxine on the peripheral metabolism of thyroxine and triiodothyronine in man. J Clin Invest. 1973;52(5):1010–7.
8. Pilo A, Iervasi G, Vitek F, Ferdeghini M, Cazzuola F, Bianchi R. Thyroidal and peripheral production of 3,5,3'-triiodothyronine in humans by multicompartmental analysis. Am J Phys. 1990;258(4 Pt 1):E715–26.
9. van de Ven AC, Netea-Maier RT, de Vegt F, Ross HA, Sweep FC, Kiemeney LA, Hermus AR, den Heijer M. Is there a relationship between fatigue perception and the serum levels of thyrotropin and free thyroxine in euthyroid subjects? Thyroid. 2012;22(12):1236–43.
10. Wekking EM, Appelhof BC, Fliers E, Schene AH, Huyser J, Tijssen JG, Wiersinga WM. Cognitive functioning and well-being in euthyroid patients on thyroxine replacement therapy for primary hypothyroidism. Eur J Endocrinol. 2005;153(6):747–53.
11. Jonklaas J, Davidson B, Bhagat S, Soldin SJ. Triiodothyronine levels in athyreotic individuals during levothyroxine therapy. JAMA. 2008;299(7):769–77.
12. Woeber KA. Levothyroxine therapy and serum free thyroxine and free triiodothyronine concentrations. J Endocrinol Investig. 2002;25(2):106–9.
13. Gullo D, Latina A, Frasca F, Le Moli R, Pellegriti G, Vigneri R. Levothyroxine monotherapy cannot guarantee euthyroidism in all athyreotic patients. PLoS One. 2011;6(8):e22552.
14. Alevizaki M, Mantzou E, Cimponeriu AT, Alevizaki CC, Koutras DA. TSH may not be a good marker for adequate thyroid hormone replacement therapy. Wien Klin Wochenschr. 2005;117(18):636–40.
15. Ito M, Miyauchi A, Morita S, Kudo T, Nishihara E, Kihara M, Takamura Y, Ito Y, Kobayashi K, Miya A, et al. TSH-suppressive doses of levothyroxine are required to achieve preoperative native serum triiodothyronine levels in patients who have undergone total thyroidectomy. Eur J Endocrinol. 2012;167(3):373–8.
16. Peterson SJ, McAninch EA, Bianco AC. Is a normal TSH synonymous with "Euthyroidism" in levothyroxine monotherapy? J Clin Endocrinol Metab. 2016;101(12):4964–73.
17. Escobar-Morreale HF, Obregón MJ, Escobar del Rey F, Morreale de Escobar G. Replacement therapy for hypothyroidism with thyroxine alone does not ensure euthyroidism in all tissues, as studied in thyroidectomized rats. J Clin Invest. 1995;96(6):2828–38.
18. Bunevicius R, Kazanavicius G, Zalinkevicius R, Prange AJ. Effects of thyroxine as compared with thyroxine plus triiodothyronine in patients with hypothyroidism. N Engl J Med. 1999;340(6):424–9.
19. Bunevicius R, Jakuboniene N, Jakubonien N, Jurkevicius R, Cernicat J, Lasas L, Prange AJ. Thyroxine vs thyroxine plus triiodothyronine in treatment of hypothyroidism after thyroidectomy for Graves' disease. Endocrine. 2002;18(2):129–33.
20. Clyde PW, Harari AE, Getka EJ, Shakir KM. Combined levothyroxine plus liothyronine compared with levothyroxine alone in primary hypothyroidism: a randomized controlled trial. JAMA. 2003;290(22):2952–8.
21. Sawka AM, Gerstein HC, Marriott MJ, MacQueen GM, Joffe RT. Does a combination regimen of thyroxine (T4) and 3,5,3'-triiodothyronine improve depressive symptoms better than T4 alone in patients with hypothyroidism? Results of a double-blind, randomized, controlled trial. J Clin Endocrinol Metab. 2003;88(10):4551–5.
22. Rodriguez T, Lavis VR, Meininger JC, Kapadia AS, Stafford LF. Substitution of liothyronine at a 1:5 ratio for a portion of levothyroxine: effect on fatigue, symptoms of depression, and working memory versus treatment with levothyroxine alone. Endocr Pract. 2005;11(4):223–33.
23. Walsh JP, Shiels L, Lim EM, Bhagat CI, Ward LC, Stuckey BG, Dhaliwal SS, Chew GT, Bhagat MC, Cussons AJ. Combined thyroxine/liothyronine treatment does not improve well-being, quality of life, or cognitive function compared to thyroxine alone: a randomized controlled trial in patients with primary hypothyroidism. J Clin Endocrinol Metab. 2003;88(10):4543–50.
24. Appelhof BC, Fliers E, Wekking EM, Schene AH, Huyser J, Tijssen JG, Endert E, van Weert HC, Wiersinga WM. Combined therapy with levothyroxine and

liothyronine in two ratios, compared with levothyroxine monotherapy in primary hypothyroidism: a double-blind, randomized, controlled clinical trial. J Clin Endocrinol Metab. 2005;90(5):2666–74.

25. Escobar-Morreale HF, Botella-Carretero JI, Gómez-Bueno M, Galán JM, Barrios V, Sancho J. Thyroid hormone replacement therapy in primary hypothyroidism: a randomized trial comparing L-thyroxine plus liothyronine with L-thyroxine alone. Ann Intern Med. 2005;142(6):412–24.

26. Saravanan P, Simmons DJ, Greenwood R, Peters TJ, Dayan CM. Partial substitution of thyroxine (T4) with tri-iodothyronine in patients on T4 replacement therapy: results of a large community-based randomized controlled trial. J Clin Endocrinol Metab. 2005;90(2):805–12.

27. Siegmund W, Spieker K, Weike AI, Giessmann T, Modess C, Dabers T, Kirsch G, Sänger E, Engel G, Hamm AO, et al. Replacement therapy with levothyroxine plus triiodothyronine (bioavailable molar ratio 14 : 1) is not superior to thyroxine alone to improve well-being and cognitive performance in hypothyroidism. Clin Endocrinol. 2004;60(6):750–7.

28. Nygaard B, Jensen EW, Kvetny J, Jarløv A, Faber J. Effect of combination therapy with thyroxine (T4) and 3,5,3'-triiodothyronine versus T4 monotherapy in patients with hypothyroidism, a double-blind, randomised cross-over study. Eur J Endocrinol. 2009;161(6):895–902.

29. Valizadeh M, Seyyed-Majidi MR, Hajibeigloo H, Momtazi S, Musavinasab N, Hayatbakhsh MR. Efficacy of combined levothyroxine and liothyronine as compared with levothyroxine monotherapy in primary hypothyroidism: a randomized controlled trial. Endocr Res. 2009;34(3):80–9.

30. Fadeyev VV, Morgunova TB, Melnichenko GA, Dedov II. Combined therapy with L-thyroxine and L-triiodothyronine compared to L-thyroxine alone in the treatment of primary hypothyroidism. Hormones (Athens). 2010;9(3):245–52.

31. Hoang TD, Olsen CH, Mai VQ, Clyde PW, Shakir MK. Desiccated thyroid extract compared with levothyroxine in the treatment of hypothyroidism: a randomized, double-blind, crossover study. J Clin Endocrinol Metab. 2013; 98(5):1982–90.

32. Grozinsky-Glasberg S, Fraser A, Nahshoni E, Weizman A, Leibovici L. Thyroxine-triiodothyronine combination therapy versus thyroxine monotherapy for clinical hypothyroidism: meta-analysis of randomized controlled trials. J Clin Endocrinol Metab. 2006;91(7):2592–9.

33. Escobar-Morreale HF, Botella-Carretero JI, Escobar del Rey F, Morreale de Escobar G. REVIEW: treatment of hypothyroidism with combinations of levothyroxine plus liothyronine. J Clin Endocrinol Metab. 2005;90(8):4946–54.

34. Joffe RT, Brimacombe M, Levitt AJ, Stagnaro-Green A. Treatment of clinical hypothyroidism with thyroxine and triiodothyronine: a literature review and metaanalysis. Psychosomatics. 2007;48(5):379–84.

35. Ma C, Xie J, Huang X, Wang G, Wang Y, Wang X, Zuo S. Thyroxine alone or thyroxine plus triiodothyronine replacement therapy for hypothyroidism. Nucl Med Commun. 2009;30(8):586–93.

36. Panicker V, Saravanan P, Vaidya B, Evans J, Hattersley AT, Frayling TM, Dayan CM. Common variation in the DIO2 gene predicts baseline psychological well-being and response to combination thyroxine plus triiodothyronine therapy in hypothyroid patients. J Clin Endocrinol Metab. 2009;94(5):1623–9.

37. Appelhof BC, Peeters RP, Wiersinga WM, Visser TJ, Wekking EM, Huyser J, Schene AH, Tijssen JG, Hoogendijk WJ, Fliers E. Polymorphisms in type 2 deiodinase are not associated with well-being, neurocognitive functioning, and preference for combined thyroxine/3,5,3'-triiodothyronine therapy. J Clin Endocrinol Metab. 2005;90(11):6296–9.

38. Carlé A, Faber J, Steffensen R, Laurberg P, Nygaard B. Hypothyroid patients encoding combined MCT10 and DIO2 gene polymorphisms may prefer L-T3 + L-T4 combination treatment - data using a blind, randomized, clinical study. Eur Thyroid J. 2017;6(3):143–51.

39. Wouters HJ, van Loon HC, van der Klauw MM, Elderson MF, Slagter SN, Kobold AM, Kema IP, Links TP, van Vliet-Ostaptchouk JV, Wolffenbuttel BH. No effect of the Thr92Ala polymorphism of Deiodinase-2 on thyroid hormone parameters, health-related quality of life, and cognitive functioning in a large population-based cohort study. Thyroid. 2017;27(2):147–55.

40. Burch HB, Burman KD, Cooper DS, Hennessey JV. A 2013 survey of clinical practice patterns in the management of primary hypothyroidism. J Clin Endocrinol Metab. 2014;99(6):2077–85.

41. de Jong NW, Baljet GM. Use of t4, t4 + t3, and t3 in the dutch population in the period 2005-2011. Eur Thyroid J. 2012;1(2):135–6.

42. Leese GP, Soto-Pedre E, Donnelly LA. Liothyronine use in a 17 year observational population-based study - the tears study. Clin Endocrinol. 2016;85(6):918–25.

43. Michaelsson LF, Medici BB, la Cour JL, Selmer C, Røder M, Perrild H, Knudsen N, Faber J, Nygaard B. Treating hypothyroidism with thyroxine/triiodothyronine

44. Leese GP, Flynn RV, Jung RT, Macdonald TM, Murphy MJ, Morris AD. Increasing prevalence and incidence of thyroid disease in Tayside, Scotland: the Thyroid Epidemiology Audit and Research Study (TEARS). Clin Endocrinol. 2008;68(2):311–6.

45. Mandel SJ, Brent GA, Larsen PR. Levothyroxine therapy in patients with thyroid disease. Ann Intern Med. 1993;119(6):492–502.

46. Singer PA, Cooper DS, Levy EG, Ladenson PW, Braverman LE, Daniels G, Greenspan FS, McDougall IR, Nikolai TF. Treatment guidelines for patients with hyperthyroidism and hypothyroidism. Standards of Care Committee, American Thyroid Association. JAMA. 1995;273(10):808–12.

47. Canaris GJ, Manowitz NR, Mayor G, Ridgway EC. The Colorado thyroid disease prevalence study. Arch Intern Med. 2000;160(4):526–34.

48. Parle JV, Franklyn JA, Cross KW, Jones SR, Sheppard MC. Thyroxine prescription in the community: serum thyroid stimulating hormone level assays as an indicator of undertreatment or overtreatment. Br J Gen Pract. 1993;43(368):107–9.

49. Wartofsky L, Dickey RA. The evidence for a narrower thyrotropin reference range is compelling. J Clin Endocrinol Metab. 2005;90(9):5483–8.

50. Andersen S, Pedersen KM, Bruun NH, Laurberg P. Narrow individual variations in serum T(4) and T(3) in normal subjects: a clue to the understanding of subclinical thyroid disease. J Clin Endocrinol Metab. 2002;87(3):1068–72.

51. Surks MI, Goswami G, Daniels GH. The thyrotropin reference range should remain unchanged. J Clin Endocrinol Metab. 2005;90(9):5489–96.

52. Walsh JP, Ward LC, Burke V, Bhagat CI, Shiels L, Henley D, Gillett MJ, Gilbert R, Tanner M, Stuckey BG. Small changes in thyroxine dosage do not produce measurable changes in hypothyroid symptoms, well-being, or quality of life: results of a double-blind, randomized clinical trial. J Clin Endocrinol Metab. 2006;91(7):2624–30.

53. Somers EC, Thomas SL, Smeeth L, Hall AJ. Are individuals with an autoimmune disease at higher risk of a second autoimmune disorder? Am J Epidemiol. 2009;169(6):749–55.

54. Boelaert K, Newby PR, Simmonds MJ, Holder RL, Carr-Smith JD, Heward JM, Manji N, Allahabadia A, Armitage M, Chatterjee KV, et al. Prevalence and relative risk of other autoimmune diseases in subjects with autoimmune thyroid disease. Am J Med. 2010;123(2):183.e181-189.

55. Weetman AP. Diseases associated with thyroid autoimmunity: explanations for the expanding spectrum. Clin Endocrinol. 2011;74(4):411–8.

56. Engum A, Bjøro T, Mykletun A, Dahl AA. Thyroid autoimmunity, depression and anxiety; are there any connections? An epidemiological study of a large population. J Psychosom Res. 2005;59(5):263–8.

57. Pop VJ, Maartens LH, Leusink G, van Son MJ, Knottnerus AA, Ward AM, Metcalfe R, Weetman AP. Are autoimmune thyroid dysfunction and depression related? J Clin Endocrinol Metab. 1998;83(9):3194–7.

58. Ott J, Promberger R, Kober F, Neuhold N, Tea M, Huber JC, Hermann M. Hashimoto's thyroiditis affects symptom load and quality of life unrelated to hypothyroidism: a prospective case-control study in women undergoing thyroidectomy for benign goiter. Thyroid. 2011;21(2):161–7.

59. Lucke C, Hehrmann R, von Mayersbach K, von zur Mühlen A. Studies on circadian variations of plasma TSH, thyroxine and triiodothyronine in man. Acta Endocrinol. 1977;86(1):81–8.

60. Weeke J, Gundersen HJ. Circadian and 30 minutes variations in serum TSH and thyroid hormones in normal subjects. Acta Endocrinol. 1978;89(4):659–72.

61. Balsam A, Dobbs CR, Leppo LE. Circadian variations in concentrations of plasma thyroxine and triiodothyronine in man. J Appl Physiol. 1975;39(2):297–9.

62. Russell W, Harrison RF, Smith N, Darzy K, Shalet S, Weetman AP, Ross RJ. Free triiodothyronine has a distinct circadian rhythm that is delayed but parallels thyrotropin levels. J Clin Endocrinol Metab. 2008;93(6):2300–6.

63. Saravanan P, Siddique H, Simmons DJ, Greenwood R, Dayan CM. Twenty-four hour hormone profiles of TSH, Free T3 and free T4 in hypothyroid patients on combined T3/T4 therapy. Exp Clin Endocrinol Diabetes. 2007;115(4):261–7.

64. Saberi M, Utiger RD. Serum thyroid hormone and thyrotropin concentrations during thyroxine and triiodothyronine therapy. J Clin Endocrinol Metab. 1974;39(5):923–7.

65. Jonklaas J, Burman KD. Daily administration of short-acting liothyronine is associated with significant triiodothyronine excursions and fails to alter thyroid-responsive parameters. Thyroid. 2016;26(6):770–8.

66. Leggio GM, Incognito T, Privitera G, Marano MR, Drago F. Comparative bioavailability of different formulations of levothyroxine and liothyronine in healthy volunteers. J Endocrinol Invest. 2006;29(11):RC35–8.

67. Fadeyev VV, Morgunova TB, Sytch JP, Melnichenko GA. TSH and thyroid hormones concentrations in patients with hypothyroidism receiving replacement therapy with L-thyroxine alone or in combination with L-triiodothyronine. Hormones (Athens). 2005;4(2):101–7.

68. Yavuz S, Linderman JD, Smith S, Zhao X, Pucino F, Celi FS. The dynamic pituitary response to escalating-dose TRH stimulation test in hypothyroid patients treated with liothyronine or levothyroxine replacement therapy. J Clin Endocrinol Metab. 2013;98(5):E862–6.

69. Cheng S-Y, Leonard JL, Davis PJ. Molecular aspects of thyroid hormone actions. Endocr Rev. 2010;31(2):139–70.

70. Hennemann G, Docter R, Visser TJ, Postema PT, Krenning EP. Thyroxine plus low-dose, slow-release triiodothyronine replacement in hypothyroidism: proof of principle. Thyroid. 2004;14(4):271–5.

71. Wartofsky L. Combined levotriiodothyronine and levothyroxine therapy for hypothyroidism: are we a step closer to the magic formula? Thyroid. 2004;14(4):247–8.

72. Boulton DW, Fawcett JP, Woods DJ. Stability of an extemporaneously compounded levothyroxine sodium oral liquid. Am J Health Syst Pharm. 1996;53(10):1157–61.

73. Jha S, Waghdhare S, Reddi R, Bhattacharya P. Thyroid storm due to inappropriate administration of a compounded thyroid hormone preparation successfully treated with plasmapheresis. Thyroid. 2012;22(12):1283–6.

74. Bains A, Brosseau AJ, Harrison D. Iatrogenic thyrotoxicosis secondary to compounded liothyronine. Can J Hosp Pharm. 2015;68(1):57–9.

75. Pappy AL, Oyesiku N, Ioachimescu A. Severe TSH elevation and pituitary enlargement after changing thyroid replacement to compounded T4/T3 therapy. J Investig Med High Impact Case Rep. 2016;4(3):2324709616661834.

76. Escobar-Morreale HF, del Rey FE, Obregón MJ, de Escobar GM. Only the combined treatment with thyroxine and triiodothyronine ensures euthyroidism in all tissues of the thyroidectomized rat. Endocrinology. 1996;137(6):2490–502.

77. Celi FS, Zemskova M, Linderman JD, Babar NI, Skarulis MC, Csako G, Wesley R, Costello R, Penzak SR, Pucino F. The pharmacodynamic equivalence of levothyroxine and liothyronine: a randomized, double blind, cross-over study in thyroidectomized patients. Clin Endocrinol. 2010;72(5):709–15.

78. Flynn RW, Bonellie SR, Jung RT, MacDonald TM, Morris AD, Leese GP. Serum thyroid-stimulating hormone concentration and morbidity from cardiovascular disease and fractures in patients on long-term thyroxine therapy. J Clin Endocrinol Metab. 2010;95(1):186–93.

79. Hennessey JV. Historical and current perspective in the use of thyroid extracts for the treatment of hypothyroidism. Endocr Pract. 2015;21(10):1161–70.

80. Penny R, Frasier SD. Elevated serum concentrations of triiodothyronine in hypothyroid patients. Values for patients receiving USP thyroid. Am J Dis Child. 1980;134(1):16–8.

81. LeBoff MS, Kaplan MM, Silva JE, Larsen PR. Bioavailability of thyroid hormones from oral replacement preparations. Metabolism. 1982;31(9):900–5.

82. Lev-Ran A. Part-of-the-day hypertriiodothyroninemia caused by desiccated thyroid. JAMA. 1983;250(20):2790–1.

83. Smith SR. Desiccated thyroid preparations. Obsolete therapy. Arch Intern Med. 1984;144(5):926–7.

84. Shrestha RT, Malabanan A, Haugen BR, Levy EG, Hennessey JV. Adverse event reporting in patients treated with thyroid hormone extract. Endocr Pract. 2017;23(5):566–75.

85. Jackson IM, Cobb WE. Why does anyone still use desiccated thyroid USP? Am J Med. 1978;64(2):284–8.

86. Surks MI, Schadlow AR, Oppenheimer JH. A new radioimmunoassay for plasma L-triiodothyronine: measurements in thyroid disease and in patients maintained on hormonal replacement. J Clin Invest. 1972;51(12):3104–13.

Permissions

The contributors of this book come from diverse backgrounds, making this book a truly international effort. This book will bring forth new frontiers with its revolutionizing research information and detailed analysis of the nascent developments around the world.

We would like to thank all the contributing authors for lending their expertise to make the book truly unique. They have played a crucial role in the development of this book. Without their invaluable contributions this book wouldn't have been possible. They have made vital efforts to compile up to date information on the varied aspects of this subject to make this book a valuable addition to the collection of many professionals and students.

This book was conceptualized with the vision of imparting up-to-date information and advanced data in this field. To ensure the same, a matchless editorial board was set up. Every individual on the board went through rigorous rounds of assessment to prove their worth. After which they invested a large part of their time researching and compiling the most relevant data for our readers.

The editorial board has been involved in producing this book since its inception. They have spent rigorous hours researching and exploring the diverse topics which have resulted in the successful publishing of this book. They have passed on their knowledge of decades through this book. To expedite this challenging task, the publisher supported the team at every step. A small team of assistant editors was also appointed to further simplify the editing procedure and attain best results for the readers.

Apart from the editorial board, the designing team has also invested a significant amount of their time in understanding the subject and creating the most relevant covers. They scrutinized every image to scout for the most suitable representation of the subject and create an appropriate cover for the book.

The publishing team has been an ardent support to the editorial, designing and production team. Their endless efforts to recruit the best for this project, has resulted in the accomplishment of this book. They are a veteran in the field of academics and their pool of knowledge is as vast as their experience in printing. Their expertise and guidance has proved useful at every step. Their uncompromising quality standards have made this book an exceptional effort. Their encouragement from time to time has been an inspiration for everyone.

The publisher and the editorial board hope that this book will prove to be a valuable piece of knowledge for researchers, students, practitioners and scholars across the globe.

List of Contributors

Caroline Jacques, Frédérique Savagner and Yves Malthièry
INSERM U694, Institut Biologie Santé (IBS), rue des Capucins, F-49100 Angers, France
University of Angers, rue de Rennes, F-49045 Angers, France

Abdelaziz Belkadi
INSERM U694, Institut Biologie Santé (IBS), rue des Capucins, F-49100 Angers, France
University of Angers, rue de Rennes, F-49045 Angers, France
Laboratory of human genetics of infectious diseases. Necker Branch, INSERM, U980 Paris, France

Katarzyna Lacka and Adam Maciejewski
Department of Endocrinology, Metabolism and Internal Medicine, University of Medical Sciences, Poznan, Poland

Sasan Mirfakhraee and Jeffrey M Zigman
Department of Internal Medicine, Division of Endocrinology and Metabolism, The University of Texas Southwestern Medical Center, Dallas, Texas 75390, USA

Dana Mathews
Department of Radiology, Neurology and Neurotherapeutics, The University of Texas Southwestern Medical Center, Dallas, TX 75390, USA

Lan Peng
Department of Pathology, The University of Texas Southwestern Medical Center, Dallas, TX, USA75390

Stacey Woodruff
Department of Surgery, The University of Texas Southwestern Medical Center, Dallas, TX 75390, USA

Monica A Ercolano, Monica L Drnovsek, Maria C Silva Croome, Monica Moos, Ana M Fuentes, Fanny Viale and Alicia T Gauna
Endocrinology Division, Hospital Ramos Mejía, Buenos Aires, Argentina

Ulla Feldt-Rasmussen
Department of Medical Endocrinology, Rigshospitalet, Copenhagen University, Copenhagen, Denmark

Claudia Campomenosi, Stefano Gay and Eleonora Monti
Endocrine Unit, IRCCS Azienda Ospedaliera Universitaria San Martino – IST Istituto Nazionale per la Ricerca sul Cancro, Genoa, Italy

Massimo Giusti
Endocrine Unit, IRCCS Azienda Ospedaliera Universitaria San Martino – IST Istituto Nazionale per la Ricerca sul Cancro, Genoa, Italy
UO Clinica Endocrinologica, Viale Benedetto XV, 6, I-16100 Genoa, Italy

Barbara Massa
Cytopathology and Pathology Unit, IRCCS Azienda Ospedaliera Universitaria San Martino – IST Istituto Nazionale per la Ricerca sul Cancro, Genoa, Italy

Enzo Silvestri and Giovanni Turtulici
Radiology Unit, Ospedale Evangelico, Genoa, Italy

Jan Stępniak
Department of Oncological Endocrinology, Medical University of Łódź, 7/9 Żeligowski St, 90-752, Łódź, Poland

Małgorzata Karbownik-Lewińska
Department of Oncological Endocrinology, Medical University of Łódź, 7/9 Żeligowski St, 90-752, Łódź, Poland
Polish Mother's Memorial Hospital - Research Institute, 281/ 289, Rzgowska St, 93-338, Łódź, Poland

Andrzej Lewińsk
Department of Endocrinology and Metabolic Diseases, Medical University of Łódź, 281/289 Rzgowska St, 93-338, Łódź, Poland
Polish Mother's Memorial Hospital - Research Institute, 281/ 289, Rzgowska St, 93-338, Łódź, Poland

Michael B. Zimmermann
Laboratory of Human Nutrition, Department of Health Sciences and Technology, ETH Zürich, Schmelzbergstrasse 7, LFV D21, CH-8092 Zürich, Switzerland

Valeria Galetti
Laboratory of Human Nutrition, Department of Health Sciences and Technology, ETH Zürich, Schmelzbergstrasse 7, LFV E14, CH-8092 Zürich, Switzerland

Mario Vaisman
Hospital Clementino Fraga Filho, Universidade Federal do Rio de Janeiro, Rua Prof. Rodolpho Paulo Rocco 255, Cidade Universitária, CEP 21941-913, Rio de Janeiro-RJ, Brazil

Rosita Fontes
Hospital Clementino Fraga Filho, Universidade
Federal do Rio de Janeiro, Rua Prof. Rodolpho Paulo
Rocco 255, Cidade Universitária, CEP 21941-913, Rio
de Janeiro-RJ, Brazil
Diagnósticos da América SA, Rio de Janeiro, Brazil

Claudia Regina Coeli and Fernanda Aguiar
Núcleo de Estudos de Saúde Coletiva, Universidade
Federal do Rio de Janeiro, Rio de Janeiro, Brazil

**Yurena Caballero, Eudaldo M. López-Tomassetti,
Julián Favre, José R. Santana and Juan R. Hernández**
General Surgery Department, Hospital Universitario
Insular de Gran Canaria, Las Palmas de Gran Canaria,
Las Palmas, Spain

Juan J. Cabrera
Pathology Department, Hospital Universitario Insular
de Gran Canaria, Las Palmas de Gran Canaria, Las
Palmas, Spain

Adam Gesing
Department of Oncological Endocrinology, Medical
University of Lodz, 7/9 Zeligowski St., 90-752, Lodz,
Poland

Małgorzata Karbownik-Lewińska
Department of Oncological Endocrinology, Medical
University of Lodz, 7/9 Zeligowski St., 90-752, Lodz,
Poland
Department of Endocrinology and Metabolic Diseases,
Polish Mother's Memorial Hospital, Research Institute,
Lodz, Poland

Paweł Szychta
Department of Oncological Endocrinology, Medical
University of Lodz, 7/9 Zeligowski St., 90-752, Lodz,
Poland
Department of Oncological Surgery and Breast
Diseases, Polish Mother's Memorial Hospital,
Research Institute, Lodz, Poland

Wojciech Szychta
Department of Oncological Endocrinology, Medical
University of Lodz, 7/9 Zeligowski St., 90-752, Lodz,
Poland
1st Department of Cardiology, Medical
University of Warsaw, Warsaw, Poland

Andrzej Lewiński
Department of Endocrinology and Metabolic Diseases,
Medical University of Lodz, Lodz, Poland
Department of Endocrinology and Metabolic Diseases,
Polish Mother's Memorial Hospital, Research Institute,
Lodz, Poland

**Janina Krupińska, Grzegorz Kulig, Elżbieta
Sowińska-Przepiera, Elżbieta Andrysiak-Mamos and
Anhelli Syrenicz**
Department of Endocrinology, Metabolic Diseases and
Internal Diseases, Pomeranian Medical University,
Szczecin, Poland

Waldemar Urbanowicz
Department of Infectious Diseases and Hepatology,
Pomeranian Medical University, Szczecin, Poland

Mariusz Kaczmarczyk
Institute of Clinical Biochemistry and Molecular
Diagnostics, Pomeranian Medical University, Szczecin,
Poland

Thierry Ragot
UMR 8203, Gustave Roussy, Laboratoire de
Vectorologie et de Thérapeutiques Anticancéreuses,
Villejuif 94805, France
UMR 8203, CNRS, Laboratoire de Vectorologie et
Thérapeutiques Anticancéreuses, Villejuif 94805,
France
UMR 8203, Univ Paris-Sud, Laboratoire de Vectorologie
et Thérapeutiques Anticancéreuses, Villejuif 94805,
France

Claire Provost, Aurélie Prignon and Sylvie Lausson
Sorbonne Universités, UPMC University Paris 06,
plateforme LIMP, Laboratoire d'Imagerie Médicale
Positonique, Hôpital Tenon, Paris 75020, France

Régis Cohen
Hopital Delafontaine, Endocrinology Unit, Saint Denis,
France

Michel Lepoivre
IBBMC, CNRS 8619, bat 430, Université Paris Sud XI,
Orsay, Paris 91405, France

Magdalena Milczarek and Jan Stępniak
Department of Oncological Endocrinology, Medical
University of Łódź, 7/9 Żeligowski Street, Łódź 90-
752, Poland

Małgorzata Karbownik-Lewińska
Department of Oncological Endocrinology, Medical
University of Łódź, 7/9 Żeligowski Street, Łódź 90-
752, Poland
Polish Mother's Memorial Hospital – Research Institute,
281/289, Rzgowska Street, Łódź 93-338, Poland

Andrzej Lewiński
Department of Endocrinology and Metabolic Diseases,
Medical University of Łódź, 281/289 Rzgowska Street,
Łódź 93-338, Poland

Polish Mother's Memorial Hospital – Research Institute, 281/289, Rzgowska Street, Łódź 93-338, Poland

Bartosz Pula and Marzena Podhorska-Okolow
Department of Histology and Embryology, Medical University in Wroclaw, Wroclaw, Poland

Piotr Dziegiel
Department of Histology and Embryology, Medical University in Wroclaw, Wroclaw, Poland
Department of Physiotherapy, Wroclaw University School of Physical Education in Wroclaw, Wroclaw, Poland

Pawel Domoslawski
Department of General, Gastroenterological and Endocrinological Surgery, Medical University in Wroclaw, Wroclaw, Poland

Kaoru Kobayashi, Mitsuyoshi Hirokawa, Tomonori Yabuta, Mitsuhiro Fukushima, Hiroo Masuoka, Takuya Higashiyama, Minoru Kihara, Yasuhiro Ito, Akihiro Miya, Nobuyuki Amino and Akira Miyauchi
Kuma Hospital, 8-2-35 Shimoyamate-dori, Chuo-ku, Kobe-City 650-0011, Japan

Zbigniew Adamczewski and Andrzej Lewiński
Department of Endocrinology and Metabolic Diseases, Medical University of Lodz, Polish Mother's Memorial Hospital – Research Institute, Rzgowska 281/ 289, 93-338, Lodz, Poland

Kwan Yee Queenie Tsui
Department of Psychiatry, Pamela Youde Nethersole Eastern Hospital, 3 Lok Man Road, Chai Wan, Hong Kong SAR, China

Beverley M. Shields
NIHR Exeter Clinical Research Facility, Royal Devon and Exeter Hospital, University of Exeter Medical School, University of Exeter, Exeter EX2 5DW, UK

Bridget A. Knight
NIHR Exeter Clinical Research Facility, Royal Devon and Exeter Hospital, University of Exeter Medical School, University of Exeter, Exeter EX2 5DW, UK
Research and Development Department, Royal Devon and Exeter Hospital NHS Foundation Trust, Exeter, UK

Xuemei He, Elizabeth N. Pearce and Lewis E. Braverman
Section of Endocrinology, Diabetes and Nutrition, Boston University School of Medicine, Boston, USA

Rachel Sturley
Centre for Women's Health, Royal Devon and Exeter Hospital NHS Foundation Trust, Exeter, UK

Bijay Vaidya
Department of Endocrinology, Royal Devon and Exeter Hospital NHS Foundation Trust, Exeter, UK. University of Exeter Medical School, Exeter, UK

Hernando Vargas-Uricoechea
Department of Internal Medicine, Division of Endocrinology and Metabolism, Universidad del Cauca, Popayán, Colombia

Ivonne Meza-Cabrera
Laboratory of Pathology, Hospital Universitario San José, Popayán, Cauca, Colombia

Jorge Herrera-Chaparro
Department of surgery, Universidad del Cauca, Carrera 6 No 41 N-135 apto 202B terrazas del campestre, Popayán, Cauca, Colombia

Christina Tugendsam, Karin Rudolph and Georg Zettinig
Schilddruesenpraxis Josefstadt, Laudongasse 12/8, Vienna AT-1080, Austria

Brigitta Schmoll-Hauer
Schilddruesenpraxis Josefstadt, Laudongasse 12/8, Vienna AT-1080, Austria
Department of Nuclear Medicine, Krankenanstalt Rudolfstiftung, Vienna, Austria

Iris Pia Schenk
Schilddruesenpraxis Josefstadt, Laudongasse 12/8, Vienna AT-1080, Austria
Department of Nuclear Medicine, Sozialmedizinisches Zentrum Hietzing, Vienna, Austria

Michael Krebs
Schilddruesenpraxis Josefstadt, Laudongasse 12/8, Vienna AT-1080, Austria
Clinical Division of Endocrinology, Department of Medicine III, Medical University of Vienna, Vienna Austria

Veronika Petz
Division of Nuclear Medicine, Department of Biomedical Imaging and Image-guided Therapy, Medical University of Vienna, Vienna, Austria

Wolfgang Buchinger
Schilddrueseninstitut Gleisdorf, Gleisdorf, Austria

Tomoe Nakao, Mitsushige Nishikawa, Mako Hisakado, Toshihiko Kasahara, Takumi Kudo, Eijun Nishihara, Mitsuru Ito, Shuji Fukata and Hirotoshi Nakamura
Department of Internal Medicine, Kuma Hospital, Centre for Excellence in Thyroid Cares, 8-2-35 Shimoyamate-dori, Chuo-ku, Kobe 650-0011, Japan

Mitsuyoshi Hirokawa
Department of Diagnostic Pathology and Cytology, Kuma Hospital, Centre for Excellence in Thyroid Cares, 8-2-35 Shimoyamate-dori, Chuo-ku, Kobe 650-0011, Japan

Akira Miyauchi
Department of Surgery, Kuma Hospital, Centre for Excellence in Thyroid Care, 8-2-35 Shimoyamate-dori, Chuo-ku, Kobe 650-0011, Japan

Simon H. S. Pearce
Institute of Genetic Medicine and Queen Elizabeth Hospital, International Centre for Life, Newcastle University, Central Parkway, Newcastle upon Tyne NE1 3BZ, UK

Salman Razvi
Institute of Genetic Medicine and Queen Elizabeth Hospital, International Centre for Life, Newcastle University, Central Parkway, Newcastle upon Tyne NE1 3BZ, UK
Department of Endocrinology, Queen Elizabeth Hospital, Gateshead NE9 6SX, UK

Lorna Ingoe
Department of Endocrinology, Queen Elizabeth Hospital, Gateshead NE9 6SX, UK

Vicky Ryan
Institute of Health and Society, Newcastle University, Baddiley Clark Building, Richardson Road, Newcastle upon Tyne NE2 4AX, UK

Scott Wilkes
Department of Pharmacy, Health and Wellbeing, Faculty of Applied Sciences, University of Sunderland, Sunderland SR1 3SD, UK

Mohamed S. Al Hassan, Tamer Saafan and Abdelrahman Abdelaal
Department of General Surgery, Hamad General Hospital, Doha, Qatar

Walid El Ansari
Department of Surgery, Hamad General Hospital, Doha, Qatar
College of Medicine, Qatar University, Doha, Qatar

Afaf A. Al Ansari
Department of Gynecologic Oncology, Hamad General Hospital, Doha, Qatar

Mahmoud A. Zirie
Department of Endocrinology, Hamad General Hospital, Doha, Qatar

Hanan Farghaly
Department of Pathology, Hamad General Hospital, Doha, Qatar

Jackline Namulema and Muhammudu Kalange
Department of Physiology, Faculty of Biomedical Sciences, Kampala International University, Ishaka, Bushenyi, Uganda

Miriam Nansunga
Department of Physiology, Faculty of Biomedical Sciences, Kampala International University, Ishaka, Bushenyi, Uganda
Department of Physiology, Faculty of Biomedical Sciences, St Augustine International University, Kampala, Uganda

Charles Drago Kato
Department of Immunology and Microbiology, Faculty of Biomedical Sciences, Kampala International University, Ishaka, Bushenyi, Uganda
School of Biosecurity, Biotechnical and Laboratory Sciences, College of Veterinary Medicine, Animal Resources and Biosecurity, Makerere University, Kampala, Uganda

Samuel Babafemi Olaleye
Laboratory for Gastrointestinal Secretion and Inflammation Research, Department of Physiology, College of Medicine, University of Ibadan, Ibadan, Nigeria

Jing Yang, Carmen Sarita-Reyes, David Kindelberger and Qing Zhao
Department of Pathology and Laboratory Medicine, Boston University Medical Center, 670 Albany St. Biosquare III, Boston, MA 02118, USA

Colin Dayan
Thyroid Research Group, School of Medicine, Cardiff University, Cardiff, UK

Vijay Panicker
Department of Endocrinology, Sir Charles Gairdner Hospital, Nedlands, WA 6009, Australia

Index